Herbal Medicine

Herbal Medicine

Editor: Holly Philips

CALLISTO REFERENCE

www.callistoreference.com

Callisto Reference,
118-35 Queens Blvd., Suite 400,
Forest Hills, NY 11375, USA

Visit us on the World Wide Web at:
www.callistoreference.com

ISBN: 978-1-63239-893-2 (Hardback)

Printed in China.

Cataloging-in-Publication Data

Herbal medicine / edited by Holly Philips.
p. cm.
Includes bibliographical references and index.
ISBN 978-1-63239-893-2
1. Herbs--Therapeutic use. 2. Herbs--Therapeutic use--China. 3. Medicine, Chinese. 4. Traditional medicine.
5. Materia medica, Vegetable. I. Philips, Holly.

RM666.H33 H47 2017
615.321--dc23

Table of Contents

Preface

The purpose of the book is to provide a glimpse into the dynamics and to present opinions and studies of some of the scientists engaged in the development of new ideas in the field from very different standpoints. This book will prove useful to students and researchers owing to its high content quality.

Herbal Medicine is a form of alternative medicine that uses plants for medical treatment. Plant-derived compounds are widely recognized for their medicinal properties and are increasingly being implemented for drug development. Topics included in this book delve into effective remedies that can improve already existing products. This book covers in detail some existent theories and innovative concepts revolving around herbal medicine. It strives to provide a fair idea about this discipline and to help develop a better understanding of the latest advances within this field. In this book, using case studies and examples, constant effort has been made to make the understanding of the difficult concepts of herbal medicine as easy and informative as possible for the readers.

At the end, I would like to appreciate all the efforts made by the authors in completing their chapters professionally. I express my deepest gratitude to all of them for contributing to this book by sharing their valuable works. A special thanks to my family and friends for their constant support in this journey.

Editor

1

Identification of Licopyranocoumarin and Glycyrurol from Herbal Medicines as Neuroprotective Compounds for Parkinson's Disease

Takahiro Fujimaki[1], Shinji Saiki[2], Etsu Tashiro[1], Daisuke Yamada[2], Mitsuhiro Kitagawa[1], Nobutaka Hattori[2]*, Masaya Imoto[1]*

1 Department of Biosciences and Informatics, Faculty of Science and Technology, Keio University, Yokohama, Japan, **2** Department of Neurology, Juntendo University School of Medicine, Bunkyo, Tokyo

Abstract

In the course of screening for the anti-Parkinsonian drugs from a library of traditional herbal medicines, we found that the extracts of *choi-joki-to* and *daio-kanzo-to* protected cells from MPP^+-induced cell death. Because *choi-joki-to* and *daio-kanzo-to* commonly contain the genus *Glycyrrhiza*, we isolated licopyranocoumarin (LPC) and glycyrurol (GCR) as potent neuroprotective principals from *Glycyrrhiza*. LPC and GCR markedly blocked MPP^+-induced neuronal PC12D cell death and disappearance of mitochondrial membrane potential, which were mediated by JNK. LPC and GCR inhibited MPP^+-induced JNK activation through the suppression of reactive oxygen species (ROS) generation, thereby inhibiting MPP^+-induced neuronal PC12D cell death. These results indicated that LPC and GCR derived from *choi-joki-to* and *daio-kanzo-to* would be promising drug leads for PD treatment in the future.

Editor: Hiroyoshi Ariga, Hokkaido University, Japan

Funding: This work was supported by Health Labour Sciences Research Grants from the Ministry of Health, Labour and Welfare of Japan. The extract powder of 128 traditional herbal (kampo) medicines (The Kampo, TJ-1~3, TJ-5~12, TJ-14~41, TJ-43, TJ-45~48, TJ-50~93, TJ-95~128, TJ-133~138) and powder of Glycyrrhiza were kindly donated from Tsumura Corporation (Tokyo, Japan). The funders had no role in study design, data collection and analysis, decision to publish, or preparation of the manuscript.

Competing Interests: The extract powder of 128 traditional herbal (kampo) medicines (The Kampo, TJ-1~3, TJ-5~12, TJ-14~41, TJ-43, TJ-45~48, TJ-50~93, TJ-95~128, TJ-133~138) and powder of Glycyrrhiza were kindly donated from Tsumura Corporation (Tokyo, Japan). This does not alter the authors' adherence to PLOS ONE policies on sharing data and materials.

* Email: nhattori@juntendo.ac.jp (NH); imoto@bio.keio.ac.jp (MI)

Introduction

Parkinson's disease (PD) is a common neurodegenerative disease characterized by progressive dopaminergic neuronal cell death in the substantia nigra par compacta of the midbrain. The main symptoms of PD are movement disorders such as tremors, bradykinesia/akinesia, rigidity, postural instability, and gait abnormalities. Although deep-brain stimulation and oral administration of L-dopa, dopamine agonists and amantadine hydrochloride have been well established as symptomatic treatments, there are no therapies to completely cure patients with the disorder [1]. Mitochondrial dysfunction, especially dysfunction of the mitochondrial electron transport chain mainly relying on complex I activity, has been implicated in the disease's pathogenesis. In addition to defects of complex I in postmortem brains, skeletal muscle and platelets of patients with PD [2,3,4,5,6], cybrid cells containing mtDNA derived from PD platelets have indicated complex I defects [7,8,9]. Because various rodents treated with mitochondrial toxins such as rotenone, 1-methyl-4-phenyl-1,2,3,6-tetrahydropyridine (MPTP), and its toxic metabolite 1-methyl-4-phenylpyridinium (MPP^+) show motor deficits associated with selective loss of dopaminergic neurons, they have been widely used as acquired PD models [10,11,12,13,14,15]. Selegiline, a medication widely used at present, has the capacity to protect dopamine neurons by inhibiting MAO-B oxidation for conversion of MPTP into MPP^+ and blocking the formation of free radicals derived from the oxidative metabolism of dopamine [16,17]. Also, MPP^+ models offer unexploited therapeutic potential for some atypical antipsychotics (olanzapine, aripiprazole, and ziprasidone) and the anticonvulsant zonisamide in PD, and new mechanisms of neuroprotective effects of FLZ (which activates HSP27/HSP70) and paeoniflorin (which modulates autophagy) have led to treatments for PD [18,19,20,21].

Herbal medicines are employed to treat PD in ancient medical systems in Asian countries such as India, China, Japan, and Korea based on anecdotal and experience-based theories [22]. The traditional herbal medicines *yi-gan san* and *modified yeoldahanso-tang* have neuroprotective effects and can rescue dopaminergic neurons from MPP^+/MPTP toxicity using both *in vitro* and *in vivo* methods [23,24]. Several compounds derived from herbal medicines also exert anti-Parkinsonian activities. For instance, ginsenoside Rb1 isolated from *Panax ginseng C. A. Meyer*, 3-*O*-demethylswertipunicoside isolated from *S. punicea*, and salidroside isolated from *Rhodiola rosea L.*, have been reported to attenuate MPP^+-induced neurotoxicity in PC12 cells *in vitro* [25,26,27]. However, clinical evidence for the efficacy and safety of these herbal medicines for PD is

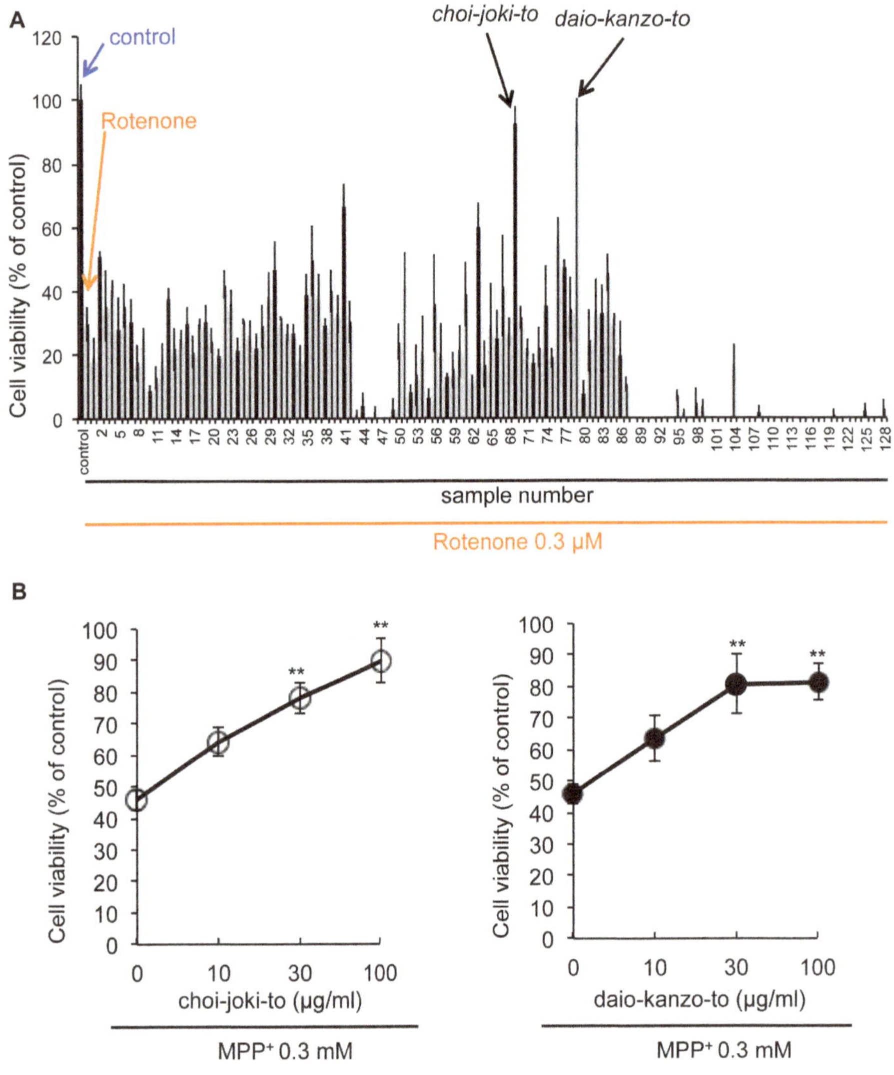

Figure 1. Two herbal medicines, *daio-kanzo-to* and *choi-joki-to*, identified as neuroprotective agents in the course of screening. (A) NGF-differentiated PC12D cells were treated with 0.3 μM rotenone and herbal medicine extract for 48 h. Cell viability was evaluated by trypan blue dye exclusion assay. (**B**) NGF-differentiated PC12D cells were treated with various concentrations of *choi-joki-to* or *daio-kanzo-to* in the presence of 0.3 mM MPP^+ for 48 h. Cell viability was evaluated by trypan blue dye exclusion assay. Values are the means of triplicate samples; bars, s.d. $^{**}p<0.01$ compared with MPP^+ group cells.

insufficient [28]. Therefore, in this study, we screened a library containing 128 traditional herbal medicines, which have been used clinically for at least 10 years in Japan, focusing on their neuroprotective effects using PD-like cellular models of cell death by mitochondrial toxins, and found the anti-Parkinsonian herbal medicines *choi-joki-to* and *daio-kanzo-to*. Moreover, we identified licopyranocoumarin and glycyrurol derived from the genus *Glycyrrhiza* as common components contained in these two herbal medicines, and found they exerted neuroprotective effects against MPP^+-induced toxicity.

Results

Identification of *choi-joki-to* and *daio-kanzo-to* as potent neuroprotective herbal medicines using *in vitro* PD-like model screening

Rotenone, a direct inhibitor of mitochondria complex I, is usually employed to mimic Parkinsonism *in vitro* and *in vivo* [29]. Treatment of NGF-differentiated PC12D cells [30] with 0.3 μM of rotenone for 48 h caused marked cell death as evaluated by the trypan blue dye exclusion assay. Using this PD-like model, we screened a library containing 128 traditional herbal medicines, which have been used clinically in Japan, focusing on preventive effects against rotenone-induced cell death of NGF-differentiated PC12D cells.

As a result, several ethyl acetate (EtOAc) extracts of herbal medicines showed suppressive effects against rotenone-induced cell death generally, but two traditional herbal medicines, *choi-joki-to* and *daio-kanzo-to* exerted significant neuroprotective effects against rotenone-induced neurotoxicity (Figure 1A). Furthermore, the EtOAc extracts of *choi-joki-to* or *daio-kanzo-to* also conferred dose-dependent protection from neuronal cell death induced by MPP^+, another well-known PD-like cellular model (Figure 1B).

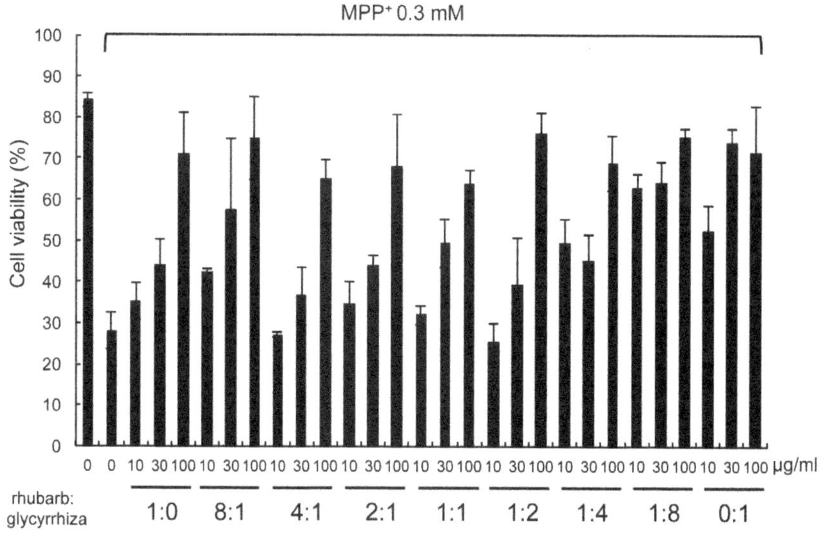

Figure 2. *Glycyrrhiza* prevented MPP$^+$-induced cell death more potently than rhubarb. NGF-differentiated PC12D cells were treated with various concentrations of rhubarb and *Glycyrrhiza* (rhubarb:*Glycyrrhiza* ratio = 1:0, 8:1, 4:1, 2:1, 1:1, 1:2, 1:4, 1:8, 0:1) in the presence of 0.3 mM MPP$^+$ for 48 h. Cell viability was evaluated by trypan blue exclusion assay. Values are the means of three independent experiments; bars, s.d. $^{**}p<0.01$ compared with MPP$^+$ group cells.

Licopyranocoumarin and glycyrurol isolated from *Glycyrrhiza* as potent neuroprotective compounds

Next, we attempted to identify the major components responsible for neuroprotective effects contained in *choi-joki-to* and *daio-kanzo-to*. First, we noted that both *choi-joki-to* and *daio-kanzo-to* commonly contain rhubarb and *Glycyrrhiza* species, at the ratio of 2:1 (Table 1). Therefore, we examined whether this 2:1 ratio of rhubarb to *Glycyrrhiza* is important for neuroprotective effects against MPP$^+$-induced toxicity. As shown in Figure 2, rhubarb and *Glycyrrhiza* contained in *choi-joki-to* and *daio-kanzo-to* at 2:1 is not a special ratio necessary for neuroprotective effects, but rather increased *Glycyrrhiza* content potentiated the neuroprotective activity against MPP$^+$-induced cell death. Thus, we attempted to isolate the active principle responsible for neuroprotective effects from EtOAc extract of *Glycyrrhiza* by monitoring the inhibitory activity of MPP$^+$-induced NGF-differentiated PC12D cell death using a trypan blue dye exclusion assay. As a result, we isolated 10.8 mg of licopyranocoumarin (LPC) and 4.0 mg of glycyrurol (GCR) from 50 g of *Glycyrrhiza* powder as potent neuroprotective compounds (Figure 3A, B). Both LPC and GCR markedly blocked MPP$^+$-induced cell death in a dose-dependent manner with IC_{50} values of 0.9 µM and 1.2 µM, respectively (Figure 3C). Furthermore, both LPC and GCR did not show cytoprotective effects against other toxins, such as taxol and cisplatin (CDDP) even at 3 µM concentration, which significantly suppressed MPP$^+$-induced cell death in PC12D cells. Therefore, cytoprotective ability of LPC and GCR may specific for mitochondrial toxins (Figure 3D). To further verify the inhibitory effect of LPC and GCR on MPP$^+$-induced cell death, PC12D cells were labeled with PI and histogram analysis-related nuclear DNA contents were ascertained by flow cytometry. By the treatment of PC12D cells with 0.3 mM of MPP$^+$, NGF-differentiated PC12D cells with DNA content below G1 phase levels (defined as hypodiploid sub-G1 peak) were distinguishable in the population as compared with control levels (49.63±6.41% versus 7.23±1.04% of cells in sub-G1, respectively) (Figure 4A,B). LPC or GCR alone did not show any effects on the overall population of cells. However, they decreased the percentage of MPP$^+$-induced cell death by 11.2–29.0% and 11.4–28.0% (values are the mean of average of three data), respectively (Figure 4A,B), confirming that LPC and GCR inhibited MPP$^+$-induced cell death.

Licopyranocoumarin and glycyrurol attenuate the MPP$^+$-induced decrease in mitochondrial membrane potential

MPP$^+$ is a well-known inhibitor of mitochondria complex I and induces mitochondrial dysfunction. Because LPC or GCR suppressed MPP$^+$-induced cell death, we next surveyed the effect of LPC and GCR on MPP$^+$-mediated loss of mitochondrial membrane potential ($\Delta\Psi_{mit}$) using JC-1 dyes. As shown in Figure 5, by the treatment of PC12D cells with 0.3 mM of MPP$^+$ for 48 h, $\Delta\Psi_{mit}$ was decreased to 45–50% as estimated from decrease of JC-1 aggregate fluorescence. LPC or GCR alone did not affect $\Delta\Psi_{mit}$. Compared with the group treated with MPP$^+$ alone, fluorescent intensities increased in a dose-dependent manner following addition of LPC and GCR individually, indicating that LPC and GCR each inhibited MPP$^+$-induced decrease of $\Delta\Psi_{mit}$.

Licopyranocoumarin and glycyrurol counteract MPP$^+$-induced ROS production

MPP$^+$ has been extensively reported to evoke generation of reactive oxygen species (ROS). Figure 6 showed cytofluorometric histograms of NGF-differentiated PC12D cells after 12 h of treatment with 0.3 mM MPP$^+$ upon staining with CMH_2DCFDA. ROS levels were significantly increased from 100±7.8% (control level) to 247±14.9% ($p<0.001$). However, the generation of intracellular ROS was reduced to 164±15.7% ($p<0.01$) and 153±13.0% ($p<0.01$) by the addition of 3 µM LPC and 3 µM GCR, respectively.

Antioxidant activities of licopyranocoumarin and glycyrurol *in vitro*

Because treatment of PC12D cells with LPC and GCR each effectively reduced MPP$^+$-induced ROS generation, the free radical scavenging activities of these two compounds were

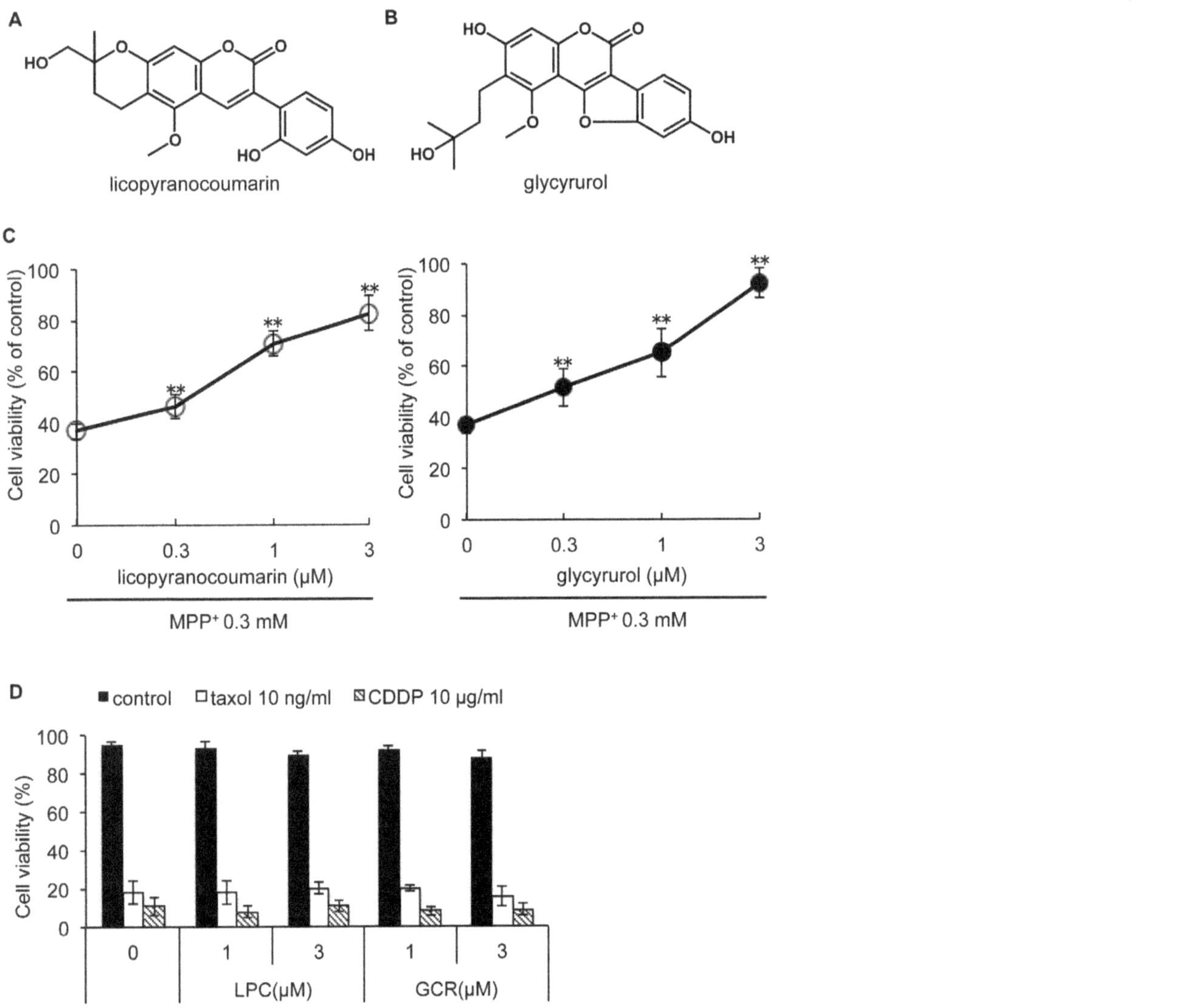

Figure 3. Licopyranocoumarin and glycyrurol prevented MPP$^+$-induced cell death. Structures of (**A**) licopyranocoumarin (LPC) and (**B**) glycyrurol (GCR). (**C**) NGF-differentiated PC12D cells were treated with various concentrations of LPC or GCR in the presence of 0.3 mM MPP$^+$ for 48 h. Cell viability was evaluated by trypan blue dye exclusion assay. (**D**) PC12D cells were treated with various concentration of LPC or GCR in the presence of 10 ng/ml taxol or 10 μg/ml cisplatin (CDDP) for 48 h. Values are the means of three independent experiments; bars, s.d. $^{**}p<0.01$ compared with MPP$^+$ group cells.

examined. When the antioxidant activity of LPC and GCR were evaluated by β-carotene bleaching assay, LPC and GCR inhibited less than 10% of the carotene bleaching even at the final concentration of 30 μM (Figure 7A). The DPPH free radical scavenging potentials of LPC and GCR at 30 μM each showed little to no scavenging activity (Figure 7B). These results indicated that LPC and GCR did not possess antioxidant activity *in vitro*.

Licopyranocoumarin and glycyrurol attenuate JNK activity induced by MPP$^+$

It is well-established that JNK plays a central role in the mediation of MPP$^+$-induced neurotoxicity [31,32,33,34]. Particularly, MPP$^+$-induced ROS generation is reported to be closely associated with JNK activation [35]. Thus, we investigated whether the ability of LPC or GCR to reduce MPP$^+$-induced cell death involves the alteration of JNK signaling in MPP$^+$-induced neurotoxicity. As shown in Figure 8A, phosphorylated JNK levels were increased after exposure to MPP$^+$ for 36 h, and treatment with LPC or GCR significantly reduced the expression levels of the phosphorylated protein. In addition, a JNK inhibitor, SP600125, led to attenuation of the MPP$^+$-induced neuronal cell death and decreased $\Delta\Psi_{mit}$ (Figure 8B, C). These results suggest that MPP$^+$-induced lowering of $\Delta\Psi_{mit}$, which leads to neuronal cell death, were mediated by JNK, and neuroprotective activity of LPC and GCR against MPP$^+$-induced neuronal cell death might be due to downregulation of ROS generation, resulting in the inhibition of JNK activation.

Discussion

Both *choi-joki-to* and *daio-kanzo-to* are traditional herbal medicines available in Japan (called *kanpo* in Japan in particular) that are usually used for laxative products. In the laboratory, *choi-joki-to* exhibited oxygen radical scavenging capacity [36] and inhibited the progression of atheroma in a KHC rabbit model [37], On the other hand, *daio-kanzo-to* has provided inhibition of amylase

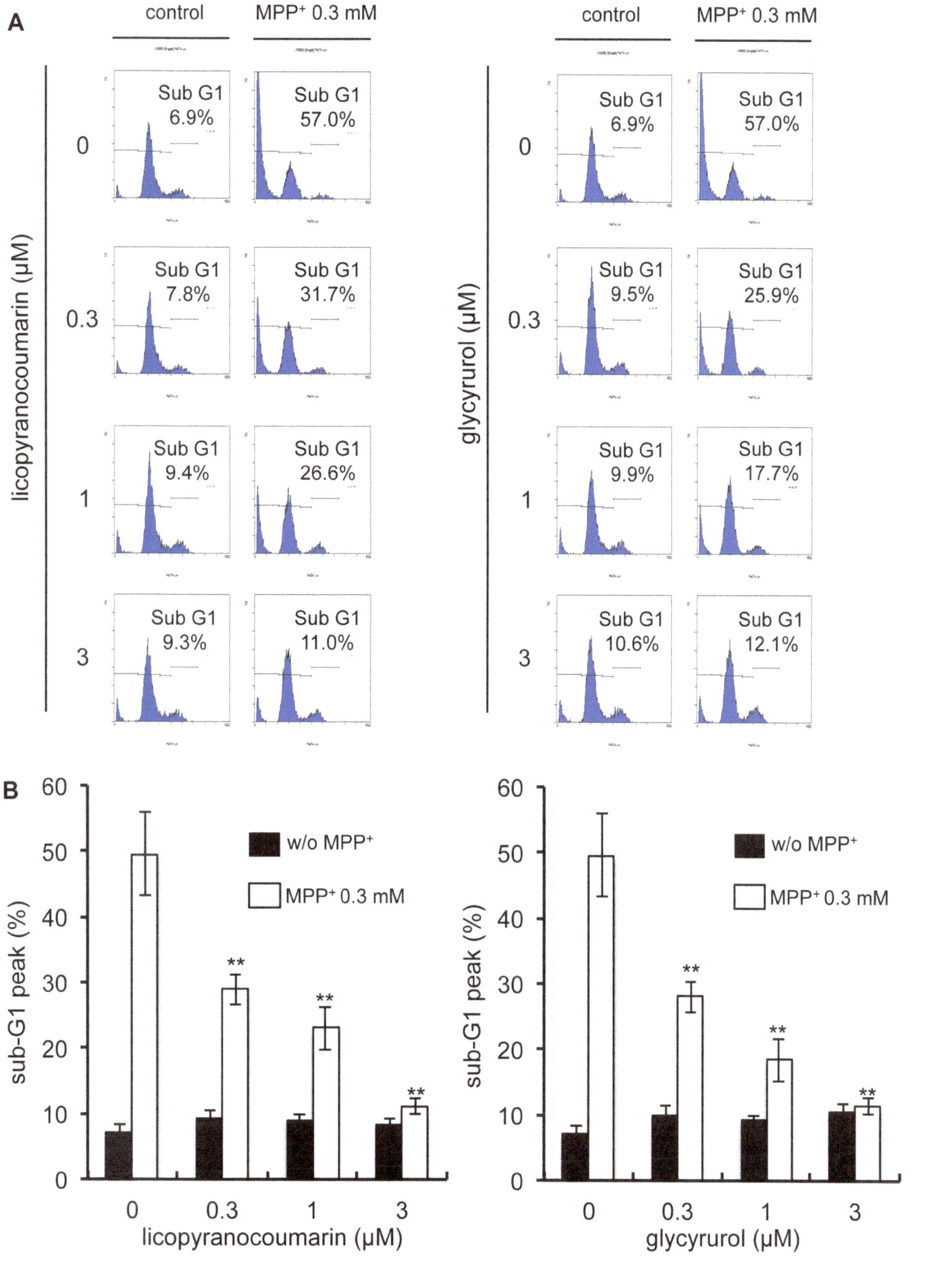
A
control
MPP+ 0.3 mM
licopyranocoumarin (μM)
0
0.3
1
3
Sub G1 6.9%
Sub G1 57.0%
Sub G1 7.8%
Sub G1 31.7%
Sub G1 9.4%
Sub G1 26.6%
Sub G1 9.3%
Sub G1 11.0%
glycyrurol (μM)
Sub G1 6.9%
Sub G1 57.0%
Sub G1 9.5%
Sub G1 25.9%
Sub G1 9.9%
Sub G1 17.7%
Sub G1 10.6%
Sub G1 12.1%
B
sub-G1 peak (%)
w/o MPP+
MPP+ 0.3 mM
**
licopyranocoumarin (μM)
glycyrurol (μM)

Figure 4. Licopyranocoumarin and glycyrurol attenuated MPP$^+$-induced apoptosis. (**A**) NGF-differentiated PC12D cells were treated with various concentrations of licopyranocoumarin or glycyrurol in the presence of 0.3 mM MPP$^+$ for 48 h. Collected cells were stained with PI and analyzed by flow cytometry. (**B**) The sub G1 ratio was analyzed. Values are the means of three independent experiments; bars, s.d. $^{**}p<0.01$ compared with MPP$^+$ group cells.

activity in mouse plasma and gastrointestinal tube [38], inhibition of cholera toxin [39], and inhibitory effects on drug oxidations [40]. In this study, we have demonstrated that *choi-joki-to* and *daio-kanzo-to* had neuroprotective effects against MPP$^+$- and rotenone-induced toxicity in NGF-differentiated neuronal PC12D cells. Furthermore, we identified that *Glycyrrhiza*, commonly contained in these two herbal medicines, possessed potent neuroprotective activity against MPP$^+$-induced toxicity. *Glycyrrhiza* is contained in a number of traditional herbal medicines including *yi-gan san* previously identified as neuroprotective agents against mitochondrial toxins, therefore, we investigated relationships between the neuroprotective effects of traditional herbal medicines and their contents of *Glycyrrhiza*. The correlation coefficient between neuroprotective effects of traditional herbal medicines and contents of *Glycyrrhiza* in each herbal medicine was calculated at 0.20 (Figure S1), indicating a very weak relationship. This weak relationship might be explained by our finding that higher concentration of *Glycyrrhiza* (300 μg/ml) showed cytotoxic effect in PC12D cells (Figure S2). Another possible explanation is that other constituent of traditional herbal medicines, such as rhubarb, also exerted neuroprotective effects in PC12D cells (Figure 2). Major components of *Glycyrrhiza* are triterpenoid saponins, and glycyrrhizin and its metabolite. These compounds show several potential health effects including anti-inflammatory, anti-viral, hepatoprotective, anti-cancer and immunomodulatory effects [41]. Therefore, at first we predicted that glycyrrhizin might be an active principle contained in *Glycyrrhiza* that suppressed MPP$^+$- and rotenone-induced toxicity, but glycyrrhizin did not show such activities. Instead, we isolated the coumarin derivatives, licopyranocoumarin (LPC) and glycyrurol (GCR), as the most potent neuroprotective compounds in *Glycyrrhiza*. LPC isolated from *Glycyrrhiza* sp. has been reported to show several bioactivities, including anti-HIV effects and inhibition of CYP3A4 and the aryl hydrocarbon receptor antagonist [42,43,44]. On the other hand, GCR, which was very recently isolated from *Glycyrrhiza uralensis*, shows antithrombotic effects [45]. However, so far the neuroprotective effects of these two compounds have not yet been reported. This study has indeed revealed, for the first time, the potent neuroprotective activity of LPC and GCR in a PD-like cellular model system. LPC and GCR also inhibited rotenone-induced cell death in HeLa cells; however, the effects in HeLa cells were quite weak when compared to that seen in PC12D cells (Figure S3). Therefore, LPC and GCR seem to prefer to exert cytoprotection in neuronal cells. Oxidative stress associated with a general dysfunction of mitochondrial homeostasis is a leading hypothesis as a potential mechanism for dopaminergic neuronal degeneration in PD [46]. Postmortem analyses of the substantia nigra from PD patients confirm several oxidative stress-related alterations [47,48,49], and several toxins (rotenone, paraquat, and MPP$^+$) used to produce PD-animal models directly and/or indirectly inhibit mitochondrial function, induce the production of ROS, and promote oxidative damage. Therefore, antioxidant ingredients are considered to be promising approach to prevent the disease progression. For example, α-tocopherol, coenzyme Q_{10} and catechols have been reported to exert neuroprotective effects by attenuating rotenone-induced oxidative stress on rotenone models *in vitro* and *in vivo* [50,51,52]. Likewise, we found that LPC and GCR attenuated the MPP$^+$-induced increase in intracellular ROS generation (Figure 6A), indicating that inhibition of MPP$^+$-mediated ROS generation is closely related to the neuroprotective effects of LPC and GCR. Several lines of evidence have suggested that ROS generation induces the activation of JNK signaling, and JNK represents one of the major signaling pathways implicated in PD pathogenesis. JNK activity is increased in MPTP animal models [53,54,55,56], MPP$^+$-treated cell culture models [35,54], and rotenone neurotoxicity [57,58]. Moreover, ROS-mediated activation of JNK almost inevitably leads to cell death. Indeed, we also confirmed that a JNK inhibitor, SP600125, suppressed MPP$^+$-induced cell death (Figure 8B), and MPP$^+$-induced activation of JNK and cell death were found to be inhibited by LPC and GCR under conditions where LPC or GCR inhibited the MPP$^+$-mediated ROS generation (Figure 8A). Although the potential mechanisms by which JNK participates in MPP$^+$-induced cell death remains to be fully determined, activation of JNK has been reported to mediate cell death by participating in the induction of mitochondrial permeability transition (mPT) and decrease of $\Delta\Psi_{mit}$ in subsets of cell types [59,60]. Because in our assay system SP600125 inhibited both cell death and the decrease in $\Delta\Psi_{mit}$ induced by MPP$^+$ (Figure. 8B and C), we consider the inhibition of the decrease in MPP$^+$-induced $\Delta\Psi_{mit}$ caused by LPC and GCR (Figure 5) to be due to the inhibition of ROS-mediated JNK activation.

Several neuroprotective compounds have significant antioxidant and free radical-scavenging activities. LPC and GCR are members of the coumarin compound family. There have been several reports on the antioxidant activities of coumarins [61,62,63], and LPC and GCR each inhibited MPP$^+$-induced ROS generation. Nevertheless, neither LPC nor GCR possessed ROS scavenging activity *in vitro*. Increased amount of ROS can be generated by an imbalance of antioxidant enzymes and activation of the oxidase

Table 1. Crude drugs constituents of "*choi-joki-to*" and "*daio-kanzo-to*".

choi-joki-to		*daio-kanzo-to*	
Scientific names	**Contents (g)**	**Scientific names**	**Contents (g)**
rhubarb	2	rhubarb	4
glycyrrhiza	1	*glycyrrhiza*	2
Salt cake	0.5		

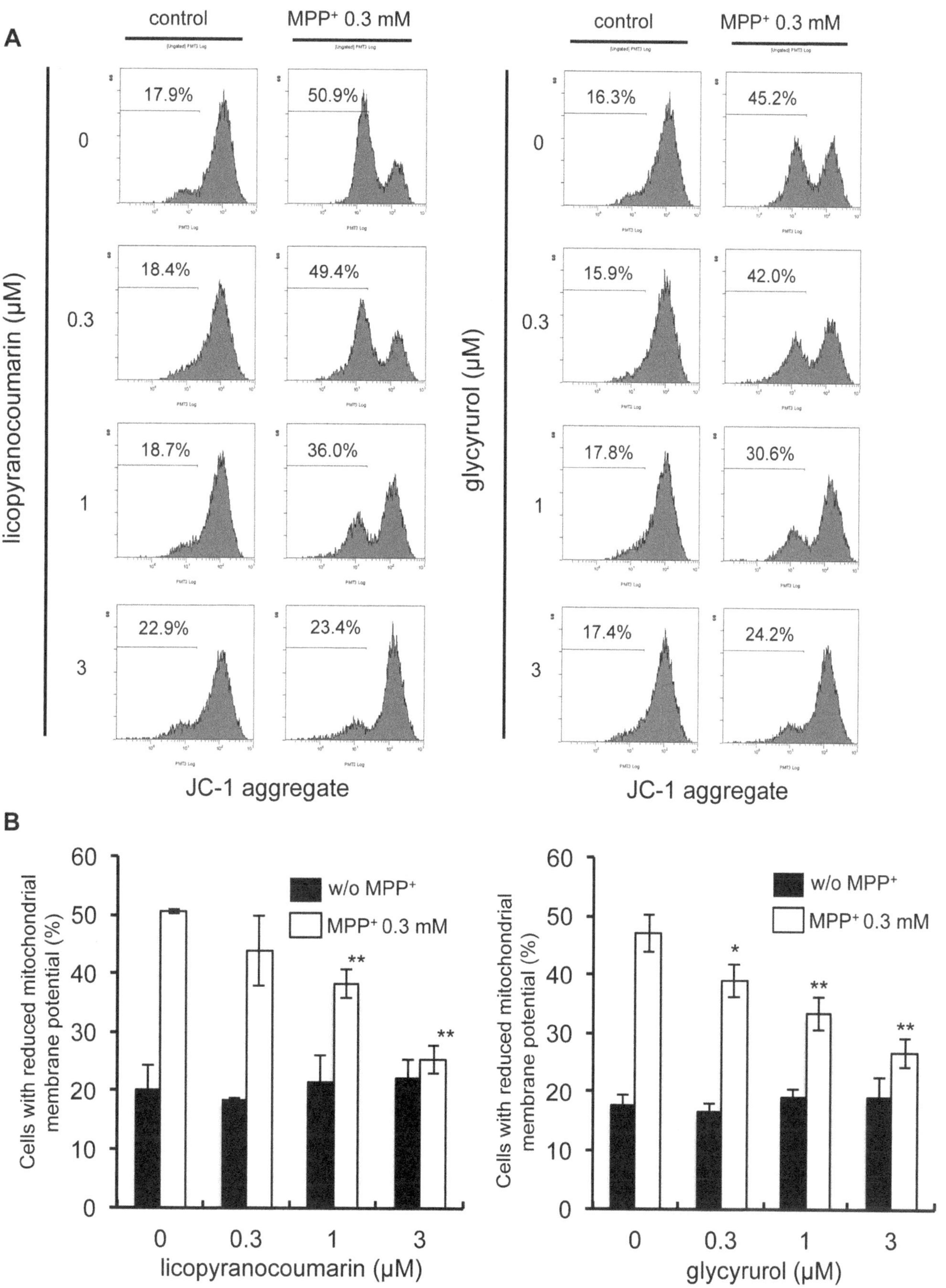
A
control
MPP+ 0.3 mM
licopyranocoumarin (μM)
glycyrurol (μM)
0
0.3
1
3
17.9%
50.9%
18.4%
49.4%
18.7%
36.0%
22.9%
23.4%
16.3%
45.2%
15.9%
42.0%
17.8%
30.6%
17.4%
24.2%
JC-1 aggregate
B
Cells with reduced mitochondrial membrane potential (%)
w/o MPP+
MPP+ 0.3 mM
licopyranocoumarin (μM)
glycyrurol (μM)

Figure 5. Licopyranocoumarin and glycyrurol protected cells against MPP$^+$-induced disappearance of mitochondrial membrane potential. (**A**) NGF-differentiated PC12D cells were treated with various concentrations of licopyranocoumarin or glycyrurol in the presence of 0.3 mM MPP$^+$ for 48 h. Collected cells were stained with JC-1 and analyzed by flow cytometry. (**B**) The ratio of cells exhibiting disappearance of mitochondrial membrane potential was analyzed. Values are the means of three independent experiments; bars, s.d. $^*p<0.05$, $^{**}p<0.01$ compared with MPP$^+$ group cells.

system. Membrane-bound nicotinamide adenine dinucleotide phosphate (NADPH) oxidase (Nox) is known to be a neurotoxin-related oxidase enzyme system [64,65], and enzymatic antioxidants include superoxide dismutase (SOD), glutathione peroxidase (GPx), thioredoxin reductase (TPx) and catalase [66]. Therefore, it is likely that LPC and GCR might induce the imbalance by inhibiting oxidase activity directly or neurotoxin-induced activation of oxidase system. Furthermore, we can't exclude the possibility that LPC and GCR could induce the expression or activation of antioxidant enzymes.

In summary, we identified *choi-joki-to* and *daio-kanzo-to* as neuroprotective herbal medicines, and both LPC and GCR were identified as neuroprotective substances from *Glycyrrhiza* contained in *choi-joki-to* and *daio-kanzo-to*. LPC or GCR exert their neuroprotective effects by inhibiting MPP$^+$-induced ROS production and thus limiting JNK activation, and causing a subsequent decrease in $\Delta\Psi_{mit}$. Our proposed mechanism is illustrated in Figure 9. Further studies are required to elucidate the molecular mechanisms for the suppression of ROS generation by LPC and GCR in PC12D cells. Our findings enliven the prospect of using LPC, GCR, *choi-joki-to* and *daio-kanzo-to* as effective and safe natural therapeutic agents in PD; *in vivo* trials in MPTP animal models are needed.

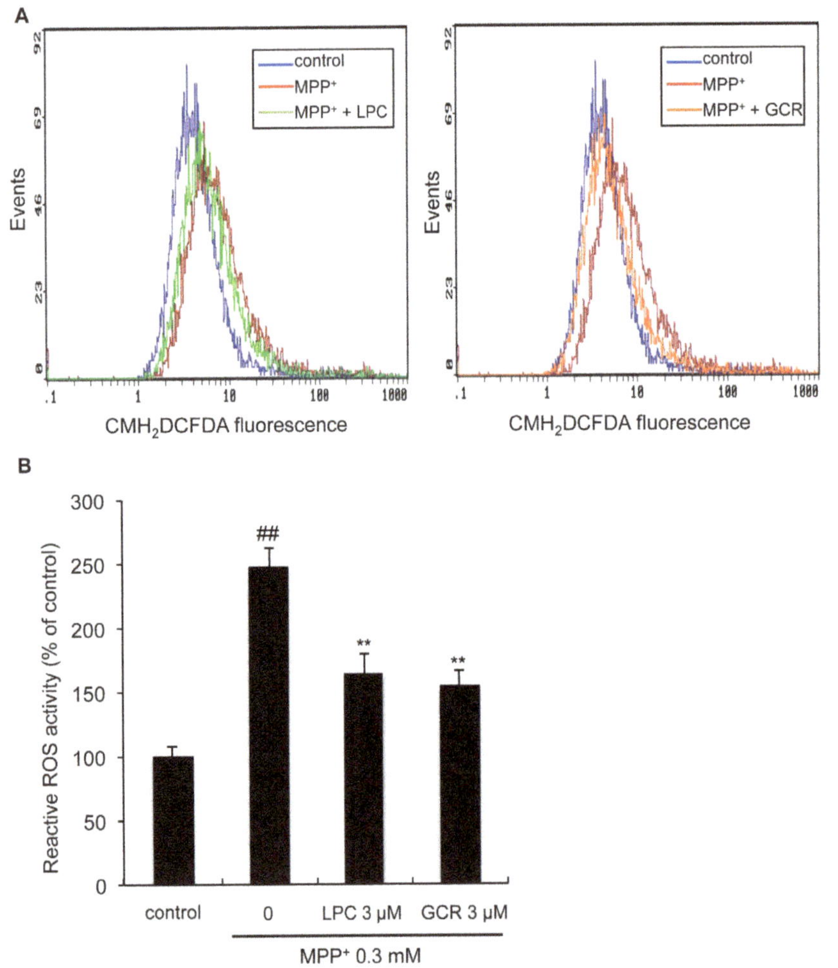

Figure 6. Licopyranocoumarin and glycyrurol decreased MPP$^+$-induced intracellular ROS generation. (**A**) NGF-differentiated PC12D cells were pre-incubated for 1 h with 3 µM licopyranocoumarin (LPC) or 3 µM glycyrurol (GCR), then treated with 0.3 mM MPP$^+$ for 12 h. Then, the samples were loaded with 2.5 µM CM-H_2DCFDA and the fluorescence intensities were measured by flow cytometry. (**B**) The ratio of cells exhibiting ROS production was analyzed. Values are the means of four independent experiments; bars, s.d. $^{\#\#}p<0.01$ compared with control cells. $^{**}p<0.01$ compared with MPP$^+$ group cells.

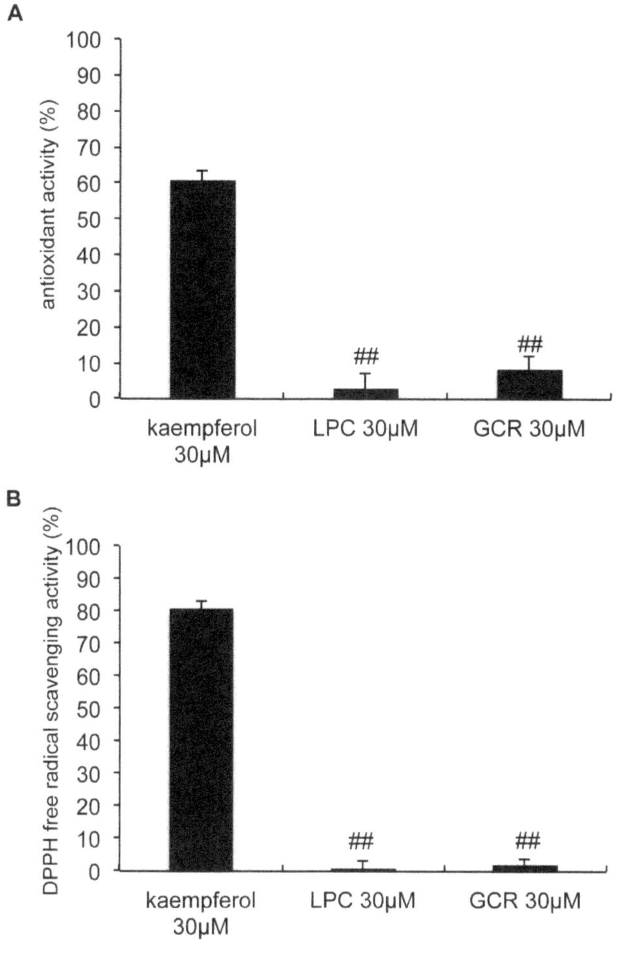

Figure 7. Licopyranocoumarin and glycyrurol lacked potency for scavenging free radicals. Antioxidant activities of licopyranocoumarin (LPC) and glycyrurol (GCR) were measured by (**A**) a β-carotene bleaching assay system and (**B**) a DPPH radical scavenging assay. Kaempferol served as the positive control. Values are the means of three independent experiments; bars, s.d. $^{\#\#}p<0.01$ compared with antioxidant activity of kaempferol.

Materials and Methods

Reagents

MPP^+, Rotenone, linoleic acid, 2,2-Diphenyl-1-pocrylhydrazyl (DPPH), SP600125 and mouse monoclonal anti-β-actin antibodies were purchased from Sigma Chemical Co. (St. Louis, MO). Taxol, cisplatin, JC-1 and pyridinium iodide were purchased from Wako Pure Chemical Industries, Ltd. (Osaka, Japan). Nerve growth factors, CM-H_2DCFDA, and β-carotene standard were purchased from Alomone Labs (Jerusalem, Israel), Life Technologies (Carlsbad, CA) and Kanto Chemical Co. (Tokyo, Japan), respectively. Rabbit polyclonal anti-JNK antibody and rabbit monoclonal anti-phospho-JNK antibody were purchased from Santa Cruz Biotechnology (Santa Cruz, CA) and Cell Signaling (Beverly, MA), respectively. Horseradish peroxidase-conjugated anti-mouse and anti-rabbit IgG used as a secondary antibodies were from GE Healthcare (Little Chalfont, UK).

Cell cultures

PC12D was identified a new subline of PC12 pheochromocytoma cells (PC12D cells) in which neurites are extended within 24 h in response to cAMP-enhancing reagents as well as in response to nerve growth factor (NGF) [30]. PC12D cells were cultured in Dulbecco's modified Eagle medium supplemented with 5% (v/v) inactivated fetal bovine serum, 10% (v/v) inactivated horse serum, 100 U/mL penicillin G, 0.6 mg/mL L-glutamine, and 0.1 mg/mL kanamycin at 37°C with 5% CO_2. PC12D cells were differentiated by 100 ng/mL NGF treatment for 48 h.

Cell viability assays

For the trypan blue dye exclusion assay, differentiated PC12D cells were cultured in 48-well dishes. Drug-treated or untreated cells were stained with trypan blue (Sigma Chemical Co.), and the ratio of viable cells was determined using a hemocytometer. Cell viability (%) means the ratio of the number of trypan blue-impermeable cells to total cell count. IC_{50} values were calculated by linear regression analysis from the inhibition of MPP^+-induced cell death at different concentrations of the drug.

Cell cycle analysis

To examine apoptosis, differentiated PC12D cells were harvested after drug treatment. The cells were washed with PBS and fixed with 70% ethanol at 4°C for more than 1 h. The cells were then stained with propidium iodide (PI) solution according to a previously reported protocol [67]. The labeled nuclei were subjected to flow cytometry (FCM, Beckman-Coulter, Miami, FL).

Measurements of mitochondrial membrane potential

Changes in mitochondrial membrane potentials were assessed JC-1 (5,5′,6,6′-tetrachloro-1,1′,3,3′-tetraehylbenzimidazolylcarbocyanineiodide) (Wako) was used according to the manufacturer's protocol. Briefly, treated cells were collected by pipetting and removing medium. Next, the cells were incubated in medium containing 2.5 μg/ml JC-1 for 20 min at 37°C. Cells were then washed with PBS. JC-1 fluorescence was measured by a flow cytometer.

Measurement of intracellular ROS

Intracellular ROS production was measured using CM-H_2DCFDA. The cells were plated at a density of 12×10^4 cells per 12-well dish. The cells were treated with MPP^+ and test compounds for 12 h, and then trypsinized and collected. After the cells were washed with PBS, incubated with 2.5 μM CM-H_2DCFDA in HBSS at 37°C for 30 min, and then washed again with PBS three times. The relative levels of fluorescence were quantified by using a flow cytometer.

β-carotene bleaching assay

This assay was carried out according to the β-carotene bleaching method [68]. A mixture of β-carotene and linoleic acid was prepared by adding a mixture of 0.3 mg of β-carotene in 3 mL chloroform, 40 mg linoleic acid and 400 mg Tween 20. Chloroform was removed and 100 mL of distilled water was added to form an emulsion with continuous shaking. Aliquots (0.1 mL) of the β-carotene/linoleic acid emulsion were mixed with 1 μL of sample solution and incubated in a water bath at 50°C. The oxidation of the emulsion was monitored spectrophotometrically by measuring absorbance at 470 nm over a 60-min period. Control samples contained 1 μL of methanol. Antioxidant activity is expressed as percent inhibition relative to control after 60 min incubation using the following equation:

$$AA(\%) = 100(DR_c - DR_s)/DR_c,$$

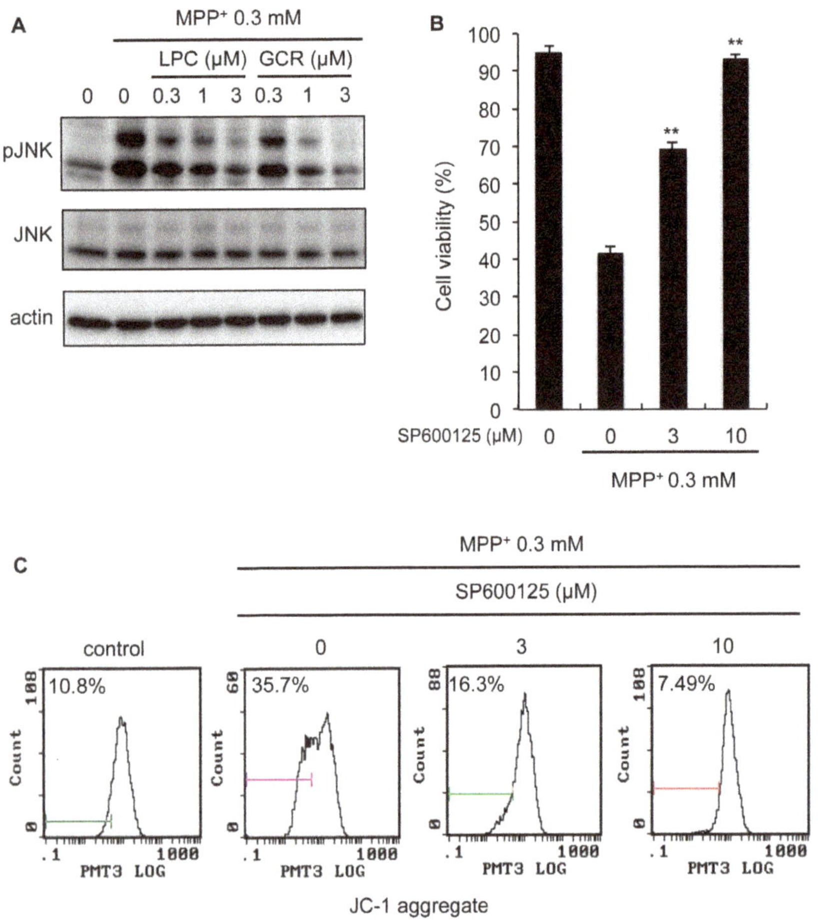

Figure 8. Licopyranocoumarin and glycyrurol attenuated MPP$^+$-induced JNK activation. (**A**) NGF-differentiated PC12D cells were treated with various concentrations of licopyranocoumarin (LPC) or glycyrurol (GCR) and 0.3 mM MPP$^+$ for 36 h, and JNK and phosphor-JNK level were detected by Western blot. NGF-differentiated PC12D cells were treated with SP600125 and 0.3 mM MPP$^+$ for 48 h. Thereafter (**B**) cell viability was measured by trypan blue dye exclusion assay and (**C**) mitochondrial membrane potentials were assessed by JC-1 assay. Values of (B) are the means of three independent experiments; $^{**}p<0.01$ compared with MPP$^+$ group cells.

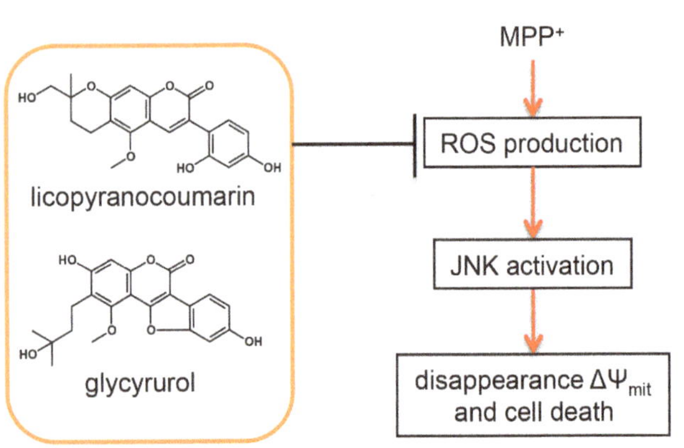

Figure 9. Suggested model for neuroprotection of licopyranocoumarin and glycyrurol against MPP$^+$-induced toxicity in PC12D cells. Both licopyranocoumarin and glycyrurol exert neuroprotective effects against MPP$^+$-induced toxicity via suppression of ROS generation and of JNK activation.

where AA = antioxidant activity; DR_c = degradation rate of the control = $[\ln(a/b)/60]$; DR_s = degradation rate in presence of the sample = $[\ln(a/b)/60]$; a = absorbance at time 0; b = absorbance at 60 min.

DPPH radical scavenging assay

The DPPH radical scavenging effect of test compounds was determined according to the previously described method [68]. The reaction mixtures contained 100 μL ethanol, 125 μM DPPH, and test compounds. After 2 min of incubation at room temperature, the absorbance was recorded at 517 nm.

Extraction and isolation of licopyranocoumarin and glycyrurol from *Glycyrrhiza*

Compounds were extracted from dried and pulverized *Glycyrrhiza* (50 g) with 90% EtOH, then filtrated and concentrated *in vacuo*. This suspension was adjusted to pH 7.0, followed by extraction with EtOAc (5 L) twice; the organic layer was concentrated to yield residue (3.76 g). The EtOAc extract was fractionated by centrifugal partition chromatography (CPC) with $CHCl_3$:MeOH:H_2O (5:6:4). The obtained crude active extract was applied on Sephadex LH20 column chromatography (Sephadex LH-20, 70 μM; GE Healthcare, NJ, USA), and eluted with MeOH. The active fraction (250.6 mg) was further purified by preparative octadecyl silyl (ODS) HPLC (YMC-Pack ODS-AQ, YMC Co. Ltd., Japan) with 40% aqueous CH_3CN to give pure licopyranocoumarin (10.8 mg) and glycyrurol (4 mg), respectively.

Western blotting

Cells were lysed in RIPA buffer (25 mM HEPES (pH 7.2), 1.5% Triton X-100 (Wako), 1% sodium deoxycholate (Wako), 0.1% SDS, 0.5 M NaCl (Wako), 5 mM EDTA, 50 mM NaF (Sigma), 0.1 mM sodium vanadate (Sigma) and 1 mM phenylmethylsulfonyl fluoride (PMSF) with sonication. The lysates were centrifuged at 13,000 rpm for 15 min to yield the soluble cell lysates. For immunoblotting, cell lysates were subjected to SDS-polyacrylamide gel electrophoresis. Proteins were transferred onto a polyvinylidene fluoride membrane (Millipore) by electroblotting and then incubated with appropriate antibodies. Immune complexes were detected with an Immobilon Western kit (Millipore), and luminescence was detected with a LAS-1000 mini (Fujifilm Co., Tokyo, Japan).

Statistical analysis

All statistical analyses in bar plots were performed with a two-tailed paired Student's *t*-test.

Supporting Information

Figure S1 The correlation between contents of *Glycyrrhiza* and neuroprotective activity in herbal medicines. (TIF)

Figure S2 Toxicity of EtOAc extract of *Glycyrrhiza*. NGF-differentiated PC12D cells were treated with various concentrations of EtOAc extract of *Glycyrrhiza* for 48 h. Cell viability was evaluated by trypan blue dye exclusion assay. (TIF)

Figure S3 Licopyranocoumarin and glycyrurol preferentially showed cytoprotective effects in neuronal cells. HeLa cells or NGF-differentiated PC12D cells were treated with various concentrations of licopyranocoumarin (LPC) or glycyrurol (GCR) in the presence of 0.3 μM Rotenone for 48 h. Cell viability was evaluated by trypan blue dye exclusion assay. (TIF)

Author Contributions

Conceived and designed the experiments: NH MI. Performed the experiments: TF DY. Analyzed the data: TF MK. Contributed reagents/materials/analysis tools: TF SS ET MI. Wrote the paper: TF SS ET NH MI.

References

1. Dawson TM, Dawson VL (2002) Neuroprotective and neurorestorative strategies for Parkinson's disease. Nature neuroscience 5 Suppl: 1058–1061.
2. Bindoff LA, Birch-Machin M, Cartlidge NE, Parker WD Jr, Turnbull DM (1989) Mitochondrial function in Parkinson's disease. Lancet 2: 49.
3. Parker WD Jr, Parks JK, Swerdlow RH (2008) Complex I deficiency in Parkinson's disease frontal cortex. Brain research 1189: 215–218.
4. Parker WD Jr, Swerdlow RH (1998) Mitochondrial dysfunction in idiopathic Parkinson disease. American journal of human genetics 62: 758–762.
5. Schapira AH, Cooper JM, Dexter D, Clark JB, Jenner P, et al. (1990) Mitochondrial complex I deficiency in Parkinson's disease. Journal of neurochemistry 54: 823–827.
6. Smigrodzki R, Parks J, Parker WD (2004) High frequency of mitochondrial complex I mutations in Parkinson's disease and aging. Neurobiology of aging 25: 1273–1281.
7. Esteves AR, Domingues AF, Ferreira IL, Januario C, Swerdlow RH, et al. (2008) Mitochondrial function in Parkinson's disease cybrids containing an nt2 neuron-like nuclear background. Mitochondrion 8: 219–228.
8. Swerdlow RH, Parks JK, Cassarino DS, Shilling AT, Bennett JP Jr, et al. (1999) Characterization of cybrid cell lines containing mtDNA from Huntington's disease patients. Biochemical and biophysical research communications 261: 701–704.
9. Trimmer PA, Borland MK, Keeney PM, Bennett JP Jr, Parker WD Jr (2004) Parkinson's disease transgenic mitochondrial cybrids generate Lewy inclusion bodies. Journal of neurochemistry 88: 800–812.
10. Heikkila RE, Hess A, Duvoisin RC (1984) Dopaminergic neurotoxicity of 1-methyl-4-phenyl-1,2,5,6-tetrahydropyridine in mice. Science 224: 1451–1453.
11. Eberhardt O, Schulz JB (2003) Apoptotic mechanisms and antiapoptotic therapy in the MPTP model of Parkinson's disease. Toxicology letters 139: 135–151.
12. Burns RS, Chiueh CC, Markey SP, Ebert MH, Jacobowitz DM, et al. (1983) A primate model of parkinsonism: selective destruction of dopaminergic neurons in the pars compacta of the substantia nigra by N-methyl-4-phenyl-1,2,3,6-tetrahydropyridine. Proceedings of the National Academy of Sciences of the United States of America 80: 4546–4550.
13. Davis GC, Williams AC, Markey SP, Ebert MH, Caine ED, et al. (1979) Chronic Parkinsonism secondary to intravenous injection of meperidine analogues. Psychiatry research 1: 249–254.
14. Betarbet R, Sherer TB, MacKenzie G, Garcia-Osuna M, Panov AV, et al. (2000) Chronic systemic pesticide exposure reproduces features of Parkinson's disease. Nature neuroscience 3: 1301–1306.
15. Martinez TN, Greenamyre JT (2012) Toxin models of mitochondrial dysfunction in Parkinson's disease. Antioxidants & redox signaling 16: 920–934.
16. Heikkila RE, Manzino L, Cabbat FS, Duvoisin RC (1984) Protection against the dopaminergic neurotoxicity of 1-methyl-4-phenyl-1,2,5,6-tetrahydropyridine by monoamine oxidase inhibitors. Nature 311: 467–469.
17. Cohen G, Pasik P, Cohen B, Leist A, Mytilineou C, et al. (1984) Pargyline and deprenyl prevent the neurotoxicity of 1-methyl-4-phenyl-1,2,3,6-tetrahydropyridine (MPTP) in monkeys. European journal of pharmacology 106: 209–210.
18. Cao BY, Yang YP, Luo WF, Mao CJ, Han R, et al. (2010) Paeoniflorin, a potent natural compound, protects PC12 cells from MPP+ and acidic damage via autophagic pathway. Journal of ethnopharmacology 131: 122–129.
19. Kong XC, Zhang D, Qian C, Liu GT, Bao XQ (2011) FLZ, a novel HSP27 and HSP70 inducer, protects SH-SY5Y cells from apoptosis caused by MPP(+). Brain research 1383: 99–107.
20. Park SW, Lee CH, Lee JG, Kim LW, Shin BS, et al. (2011) Protective effects of atypical antipsychotic drugs against MPP(+)-induced oxidative stress in PC12 cells. Neuroscience research 69: 283–290.
21. Yurekli VA, Gurler S, Naziroglu M, Uguz AC, Koyuncuoglu HR (2013) Zonisamide attenuates MPP+-induced oxidative toxicity through modulation of Ca2+ signaling and caspase-3 activity in neuronal PC12 cells. Cellular and molecular neurobiology 33: 205–212.
22. Manyam BV, Sanchez-Ramos JR (1999) Traditional and complementary therapies in Parkinson's disease. Advances in neurology 80: 565–574.
23. Bae N, Ahn T, Chung S, Oh MS, Ko H, et al. (2011) The neuroprotective effect of modified Yeoldahanso-tang via autophagy enhancement in models of Parkinson's disease. Journal of ethnopharmacology 134: 313–322.
24. Doo AR, Kim SN, Park JY, Cho KH, Hong J, et al. (2010) Neuroprotective effects of an herbal medicine, Yi-Gan San on MPP+/MPTP-induced cytotoxicity in vitro and in vivo. Journal of ethnopharmacology 131: 433–442.
25. Hashimoto R, Yu J, Koizumi H, Ouchi Y, Okabe T (2012) Ginsenoside Rb1 Prevents MPP(+)-Induced Apoptosis in PC12 Cells by Stimulating Estrogen Receptors with Consequent Activation of ERK1/2, Akt and Inhibition of SAPK/JNK, p38 MAPK. Evidence-based complementary and alternative medicine: eCAM 2012: 693717.
26. Li X, Ye X, Sun X, Liang Q, Tao L, et al. (2011) Salidroside protects against MPP(+)-induced apoptosis in PC12 cells by inhibiting the NO pathway. Brain research 1382: 9–18.
27. Zhou J, Sun Y, Zhao X, Deng Z, Pu X (2013) 3-O-demethylswertipunicoside inhibits MPP(+)-induced oxidative stress and apoptosis in PC12 cells. Brain research 1508: 53–62.
28. Chung V, Liu L, Bian Z, Zhao Z, Leuk Fong W, et al. (2006) Efficacy and safety of herbal medicines for idiopathic Parkinson's disease: a systematic review. Movement disorders: official journal of the Movement Disorder Society 21: 1709–1715.
29. Beal MF (2001) Experimental models of Parkinson's disease. Nature reviews Neuroscience 2: 325–334.
30. Katoh-Semba R, Kitajima S, Yamazaki Y, Sano M (1987) Neuritic growth from a new subline of PC12 pheochromocytoma cells: cyclic AMP mimics the action of nerve growth factor. Journal of neuroscience research 17: 36–44.

31. Yao S, Li Y, Kong L (2006) Preparative isolation and purification of chemical constituents from the root of Polygonum multiflorum by high-speed counter-current chromatography. Journal of chromatography A 1115: 64–71.
32. Mielke K, Herdegen T (2000) JNK and p38 stresskinases—degenerative effectors of signal-transduction-cascades in the nervous system. Progress in neurobiology 61: 45–60.
33. Tatton WG, Chalmers-Redman R, Brown D, Tatton N (2003) Apoptosis in Parkinson's disease: signals for neuronal degradation. Annals of neurology 53 Suppl 3: S61-70; discussion S70–62.
34. Voss T, Ravina B (2008) Neuroprotection in Parkinson's disease: myth or reality? Current neurology and neuroscience reports 8: 304–309.
35. Kim SY, Kim MY, Mo JS, Park JW, Park HS (2007) SAG protects human neuroblastoma SH-SY5Y cells against 1-methyl-4-phenylpyridinium ion (MPP+)-induced cytotoxicity via the downregulation of ROS generation and JNK signaling. Neuroscience letters 413: 132–136.
36. Nishimura K, Osawa T, Watanabe K (2011) Evaluation of oxygen radical absorbance capacity in kampo medicine. Evidence-based complementary and alternative medicine: eCAM 2011: 812163.
37. Iizuka A, Iijima OT, Kondo K, Matsumoto A, Itakura H, et al. (2000) Antioxidative effects of Choi-oki-to and its ability to inhibit the progression of atheroma in KHC rabbits. Journal of atherosclerosis and thrombosis 6: 49–54.
38. Kobayashi K, Funayama N, Suzuki R, Yoshizaki F (2002) Survey of the influence of Chinese medicinal prescriptions on amylase activity in mouse plasma and gastrointestinal tube. Biological & pharmaceutical bulletin 25: 1108–1111.
39. Oi H, Matsuura D, Miyake M, Ueno M, Takai I, et al. (2002) Identification in traditional herbal medications and confirmation by synthesis of factors that inhibit cholera toxin-induced fluid accumulation. Proceedings of the National Academy of Sciences of the United States of America 99: 3042–3046.
40. Hasegawa A, Kawaguchi Y, Nakasa H, Nakamura H, Ohmori S, et al. (2002) Effects of Kampo extracts on drug metabolism in rat liver microsomes: Rhei Rhizoma extract and Glycyrrhizae Radix extract inhibit drug oxidation. Japanese journal of pharmacology 89: 164–170.
41. Asl MN, Hosseinzadeh H (2008) Review of pharmacological effects of Glycyrrhiza sp. and its bioactive compounds. Phytotherapy research: PTR 22: 709–724.
42. Hatano T, Yasuhara T, Fukuda T, Noro T, Okuda T (1989) Phenolic constituents of licorice. II. Structures of licopyranocoumarin, licoarylcoumarin and glisoflavone, and inhibitory effects of licorice phenolics on xanthine oxidase. Chemical & pharmaceutical bulletin 37: 3005–3009.
43. Tsukamoto S, Aburatani M, Yoshida T, Yamashita Y, El-Beih AA, et al. (2005) CYP3A4 inhibitors isolated from Licorice. Biological & pharmaceutical bulletin 28: 2000–2002.
44. Kasai A, Hiramatsu N, Hayakawa K, Yao J, Kitamura M (2008) Blockade of the dioxin pathway by herbal medicine Formula Bupleuri Minor: identification of active entities for suppression of AhR activation. Biological & pharmaceutical bulletin 31: 838–846.
45. Tao WW, Duan JA, Yang NY, Tang YP, Liu MZ, et al. (2012) Antithrombotic phenolic compounds from Glycyrrhiza uralensis. Fitoterapia 83: 422–425.
46. Seaton TA, Cooper JM, Schapira AH (1997) Free radical scavengers protect dopaminergic cell lines from apoptosis induced by complex I inhibitors. Brain research 777: 110–118.
47. Alam ZI, Jenner A, Daniel SE, Lees AJ, Cairns N, et al. (1997) Oxidative DNA damage in the parkinsonian brain: an apparent selective increase in 8-hydroxyguanine levels in substantia nigra. Journal of neurochemistry 69: 1196–1203.
48. Dexter DT, Carter CJ, Wells FR, Javoy-Agid F, Agid Y, et al. (1989) Basal lipid peroxidation in substantia nigra is increased in Parkinson's disease. Journal of neurochemistry 52: 381–389.
49. Floor E, Wetzel MG (1998) Increased protein oxidation in human substantia nigra pars compacta in comparison with basal ganglia and prefrontal cortex measured with an improved dinitrophenylhydrazine assay. Journal of neurochemistry 70: 268–275.
50. Song JX, Sze SC, Ng TB, Lee CK, Leung GP, et al. (2012) Anti-Parkinsonian drug discovery from herbal medicines: what have we got from neurotoxic models? Journal of ethnopharmacology 139: 698–711.
51. Testa CM, Sherer TB, Greenamyre JT (2005) Rotenone induces oxidative stress and dopaminergic neuron damage in organotypic substantia nigra cultures. Brain research Molecular brain research 134: 109–118.
52. Yang L, Calingasan NY, Wille EJ, Cormier K, Smith K, et al. (2009) Combination therapy with coenzyme Q10 and creatine produces additive neuroprotective effects in models of Parkinson's and Huntington's diseases. Journal of neurochemistry 109: 1427–1439.
53. Saporito MS, Brown EM, Miller MS, Carswell S (1999) CEP-1347/KT-7515, an inhibitor of c-jun N-terminal kinase activation, attenuates the 1-methyl-4-phenyl tetrahydropyridine-mediated loss of nigrostriatal dopaminergic neurons In vivo. The Journal of pharmacology and experimental therapeutics 288: 421–427.
54. Xia XG, Harding T, Weller M, Bieneman A, Uney JB, et al. (2001) Gene transfer of the JNK interacting protein-1 protects dopaminergic neurons in the MPTP model of Parkinson's disease. Proceedings of the National Academy of Sciences of the United States of America 98: 10433–10438.
55. Hunot S, Vila M, Teismann P, Davis RJ, Hirsch EC, et al. (2004) JNK-mediated induction of cyclooxygenase 2 is required for neurodegeneration in a mouse model of Parkinson's disease. Proceedings of the National Academy of Sciences of the United States of America 101: 665–670.
56. Park SW, Kim SH, Park KH, Kim SD, Kim JY, et al. (2004) Preventive effect of antioxidants in MPTP-induced mouse model of Parkinson's disease. Neuroscience letters 363: 243–246.
57. Newhouse K, Hsuan SL, Chang SH, Cai B, Wang Y, et al. (2004) Rotenone-induced apoptosis is mediated by p38 and JNK MAP kinases in human dopaminergic SH-SY5Y cells. Toxicological sciences: an official journal of the Society of Toxicology 79: 137–146.
58. Klintworth H, Newhouse K, Li T, Choi WS, Faigle R, et al. (2007) Activation of c-Jun N-terminal protein kinase is a common mechanism underlying paraquat- and rotenone-induced dopaminergic cell apoptosis. Toxicological sciences: an official journal of the Society of Toxicology 97: 149–162.
59. Hanawa N, Shinohara M, Saberi B, Gaarde WA, Han D, et al. (2008) Role of JNK translocation to mitochondria leading to inhibition of mitochondria bioenergetics in acetaminophen-induced liver injury. The Journal of biological chemistry 283: 13565–13577.
60. Lin X, Wang YJ, Li Q, Hou YY, Hong MH, et al. (2009) Chronic high-dose morphine treatment promotes SH-SY5Y cell apoptosis via c-Jun N-terminal kinase-mediated activation of mitochondria-dependent pathway. The FEBS journal 276: 2022–2036.
61. Ng TB, Liu F, Wang ZT (2000) Antioxidative activity of natural products from plants. Life sciences 66: 709–723.
62. Fernandez-Puntero B, Barroso I, Iglesias I, Benedi J, Villar A (2001) Antioxidant activity of Fraxetin: in vivo and ex vivo parameters in normal situation versus induced stress. Biological & pharmaceutical bulletin 24: 777–784.
63. Vladimirov Iu A, Parfenov EA, Epanchintseva OM, Smirnov LD (1991) [The antiradical activity of coumarin reductones]. Biulleten' eksperimental'noi biologii i meditsiny 112: 472–475.
64. Infanger DW, Sharma RV, Davisson RL (2006) NADPH oxidases of the brain: distribution, regulation, and function. Antioxidants & redox signaling 8: 1583–1596.
65. Sawada M, Imamura K, Nagatsu T (2006) Role of cytokines in inflammatory process in Parkinson's disease. Journal of neural transmission Supplementum: 373–381.
66. Jin H, Kanthasamy A, Ghosh A, Anantharam V, Kalyanaraman B, et al. (2013) Mitochondria-targeted antioxidants for treatment of Parkinson's disease: Preclinical and clinical outcomes. Biochimica et biophysica acta.
67. Kawatani M, Uchi M, Simizu S, Osada H, Imoto M (2003) Transmembrane domain of Bcl-2 is required for inhibition of ceramide synthesis, but not cytochrome c release in the pathway of inostamycin-induced apoptosis. Experimental cell research 286: 57-66.
68. Kumazawa S, Taniguchi M, Suzuki Y, Shimura M, Kwon MS, et al. (2002) Antioxidant activity of polyphenols in carob pods. Journal of agricultural and food chemistry 50: 373–377.

2

Microbial Diversity Analysis of Fermented Mung Beans (Lu-Doh-Huang) by Using Pyrosequencing and Culture Methods

Shiou-Huei Chao[1], Hui-Yu Huang[2], Chuan-Hsiung Chang[3,4], Chih-Hsien Yang[3,4], Wei-Shen Cheng[4], Ya-Huei Kang[1], Koichi Watanabe[5], Ying-Chieh Tsai[1]*

1 Institute of Biochemistry and Molecular Biology, National Yang-Ming University, Taipei, Taiwan, **2** Department of Food Science, Nutrition and Nutraceutical Biotechnology, Shih Chien University, Taipei, Taiwan, **3** Center for Systems and Synthetic Biology, National Yang-Ming University, Taipei, Taiwan, **4** Institute of Biomedical Informatics, National Yang-Ming University, Taipei, Taiwan, **5** Yakult Central Institute for Microbiological Research, Tokyo, Japan

Abstract

In Taiwanese alternative medicine Lu-doh-huang (also called *Pracparatum mungo*), mung beans are mixed with various herbal medicines and undergo a 4-stage process of anaerobic fermentation. Here we used high-throughput sequencing of the 16S rRNA gene to profile the bacterial community structure of Lu-doh-huang samples. Pyrosequencing of samples obtained at 7 points during fermentation revealed 9 phyla, 264 genera, and 586 species of bacteria. While mung beans were inside bamboo sections (stages 1 and 2 of the fermentation process), family *Lactobacillaceae* and genus *Lactobacillus* emerged in highest abundance; *Lactobacillus plantarum* was broadly distributed among these samples. During stage 3, the bacterial distribution shifted to family *Porphyromonadaceae*, and *Butyricimonas virosa* became the predominant microbial component. Thereafter, bacterial counts decreased dramatically, and organisms were too few to be detected during stage 4. In addition, the microbial compositions of the liquids used for soaking bamboo sections were dramatically different: *Exiguobacterium mexicanum* predominated in the fermented soybean solution whereas *B. virosa* was predominant in running spring water. Furthermore, our results from pyrosequencing paralleled those we obtained by using the traditional culture method, which targets lactic acid bacteria. In conclusion, the microbial communities during Lu-doh-huang fermentation were markedly diverse, and pyrosequencing revealed a complete picture of the microbial consortium.

Editor: Stefan Bereswill, Charité-University Medicine Berlin, Germany

Funding: This work was supported by the National Science Council (NSC 99-2321-B-010-001-MY3), and High-throughput Genome Analysis Core Facility (NSC-100-2319-B-010-001) for pyrosequencing and Bioinformatics Consortium of Taiwan (NSC 100-2319-B-010-002) for bioinformatics analysis of National Core Facility Program for Biotechnology in Taiwan. The funders had no role in study design, data collection and analysis, decision to publish, or preparation of the manuscript.

Competing Interests: The authors have declared that no competing interests exist.

* E-mail: tsaiyc@ym.edu.tw

Introduction

Lu-doh-huang (also called *Pracparatum mungo*), which is based on fermented mung beans (*Vigna radiata*), is a Taiwanese alternative medicine. In this setting, Lu-doh-huang is used for its antipyretic and diuretic effects and for detoxification, reduction of swelling, and gut decontamination as empiric treatment. In addition, Lu-doh-huang induces apoptosis of Hep3B hepatoma cells [1], reduces inflammation in lipopolysaccharide-induced RAW264.7 cells [2], and has antioxidative properties [2–4]. In animal models, Lu-doh-huang exerts a protective effect on CCl_4-induced hepatotoxicity in rats [5]; induces the activities of NADPH-CYP reductase, glutathione S-transferase, superoxide dismutase, glutathione peroxidase, and catalase in Balb/c mice [2,3]; significantly decreases plasma glucose, total cholesterol, and triglycerides [3]; and inhibits tyrosinase activity in MDCK and A375 cells [3].

The manufacturing process of Lu-doh-huang is divided into 4 stages, and each stage lasts for 4 months (Fig. 1 and 2). Stage 1 runs from about the beginning of September to the end of the following January. During this stage, mung beans are mixed with various Chinese herbal medicines, including powdered *Ganoderma lucidum*, *Taiwanofungus camphoratus*, *Coptis chinensis* Franch., *Houttuynia cordata* Thunb., and *Glycyrrhiza uralensis* Fisch. Small- diameter holes are drilled into sections of live bamboo. The mixture of mung beans then is stuffed through these holes in the bamboo by using a funnel; once the section is filled, these holes are corked and sealed tightly with tape. During stage 2, the bean-filled bamboo sections are sawn open and soaked in a spontaneously fermented soybean solution; these bamboo sections are transferred to a pool of slowly running spring water to soak during stage 3. At stage 4, the bamboo sections are cleaved into two so that the mung beans can be removed, rinsed in spring water, and sun-dried during the day. At night, the mung beans are soaked in an aqueous mixture of Chinese herbal medicines or put outside to expose them to the dew. These steps are repeated several times until the mung beans are dried completely to become the final product. Although a wide variety of fermented soybean products are used worldwide–including chungkokjang (Korea), kinema (India), miso (Japan), natto (Japan), shoyu (China and Japan), and tempeh (Indonesia)–none results from a fermentation process similar to that for Lu-doh-huang. Whereas the medical applications of Lu-doh-huang have been explored in several studies, the composition of the bacterial communities during its manufacture remains unknown.

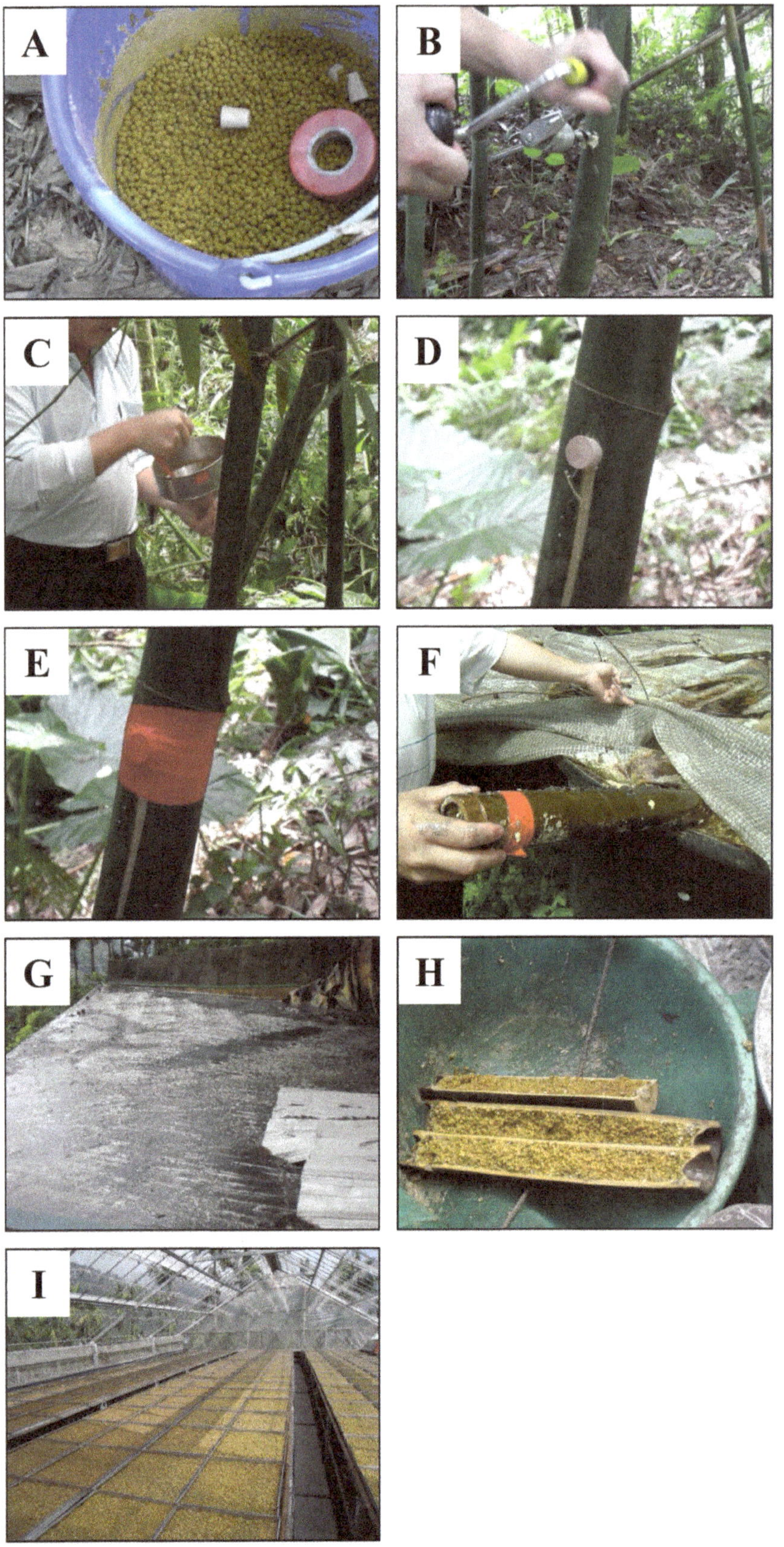

Figure 1. Lu-doh-huang manufacture processes. Images (a) through (e) represent stage 1 in Figure 2. Image (f) represents stage 2, (g) illustrates stage 3, and (h) and (i) correspond to stage 4.

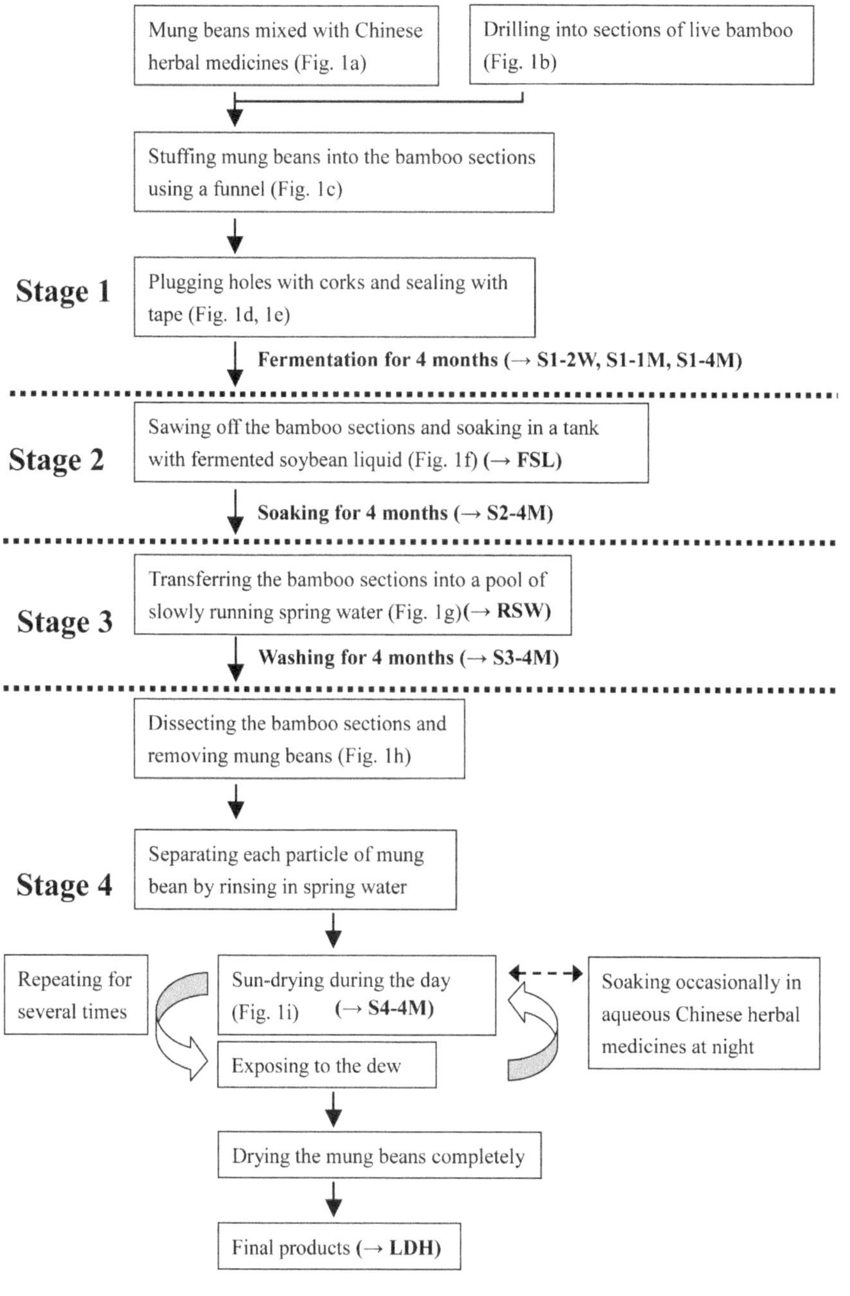

Figure 2. Flowchart of the Lu-doh-huang manufacturing process. Sampling points (in bold) are shown in brackets.

In the current study, we used pyrosequencing to assess the microbial diversity of Lu-doh-huang during its production by fermentation and applied the traditional culture method to identify the predominant lactic acid bacteria (LAB) during Lu-doh-huang fermentation.

Materials and Methods

Sample Collection and pH Analysis

Throughout the 4-stage process, we collected samples of the mung beans inside bamboo sections and the liquids in which the bamboo sections were soaked. At least 3 samples each of beans and liquid were collected at each of 7 points during the manufacturing process; like samples were pooled for further analysis. During stage 1, mung beans were fermented in sections of live bamboo; samples were collected after 2 weeks (S1–2W), 1 month (S1–1M), and 4 months (S1–4M) of fermentation. During stage 2, the bamboo sections containing mung beans were soaked in fermented soybean liquid (FSL) for 4 months (the S2–4M sample); during stage 3, the bamboo sections were soaked in slowly running spring water (RSW) for 4 months (the S3–4M sample). During stage 4, the mung beans were removed from the bamboo sections and then repeatedly sun-dried during the day and exposed to dew (or Chinese herbal medicine) during the night for 4 months (S4–4M). The fermented mung beans then were dried to yield the final product, Lu-doh-huang (LDH). Samples of the unfermented material (UFM) and the FSL and RSW in which the filled bamboo sections were soaked were collected also. The samples were stored on ice during transport to the laboratory for analysis within 7 days of sampling. The pH of the samples was measured (model PHB-9901, DO Microelectronic pH-Vision meter, Ai-On Industrial Corporation, Taipei, Taiwan).

PCR Amplification for Pyrosequencing

The V1–V2 hypervariable regions of the 16S rRNA genes of bacteria present at each sampling point were amplified individually by using nested PCR as previously described [6]. For the first round of amplification, primers 27f (5′-AGRGTTTGATYMTGGCTCAG-3′) and 338r (5′- TGCTGCCTCCCGTAGGAGT-3′) were used. Each reaction (volume, 25 µL) contained 10 ng of extracted DNA, 10 mM Tris-HCl (pH 8.3), 50 mM KCl, 1.5 mM $MgCl_2$, 200 µM deoxynucleoside triphosphate (dNTP) mixture, 5 pmol of each primer, and 0.625 U ExTaq HS (Takara Bio, Shiga, Japan). Thermocycling conditions were: 1 cycle of 98°C for 2.5 min; 15 cycles of 98°C for 15 s, 50°C for 30 s, and 72°C for 20 s; and a final cycle of 72°C for 5 min. The second round of PCR was performed by using the primers Pyro-27f (5′-CCATCTCATCCCTGCGTGTCTCCGACtcagN_{10}*AGRGTTTGATYMTGGCTCAG*-3′) and Pyro-338r (5′-CCTATCCCCTGTGTGCCTTGGCAGTCtcag*TGCTGCCTCCCGTAGGAGT*-3′). The underlined sequences are dictated by the requirements of the 454 Sequencing System (Roche Diagnostics, Branford, CT, USA); the nucleotides in lowercase letters are sequence keys used for amplicon sequencing; italicized sequences are those for universal primers for bacteria; and N_{10} designates the 10-base multiplex identifiers (Roche Diagnostics) used to label each PCR product. The second round of PCR amplification was performed in a 50-µL volume containing 0.5 µL of the product of the first-round of PCR, 10 pmol of each primer, and 1.25 U Ex Taq HS (TaKaRa Bio., Shiga, Japan); all other components were the same as for the first round of PCR. Cycling conditions for the second round of PCR were: 1 cycle of 98°C for 2.5 min; 15 cycles at 98°C for 15 s, 54°C for 30 s, and 72°C for 20 s; and a final cycle of 72°C for 5 min.

The quantity and quality of amplicons were determined by using the Quant-iT PicoGreen dsDNA Assay Kit (Molecular Probes, OR. USA) and Agilent DNA 1000 chip, respectively, on a BioAnalyzer 2100 (Agilent Technologies, CA, USA). Each amplicon was purified separately by using Agencourt AMPure XP beads (Beckman Coulter, Brea, CA, USA) according to the manufacturer's protocol. Purified amplicons were quantified, diluted to 1×10^9 molecules/µL, and underwent a second purification step by using Agencourt AMPure XP beads (Beckman Coulter). Samples with different sample-specific barcode sequences were quantified and diluted to 1×10^8 molecules/µL each and pooled proportionally. The quality of the amplicon pool was assessed by using a High-Sensitivity DNA chip (Agilent Technologies) and subsequently subjected to emulsion PCR by using a GS emPCR Lib-L Kit (Roche Diagnostics). Pyrosequencing was performed on a GS Junior System (Roche Diagnostics) by using Titanium chemistry (Roche Diagnostics) according to the manufacturer's instructions.

Analysis of Pyrosequencing Data

Raw Fasta data were trimmed by using FASTX-Toolkit [7] (Q>25); reads were recognized as derived from specific samples by their unique multiplex identifier. After removing the multiplex identifier and primer sequences for each read, only reads longer than 310 nucleotides were chosen for taxonomic assignment by using BLASTn [8]. High-quality trimmed reads were used as BLASTn queries against the 9701 full-length (≥1200 nucleotides) high-quality 16S rRNA sequences from isolated typed strains (September 2012, RDP release 10, update 30) [9]. In BLASTn results, only the best hit queried by each read was considered. Only reads with more than 97% sequence identity were assigned to the corresponding species. Aligned sequences were clustered into operational taxonomic units (OTU) defined at 3% sequence distance by using the complete-linkage clustering tool in RDP [9]. The Shannon–Weaver index [10], Chao1 index, and evenness and rarefaction analyses also were completed by using the web-based services of RDP.

The relative abundance of sequence reads at the bacterial genus level for seven samples were studied by principal component analysis (PCA). Hierarchical clustering was performed according to the Euclidean distance and complete linkage method. The data used for the clustering analysis were the relative abundance matrix, in which each row corresponds to a genus, and each column corresponds to a sample. Before clustering, data were filtered to eliminate genera with the sum of relative abundance across seven samples lower than 1%; remaining data were $\log_{10}$-transformed. A heatmap of the results of the clustering analysis and PCA were generated by using R/Bioconductor (www.R-project.org; www.bioconductor.org).

Isolation and Enumeration of LAB

Mung beans collected from the various processing stages were washed with 9-fold volume of phosphate buffered saline. After vigorous vortexing, serial 10-fold dilutions were performed, and 0.1-mL aliquots of the appropriate dilutions were plated onto acidic MRS agar plates (pH 5.4; Diagnostic Systems, MD, USA) supplemented with 0.001% sodium azide and cycloheximide for LAB analysis. The plates were incubated at 30°C for 3 days in an anaerobic chamber (Coy Laboratory Products, Grass Lake, MI, USA; atmosphere comprising 85:5:10 N_2:CO_2:H_2). Colonies with distinct morphologies (that is, color, shape, and size) were selected and purified by streaking at least twice on MRS (pH 6.8) agar plates. The isolates were stored at −80°C in Nutrient Broth (Diagnostic Systems) containing 10% dimethyl sulfoxide.

DNA Extraction

LAB isolates were cultured in MRS broth (pH 6.8) at 30°C for 1 to 2 days in an anaerobic chamber (Coy Laboratory Products) and harvested by centrifugation at 14,000×*g* for 3 min. For the genomic DNA extraction, the solid samples collected at the different processing stages were ground into powder, and diluted with 9-fold sterile saline (0.85% NaCl). After vigorous vortexing, 0.2-ml aliquots were used, as well as the liquid samples. The genomic DNA of LAB isolates or the total DNA of these samples was extracted as previously described [11]. Extracted DNA was dissolved in TE buffer (10 mM Tris-HCl, 1 mM EDTA, pH 8.0) for further analyses. To obtain total DNA, mung beans were suspended with 9-fold volume of phosphate buffered saline; total DNA was extracted from 200-µL aliquots of the suspension.

RAPD Fingerprinting

RAPD-PCR analysis using random primers A (5′-CCGCAGCCAA-3′), B (5′-AACGCGCAAC-3′), and C (5′-GCGGAAATAG-3′) was performed as previously described [11]. The PCR products were separated by electrophoresis on a 1% agarose gel. Isolates with the same pattern were grouped, and a single representative strain from each group was chosen for subsequent gene analyses.

Sequencing and Phylogenetic Analyses of 16S rRNA, pheS, and recA Genes

Approximately 1500 bases of each 16S rRNA gene sequence was amplified as previously described [11]. The primer sets and reaction conditions used for *pheS* gene amplification were those previously described [12,13]. To identify strains in the *Lactobacillus plantarum* group (including *L. paraplantarum*, *L. pentosus*, and *L. plantarum*), *recA* sequences were used [14]. The PCR products were sequenced at the National Yang-Ming University Genome Research Centre. The methods for sequence assembly, similarity searches, and phylogenetic analyses have been described previously [15].

Results

Pyrosequencing-based 16S rRNA Profiling of Lu-doh-huang

High-throughput DNA analysis was applied to analyze changes in the total microbial composition during the manufacture of Lu-doh-huang. PCR yields from the UFM, S4–4M, and LDH samples were insufficient for further analysis due to the submarginal DNA-yield. A total of 71,792 sequence reads of the 16S rRNA gene were obtained from a single run by using barcoded pyrosequencing. We obtained a total of 71,623 high-quality reads, which had an average length of 340 bases and yielded approximately 24 Mb of sequence information. After barcode sorting, the read number of each sample varied from 6,622 to 14,473, with an average of 10,232 (Table 1). According to the Shannon–Weaver index, microbial diversity decreased as fermentation progressed during stage 1. However, the indices from S2–4M and S3–4M, corresponding to stages 2 and 3, respectively, were higher than those from stage 1. The microbial diversities of FSL and RSW were both higher than those of the samples that soaked in these liquids. The species evenness and rarefaction curves supported this finding (Fig. S1). We used rarefaction curves of reads at the 97% similarity level to estimate the richness of the bacterial communities. Except for the FSL and RSW samples, the OTUs detected were sufficient to represent the microbial composition present. In FSL, the numbers of genera and species detected were as many as 162 and 291, whereas RSW yielded 116 genera and 189 species. However, the sequence reads of these two samples were not sufficient to describe the entire microbial community, given that neither of the rarefaction curves reached a plateau.

Bacterial Community Structures of Lu-doh-huang Samples

After classification, some sequences belonged to kingdom Plantae; phylum *Magnoliphyta* or *Prasinophyta*; genus *Agrostis*, *Glycine*, *Nephroselmis*, or *Nymphaea*. We concluded that chloroplast 16S rRNA genes that originated from the herbal medicines used during the production process or from the mung beans themselves were the source of these 'outlier' sequences, which were deleted from further analysis. Nine phyla (*Actinobacteria*, *Bacteroidetes*, *Chlorobi*, *Firmicutes*, *Proteobacteria*, *Synergistetes*, *Tenericutes*, *Thermotogae*, and *Verrucomicrobia*) were detected among all samples. Of these, phyla *Firmicutes*, *Proteobacteria*, and *Bacteroidetes* predominated. Sample FSL had the highest diversity, with 8 phyla, 162 genera, and 291 species of bacteria detected (Table 1).

Figure 3 presents the relative abundance of microbial components at family level in the Lu-doh-huang samples. In the earliest sample during fermentation (S1–2W), phylum *Proteobacteria* accounted for 71.9% of the bacterial community, in which family

Table 1. Pyrosequencing-based data from Lu-doh-huang samples.

	Sample	Total no. of reads	No. of high-quality reads	Average length (nt) of read	OTU	Shannon-Weaver index	Chao1	Evenness	No. of phyla	No. of genera	Total no. of species	No. of LAB species
Stage 1	S1–2W	11568	11560	330	124	2.73	149.59	0.57	3	49	84	21
	S1–1M	14486	14473	343	125	2.65	166.63	0.55	4	54	102	41
	S1–4M	7949	7937	348	61	2.09	71.91	0.51	4	39	66	26
Stage 2	FSL	10066	10052	336	485	4.13	616.47	0.67	8	162	291	36
	S2–4M	6626	6622	352	82	2.39	110.11	0.54	5	32	64	37
Stage 3	RSW	8999	8890	329	453	3.70	664.41	0.61	6	116	189	9
	S3–4M	12098	12089	339	213	2.45	288.30	0.46	6	79	170	63

Abbreviations: OTU, operational taxonomic unit. Chao1,
Shannon and evenness were calculated with Mothur at the 3% distance level.

Enterobacteriaceae (69.3%) was predominant. The contribution of phylum *Firmicutes* increased as fermentation progressed during stage 1. In S1–1M and S1–4M, bacteria belonging to *Firmicutes* substituted for *Proteobacteria* and accounted for 82.8% and 93.1%, respectively, of the total population. In addition, the dominant bacteria shifted to *Lactobacillaceae* (73.5% and 53.9%, respectively) in these 2 samples. In S2–4M, phylum *Firmicutes* remained predominant (98.8%), in which the contribution from *Lactobacillaceae* increased to 81.6%. The bacterial composition of S3–4M was distinct, in that phylum *Firmicutes* (51.8%) decreased dramatically and was replaced by phylum *Bacteroidetes* (45.5%). The predominant family in S3–4M was *Porphyromonadaceae* (44.4%). The FSL was dominated by *Firmicutes* (82.1%), in which no particular bacteria was dominant and unclassified *Bacillales* (27.5%) and family *Veillonellaceae* (18.0%) were slightly more abundant than other families. In the RSW sample, phylum *Firmicutes* (62.7%) was dominant, followed by *Proteobacteria* (33.9%); the main family was *Bacillaceae* (45.5%).

Because the family *Lactobacilliaceae* (to which LAB belong) was the major bacteria, especially in samples collected within the bamboo sections, we performed a detailed analysis of these organisms at the species level (Table 2). A total of 264 genera and 586 species were obtained from all samples, among which 20 genera and 112 species were LAB and included *Aerococcus* (1 species), *Atopostipes* (1 species), *Bifidobacterium* (3 species), *Carnobacterium* (2 species), *Desemzia* (1 species), *Enterococcus* (14 species), *Facklamia* (3 species), *Globicatella* (1 species), *Ignavigranum* (1 species), *Lactobacillus* (54 species), *Lacticigenium* (1 species), *Lactococcus* (2 species), *Leuconostoc* (6 species), *Paralactobacillus* (1 species), *Pediococcus* (8 species), *Streptococcus* (2 species), *Tetragenococcus* (1 species), *Trichococcus* (1 species), *Vagococcus* (3 species), and *Weissella* (6 species). LAB abundances were 27.4%, 82.6%, 92.8%, 98.3%, and 43.2% in S1–2W, S1–1M, S1–4M, S2–4M, and S3–4M, respectively. The dominant LAB in these samples were *Enterococcus casselifavus* (11.7%) and *L. lactis* (8.2%) initially; these were replaced gradually by *Lactobacillus cacaonum* (33.2%) and *L. pentosus* (24.3%). Because *L. plantarum* and *L. pentosus* cannot be discriminated by use of their 16S rRNA gene sequences, *L. plantarum* should also contain according to culturing result. The contribution of these two bacteria increased as fermentation proceeded, reaching a maximum of 36.4% in S2–4M. *L. brevis* similarly increased over time, from 0.1% (S1–2W) to 30.7% (S2–4M). In S3–4M, the combined abundance of all LAB decreased to less than 10%. The abundance of LAB was only 6.0% in FSL and 4.4% in RSW. For samples in which family *Lactobacilliaceae* was not the main component, the dominant species were *Pragia fontium* (35.4%) in S1–2W, *Exiguobacterium mexicanum* (27.4%) in FSL, *Gracilibacillus boraciitolerans* (37.3%) in RSW, and *B. virosa* (40.4%) in S3–4M.

For all genera detected, 48 genera occupied 84.8% to 99.2% of the total bacterial community which the minimum incidence of 1% in a genus in each sample. To analyze the bacterial community associated with Lu-doh-huang fermentation in detail, we performed hierarchical clustering by using the relative abundance of genera (Fig. 4). The microflora of the environmental

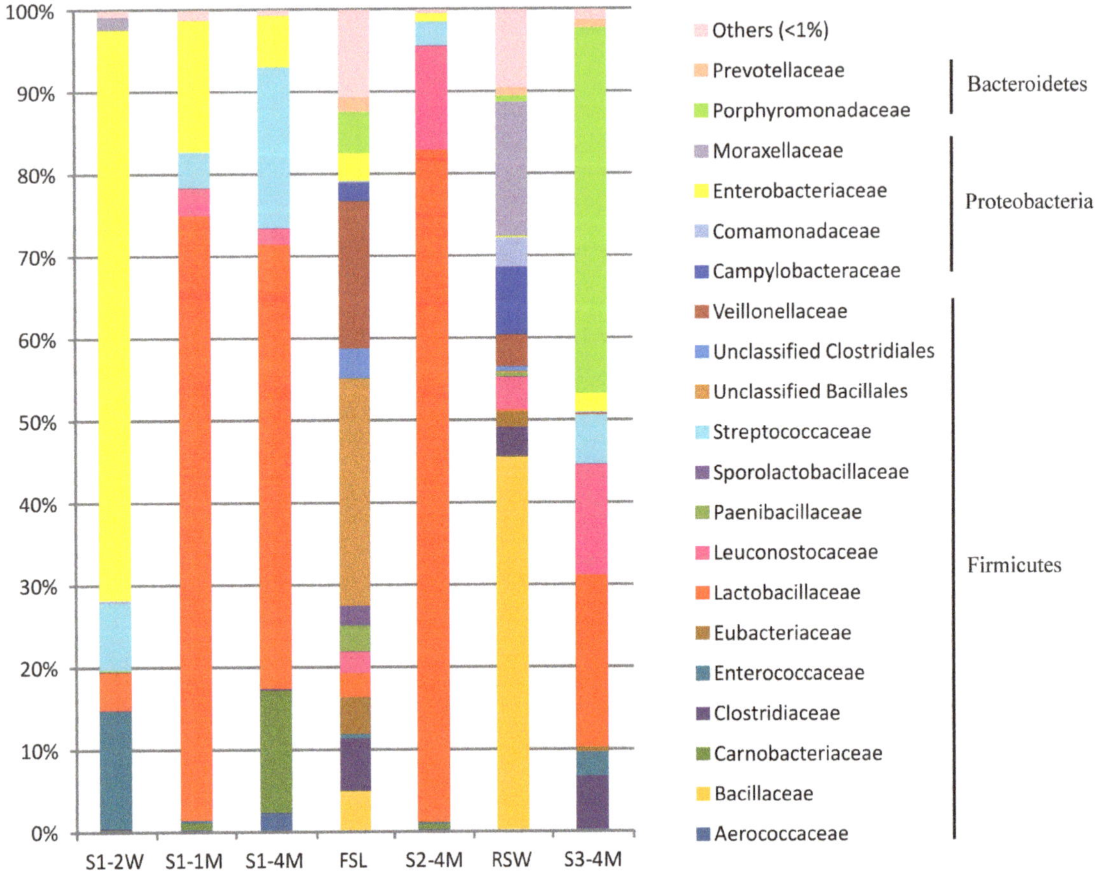

Figure 3. Bacterial community diversity during the fermentation of Lu-doh-huang. The relative abundance of bacterial 16S rRNA genes was estimated through classification at the family level.

Table 2. Represented species composition of Lu-doh-huang.

	Species name	Stage 1			Stage 2		Stage 3	
		S1–2W	S1–1M	S1–4M	FSL	S2–4M	RSW	S3–4M
LAB	*Enterococcus casseliflavus*	11.7	0.2	–	0.1	–	–	<0.1
	Enterococcus hirae	–	<0.1	–	–	<0.1	–	1.5
	Enterococcus mundtii	1.0	–	–	–	–	–	–
	Ignavigranum ruoffiae	<0.1	0.1	2.2	–	0.2	–	<0.1
	Lactobacillus brevis	0.1	4.8	16.3	–	30.7	–	7.9
	Lactobacillus cacaonum	2.2	33.2	1.6	<0.1	0.2	–	0.1
	Lactobacillus collinoides	–	<0.1	–	–	11.2	–	0.3
	Lactobacillus coryniformis	–	–	–	<0.1	–	–	1.8
	Lactobacillus hordei	0.4	4.9	0.2	–	–	–	<0.1
	Lactobacillus kimchii	–	4.4	–	–	0.6	–	–
	Lactobacillus mali	0.0	0.3	3.2	–	0.1	–	<0.1
	Lactobacillus pentosus	1.9	24.3	31.8	0.1	36.4	–	6.7
	Lactococcus lactis	8.2	4.4	19.5	<0.1	2.7	–	5.9
	Leuconostoc kimchii	0.1	2.1	–	–	–	–	–
	Leuconostoc mesenteroides	<0.1	0.9	1.6	–	2.4	–	2.0
	Pediococcus acidilactici	–	–	–	–	–	–	1.5
	Weissella fabaria	–	–	–	2.3	–	4.0	8.7
	Weissella hellenica	<0.1	<0.1	<0.1	0.1	10.0	–	2.2
	Other LAB[a]	2.4	4.6	16.7	3.6	14.9	0.5	4.9
Other bacteria	*Acinetobacter baumannii*	–	–	<0.1	–	–	10.3	–
	Anaerovibrio lipolyticus	–	<0.1	–	6.6	–	1.4	0.1
	Butyricimonas virosa	<0.1	<0.1	–	2.2	<0.1	0.6	40.4
	Enterobacter asburiae	12.2	0.4	0.8	<0.1	–	–	0.1
	Exiguobacterium mexicanum	–	–	–	27.4	–	0.1	<0.1
	Gracilibacillus boraciitolerans	–	–	–	<0.1	–	37.3	–
	Klebsiella pneumoniae	9.9	1.6	0.1	0.1	<0.1	–	<0.1
	Pragia fontium	35.4	5.0	0.1	0.1	–	–	0.1
	Other bacteria[b]	15.1	12.4	7.2	60.1	1.7	48.0	16.4

[a]Sum of LAB for which relative abundance was less than 1% each.
[b]Sum of all other bacteria for which relative abundance was less than 5% each.

samples, FSL and RSW, formed a cluster separate from those representing the bacterial communities in mung bean samples obtained from bamboo sections (that is, S1–2W, S1–1M, S1–4M, S2–4M, and S3–4M). The dominant OTUs inside the bamboo sections were clearly dissimilar to those of environmental samples. Samples S1–1M, S1–4M, and S2–4M were close to each other in the hierarchical clustering, and the genus *Lactobacillus* was the strongest influencing factor for clustering. The remaining samples (S1–2W, FSL, RSW, and S3–4M) were well separated from other clusters. In addition, we performed PCA to characterize the microbial community succession of Lu-doh-huang (Fig. 5). A projection of the first two principal components explained about 75% (61.3% and 13.6%) of the total variance, with strong separation by region.

pH and Cell Counts of LAB of Lu-doh-huang Samples

The pH of the unfermented starting material (UFM), which contained mung beans and various Chinese medicines, was 5.4 (Table 3). After this mixture was stuffed into bamboo sections for 2 weeks (S1–2W), the pH increased slightly to 5.9. However, pH started to decrease gradually and 4 months later, it was 3.9 (S1–4W). During stages 2 and 3 (S2–4M and S3–4M), pH increased to approximately 5.0. The pH of the FSL and RSW samples was 5.5 and 6.9, respectively.

The traditional culture method detected no LAB in the UFM, S4–4M, and LDH samples (Table 3). After anaerobic fermentation for 2 weeks inside bamboo sections, the cell counts of LAB increased to the level of 10^8 cfu/g. This cell count remained stable throughout the manufacturing process, until the fermented mung beans were removed from the bamboo sections. However, sample S4–4M lacked LAB, which were isolated from FSL and RSW at a level of about 10^4 cfu/mL.

Identification and Distribution of LAB

LAB strains were then isolated from each sample according to their colony morphologies and analyzed by RAPD-PCR for grouping and 16S rRNA gene sequencing for identification. In total, 218 strains were isolated (7 from UFM, 35 from S1–2W, 16 from S1–1M, 24 from S1–4M, 16 from FSL, 72 from S2–4M, 16 from RSW, and 32 from S3–4M). No colonies grew on MSR agar

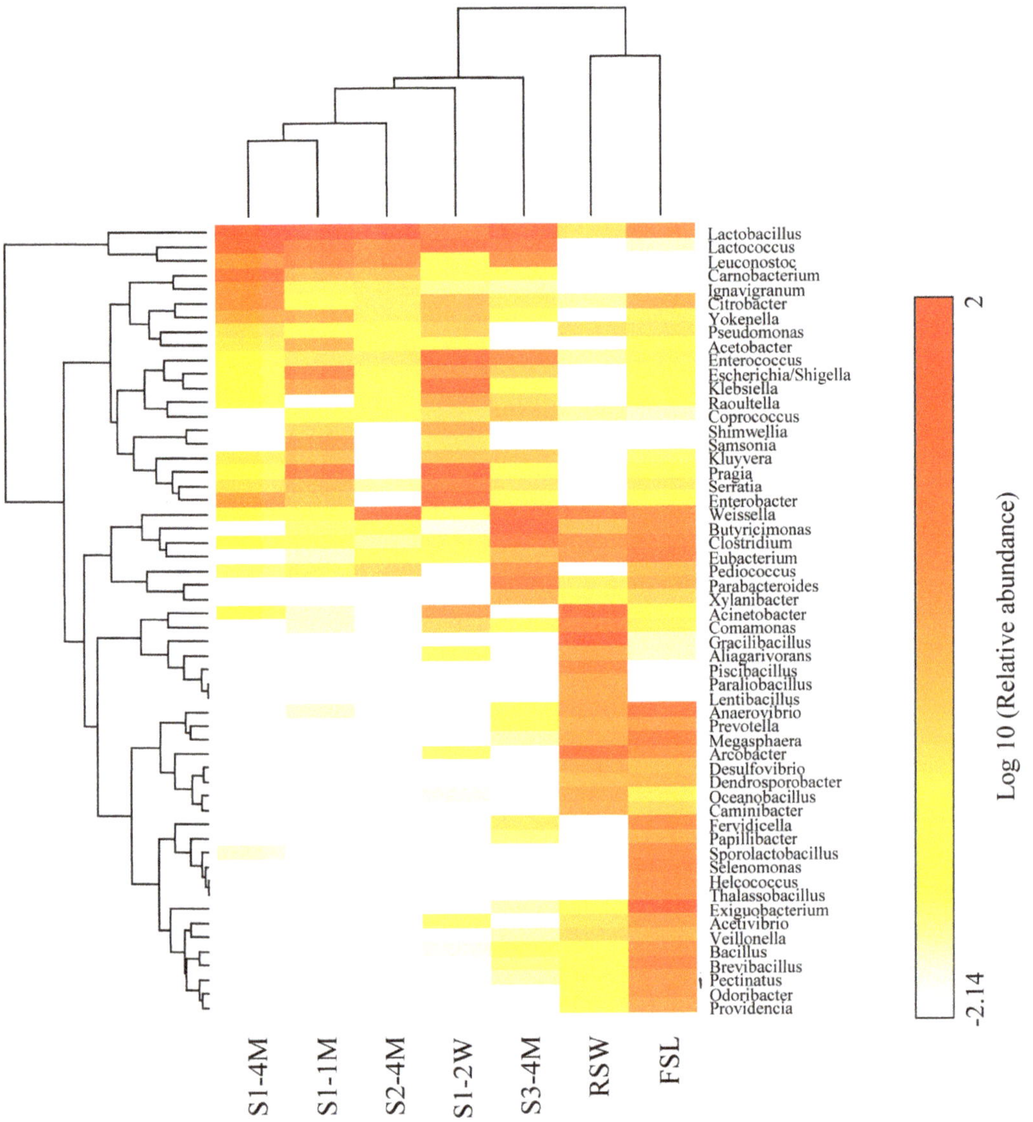

Figure 4. Phylogenetic tree and representative reads from the pyrosequencing analysis that only organisms with the sum of at least 1% relative abundance in all samples were included. Each column represents 1 sampling point; rows indicate different genera. The color intensity of the panel is proportional to the abundance of Log_{10} OTU.

streaked with the LDH sample. On the basis of the resulting RAPD profiles, 218 isolates were categorized into 82 different groups (5 from UFM, 10 from S1–2W, 9 from S1–1M, 4 from S1–4M, 9 from FSL, 25 from S2–4M, 9 from RSW, and 11 from S3–4M). A representative strain was chosen from each of the 82 groups for partial sequencing of the 16S rRNA gene (500 nucleotides containing the V1 to V3 regions) [16]; the sequences obtained were identified as belonging to 4 genera (*Enterococcus*, *Lactobacillus*, *Lactococcus*, and *Pediococcus*) and 24 species. Most of the isolates were *Lactobacillus*, comprising 19 different species. The strains from UFM were not LAB.

Sample S1–2W contained 6 different LAB species; *Enterococcus casseliflavus* and *Lactococcus lactis* were the dominant species, with cell counts as high as 10^8 cfu/g (Table 4). As the fermentation proceeded, the number of LAB species decreased, and the main species shifted to *Lactobacillus brevis* and *L. plantarum* (S1–1M and S1–4M). After the bamboo sections had been opened to soak in the fermented soybean liquid for 4 months (S2–4M), the diversity of LAB had changed dramatically. The 10 LAB species obtained were present in similar numbers, and *L. plantarum* was the only species that remained from stage 1. None of the LAB species isolated from FSL was present in S2–4M. Similarly, except for *L. brevis*, none of the LAB in RSW was found in S3–4M. LAB cell counts increased slightly between stages 2 and 3, and *L. brevis* and *L. pentosus* predominated during both stages.

Among the *Lactobacillus* species identified, 6 representative strains isolated from S1–2W and S3–4W could not be identified conclusively by using the full-length 16S rRNA gene sequences because these sequences were more than 99% or less than 97% similar to those of known species in the databases. Therefore, we compared *pheS* gene sequences of these 6 strains. Because the *pheS* sequence identities of these strains were all lower than 90% with recognized species (data not shown), these isolates were tentatively identified as *Lactobacillus* sp. A, B, C, and D.

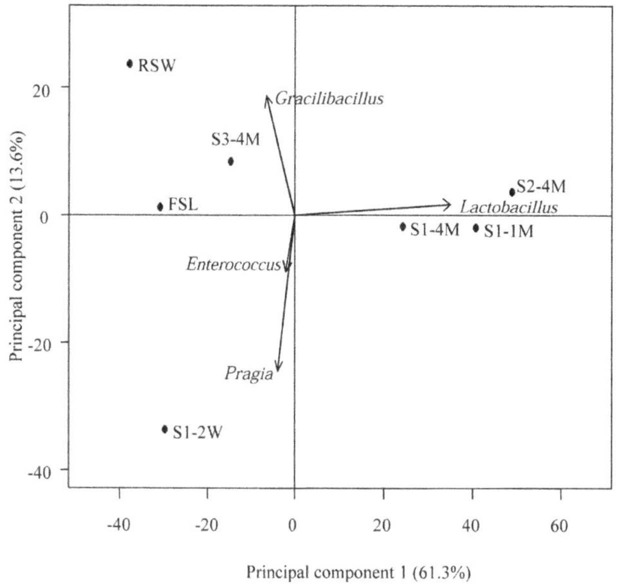

Figure 5. Principal component analysis plot derived from the relative abundance of bacterial communities at the genus level during Lu-doh-huang fermentation. The directions of arrows indicate the relative loading during the first and second principal components.

Discussion

In this study, we used pyrosequencing of tagged 16S rRNA gene amplicons and the traditional culture method to reveal changes in microbioflora of Lu-doh-huang during its production. Lu-doh-huang is a unique regional and alternative medicine that is especially popular in southern Taiwan. To produce Lu-doh-huang, mung beans are mixed with other Chinese herbal medicines, fermented anaerobically, soaked in liquid herbal medicines repeatedly, and then dried completely. A similar product is Semen Sojae Praeparatum in mainland China. The processing of Lu-doh-huang and Semen Sojae Praeparatum is comparable: both combine a type of bean (mung beans and black beans, respectively) with other herbal medicines and undergo natural fermentation. A key difference between these products is the type of fermentation used in their manufacture, that is, Lu-doh-huang undergoes strictly anaerobic fermentation (inside bamboo sections), whereas the production of Semen Sojae Praeparatum involves aerobic fermentation. However, the microflora of Semen Sojae Praeparatum has not been analyzed extensively [17].

Natural fermentation is a common production method for Chinese herbal medicines that has been used for almost 2,000 years. Many medicines produced through natural fermentation are still popular, including Massa Medicata Fermentata, medicated leaven, Semen Sojae Praeparatum, and Chinese gall leaven [18]. Microbial enzymes present during fermentation are thought to convert or detoxify bioactive compounds in the medicinal herbs to enhance the health benefits of the final product [18,19]. For example, gastrointestinal bacteria transform bioactive ingredients of herbal medicines so that they become easily absorbed or

Table 4. Lactic acid bacteria (LAB) composition in the different stages of Lu-doh-huang.

LAB species	1st stage			2nd stage		3rd stage	
	S1–2W	S1–1M	S1–4M	FSL	S2–4M	RSW	S3–4M
Enterococcus casseliflavus	8.18[a]	–	–	–	–	–	–
Lactobacillus acidipiscis	–	–	–	2.48	–	3.91	–
Lactobacillus brevis	6.27	6.60	7.79	–	–	2.00	7.23
Lactobacillus buchneri	–	–	–	3.88	–	3.45	–
Lactobacillus casei	–	–	–	–	5.04	–	–
Lactobacillus collinoides	–	–	–	–	5.51	–	–
Lactobacillus concavus	–	–	–	–	–	2.70	–
Lactobacillus farciminis	–	–	–	–	5.88	–	–
Lactobacillus hilgardii	–	–	–	3.13	–	–	–
Lactobacillus kimchii	–	–	–	–	–	–	–
Lactobacillus paralimentarius	–	6.78	–	–	–	–	–
Lactobacillus pentosus	–	–	–	–	–	–	7.09
Lactobacillus perolens	–	–	–	–	–	–	–
Lactobacillus plantarum	6.85	7.59	7.89	–	–	–	–
Lactobacillus similis	–	–	–	2.93	–	–	–
Lactobacillus vaccinostercus	–	–	–	–	–	–	–
Lactobacillus sp. A	6.56	–	–	–	–	–	–
Lactobacillus sp. B	7.13	–	–	–	–	–	–
Lactobacillus sp. C	–	–	–	–	–	–	5.56
Lactobacillus sp. D	–	–	–	–	–	–	6.47
Lactococcus lactis	8.23	–	–	–	–	–	–
Pediococcus acidilactici	–	–	–	–	–	–	–
Pediococcus cellicola	–	–	–	–	6.08	–	–
Pediococcus parvulus	–	–	–	–	6.08	–	–
							–
							–

[a]cfu/g (ml). Cell counts are given as Log10 cfu/g or cfu/mL, depending on the sample (mung beans or soaking liquid).

Table 3. The pH values and cell counts of lactic acid bacteria (LAB) in Lu-doh-huang.

	Stage 1				Stage 2		Stage 3		Stage 4	
	UFM	S1–2W	S1–1M	S1–4M	FSL	S2–4M	RSW	S3–4M	S4–4M	LDH
pH value	5.4	5.9	5.3	3.9	5.5	4.8	6.9	5.1	5.3	4.9
LAB	–[a]	3.5×10^{8}[b]	4.9×10^{7}	1.6×10^{8}	1.1×10^{4}	6.3×10^{7}	1.4×10^{4}	3.5×10^{7}	–	–

[a]Not detected.
[b]No. of LAB cfu/g or cfu/mL.

pharmacologically active [20–24]. *Aspergillus* spp. present in fermented *Radix astragalus* significantly increased the phenolic content and antioxidant activity of the product compared with those of the unfermented form [25]. *Bacillus subtilis* natto and fermented *Radix astragali* stimulated hyaluronic acid production and increased the mRNA expression of hyaluronan synthase 3 and hyaluronan synthase 2 in HaCaT cells and human fibroblasts, respectively [26]. Semen Sojae Praeparatum had greater quantities of isoflavone glucosides and aglycones, which show extensive pharmacologic activities, than did natural soy materials [27]. In our study, LAB were the major bacterial components of Lu-doh-huang, especially in samples S1–1M, S1–4M, and S2–4M, which were obtained while the mung beans were fermenting inside the bamboo sections. Fermentation by LAB reportedly increased the pharmacologic effects of several herbal medicines and detoxified various dietary carcinogens [28–33]. Therefore, we speculate that the main purpose of the unique production process of Lu-doh-huang is to enable microbial enzymes secreted during fermentation to biotransform various components of the product.

Genus *Lactobacillus* was the most frequent and predominant LAB detected by both pyrosequencing and culturing. Pyrosequencing revealed greater diversity in *Lactobacillus* (54 species) than did culturing (19 species). However, culturing–but not pyrosequencing–detected *L. acidipiscis* (at $10^{3.91}$ cfu/g in RSW), *L. brevis* (at $10^{2.00}$ cfu/g in RSW), *L. casei* (at $10^{5.04}$ cfu/g in S2–4M), *L. concavus* (at $10^{2.70}$ cfu/g in RSW), *L. farciminis* (at $10^{5.88}$ cfu/g in S2–4M), *L. hilgardii* (at $10^{3.13}$ cfu/g in FSL), *L. plantarum* (at $10^{6.85}$, $10^{7.59}$, $10^{7.89}$, and $10^{5.04}$ cfu/g in S1–2W, S1–1M, S1–4M, and S2–4M, respectively), and *L. similis* (at $10^{2.93}$ cfu/g in FSL). The dissimilarity in the results obtained by using culturing and pyrosequencing may reflect the fact that the V1–V2 region of 16S rRNA does not sufficiently discriminate some species to enable their precise classification. For example, members of the *L. plantarum* group–*L. fabifermentans*, *L. pentosus*, *L. paraplantarum*, and *L. plantarum*–showed high sequence similarity (97.2%–99.7%). In fact, these values generally were considerably higher than the threshold level typically recommended for species differentiation (97%) [34]. Therefore, additional genetic biomarkers were needed to accurately speciate members of the *L. plantarum* group that were identified by BLAST searching of the pyrosequencing reads [14,35].

Additional data garnered through sequencing of *recA* and culturing indicated that the species *L. fabifermentans*, *L. paraplantarum*, and *L. pentosus* that were identified through pyrosequencing (data not shown) should be classified instead as *L. plantarum*, whereas *L. pentosus* in S2–4M actually comprises both *L. pentosus* and *L. plantarum* (data not shown). In contrast, *L. hilgardii* and *L. parakefiri* in the *L. buchneri* group; *L. farciminis* in the *L. farciminis* group, could be identified appropriately on the basis of the similarity values of the V1–V2 region of the 16S rRNA gene (which were lower than 97%) that were obtained by pyrosequencing (except in the pairs, *L. casei* and *L. paracasei* in the *L. casei* group, and *L. bobalius* and *L. paralimentarius* in the *L. farciminis* group), even though similarity values of the full-length 16S rRNA sequences were considerably higher (>97.3%) (data not shown).

Another possible reason for the dissimilarities between the results of culturing and pyrosequencing may be in the different detection limits of the two methods: 10^2 cfu/g (or cfu/mL, depending on the type of sample) for culturing compared with 10^5–10^6 cfu/g (or cfu/mL) for pyrosequencing (estimated the concentration of isolated bacteria from the conversion of the abundance of pyrosequencing reads). The different limits of detection account for why *L. acidipiscis, L. brevis, L. concavus* and *L. similis* were not identified through pyrosequencing of FSL or RSW, whereas these organisms were isolated in concentrations ranging from 10^2 to $10^{3.91}$ cfu/mL through culturing. In contrast, *L. cacaonum* was detected as the predominant species (33.2%) in S1–1M by pyrosequencing, but culturing failed to yield this organism. Perhaps only dead (and therefore unculturable) cells were present at this stage: DNA-based methods such as pyrosequencing do not distinguish viable from dead cells.

The results of heatmap and PCA plot indicated that the microbial communities of S1–2W and S3–4M were markedly different from those of S1–1M, S1–4M, and S2–4M. Early during fermentation of the mung beans inside bamboo sections, air was consumed gradually to form an anaerobic environment. In addition, various compounds derived from the herbal medicines that were mixed with the mung beans have antimicrobial activity [36–38]. These features caused the microbial composition during stage 1 to be more unstable than those at later sampling points. By the end of production, facultative or obligate anaerobes, such as *Lactobacillaceae*, *P. fontium* and *B. virosa*, had become predominant. The predominant microflora inside the bamboo sections began as phylum *Proteobacteria* (S1–2W, 71.9%) and then gradually shifted to phylum *Firmicutes* (28.1%, 82.8%, 93.1%, and 98.8% in S1–2W, S1–1M, S1–4M, and S2–4M, respectively). However, in S3–4M, the microbial composition was distinct in that phylum *Bacteroidetes* (45.5%) substituted *Firmicutes*. Given that the microbial composition of the environmental samples (FSL and RSW) differed markedly from those collected from inside the bamboo sections according to the pyrosequencing and culture results, bacteria seem to be unable to pass from the solutions, through the bamboo sections, and into the mung beans. Instead, perhaps the pH of or small molecules in the soaking solutions influence the bacterial succession inside the bamboo sections.

In conclusion, we used culturing and high-throughput pyrosequencing analyses to characterize the microbial community of the Lu-doh-huang fermentation ecosystem. Our work provides a detailed picture of the structures of the microbiomes of 7 samples obtained at different points during the manufacturing process. Results from pyrosequencing generally were consistent with the culture-dependent analysis and provided deeper insight into the entire prokaryotic microbial communities at the various time points. The details of relationship the microbes in Lu-doh-huang and its functions are still unclear. Further investigations are needed to shed light on the microbial dynamics, and the analysis of bioactive components would contribute to a better understanding of this Taiwanese alternative medicine.

Supporting Information

Figure S1 Rarefaction curves for each sample were calculated at 3% distance by using the RDP pipeline data of the 16S rRNA gene sequences.
(TIF)

Acknowledgments

We acknowledge the Cao-De-Zhuang-Yuan Company for their generous contribution of Lu-doh-huang samples. We thank Professor Chia-Li Wei (Department of Biochemical Science and Technology, National Chiayi University) for support during sampling. We are grateful to Miss Ying-Hsueh Huang (Institute of Biomedical Informatics, National Yang-Ming University) for statistic support.

Author Contributions

Conceived and designed the experiments: SHC YCT. Performed the experiments: SHC HYH CHC YHK. Analyzed the data: SHC CHY WSC

KW. Contributed reagents/materials/analysis tools: SHC CHY WSC. Wrote the paper: SHC CHC WSC KW.

References

1. Liu C-W (2007) *Phellinus linteus* and *Pracparatum mungo* induce apoptosis and anti-angiogenesis in Hep3B hepatoma cells. Taiwan: Shih Chieh University.
2. Chu H-C (2007) Safety evaluation, liver detoxification, and anti-inflammation effect of lvdou huang. Taiwan: Shih Chieh University.
3. Wang Y-C (2007) Functional studies of lvdou huang and *Phellinus linteus*. Taiwan: Shih Chien University.
4. Peng H-P (2007) Antioxidant activities of *Houttuynia cordata*, *Saussurea involucrate*, liu-dou-huang, and *Camellia sinensis*. Taiwan: National Chung-Hsing University.
5. Kuo D-H, Kang W-H, Shieh P-C, Chen F-A, Chang C-D, et al. (2010) Protective effect of *Pracparatum mungo* extract on carbon tetrachloride-induced hepatotoxicity in rats. Food Chem 123: 1007–1012.
6. Sakamoto N, Tanaka S, Sonomoto K, Nakayama J (2011) 16S rRNA pyrosequencing-based investigation of the bacterial community in nukadoko, a pickling bed of fermented rice bran. Int J Food Microbiol 144: 352–359.
7. Goecks J, Nekrutenko A, Taylor J (2010) Galaxy: a comprehensive approach for supporting accessible, reproducible, and transparent computational research in the life sciences. Genome Biol 11: R86.
8. Altschul SF, Gish W, Miller W, Myers EW, Lipman DJ (1990) Basic local alignment search tool. J Mol Biol 215: 403–410.
9. Cole JR, Wang Q, Cardenas E, Fish J, Chai B, et al. (2009) The Ribosomal Database Project: improved alignments and new tools for rRNA analysis. Nucleic Acids Res 37: D141–145.
10. Longuet-Higgins MS (1971) On the Shannon–Weaver index of diversity, in relation to the distribution of species in bird censuses. Theor Popul Biol 2: 271–289.
11. Chao SH, Tomii Y, Watanabe K, Tsai YC (2008) Diversity of lactic acid bacteria in fermented brines used to make stinky tofu. Int J Food Microbiol 123: 134–141.
12. Berger B, Pridmore RD, Barretto C, Delmas-Julien F, Schreiber K, et al. (2007) Similarity and differences in the *Lactobacillus acidophilus* group identified by polyphasic analysis and comparative genomics. J Bacteriol 189: 1311–1321.
13. Naser SM, Thompson FL, Hoste B, Gevers D, Dawyndt P, et al. (2005) Application of multilocus sequence analysis (MLSA) for rapid identification of *Enterococcus* species based on *rpoA* and *pheS* genes. Microbiology 151: 2141–2150.
14. Torriani S, Felis GE, Dellaglio F (2001) Differentiation of *Lactobacillus plantarum*, *L. pentosus*, and *L. paraplantarum* by *recA* gene sequence analysis and multiplex PCR assay with *recA* gene-derived primers. Appl Environ Microbiol 67: 3450–3454.
15. Chao S-H, Wu R-J, Watanabe K, Tsai Y-C (2009) Diversity of lactic acid bacteria in suan-tsai and fu-tsai, traditional fermented mustard products of Taiwan. Int J Food Microbiol 135: 203–210.
16. Huysman E, DeWachter R (1986) Compilation of small subunit RNA sequences. Nucleic Acids Res 14(Suppl.): r73-r118.
17. Cai Q-Y, Zheng H-Z, Want M (2012) Initial study on microbial of four kinds of Chinese medicinal materials processed by fermented method. Chinese J Exp Traditional Med Formulae 18: 119–121.
18. Li Y, Wan DG (2010) Discussion on processed traditional Chinese medicine by fermentation. J Chengdu Univ Tradit Chin Med 33: 69–71.
19. Wang Y, Dong X, Qiao Y, Shi X (2010) Fermentation of traditional Chinese medicine. World Sci Technol Mod Tradit Chin Med 12: 437–441.
20. Kobashi K, Akao T (1997) Relation of intestinal bacteria to pharmacological effect of glycosides. Biosci Microflora 16: 1–7.
21. Kim DH, Yu KW, Bae EA, Park HJ, Choi JW (1998) Metabolism of kalopanaxsaponin B and H by human intestinal bacteria and antidiabetic activity of their metabolites. Biol Pharm Bull 21: 360–365.
22. Sato Y, He JX, Nagai H, Tani T, Akao T (2007) Isoliquiritigenin, one of the antispasmodic principles of *Glycyrrhiza ularensis* roots, acts in the lower part of intestine. Biol Pharm Bull 30: 145–149.
23. Kim DH, Lee KT, Bae EA, Han MJ, Park HJ (1999) Metabolism of liriodendrin and syringin by human intestinal bacteria and their relation to in vitro cytotoxicity. Arch Pharm Res 22: 30–34.
24. Lee DS, Kim YS, Ko CN, Cho KH, Bae HS, et al. (2002) Fecal metabolic activities of herbal components to bioactive compounds. Arch Pharm Res 25: 165–169.
25. Sheih I-C, Fang TJ, Wu T-K, Chang C-H, Chen R-Y (2011) Purification and properties of a novel phenolic antioxidant from *Radix astragali* fermented by *Aspergillus oryzae* M29. J Agric Food Chem 59: 6520–6525.
26. Hsu M-F, Chiang B-H (2009) Stimulating effects of *Bacillus subtilis* natto-fermented *Radix astragali* on hyaluronic acid production in human skin cells. J Ethnopharmacol 125: 474–481.
27. Yuan D, Pan Y, Chen Y, Uno T, Zhang S, et al. (2008) An improved method for basic hydrolysis of isoflavone malonylglucosides and quality evaluation of Chinese soy materials. Chem Pharm Bull (Tokyo) 56: 1–6.
28. Eum HA, Lee JH, Yang MC, Shim KS, Ma JY (2011) Protective effect of Ssanghwa-tang fermented by *Lactobacillus fermentum* against carbon tetrachloride-induced acute hepatotoxicity in rats. Afr J Tradit Complement Altern Med 8: 312–321.
29. Trinh HT, Han SJ, Kim SW, Lee YC, Kim DH (2007) *Bifidus* fermentation increases hypolipidemic and hypoglycemic effects of red ginseng. J Microbiol Biotechnol 17: 1127–1133.
30. Vanhaecke L, Vercruysse F, Boon N, Verstraete W, Cleenwerck I, et al. (2008) Isolation and characterization of human intestinal bacteria capable of transforming the dietary carcinogen 2-amino-1-methyl-6-phenylimidazo[4,5-b]pyridine. Appl Environ Microbiol 74: 1469–1477.
31. Kim BG, Shin KS, Yoon TJ, Yu KW, Ra KS, et al. (2011) Fermentation of Korean red ginseng by *Lactobacillus plantarum* M-2 and its immunological activities. Appl Biochem Biotechnol 165: 1107–1119.
32. Otieno DO, Shah NP (2007) A comparison of changes in the transformation of isoflavones in soymilk using varying concentrations of exogenous and probiotic-derived endogenous beta-glucosidases. J Appl Microbiol 103: 601–612.
33. Chi H, Kim DH, Ji GE (2005) Transformation of ginsenosides Rb2 and Rc from *Panax ginseng* by food microorganisms. Biol Pharm Bull 28: 2102–2105.
34. Stackebrandt E, Goebel BM (1994) Taxonomic note: a place for DNA-DNA reassociation and 16S rRNA sequence analysis in the present species definition in bacteriology. Int J Syst Bacteriol 44: 846–849.
35. Naser SM, Dawyndt P, Hoste B, Gevers D, Vandemeulebroecke K, et al. (2007) Identification of lactobacilli by *pheS* and *rpoA* gene sequence analyses. Int J Syst Evol Microbiol 57: 2777–2789.
36. Yoon SY, Eo SK, Kim YS, Lee CK, Han SS (1994) Antimicrobial activity of *Ganoderma lucidum* extract alone and in combination with some antibiotics. Arch Pharm Res 17: 438–442.
37. Mekseepralard C, Kamkaen N, Wilkinson JM (2010) Antimicrobial and antioxidant activities of traditional Thai herbal remedies for aphthous ulcers. Phytother Res 24: 1514–1519.
38. Lu H, Wu X, Liang Y, Zhang J (2006) Variation in chemical composition and antibacterial activities of essential oils from two species of *Houttuynia* THUNB. Chem Pharm Bull (Tokyo) 54: 936–940.

3

Herbal Medicines for Parkinson's Disease: A Systematic Review of Randomized Controlled Trials

Tae-Hun Kim[1,2], Ki-Ho Cho[1]*, Woo-Sang Jung[1], Myeong Soo Lee[2]

1 Department of Cardiovascular & Neurologic Diseases, College of Oriental Medicine, Kyung Hee University, Seoul, South Korea, **2** Korea Institute of Oriental Medicine, Daejeon, South Korea

Abstract

Objective: We conducted systematic review to evaluate current evidence of herbal medicines (HMs) for Parkinson's disease (PD).

Methods: Along with hand searches, relevant literatures were located from the electronic databases including CENTRAL, MEDLINE, EMBASE, CINAHL, AMED, PsycInfo, CNKI, 7 Korean Medical Databases and J-East until August, 2010 without language and publication status. Randomized controlled trials (RCTs), quasi-randomized controlled trials and randomized crossover trials, which evaluate HMs for idiopathic PD were selected for this review. Two independent authors extracted data from the relevant literatures and any disagreement was solved by discussion.

Results: From the 3432 of relevant literatures, 64 were included. We failed to suggest overall estimates of treatment effects on PD because of the wide heterogeneity of used herbal recipes and study designs in the included studies. When compared with placebo, specific effects were not observed in favor of HMs definitely. Direct comparison with conventional drugs suggested that there was no evidence of better effect for HMs. Many studies compared combination therapy with single active drugs and combination therapy showed significant improvement in PD related outcomes and decrease in the dose of anti-Parkinson's drugs with low adverse events rate.

Conclusion: Currently, there is no conclusive evidence about the effectiveness and efficacy of HMs on PD. For establishing clinical evidence of HMs on PD, rigorous RCTs with sufficient statistical power should be promoted in future.

Editor: Mark R. Cookson, National Institutes of Health, United States of America

Funding: The authors have no support or funding to report.

Competing Interests: The authors have declared that no competing interests exist.

* E-mail: johkiho@khmc.or.kr

Introduction

Parkinson's disease (PD) is an age-related neurodegenerative disorder that pathological feature is basically related on the progressive degradation of dopamine production in substantia nigra. The clinical manifestation includes bradykinesia (especially having difficulties in initiating movement), hypokinesia (lose of facial expression), rigidity, rest tremor (pill-rolling movement of the forearm) and non-motor features including depression, psychosis autonomic dysfunction [1].

Because of diversity of the studies with different population and methodology, the prevalence rate and incidence varies broadly in difference studies. In the European countries, crude prevalence rate estimates ranged from 65.6 per 100,000 to 12,500 per 100,000 and annual incidence estimates ranged from 5 per 100,000 to 26 per 100,000 [2]. On the contrary, prevalence rate and incidence rate is slightly lower in Asian countries. It was reported that a standardized all-age prevalence of was 51.3 to 176.9 per 100,000 and the standardized incidence rates were 8.7 per 100,000 person-years [3]. The prevalence increases progressively along with the age. According to the cross-sectional study of United Kingdom in 2000, the prevalence was only 20/100,000 in below 50 years old, but 342/100,000 in sixties and 1265/100,000 in over eighties [4]. Considering that medical expenditure for PD is one of the highest ranked neurologic diseases, PD might be a serious socioeconomic burden in future aging society [5–7].

Herbal products for PD have been used worldwide in traditional medicine [8]. Especially in China, records of herbal prescriptions for treating PD might date back to about 2200 years ago [9] and current literatures reflect active use of HM for PD until now [10,11]. Practitioners and patients employ HM as an adjuvant therapy of conventional treatment for the purpose of reducing dose of dopaminergic drugs, adverse event related to prolonged usage of dopaminergic agents and improving PD symptoms [10].

Previous literature reviews have been evaluated the clinical evidence of HM including traditional Chinese medicine (TCM) [9,10,12,13]. However these reviews did not adopt explicit search strategy so all the possible studies might not be located. Information on the herbal remedies was not presented in details. In addition, any results on the effect size were not reported. From these limitations, these reviews failed to suggest the global picture of HMs for treating PD [9,10,12,13].

The purpose of this review is to evaluate the current evidence level thorough explicit systematic review method and to present necessary information to outline the benefit and harmfulness of HMs for PD patients.

Methods

Types of studies

Randomized controlled trials (RCTs), quasi-randomized controlled trials and randomized crossover trials, which evaluate HMs for idiopathic PD were included in this review.

Types of participants

Participants of any age and sex with idiopathic PD were considered to be included. Diagnosis of PD is necessary to be done considering clinical symptoms and radiological examinations through the standard diagnostic criteria such as UK Parkinson's Disease Brain Bank criteria [14] or the Diagnosis and Differential Diagnosis of Parkinson's Disease and Parkinsonism from the Chinese Colloquium of Extracorticospinal Tract Diseases [15].

Types of intervention

Studies which used HMs as the only intervention or combination therapy with conventional medicine were included. In this review, HMs was defined as products originated from botanical sources such as whole plants or their adjuncts: seed, root, flower, bud and leaf [16]. In the boundary of HM, low or manufactured single or complex medicinal plants, plants extracts and plant preparations for the purpose of treatment were included regardless of drug preparation: extracts, decoction, tablet, capsule, pill, powder, injection and etc [17]. However, drugs, which were consisted of synthesized compounds, were excluded. Complex intervention with acupuncture, moxibustion and other CAM treatments was excluded. There is no restriction on dosage including frequency, dose, intensity and duration. Comparator interventions were conventional drugs or treatment, surgery, placebo, usual care or no treatment. Comparison between different types of HMs was excluded. Conventional drugs include levodopa (both of the immediate-release and modified-release), dopamine agonists, monoamine oxidase B inhibitors, catecho-O methyltransferase inhibitor (COMT) and amatadine etc.

Types of outcome measures

Following primary and secondary outcomes were pre-identified at the protocol stage:

Primary outcomes. Total Unified Parkinson's Disease Rating Scale score (Total UPDRS score)

Global improvement of symptoms

Secondary outcomes. UPDRS I, II, III and IV sub-scores

Webster scale

Hoehn and Yahr (H&Y) staging

Non-movement problems: total non-motor symptoms score value (NMSQuest), frequency of Nausea & vomiting or constipation

Mean levodopa or bromocriptine usage

Depression scales: Hamilton depression rating scale (HAM-D)

Quality of life measures: Parkinson's Disease Questionnaire–39 (PDQ-39) and EuroQol (EQ-5D)

Adverse events rate

Search methods for identification of studies

The following databases were searched until August, 2010. Any language, document format and date restrictions didn't included in the search strategy to minimize possible bias: Cochrane Central Register of Controlled Trials (CENTRAL), MEDLINE, EMBASE, CINAHL (Cumulative Index of Nursing and Allied Health Medicine), AMED (Allied and Complementary Medicine Database), PsycInfo, China Academic Journal in China National Knowledge Infrastructure (CNKI), China Doctor/Master's Dissertation Database in CNKI, China Proceedings of Conference Database in CNKI, Korean Medical Databases (Korean Studies Information, DBPIA, Korea Institute of Science and Technology Information, Research Information Centre for Health Database, KoreaMed and the Korean National Assembly Library, Korean traditional knowledge portal) and J-East. Related gray literature and references of included studies were hand searched. Searching strategy for medline was as follows:

Medline (Pubmed) search strategy.

#1 Parkinson Disease [mh]
#2 Parkinson$ [tiab]
#3 or/1-2
#4 Medicine, African Traditional [mh]
#5 Medicine, Arabic [mh]
#6 Medicine, Ayurvedic [mh]
#7 Medicine, Kampo [mh]
#8 Medicine, Korean Traditional [mh]
#9 Medicine, Tibetan Traditional [mh]
#10 Medicine, Mongolian Traditional [mh]
#11 Herbal Medicine [mh]
#12 Phytotherapy [mh]
#13 Drugs, Chinese Herbal [mh]
#14 Plants, Medicinal [mh]
#15 Plant Extracts [mh]
#16 Ethnobotany [mh]
#17 Ethnopharmacology [mh]
#18 Plants [mh]
#19 herb$ [tiab]
#20 (Plant Leave$ or Flower$ or Plant Root$ or Fruit$ or Seed$) [tiab]
#21 or/4-20
#22 3 and 21
#23 randomized controlled trial [pt]
#24 controlled clinical trial [pt]
#25 randomized [tiab]
#26 placebo [tiab]
#27 drug therapy [sh]
#28 randomly [tiab]
#29 groups [tiab]
#30 or/23-29
#31 animals [mh] not (humans [mh] and animals [mh])
#32 30 not 31

Data extraction, risk of bias assessment and analysis

From the included studies, data describing disease duration and severity, interventions for the treatment and control groups, summary of the outcomes, last follow up period and recipes of HMs were extracted according to the pre-defined data extraction form by two independent authors (THK and WSJ). Any disagreement between two authors was solved by discussion. Risk of bias was assessed in 6 domains: random sequence generation, allocation concealment, blinding of participants, incomplete outcome data, selective reporting and other bias. Two independent authors (THK and KHC) assessed the risk of bias according to the criteria of Cochrane collaboration [18]. Any conflict was discussed and there was no disagreement between two authors.

Estimated effect size for each outcome of included HM was calculated comparing with each control intervention individually. Individual data were combined for meta-analysis if the studies adopted the same HM and control intervention. Dichotomous data were presented as relative risk (RR) and continuous outcomes as mean difference (MD) with 95% CI. Analysis was conducted with Review manager 5.1 (Copenhagen: The Nordic Cochrane Centre, The Cochrane Collaboration, 2011).

Results

Description of included studies

Total 3432 of relevant literature were identified from electronic databases and hand searching. Among them, 64 studies (total 4024 PD patients) were included based on the predefined criteria (figure 1).

All the included studies were classified into one of four types according to the trial design: HM versus placebo [19,34], HM versus conventional medicine [30,43,44,53,57,71,73,77], HM plus active drug versus active drug [20–23,25–27,29,31–33,35–38,41,42,45,48–50,52,54,55,56,58–62,64–69,72,74–76,79–82] or HM plus active drug versus placebo plus active drug [11,24,28,34,39,40,46,47,51,63,70,78]. Among the 64 studies, one was conducted in Ecuador [19], another was in UK [24] and other 62 were in China. All the included studies were RCTs except two quasi-RCTs [31,54] and one cross-over study [24].

Interventions

A total 59 kinds of herbal preparations were identified in the included studies (table S1). Among them, several different herbal recipes which were prescribed individually according to each patient were used in three studies [80–82]. All the identified interventions were complex medications which were composed of three to twenty herbs. Only in two studies, single herbal extracts were tested [19,24]. In majority of included studies, treatment was provided during 3 or 6 months (ranging 1 month to 1 year). One study assessed the short term effect of herbal extract, tested shortly after taking medication once [19]. Control interventions were mainly conventional treatment with anti-Parkinson drugs or Placebo [11,19,24,28,34,39,40,46,47,51,63,70,78]. In 58 trials, several anti-Parkinson drugs were provided to PD patients, combined with HMs and 8 studies tested single HMs without conventional treatment (table S2) [30,43,44,53,57,71,73,77].

Risk of bias

There is no study with row risk of bias in all the 6 domains and no study showed low risk of biases in 5 domains. There were 14 studies which showed low risk of bias in the domain of random sequence generation [21,24,28,34,46–50,55,70,74,78,83]. Allocation concealment was conducted adequately in 5 studies [21,24,50,55,78]. 13 studies described about blinding issues [19,24,28,34,39,40,46,47,51,63,68,70,78]. In 10 studies [24,25,47,53–55,65,70,75,83], incomplete outcome data such as numbers of participants who were included, finished treatment and were dropped out were well described. The selective reporting domain was not evaluated clearly because we could not locate any registered protocol for all the included studies. Other risk of bias such as baseline imbalances were properly described in the included studies except in 12 studies [19,22,24,31,36,41,47,49,59,66,72,76].

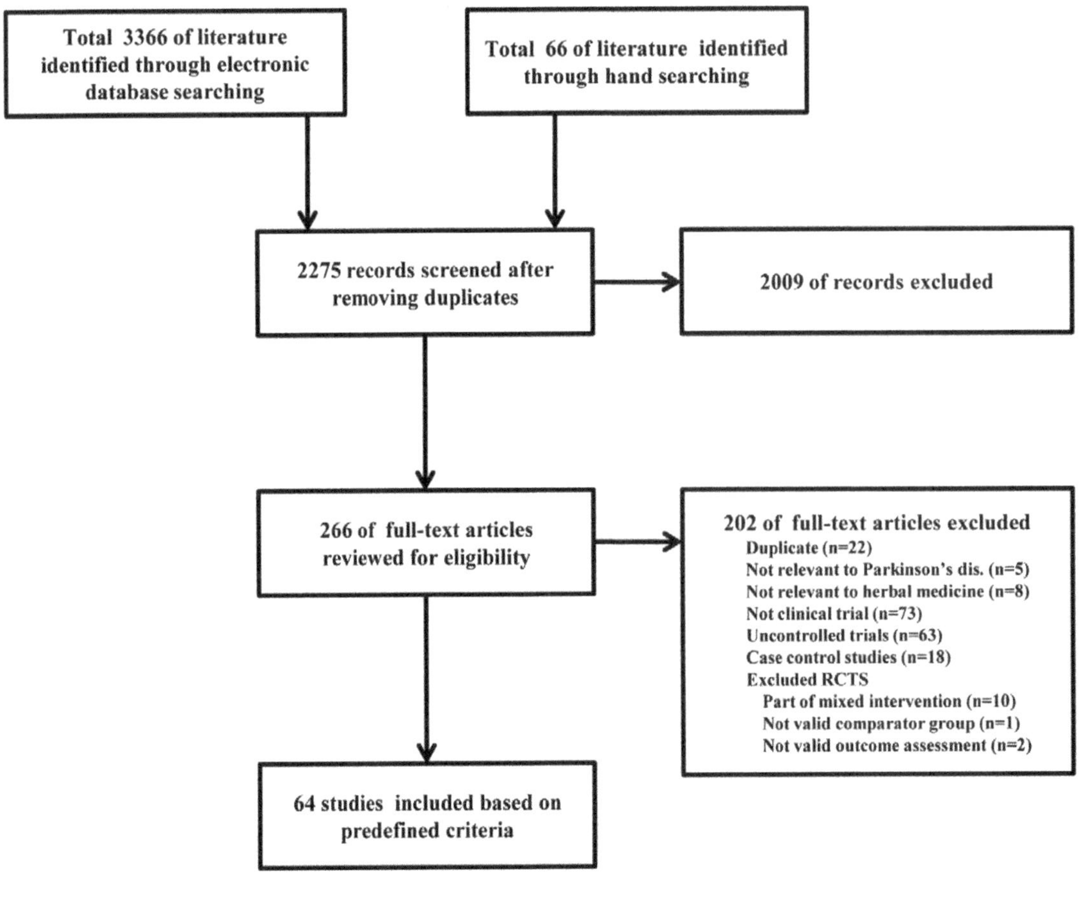

Figure 1. Flow chart of information for this systematic review.

In addition to this, several details were also evaluated to describe the methodological quality of the included studies. No study did statistical analysis on intention-to-treat basis. In only one study, sample size calculation was conducted for enough statistical power [24]. 8 studies referred to the ethical issues such as prior review by institutional review board [19,24] or written informed consent from participants [19,21,24,34,55,65,83].

Effects of interventions 1: HM versus placebo [19,34]

2 HMs were compared with placebo in 2 studies [19,34]. Global improvement of symptoms and total UPDRS score were assessed for the efficacy of HMs in 2 studies (figure 2) [19,34]. Banisteriopsis caapi extract showed significant improvement in total UPDRS score 4 hrs after the one time treatment (MD −27.40, [−28.19, −26.61]) [19]. 3 months of Guilingpaan capsule treatment did not show statistically significant difference in global symptoms (RR 1.30, [0.93, 2.06]) and total UPDRS score (MD −3.45, [−14.99, 8.09]), compared with placebo control [34].

Effects of interventions 2: HM versus conventional medicine [30,43,44,53,57,71,73,77]

8 different HMs were tested compared with conventional drug therapy [30,43,44,53,57,71,73,77]. Global improvement of symptoms, Webster scale and total UPDRS score were evaluated in these studies. Among them, herbal formula Qingxinhuatan tang only showed statistically significant improvement in global symptoms (RR 1.33, 95% CI [1.04, 1.72]) compared with madopar therapy [53]. Herbal formula Kangzhenzhijing capsule [43], Kanli tang [44] and Ziyinxifeng granule [77] reported significant improvement in Webster score (MD −1.80, [−3.40, −0.20], −2.40, [−4.29, −0.51] and −0.50, [−0.90, −0.10], respectively). Herbal formula Zhichanshudu tang showed significant improvement in total UPDRS score (MD −9.16, [−10.68, −7.64]) [73].

Effects of interventions 3: HM plus active drug versus active drug [20–23,25–27,29,31–33,35–38,41,42,45,48–50,52,54,55,56,58–62,64–69,72,74–76,79–82]

In 44 studies, HM combined with conventional drug therapy was compared with conventional drug treatment [20–23,25–27,29,31–33,35–38,41,42,45,48–50,52,54,55,56,58–62,64–69,72,74–76,79–82]. Herbal formula Guilingpaan wan was evaluated in 3 studies [35–37], Xifengdingzhan wan in 3 studies [61,63,84] and other HMs was used once:

Three months of Guilingpaan wan medication with madopar showed significant improvement in global symptoms (RR 1.45, [1.20, 1.77]) [35–37] and total UPDRS score (MD −9.97, [−16.68, −3.25] [35,36] compared with madopar alone.

Xifengdingzhan wan with madopar was administered for 3 months [61,84] and for 1 month [63], respectively. Xifengdingzhan wan combination therapy improved significantly in global symptoms (RR 1.47, [1.20, 1.81]) [61,63] and total UPDRS score (MD −5.41, [−6.96, −3.86]) [61,84].

Global improvement of symptoms. 33 studies assessed global improvement of symptoms. Among them, 3 studies [80–82] compared the effectiveness of combination treatment on global symptoms with individualized herbal recipes plus conventional drug therapy versus single drug therapy, and significant improvement was observed in 1 study only [79] (RR 2.88, [1.90, 4.34]). The other studies tested different HMs with conventional drug therapies and 10 herbal recipes including those described earlier, showed statistically significant improvement in global symptoms [33,35–37,41,50,52,55,60,61,63,65,79]: Fufangjangzhan wan plus madopar (RR 1.40, [1.16, 1.70]) [33], Kanapa granule with madopar (RR 3.13, [1.79, 5.46]) [41], Pabing formula 2 plus madopar (RR 2.80, [1.15, 6.80]) [50], Peibuganshen recipe plus madopar and artane (RR 1.89, [1.01, 3.55]) [52], Shudipingzhan tang plus Xiewu capsule plus levodopa (RR 2.27, [1.60, 3.23]) [55], Xifengdinzhan tang with madopar (RR 1.32, [1.01, 1.72]) [60] and Xifengzhizhan tang plus madopar (RR 1.50, [1.08, 2.08]) [65].

Total UPDRS score. In total 12 studies [20,21,35,36,42,45,48,61,65,74,75,84], 10 HM plus conventional drug therapies were compared with single drug therapy for the total UPDRS score and among them, 9 HMs including Guilingpaan wan and Xifengdingzhan wan showed significant improvement in the score: Bushenyanggan recipe plus levodopa (MD −5.10, [−6.01, −4.19]) [21], Kangzhanning plus madopar (MD −7.00, [−8.88, −5.12]) [42], Lemai granule plus madopar and Vit B6 (MD −5.40, [−10.05, −0.75]) [45], Pabing formula 1 plus madopar (MD −9.04, [−17.11, −0.97]) [48], Xifengzhizhan tang plus madopar (MD −8.89, [−13.29, −4.49]), Zhizhan tang plus madopar (MD −1.30, [−2.36, −0.24]) [74] and Zibuganshen recipe plus madopar, sinemet or artane (MD −10.74, [−20.74, −0.74], figure 3) [75].

Webster scale. Webster scale was assessed in 4 studies [26,52,66,75] and combination therapy showed better effect than conventional therapy alone in 3 studies: Peibuganshen recipe plus

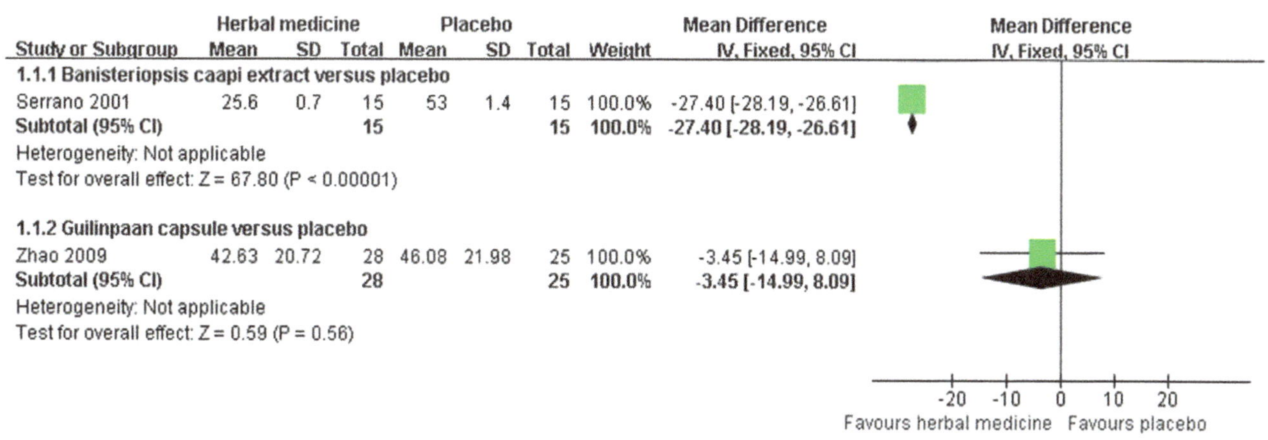

Figure 2. Herbal medicine versus placebo, total UPDRS score.

Study or Subgroup	Herb plus active drug Mean	SD	Total	Active drug Mean	SD	Total	Weight	Mean Difference IV, Fixed, 95% CI
3.2.1 Bushenpingchan formula plus madopar versus madopar								
Cui 2003	41.2	28.5	35	44.5	29.1	35	100.0%	-3.30 [-16.79, 10.19]
Subtotal (95% CI)			**35**			**35**	**100.0%**	**-3.30 [-16.79, 10.19]**
Heterogeneity: Not applicable								
Test for overall effect: Z = 0.48 (P = 0.63)								
3.2.2 Bushenyanggan recipe plus levodopa versus levodopa								
Zhao 2007	32.4	2.1	55	37.5	2.8	58	100.0%	-5.10 [-6.01, -4.19]
Subtotal (95% CI)			**55**			**58**	**100.0%**	**-5.10 [-6.01, -4.19]**
Heterogeneity: Not applicable								
Test for overall effect: Z = 10.99 (P < 0.00001)								
3.2.3 Guilinpaan wan plus madopar versus madopar								
Chang 2008	44.76	16.27	30	54.25	18.43	30	58.2%	-9.49 [-18.29, -0.69]
Jiang 2009	34.6	22.04	30	45.23	18.88	30	41.8%	-10.63 [-21.01, -0.25]
Subtotal (95% CI)			**60**			**60**	**100.0%**	**-9.97 [-16.68, -3.25]**
Heterogeneity: $Chi^2 = 0.03$, df = 1 (P = 0.87); $I^2 = 0\%$								
Test for overall effect: Z = 2.91 (P = 0.004)								
3.2.4 Kangzhanning plus madopar versus madopar								
Yang 2009	23.76	3.46	24	30.76	3.18	24	100.0%	-7.00 [-8.88, -5.12]
Subtotal (95% CI)			**24**			**24**	**100.0%**	**-7.00 [-8.88, -5.12]**
Heterogeneity: Not applicable								
Test for overall effect: Z = 7.30 (P < 0.00001)								
3.2.5 Lemai granule plus madopar and Vit B6 versus madopar and Vit B6								
Luo 2001	25.2	6.7	32	30.6	9.2	20	100.0%	-5.40 [-10.05, -0.75]
Subtotal (95% CI)			**32**			**20**	**100.0%**	**-5.40 [-10.05, -0.75]**
Heterogeneity: Not applicable								
Test for overall effect: Z = 2.27 (P = 0.02)								
3.2.6 Pabing formula 1 plus madopar versus madopar								
Sun 2005	22.96	11.84	22	32	14.19	19	100.0%	-9.04 [-17.11, -0.97]
Subtotal (95% CI)			**22**			**19**	**100.0%**	**-9.04 [-17.11, -0.97]**
Heterogeneity: Not applicable								
Test for overall effect: Z = 2.19 (P = 0.03)								
3.2.7 Xifengdingzhan wan plus madopar versus madopar								
Cheng 2007	43.2	6.74	20	50.2	5.62	20	16.3%	-7.00 [-10.85, -3.15]
Ma 2005	10.11	3.98	30	15.21	2.57	30	83.7%	-5.10 [-6.80, -3.40]
Subtotal (95% CI)			**50**			**50**	**100.0%**	**-5.41 [-6.96, -3.86]**
Heterogeneity: $Chi^2 = 0.78$, df = 1 (P = 0.38); $I^2 = 0\%$								
Test for overall effect: Z = 6.83 (P < 0.00001)								
3.2.8 Xifengzhizhan tang plus madopar versus madopar								
Lu 2009	22.82	8.62	31	31.71	9.05	31	100.0%	-8.89 [-13.29, -4.49]
Subtotal (95% CI)			**31**			**31**	**100.0%**	**-8.89 [-13.29, -4.49]**
Heterogeneity: Not applicable								
Test for overall effect: Z = 3.96 (P < 0.0001)								
3.2.9 Zhizhan tang plus madopar versus madopar								
Wang 2010	-7.63	1.97	30	-6.33	2.22	30	100.0%	-1.30 [-2.36, -0.24]
Subtotal (95% CI)			**30**			**30**	**100.0%**	**-1.30 [-2.36, -0.24]**
Heterogeneity: Not applicable								
Test for overall effect: Z = 2.40 (P = 0.02)								
3.2.10 Zibuganshen recipe plus madopar, sinemet or artane versus madopar, sinemet or artane								
Shen 2006	61.35	26.41	40	72.09	16.6	32	100.0%	-10.74 [-20.74, -0.74]
Subtotal (95% CI)			**40**			**32**	**100.0%**	**-10.74 [-20.74, -0.74]**
Heterogeneity: Not applicable								
Test for overall effect: Z = 2.10 (P = 0.04)								

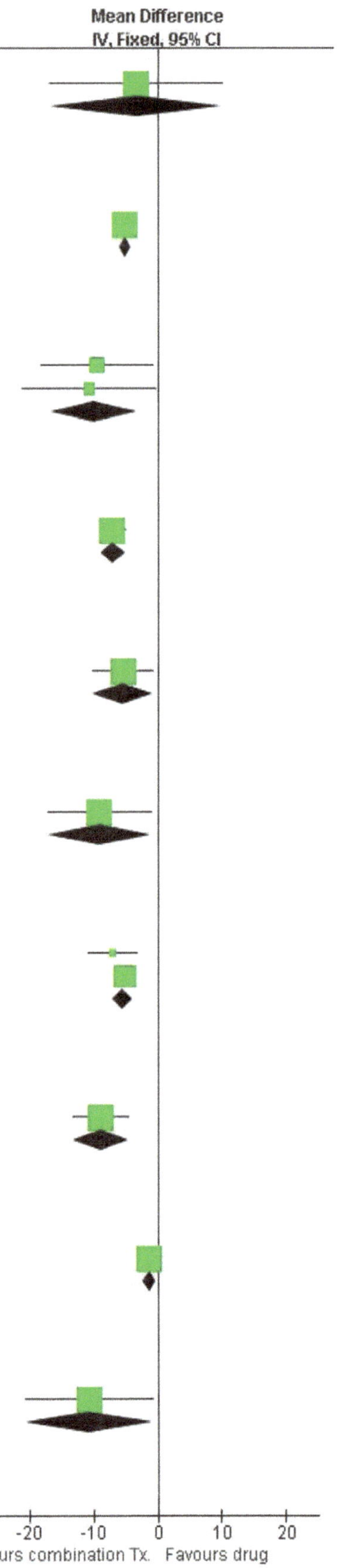

Figure 3. Herbal medicine plus active drug versus active drug, total UPDRS score.

madopar and artane (MD −3.10, [−5.00, −1.20]) [52], Yangganxifeng recipe plus madopar (MD −3.00, [−4.14, −1.86]) [66] and Zibuganshen recipe plus madopar, sinemet or artane (MD −2.86, [−5.68, −0.04]) [75].

Hoehn & Yahr score. Hoehn & Yahr score was assessed in 2 studies [21,38]. However there was no significant improvement in these studies.

The dose of anti-Parkinson drug. The dose of anti-Parkinson drug including levodopa (madopar) or bromocriptine was compared between combination treatment and conventional drug therapy groups (figure 4). Mean dose of levodopa (madopar) was assessed in 10 studies [20,21,55,60,65,67–69,83,84] and combination therapies decreased the dose significantly in 8 studies: Bushenpingchan formula (MD −199.30, [−367.65, −30.95]) [20], Bushenhuoxie recipe (MD −121.20, [−149.04, −93.36]) [83], Bushenyanggan recipe (MD −80.03, [−113.25, −46.81]) [21], Xifengdingzhan tang (MD −187.01, [−247.25, −126.77]) [60], Xifengdingzhan wan (MD −165.63, [−304.10, −27.16]) [84], Xifengzhizhan tang (MD −185.24, [−245.56, −124.92]) [65], Yiguan jian plus dabuyin wan (MD −187.01, [−257.00, −117.02]) [67] and Yizhan tang (MD −120.00, [−148.48, −91.52]) [69].

Non-movement problems. Non-movement problems such as nausea and constipation were evaluated in several studies. 1 study adopted a validated systemic tool i.e. Parkinson's disease non-movement questionnaire (NMSQuest) for non-movement symptoms: Yiyuan yin plus madopar was compared with single madopar therapy. However, there was no significant difference between 2 groups in NMSQest value (MD −1.00, [−3.19, 1.19]) [68]. 4 HMs plus conventional drug therapies were tested for the effect of reducing nausea and vomiting [35–37,55,75,83]. Among them, 2 HMs showed favorable results: Bushenhuoxie recipe plus madopar and bromocriptine (RR 0.40, [0.20, 0.81]) [83], Zibuganshen recipe plus madopar and sinemet or artane (RR 0.36, [0.14, 0.94]) [75].

7 herbal remedies with anti-Parkinson drugs were evaluated on constipation in PD patients [29,36,42,55,68,75,83] and 3 recipes showed better results: Bushenhuoxie recipe plus madopar and bromocriptine (RR 0.11, [0.03, 0.46]) [83], Dingzhen tang_2 plus conventional treatment (RR 0.48, [0.29, 0.78]) [29] and Kangzhanning plus madopar (RR 0.50, [0.28, 0.88]) [42].

Anti-depressive effect. Anti-depressive effect of combination therapy in PD patients was tested in 1 study. Compared with paroxetine treatment alone, Chaihushugan san plus paroxetine showed significant improvement in HAM-D score (MD −4.10, [−5.17, −3.03]) after 8 weeks of treatment with low adverse event rate (RR 0.48, [0.31, 0.74]) [25].

Total adverse event rate. Total adverse event rate was assessed in 8 studies [25,31,38,45,54,56,61,84] and 5 studies (4 HMs) reported significantly low rate of adverse event: Chaihushugan san plus paroxetine (RR 0.48, [0.31, 0.74]) [25], Dingzhen tang_4 plus madopar and artane (RR 0.39, [0.18, 0.83]) [31], Ruogantongluo tang plus madopar (RR 0.36, [0.14, 0.89]) [45] and Xifengdingzhan wan plus madopar (RR 0.41, [0.21, 0.80]) [61,84].

Effects of interventions 4: HM plus active drug versus placebo plus active drug [11,24,28,34,39,40,46,47,51,63,70,78]

12 studies compared the effect of HM plus active drug and those of placebo plus active drug [11,24,28,34,39,40,46,47,51,63,70,78]. In 8 studies, global improvement of symptoms was compared between HMs and placebo controls both of which were combined with active drugs [28,34,39,46,47,51,63,78]. Among them, significant improvement was observed in 5 studies: Jiaweidadingfeng zhu plus madopar (RR 3.83, [1.82, 8.05]) [39], Naokangning capsule plus madopar (RR 1.53, [1.02, 2.31]) [46], Nuzhenyangyin granule plus madopar and artane (RR 1.53, [1.09, 2.16]) [47], Pabing formula 3 plus madopar (RR 2.60, [1.06, 6.39]) [51] and Xifengdingzhan wan plus madopar (RR 1.44, [1.11, 1.87]) [63].

Total UPDRS score was evaluated in 5 studies [29,46,63,70,78] and 2 HMs showed significant improvement comparing with placebo plus active drug treatment: Naokangning capsule plus madopar (MD −6.00, [−11.24, −0.76]) [46] and Xifengdingzhan wan plus madopar (MD −5.10, [−6.57, −3.63]) [63].

SF-36 questionnaires were assessed for evaluating quality of life for PD patients in 1 study [46]. Compared with placebo plus active treatment, Naokangning capsule plus madopar improved significantly in the subsections for the physical functioning (58.74 (14.16) in Naokangning plus madopar group, 46.83 (16.43) in placebo plus madopar, $P<0.05$), social functioning (77.26 (27.57), 64.63 (20.39), $P<0.05$), role limitations due to physical health (68.59 (16.33), 49.62 (18.25), $P<0.05$) and vitality (67.21 (18.05), 48.92 (23.49), $P<0.05$) [46].

Discussion

Among the included 64 RCTs, 59 herbal preparations were used for treating PD. Majority of studies were conducted in China and HMs were composed of multiple herbs in almost all studies. Only 5 HMs were used several times but other studies were conducted with high heterogeneities in herbal preparations and study design. HMs was used with conventional drugs concomitantly in majority of the included studies. Efficacy of HMs was tested in 2 studies by comparing with placebo control. Banisteriopsis caapi extract showed short-term effect in improving UPDRS score but 3 months of Guilingpaan capsule medication did not have statistically significant differences in PD symptoms [19,34]. HMs were directly compared with conventional drug therapy in 8 studies and only Qingxinhuatan tang improved general symptoms of PD significantly in one study [53]. Combination therapy with HMs and anti-Parkinson drugs showed significant improvement in the assessment of general symptoms and UPDRS scores and decrease in the dose of anti-Parkinson drugs generally. Adverse events rate also decreased significantly in combination therapies.

Compared with the previous systematic review in 2006 [85], the number of conducted RCTs increased steeply from 9 to 64. However, as with before, the result of this systematic review cannot suggest conclusive evidence of HMs because of several limitations the included studies had. Firstly, only a small number of preparations were used twice or more and most of the HMs were tested only once. A huge heterogeneity in the herbal composition, drug formulation, dose, duration, combined therapy and control interventions was observed between the studies, which were the main obstacles to estimate the general effect size of herbal remedies. Secondly, significant improvement in the methodological qualities of included studies was not observed compared with the previous review. As pointed out before, most of the studies did not report about allocation concealment process. Incomplete outcome data including drop out were not reported in 53 studies. Because any pre-registered protocols of included trials were not located, selective outcome reporting could not be judged clearly in all the studies. Only one studies adopted ITT analysis for statistics. In this review, except 2 studies, all the searched studies were conducted in China. There have been debates about the results of clinical trials in some countries including China, which may be originated from their methodological flaws and publication bias

Study or Subgroup	Herb plus active drug Mean	SD	Total	Active drug Mean	SD	Total	Weight	Mean Difference IV, Fixed, 95% CI
3.14.1 Bushenhuoxie recipe plus madopar and bromocriptine versus madopa and bromocriptine								
Dou 2006	252.2	62.3	52	373.4	68.6	37	100.0%	-121.20 [-149.04, -93.36]
Subtotal (95% CI)			**52**			**37**	**100.0%**	**-121.20 [-149.04, -93.36]**
Heterogeneity: Not applicable								
Test for overall effect: Z = 8.53 (P < 0.00001)								
3.14.2 Bushenpingchan formula plus madopar versus madopar								
Cui 2003	496.5	285.3	35	695.8	420.5	35	100.0%	-199.30 [-367.65, -30.95]
Subtotal (95% CI)			**35**			**35**	**100.0%**	**-199.30 [-367.65, -30.95]**
Heterogeneity: Not applicable								
Test for overall effect: Z = 2.32 (P = 0.02)								
3.14.3 Bushenyanggan recipe plus levodopa versus levodopa								
Zhao 2007	340.63	98.2	55	420.66	80.58	58	100.0%	-80.03 [-113.25, -46.81]
Subtotal (95% CI)			**55**			**58**	**100.0%**	**-80.03 [-113.25, -46.81]**
Heterogeneity: Not applicable								
Test for overall effect: Z = 4.72 (P < 0.00001)								
3.14.4 Shudipingzhan tang plus Xiewu capsule plus levodopa versus levodopa								
Yuan 2010	562.2	126.4	60	555.3	132.4	60	100.0%	6.90 [-39.42, 53.22]
Subtotal (95% CI)			**60**			**60**	**100.0%**	**6.90 [-39.42, 53.22]**
Heterogeneity: Not applicable								
Test for overall effect: Z = 0.29 (P = 0.77)								
3.14.5 Xifengdingzhan tang plus madopar versus madopar								
Li 2008	396.4	141.57	27	583.41	73.89	27	100.0%	-187.01 [-247.25, -126.77]
Subtotal (95% CI)			**27**			**27**	**100.0%**	**-187.01 [-247.25, -126.77]**
Heterogeneity: Not applicable								
Test for overall effect: Z = 6.09 (P < 0.00001)								
3.14.6 Xifengdingzhan wan plus madopar versus madopar								
Cheng 2007	365.62	188.37	20	531.25	253.67	20	100.0%	-165.63 [-304.10, -27.16]
Subtotal (95% CI)			**20**			**20**	**100.0%**	**-165.63 [-304.10, -27.16]**
Heterogeneity: Not applicable								
Test for overall effect: Z = 2.34 (P = 0.02)								
3.14.7 Xifengzhizhan tang plus madopar versus madopar								
Lu 2009	426.62	136.19	31	611.86	103.97	31	100.0%	-185.24 [-245.56, -124.92]
Subtotal (95% CI)			**31**			**31**	**100.0%**	**-185.24 [-245.56, -124.92]**
Heterogeneity: Not applicable								
Test for overall effect: Z = 6.02 (P < 0.00001)								
3.14.8 Yiguan jian plus dabuyin wan plus madopar versus madopar								
Li 2009	396.4	141.57	20	583.41	73.89	20	100.0%	-187.01 [-257.00, -117.02]
Subtotal (95% CI)			**20**			**20**	**100.0%**	**-187.01 [-257.00, -117.02]**
Heterogeneity: Not applicable								
Test for overall effect: Z = 5.24 (P < 0.00001)								
3.14.9 Yiyuan yin plus madopar versus madopar								
Chen 2009	590	160	46	655	165	25	100.0%	-65.00 [-144.51, 14.51]
Subtotal (95% CI)			**46**			**25**	**100.0%**	**-65.00 [-144.51, 14.51]**
Heterogeneity: Not applicable								
Test for overall effect: Z = 1.60 (P = 0.11)								
3.14.10 Yizhan tang plus madopar and bromocriptine versus madopar and bromocriptine								
Yang 2002	245.5	55.5	40	365.5	65.5	32	100.0%	-120.00 [-148.48, -91.52]
Subtotal (95% CI)			**40**			**32**	**100.0%**	**-120.00 [-148.48, -91.52]**
Heterogeneity: Not applicable								
Test for overall effect: Z = 8.26 (P < 0.00001)								

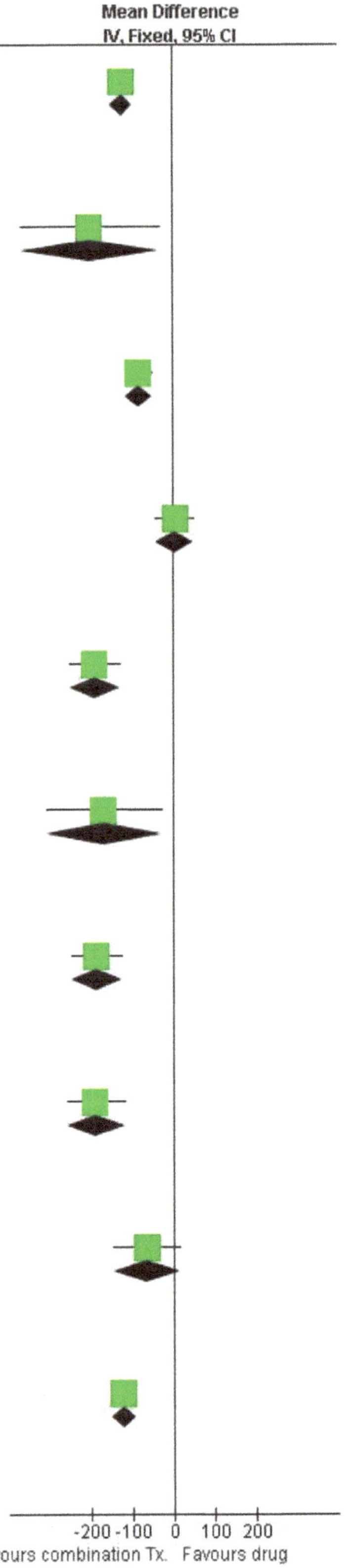

Figure 4. Herbal medicine plus active drug versus active drug, mean dose of levodopa (madopar).

[86]. Trials with less methodological rigor prone to exaggerate treatment effect than rigorous studies [87]. Thirdly all the included studies tested only small sample size without proper power calculation. Generally studies with small sample may not detect clinically important difference between interventions [88]. Among the included studies in this review, some HMs did not show statistically significant effect in favor of herbal preparations compared with placebo or conventional treatment which may be originated from their insufficient sample size. Fourthly there may be a possibility of publication bias in this review. We checked funnel plots of two key outcomes i.e. total UPDRS scores and mean dose of levodopa in the comparison of HM plus active drug and active drug only. Both of the funnel plots appeared asymmetric, which might be originated from publication bias or poor methodological qualities of the included studies (figure 5 and 6).

In these points, the findings of this systematic review should be interpreted carefully.

Even with several limitations, this review also has strength as well. We did comprehensive search regardless of language and publication types to locate every possible RCT. We failed to suggest overall estimates of treatment effects on PD but herbal recipes and estimates of effect measures on the separate outcomes for individual HMs were presented to provide information in detail, which may be available to suggest a basic source for judging the possibility of treating PD and after all may offer a principle data to find out new drug candidates for PD [89].

There are several issues on the HMs for the treatment of PD, which should be discussed more. We found that herbal recipes were generally used as adjuvant treatments to conventional drug therapy which may contribute to improve the PD symptoms and to decrease dose of anti-Parkinson drugs and adverse events rate. Many PD patients experience dyskinesia and symptom fluctuation from the long-term treatment with levodopa [90]. Combination therapy with some HMs showed significant or marginal effect in reducing complications of levodopa (UPDRS IV) [41]. The dose of levodopa is also one of the important clinical considerations because PD needs lifelong treatment generally. Considering wearing-off symptoms, it would be helpful for both patients and clinicians to reduce dose of levodopa for managing PD symptoms [1]. In this point, HM may be considered as a good adjunctive treatment to conventional drugs for PD. On the contrary, HMs for treating PD needs to equip standardized criteria for use to ensure the good quality of the products. It includes the problems related to the original species of individual herbs, chemical compositions and indexes, preparations and indications for herbal products. Chinese formulas were composed of many herbs and there were a wide heterogeneity in the HMs between the studies included in this review. In this situation, standardization of natural products used in the clinical trials is one of the most necessary factors for demonstrating good reproducibility of the research result in real clinical practices. Pharmacological researches including in vivo and in vitro studies should be promoted to support biological mechanism of herbal products as well. Adverse effects (AE) relevant to herbal recipes also need to be described clearly. AEs of the drugs for PD are well documented and are frequently reported of high occurrence rate in conventional medicine [1]. For example, in one study, dyskinesia was experienced in up to 40% of PD patients after 4 to 6 years of levodopa treatment [90]. In this review, occurrence of adverse events was relatively low in the combination therapies. This result may be originated from the fact that observation periods of the included studies were relatively short. Safety issues need to be one of the primary outcomes and clearly be described in future trials with long term observational period.

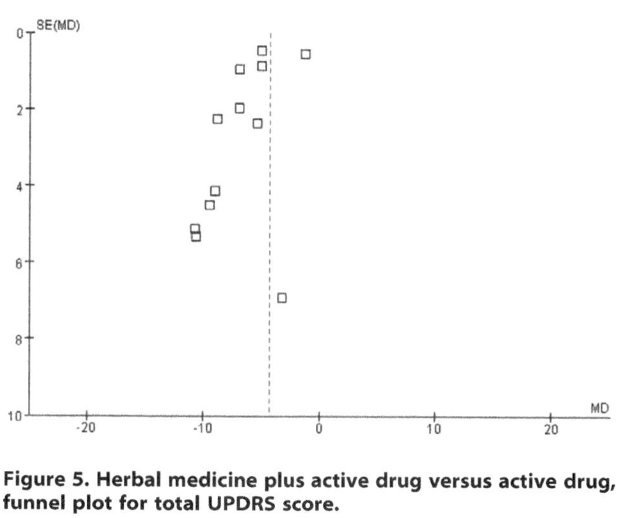

Figure 5. Herbal medicine plus active drug versus active drug, funnel plot for total UPDRS score.

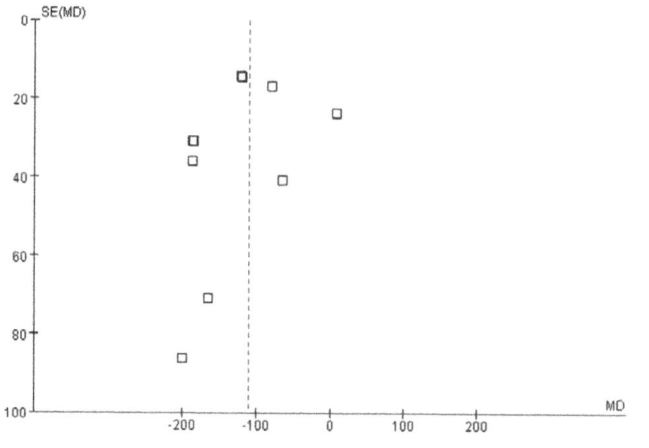

Figure 6. Herbal medicine plus active drug versus active drug, funnel plot for mean dose of levodopa (madopar).

Future clinical trials of HMs on PD need to improve methodological quality to evaluate clinical benefit and harm properly. Random sequence generation and double blinding should be ensured in study design and results need to be reported well according to the CONSORT statement [91]. Protocol registration before start of clinical trials is also important to guarantee the transparency of the study finding through avoiding selective outcome reporting and publication bias [92]. Along with trials for efficacy in which single HM is compared with placebo control, comparative effectiveness studies using combination therapy with conventional drug therapies also need to be conducted to reflect clinical situation as it is.

Supporting Information

Table S1 The preparation of the herbal medicines of the included studies.
(DOCX)

Table S2 Summary of the included studies on herbal medicines for Parkinson's disease.
(DOCX)

Acknowledgments

The authors especially thank Dr. Toru Naito for offering Japanese literature.

Author Contributions

Conceived and designed the experiments: THK KHC. Performed the experiments: THK WSJ. Analyzed the data: THK MSL. Contributed reagents/materials/analysis tools: THK. Wrote the paper: THK.

References

1. Rao SS, Hofmann LA, Shakil A (2006) Parkinson's disease: diagnosis and treatment. American Family Physician 74: 2046–2054.
2. von Campenhausen S, Bornschein B, Wick R, Bötzel K, Sampaio C, et al. (2005) Prevalence and incidence of Parkinson's disease in Europe. The Journal Of The European College Of Neuropsychopharmacology 15: 473–490.
3. Muangpaisan W, Hori H, Brayne C (2009) Systematic review of the prevalence and incidence of Parkinson's disease in Asia. Journal of epidemiology 19: 281–293.
4. Schrag A, Quinn NP, Ben-Shlomo Y (2000) Cross sectional prevalence survey of idiopathic Parkinson's disease and parkinsonism in London. British Medical Journal 321: 21–22.
5. Dowding CH, Shenton CL, Salek SS (2006) A Review of the Health-Related Quality of Life and Economic Impact of Parkinson's Disease. Drugs & Aging 23: 693–721.
6. Lokk J (2008) Caregiver strain in Parkinson's disease and the impact of disease duration. European Journal of Physical and Rehabilitation Medicine 44: 39.
7. Winter Y, von Campenhausen S, Brozova H, Skoupa J, Reese JP, et al. (2010) Costs of Parkinson's disease in Eastern Europe: A Czech cohort study. Parkinsonism & Related Disorders 16: 51–56.
8. Manyam BV, Sanchez-Ramos JR (1999) Traditional and complementary therapies in Parkinson's disease. Advances in Neurology 80: 565–574.
9. Zheng GQ (2009) Therapeutic history of Parkinson's disease in Chinese medical treatises. Journal of Alternative and Complementary Medicine 15: 1223–1230.
10. Li Q, Zhao D, Bezard E (2006) Traditional Chinese medicine for Parkinson's disease: a review of Chinese literature. Behavioural Pharmacology 17: 403–410.
11. Zhang L, Liu SM (2006) Recent developments of traditional Chinese medicine in treatment of Parkinson disease. Chinese Journal of Clinical Rehabilitation 10: 152–154.
12. Chung V, Liu L, Bian Z, Zhao Z, Fong WL, et al. (2006) Efficacy and safety of herbal medicines for idiopathic Parkinson's disease: A systematic review. Movement Disorders 21: 1709–1715.
13. Yang ZM, Tang XJ, Lao YR (2005) Systematic evaluation on clinical literature related with treatment of Parkinson's disease with traditional Chinese medicine. Chinese Journal of Integrated Traditional and Western Medicine 25: 612–615.
14. Gibb WR, Lees AJ (1988) The relevance of the Lewy body to the pathogenesis of idiopathic Parkinson's disease. Journal of Neurology, Neurosurgery & Psychiatry 51: 745–752.
15. Wang XD (1985) Diagnosis and differential diagnosis for Parkinson's disease and Parkinsonism. Chinese Journal of Neurology and Psychiatry 18: 256.
16. Ernst E, Pittler MH, Wider B, Boddy K (2008) CHAPTER 1 General issues. Oxford Handbook of Complementary Medicine: Oxford University Press.
17. Ernst E, Pittler MH, Wider B, Boddy K (2006) SECTION 3 Therapies. The Desktop Guide to Complementary and Alternative Medicine: Elsevier Ltd.
18. Higgins J, Green Se (2008) Cochrane Handbook for Systematic Reviews of Interventions Version 5.0.0 [updated February 2008]: The Cochrane Collo-boration.
19. Serrano-Duenas M, Cardozo-Pelaez F, Sanchez-Ramos JR (2001) Effects of Banisteriopsis caapi extract on Parkinson's disease. Scientific Review of Alternative Medicine 5: 127–132.
20. Cui L, Yu X-d, Cui J (2003) Clinical Observation on Effect of Combined Therapy of Bushen Pingchan Recipe and Medopa Tablet in Treating Parkinson's Disease. Chinese Journal of Integrated Traditional and Western Medicine 23: 504–507.
21. Zhao H, Li WW, Gao JP (2007) Clinical trial on treatment of Parkinson's disease of Gan-Shen yin deficiency type by recipe for nourishing Gan-Shen. Chinese Journal of Integrated Traditional and Western Medicine 27: 780–784.
22. Liu H (1994) Clinical observation on the 45 cases of Parkinson's Disease patients treated by Budushujingxifengtang with integrative medicine. Yellow River Medicine 3: 72–73.
23. Dou YQ, Yang MH, Liu Y, Wei ZM (2006) Curative effect of integrated traditional Chinese medicine and western medicine for treatment of patients with Parkinson disease:A control study. Chinese Journal of Clinical Rehabili-tation 10: 6–8.
24. Carroll CB, Wroath C, Parkin SG, Hobart J, Teare L, et al. (2004) Cannabis for dyskinesia in Parkinson disease: A randomized double-blind crossover study. Neurology 63: 1245–1250.
25. Yang MJ (2010) Clinical assessment of the effectiveness of Chaihushugansan for the depressive symptoms in Parkinson's disease. Guangming Journal of Chinese Medicine 25: 31–32.
26. Zhang JP (2009) Observational study for Chuzhantang combined with Western treatment in 34 cases of Parkinson disease. Yunnan Journal of Traditional Chinese Medicine and Materia Medica 30: 37.
27. Zhang Y, Liang WB, Luo XD (2008) Chinese drug, Dingzhentang for the treatment of Parkinson's disease: a randomized controlled clinical trial. Liaoning Journal of Traditional Chinese Medicine 35: 728–729.
28. Zhang Y, Luo XD (2006) Clinical research on Ding-Zhen-Tang. Guangzhou: Guangzhou University of Traditional Chinese Medicine.
29. Zhu XY, Fang ZL, Liu Y, Li CS (2009) Clinical Trial Treatment of Parkinson's Disease with Dingzhentang. Journal of Neurology and Neurorehabilitation 6: 114–116.
30. Teng SW, Shui RY (2000) Observation of clinical effectiveness of Dingzhentang in 32 casese of Parkinson's disease. Journal of Zhenjiang College of Traditional Chinese Medicine 24: 34.
31. Ai Lx (2004) Clinical Obsebation for the effectiveness of Dingzhentang on Parkinson's disease. Journal Traditional Chinese Medicine 19: 31–33.
32. Gu XZ (2002) Clinical Observation on Treatment of 30 Cases of Parkinsonian Syndrome with Western Medicines Combined with Dingchan Liquid. Journal of Nanjing University of Traditional Chinese Medicine 18: 275–276.
33. Yuan JP, Wang XL, Chen D (2005) On Treating 60 Cases of Parkinson' s Disease by Combination of Chinese and Western Medicine. Jilin Journal Of Traditional Chinese Medicine 25: 47.
34. Zhao GH, Meng QG, Yu XDea (2009) A multi-centered randomized double-blinded controlled clinical study on efficacy of guiling pa'an capsule in treating Parkinson's disease. Chinese Journal of Integrated Traditional and Western Medicine 29: 590–594.
35. Chang XH, Zhang LZ, Li YJ (2008) Clinical obserbation on the effectiveness of Guilingpaanwan with Madopar tablets in the treatment of 30 cases of Parkinson's disease. Journal of New Chinese Medicine 4: 62–63.
36. Jiang SY (2009) Guiling Pa an Pill in 30 Cases of Pakinson Disease Treatment. Journal of Liaoning University of Traditional Chinese Medicine 11: 118–119.
37. Wang ZY (2005) Treatment of 38 cases Parkinson disease patients with Gui Ling Pa An Wan. Tradiaitonal Chinese Medicinal Research 18: 37–38.
38. Yang YF, Fang WJ, Wan TM (2008) 32 cases of Parkinson's disease treated with Jianpiyishenfang plus western drugs. Journal of Anhui Traditional Chinese Medical College 27: 16–18.
39. Ming KW, Hong CX (2010) Clinical Research on Da Dingfeng Zhu. Journal of New Chinese Medicine 42: 23–24.
40. Lian XF, Luo XD (2008) Clinical trial for tremor type Parkinson's disease with integrative medicine. Journal of New Chinese Medicine 40: 37–38.
41. Zhao XH, Gu CZ, Huang HY, Huang ZD (2003) Study of Parkinson's disease treated with integrated tradition al Chinese and western medicine. Modern Jorunal of Integrated Traditional Chinese and Western Medicine 12: 1923–1927.
42. Yang LJ, Tian JB, Jiang GQ (2009) Chinese drug, Kangzhanning united Madopar for the treatment of Parkinson's Disease: clinical analysis of 48 cases. Chinese Journal of Gerontology 6: 1554–1555.
43. Bao YC, Zhou HG, Wang H, Zhang B, Chen HZ, et al. (2001) Effect of Kangzhen Zhijing capsule combined with Glutathione on blood antioxidase in Parkinson's disease patients. Journal of Anhui Traditional Chinese Medical College 20: 11–15.
44. Guo SR, Fu WY, Qi CY, Zhang CY, Lu E, et al. (2004) Clinical assessment of Kanlitang for Parkinson's disease. Liaoning Journal of Traditional Chinese Medicine 31: 750–751.
45. Luo ZM, Luo Y, Zhou L, Shang HF (2001) Clinical effect of Lemaikeli on patients with Parkinson's disease. West China Medical Journal 16: 40–41.
46. Kim IK (2004) The Efficacy and the underlying mechanism of Traditional Chinese Formula NaoKangNing in Patients with Parkinson's Disease. Jinan: Shandong University of Traditional Chinese Medicine.
47. Hu XJ, Yang XS, Yang XG (2003) Clinical observation on the efficacy enhancing and toxicity attenuating effect of nuzhen yangyin granule to the anti-parkinsonism therapy mainly with Medopa. Chinese Journal of Integrated Traditional and Western Medicine 23: 811–814.
48. Sun YZ (2005) Clinical research of treating hypokinesia type and rigid type Parkinson's disease with PD No. 1. Guangzhou: Guangzhou University of Traditional Chinese Medicine.
49. Zhang H, Luo XD (2008) Clinical study of TCM six Jueyin differential diagnosis for the treatment of early and mid-term Parkinson's disease. Acta Chinese Medicine and Pharmacology 36: 34–36.
50. Fan YP (2006) Clinical Research of Tremor Type Parkinson's Disease with PD NO. 2. Guangzhou: Guangzhou University of Traditional Chinese Medicine.
51. Zheng CY, Luo XD (2006) Clinical Study on Pabing Recipe III for Treatment of 30 Cases of Parkinson's Disease. Journal of Traditional Chinese Medicine 47: 516–518.
52. Chen JZ, Jian W, Shi J, Li B, Wu SH (1999) Preliminary Clinical Observation of 60 Cases of Parkinson' s Disease Mainly Treated by Tonifying Spleen and Kidney. Journal of Chengdu University of Traditional Chinese Medicine 22: 14–15, 19.
53. An LZ (2009) Clinical trial for the treatment of Parkinson's disease with clearing the heart and resolving phlegm method. Journal of Sichuan of Traditional Chinese Medicine 27: 81–82.

54. Wu DH, Zhao RC, Long HJ, Jiang JL, Tang PL, et al. (2008) Clinical observation of the effect of Ruogantongluotang: 36 Cases of Parkinson Disease. Guiding Journal of Traditional Chinese Medicine and Pharmacy 14: 24–26.
55. Yuan CX, Zhi HP, Chen SZ, Chen Y, Li J, et al. (2010) Clinical multicenter randomized controlled study on treatment of Parkinson's disease with "Shudi Pingchan Decoction" and western medicine. Shanghai Journal of Traditional Chinese Medicine 44: 3–6.
56. Wang D (2009) Clinical study of Integrative Medicine for treating 31 cases of Parkinson disease. Practical Clinical Journal of Integrated Traditional Chinese and Western Medicine 9: 27–28.
57. Wang YL (2009) Clininical trial on Shujinjiedutang for the treatment of Parkinson's disease. Journal of Shandong University of Traditional Chinese Medicine 33: 26–27.
58. Shen Y, Luo LL (2008) Parkinson's Disease Treated with Tongxinluo Capsule, Liuwei Rehmannia Root Pill and Madopar. Journal of Zhejiang University of Traditional Chinese Medicine 32: 197–198.
59. Liang JF, Yang LL, Li F (2008) Clinical obserbation of the effectiveness of WuhuZhuifengsan for the treatment of levodopa induced dyskinesia in 30 cases. Liaoning Journal of Traditional Chinese Medicine 35: 82–83.
60. Li XX (2008) Clinical study on 27 cases of Parkinson's disease treated with Xifengdingzhantang and Madopar. Traditional Chinese Medicinal Research 21: 32–33.
61. Ma YZ, Li SF, Shen XM, Jia K (2005) Clinical observation on the 30 cases of Parkinson's disease with integrative medicine. New Journal of Traditional Chinese Medicine 37: 55–56.
62. Ma YZ, Jian YP (2008) Integrative Medicine treated 30 patients with Parkinson's disease. Henan Traditional Chinese Medicine 27: 73–74.
63. Ma L (2008) 40 cases of Parkinson's disease treated with Xifengdingzhanwan. Traditional Chinese Medicinal Research 21: 39–42.
64. Cheng CH, Ma YZ, Ma L, Wang JF (2007) Study on the Effect of Xifeng Dingchan Pill on the Madopar Dosage on Parkinson's Disease. Shanxi Journal of Traditional Chinese Medicine 23: 35–36.
65. Lu Y (2009) Clinical Study on Parkinson's Disease Treated with "Xifeng Zhichan Decoction" and Madopar. Shanghai Journal of Traditional Chinese Medicine 43: 20–22.
66. Wang EL, Jian W, Zhou HF (2008) The Clinical Research of Yanggan Xifeng Chinese Medicine Treating the Parkinson Disease. Liaoning Journal of Traditional Chinese Medicine 35: 227.
67. Li N (2009) Clinical observation for TCM treatment of Parkinson's disease Chinese. Journal of Geriatric Care 7: 100–101.
68. Chen LH, Tan YF (2009) 46 cases of Yiyuanyin for Parkinson's disease with non-motor symptoms. Journal of Nanjing University of Traditional Chinese Medicine 25: 472–473.
69. Yang MH, Dou YQ, LIU Y, Zhao GY, Luo Y (2002) Contrast clinical observation in the treatment of Parkinson's disease with Yichan decoction. Integrated Traditional Chinese and Western Medicine In Practice of Critical Care Medicine 9: 256–257.
70. Pan WD, Yuan WA, Fang ZL, Liu Y, Kwak S (2009) Effects of "Zengxiao Anshen Zhichan 2 Decoction" on Motor and Non-Motor Symptoms in Parkinson's Disease. Acta Universitatis Traditionis Medicalis Sinensis Pharmacologiaeque Shanghai 23: 29–34.
71. Feng GK, Shao FY, Li JB, Chen YY, Li JL, et al. (2002) Clinical treatment of Parkinson syndrome with ZhenChanShu capsule. Modern Rehabilitation 6: 334–335.
72. Wu CH, Wu SY, Wang JM, Lin JS, Yang ZB, et al. (2008) Zhenchan Decoction with Madopar for Vibration Syndrome of Gan-Shen Deficiency Syndrome. Chinese Journal of Integrative Medicine on Cardio-/Cerebrovascular Disease 6: 397–399.
73. Wang YL (2008) Clinical Effect of Zhichanshudu Prescription Treatment Parkinson's Disease. Modern Traditional Chinese Medicine 28: 1–3.
74. Wang HX, Liu Y, Li RK (2010) Clinical study of Zhizhantang combined with Western treatment for Parkinson's disease. Guiding Journal of Traditional Chinese Medicine and Pharmacy 16: 17–18.
75. Shen W, Yuan CX (2006) Clinical Observation on Treatment of Parkinson's Disease by Nourishing Liver and Kidney. Shanghai Journal of Traditional Chinese Medicine 40: 21–22.
76. Jiang XC (2003) Clinical observation on 15 cases of Parkinson's disease with integrative medcine. Modern Jorunal of Integrated Traditional Chinese and Western Medicine 12: 934–935.
77. Tang XJ, Luo XD, Cai YF, Huang PX (2005) A Clinical Study on the Treatment of Early Stage of Parkinson's Disease by Zhiyin Xifeng Granules. New Journal Of Traditional Chinese Medicine 37: 25–26.
78. Wang WT, Luo XD, Wu W (2004) Clinical Control Study on Ziyin Xifeng Huoxue Decoction for Treatment of Parkinson's Disease at Early Stage. Journal of Traditional Chinese Medicine 45: 274–276.
79. Cui RT (2004) Clinical observation on 50 cases of Parkinson's disease with integrative medcine. Capital Mdeicine. 26 p.
80. Qiu CL (1998) Treatment with integrative medicine in Parkinson's disease. Zhejiang Journal of Integrated Traditional Chinese and Western Medicine 8: 224–225.
81. Ma QM, Du LP (2003) Clinical observation of 42 cases of Parkinson's disease with Integrative Medicine. Chinese Journal of Integrative Medicine on Cardio-/Cerebrovascular Disease 1: 614–615.
82. Wang ZY, Zhao YL, Li YJ, Li HM (2005) Clinical observation on the treatment of Parkinson's disease using integrative medicine. Capital Medicine 12: 32–33.
83. Dou YQ, Yang MH, Liu Y, Wei ZM (2006) Curative effect of integrated traditional Chinese medicine and western medicine for treatment of patients with Parkinson disease: A control study. Chinese Journal of Clinical Rehabilitation 10: 6–8.
84. Cheng CH, Ma YZ, Ma L, Wang JF (2007) Study on the Effect of Xifeng Dingchan Pill on the Madopar Dosage on Parkinson's Disease. Shanxi Journal of Traditional Chinese Medicine 23: 35–36.
85. Chung V, Liu L, Bian Z, Zhao Z, Leuk Fong W, et al. (2006) Efficacy and safety of herbal medicines for idiopathic Parkinson's disease: a systematic review. Movement Disorders 21: 1709–1715.
86. Vickers A, Goyal N, Harland R, Rees R (1998) Do certain countries produce only positive results? A systematic review of controlled trials. Controlled Clinical Trials 19: 159–166.
87. Egger M, Juni P, Bartlett C, Holenstein F, Sterne J (2003) How important are comprehensive literature searches and the assessment of trial quality in systematic reviews? Empirical study. Health Technology Assessment 7: 1–76.
88. Altman DG (1980) Statistics and ethics in medical research: III How large a sample? British Medical Journal 281: 1336–1338.
89. Campos HC, da Rocha MD, Viegas FP, Nicastro PC, Fossaluzza PC, et al. (2011) The role of natural products in the discovery of new drug candidates for the treatment of neurodegenerative disorders I: Parkinson's disease. CNS & Neurological Disorders - Drug Targets 10: 239–250.
90. Ahlskog JE, Muenter MD (2001) Frequency of levodopa-related dyskinesias and motor fluctuations as estimated from the cumulative literature. Movement Disorders 16: 448–458.
91. Schulz KF, Altman DG, Moher D (2010) CONSORT 2010 statement: Updated guidelines for reporting parallel group randomised trials. Journal of Pharmacology and Pharmacotherapeutics 1: 100–107.
92. Ross JS, Mulvey GK, Hines EM, Nissen SE, Krumholz HM (2009) Trial publication after registration in ClinicalTrials.Gov: a cross-sectional analysis. PLoS Med 6: e1000144.

4

Colorimetric Grading Scale Can Promote the Standardization of Experiential and Sensory Evaluation in Quality Control of Traditional Chinese Medicines

Jia-bo Wang[1]§, Ling-na Zeng[1,2]§, Qing-ce Zang[1,3]§, Qian-feng Gong[3], Bao-cai Li[2], Xue-ru Zhang[1], Xiao-hui Chu[1], Ping Zhang[1], Yan-ling Zhao[1], Xiao-he Xiao[4]*

1 China Military Institute of Chinese Medicine, 302 Military Hospital, Beijing, China, **2** Faculty of Life Science and Technology, Kunming University of Science and Technology, Kunming, China, **3** Pharmacy College, Jiangxi University of Traditional Chinese Medicine, Nanchang, China, **4** Integrative Medicine Center, 302 Military Hospital, Beijing, China

Abstract

Experiential and sensory evaluation is an ancient method that remains important in the current quality control system of Traditional Chinese Medicines (TCMs). The process is rapid and convenient when evaluating the quality of crude materials in TCM markets. However, sensory evaluation has been met with skepticism because it is mainly based on experience and lacks a scientific basis. In this study, rhubarb was selected to demonstrate how color-based sensory evaluation could differentiate the quality of herbal medicines objectively. The colors of the rhubarb samples, expressed as RGB values, were obtained from different parts and forms of the plant, including the plant's surface, fracture surface color, and a powdered form with or without treatment with a color-developing reagent. We first divided the rhubarb samples into three grades based on the total content of five hydroxyanthraquinone derivatives, the major pharmacological components in rhubarb. Then, a three-layer back-propagation artificial neural network (BP-ANN), calibrated with selected training samples, was used to correlate the quality of the rhubarb with its color. The color of the rhubarb powder after coloration attained the highest accuracy (92.3%) in predicting the quality grade of the test samples with the established artificial neural networks. Finally, a standardized colorimetric grading scale was created based on the spatial distribution of the rhubarb samples in a two-dimensional chromaticity diagram according to the colors of the powdered rhubarb after color enhancement. By comparing the color between the scale and the tested samples, similar to performing a pH test with indicator paper, subjects without sensory evaluation experience could quickly determine the quality grade of rhubarb. This work illustrates the technical feasibility of the color-based grading of rhubarb quality and offers references for quantifying and standardizing the sensory evaluation of TCMs, foods and other products.

Editor: Pratibha V. Nerurkar, College of Tropical Agriculture and Human Resources, University of Hawaii, United States of America

Funding: This research is supported by the Industry Research Program of Traditional Chinese Medicine (Nos. 200807020 and 201207002), the National Key Technology Research and Development Program (No. 2012BAI29B02), and the National Science Foundation of China (Nos. 81274026 and 30973947). The funders had no role in study design, data collection and analysis, decision to publish, or preparation of the manuscript.

Competing Interests: The authors have declared that no competing interests exist.

* E-mail: pharmacy302@126.com

§ These authors contributed equally to this work.

Introduction

Experiential and sensory evaluation is a rapid and effective evaluation method that has been used widely in various fields [1–3]. The technique has been used for more than 30 years in the food industry as a quality control test, characterizing the taste and colors of foods, and is becoming increasingly important in food markets [4–6]. A set of unique methods of sensory evaluation have been developed as Traditional Chinese Medicines (TCMs) evolves. Traditional sensory evaluation is based primarily on the human senses to assess shape, size, texture, color, odor and taste. Sensory evaluation remains one of the most effective methods to assess the raw materials used in TCM. Compared with modern quality control methods that involve spectroscopy, chromatography, mass spectrometry and cutting-edge biotechnology, sensory evaluation is convenient, fast and effective [7]. Nevertheless, these high-tech modern methods have been greatly researched, whereas the conventional sensory evaluation methods interest few modern researchers. In China, quality evaluation based on sensory characteristics is widely used in the TCM markets. There are some commercial specifications of TCMs conventionally accepted by the growers, medicinal vendors, TCM physicians and consumers. Also there are *Dao-di* herbs (good quality herbs produced in the native areas) conventionally accepted by practitioners to differentiate the quality of TCMs. Those commercial specifications and the concept of *Dao-di* herbs are generally defined by a set of specific morphological features. Growers of medicinal herbs typically select a superior species or variety to cultivate based on those specific morphological features. Similarly, medicinal vendors classify and price TCMs based on different specifications, and consumers primarily evaluate the quality of a TCM on the basis of sensory characteristics [8]. The repeatabilities of the experiential and sensory assessment by practitioners for the TCMs, like rhubarb and *Coptis chinensis*, etc., have been demonstrated in our previous studies [9,10]. Although traditional sensory evaluation has been regularly applied in China, there are some disadvantages. One concern is whether the sensory evaluation has a scientific foundation and chemical basis. A second issue is how the practice can be applied by people with little sensory evaluation experience, specifically users in the Western world.

Color is one of the most important characteristics in sensory evaluation for TCMs. Some ancient Chinese herbal medicine literature, such as the *Origins of the Materia Medica* (*Ben Cao Yuan Shi*), emphasize the importance of color as an identifier of high quality herbal materials (Figure 1). For example, an *Aucklandia* root (*muxiang* in Chinese) that is cadet blue in color is considered to be superior, mid-grade if yellowish-white, and inferior in quality when characterized by an oleaginous black color [11]. The correlation between color and chemical composition, however, is not well studied. Furthermore, sensory evaluation relies greatly on personal experiences, which are difficult to quantify and standardize. Thus, its application has been restricted. To our knowledge, no previous quantification and standardization of color evaluation for Chinese herbal medicine has been reported.

Rhubarb, an ancient and one of the best known Chinese herbal medicines, has been recognized for centuries in traditional medicine for its pharmacological properties, including its purgative [12], nephric protecting [13,14], liver protecting [15], antimicrobial and hemostatic properties [16]. The major pharmacological components in rhubarb are five hydroxyanthraquinones (HAQs) – aloe-emodin, rhein, emodin, chrysophanol and physcion – which are also quality control markers in the Chinese pharmacopoeia [17]. The quality of rhubarb correlates directly with the content of the five HAQs. Rhubarbs of different grades usually exhibit different colors, such as dark red, brown yellow or yellow. According to traditional sensory evaluation, rhubarbs of good quality are often bright yellow and those of poor quality were often dark yellow or brown. The objectivity and reproducibility of sensory evaluation for rhubarb have been demonstrated using the Delphi method [9]. In this study, rhubarb has been selected as a model drug for its representative color in sensory evaluation.

The overall flowchart of this study is shown in Figure 2. First, we divided the rhubarb samples into three grades based on the total content of the five HAQs. Second, we used the three-layer back-propagation artificial neural network (BP-ANN) to find relationships between the quality and the color of the samples. Finally, we defined a colorimetric grading scale for the quality of rhubarb. By comparing the color of a sample with this scale, similar to matching the color of litmus paper with a color scale to ascertain pH, customers can quickly determine rhubarb quality. To investigate which kind of sample produced the best colors to use for grading rhubarb, colors from the plant surface, fracture surface color and powder, with or without coloration by a color-developing reagent, were analyzed. Through this work, we illustrated the feasibility of color-based grading for rhubarb and developed a practical tool, a standardized colorimetric grading scale, to classify the rhubarb. Furthermore, we provided some references for the quantification and standardization of sensory evaluation of TCMs.

Materials and Methods

Materials

Thirty-four batches of rhubarb were collected from various sources in China (Table 1). All of the voucher specimens were deposited at the China Military Institute of Chinese Materia Medica. The samples were identified by Professor Xiao-He Xiao as the dried roots and rhizomes of *Rheum palmatum* L., *Rheum tanguticum* Maxim. ex Balf. and *Rheum offcinale* Baill. The chemical reagents were analytical grade and obtained from the Beijing Chemical Factory (Beijing, China).

Ethics

No specific permits were required for the described field studies. The aforementioned locations are neither privately-owned nor protected by the Chinese government. And there is no endangered or protected species involved in the specific locations where we collected the rhubarb samples.

Camera System

Images were acquired using a camera system equipped with a standard lightbox, camera, computer, ZoomBrowser EX software, data lines and digital camera (PowerShot G5 Pro 5.0 Megapixel, Canon Inc., Nagasaki, Japan). The standard lightbox consists of a steel framework, fluorescent lamp (LUMILUX, FH14W/865HE, OSRAM Company, München, Germany), ballast and shading-cloth.

Optimization of Shooting Conditions

Exposure time, aperture size, and light sensitivity were optimized to obtain clear images. The optimal camera performance parameters were determined by varying exposure time (1/4, 1/6, 1/8, 1/10, 1/13, 1/15, 1/20, 1/30, 1/40, 1/60, 1/80, 1/100), aperture size (8.0, 7.1, 6.3, 5.6) and ISO light sensitivity value (50 and 100). The results showed that the clearest image with well-balanced brightness and contrast was acquired using the following conditions: an exposure time of 1/10 second, an aperture size of 8.0 and an ISO light sensitivity value of 50.

Sample Coloration and Obtainment of RGB Values

Powder coloration: The powdered rhubarb samples of 0.3 g were weighed respectively and then dispersed into a 96-well plate which is generally used in cell culture and molecular biology experiments. Then an aqueous solution of 0.5% NaOH (0.6 ml) was added to each well to develop the color of the sample. After coloration, pieces of square filter paper (1.5×1.5 cm) were then inserted into the colored powder to absorb the rhubarb solution in the wells, and the filter papers were transferred to the standard lightbox for immediate imaging.

Fractured surface coloration: NaOH solution (0.5%, 0.2 ml) was sprayed onto the fractured surface of each sample of rhubarb. These samples were photographed immediately in the lightbox.

All samples, with or without coloration, were placed in the standard lightbox, and photographs were taken using the optimized shooting conditions described above. Some representative images are shown in Figure 3. All images were saved in the.jpg format. The RGB values were extracted from the images using Photoshop CS4 (Adobe Systems Inc., USA) image processing software.

BP Neural Network Analysis

A BP neural network with one input layer, one hidden layer, and one output layer was established in this study. According to the experimental results, the RGB values were set as three of the evaluation parameters. In this experiment, there were seven initial nodes in the hidden layer, and the number of nodes was defined to be 2N+1, where N is the number of input layer nodes. In the output layer, three nodes were designated to represent the three grades of rhubarb. The hidden layer and input vectors were

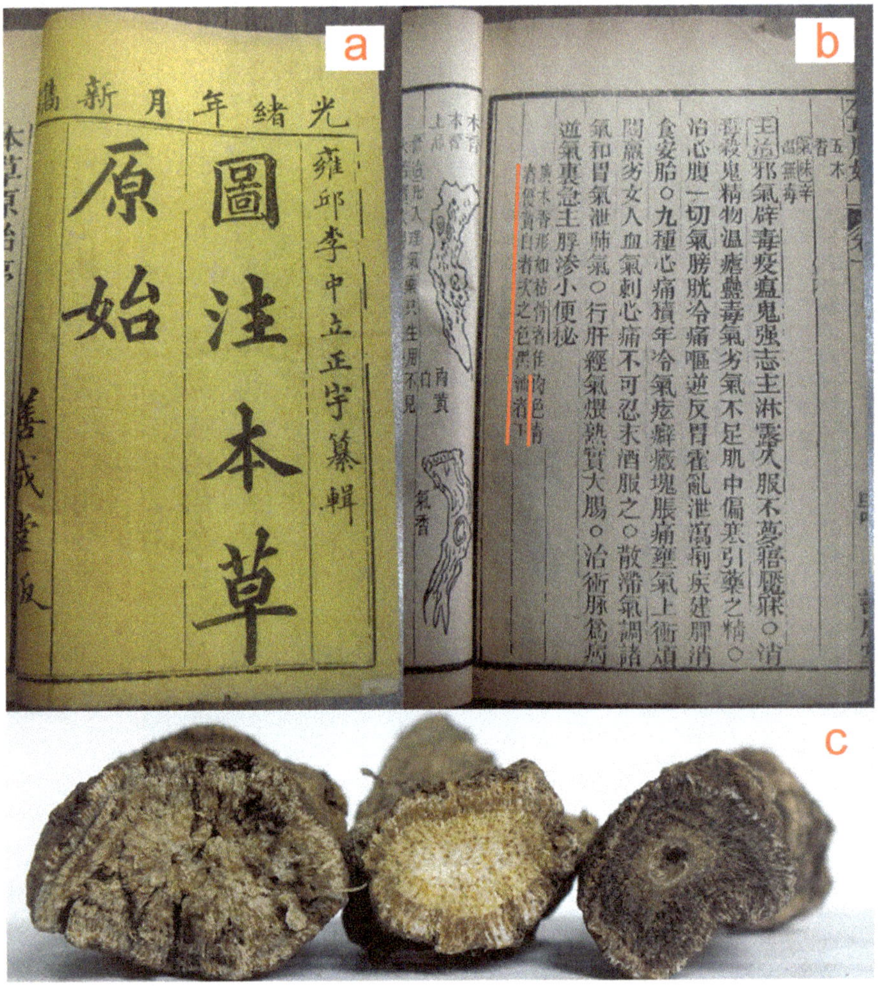

Figure 1. The herbal classic *Origin of the Materia Medica* (*Ben Cao Yuan Shi*) describes the color-based quality evaluation of Chinese herbal materials. a) *Origin of the Materia Medica*, written by Zhong-li Li in 1612 during the Ming Dynasty, has been considered the first of the herbal classics in China, which described the sensory characteristics for identification of commercial herbal materials (the medicinal parts of the plants) in detail rather than the plant morphology. b) The original description in the book for the color-based quality evaluation of *Aucklandia* root (*Aucklandia lappa* Decne, *muxiang* in Chinese). *Aucklandia* root is an herb that has been commonly used to treat gastroenterological diseases in China for over two thousand years. c) Photographs of the *Aucklandia* root samples in different color. The quality of *Aucklandia* root can be placed into three grades based on the color of its fracture surfaces: cadet blue denotes superior quality (left); yellowish-white indicates ordinary quality (middle); and an oleaginous black color suggests inferior quality (right).

connected, and the output layer and input vectors were not. In addition, the training sample set and the desired values were normalized with *Premnmx* from the Matlab toolbox. Finally, the BP network was established using the *Newcf* function and the transfer function of neurons in each layer was *tansig* and *purelin*. The network training function was *trainParam*. After training, the

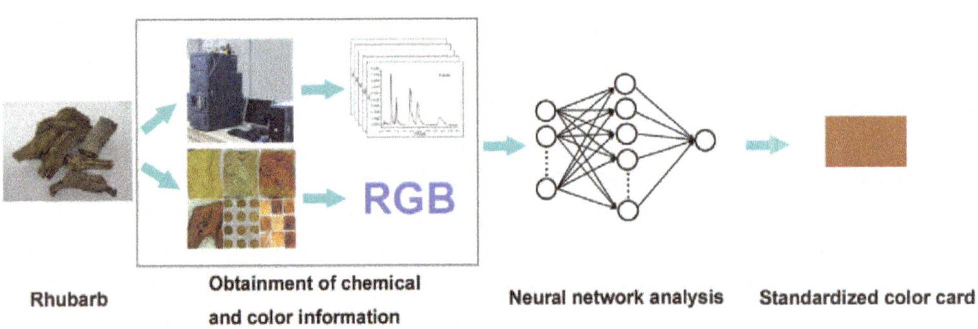

Figure 2. The flowchart for this study.

Table 1. RGB values of the color of the surface, the fracture surface and powder with or without further color development.

No.	Collection place	Grade	Surface color			Fractured surface color						Powder color					
			Without coloration			Without coloration			With coloration			Without coloration			With coloration		
			R	G	B	R	G	B	R	G	B	R	G	B	R	G	B
1	Li, Gansu	2nd	176	141	42	162	142	78	125	38	34	195	148	38	203	85	26
2	Li, Gansu	2nd	159	132	37	152	151	116	127	55	37	154	123	33	167	74	46
3	Li, Gansu	2nd	181	150	47	166	151	100	147	52	31	175	135	27	196	83	35
4	Li, Gansu	2nd	110	82	32	153	154	101	136	54	31	123	88	33	181	79	43
5	Li, Gansu	3rd	90	72	37	202	181	112	198	79	34	144	113	43	216	120	44
6	Li, Gansu	1st	149	125	33	165	150	85	144	80	31	171	131	34	240	163	69
7	Li, Gansu	1st	102	86	47	105	91	42	44	42	44	118	90	31	173	85	46
8	Dali, Yunnan	2nd	146	115	36	155	154	103	119	57	39	166	134	27	233	159	63
9	Dali, Yunnan	3rd	84	70	37	115	107	70	80	42	43	116	87	29	233	172	92
10	Dali, Yunnan	3rd	127	97	34	162	170	130	146	74	28	150	112	12	231	144	46
11	Gansu	2nd	103	86	44	117	107	55	92	47	39	119	92	31	197	114	61
12	Qinghai	1st	128	95	28	126	93	31	94	47	33	132	101	21	143	64	45
13	Xining, Qinghai	2nd	143	112	37	145	142	110	126	57	35	174	125	25	182	95	41
14	Fengjie, Chongqing	3rd	104	84	33	112	109	47	57	53	39	103	81	36	180	101	49
15	Xining,Qinghai	1st	128	97	33	141	140	119	103	53	45	148	101	32	128	58	51
16	Gansu	3rd	129	95	30	158	156	86	115	64	31	145	105	17	188	85	41
17	Shanxi	2nd	142	114	42	124	111	77	132	50	44	170	125	41	181	89	43
18	Gansu	3rd	108	92	53	114	110	42	88	56	36	108	79	27	166	83	46
19	Tibet	1st	106	83	44	127	120	61	101	54	47	126	86	18	156	58	42
20	Shiqu, Sichuan	1st	104	88	47	151	140	92	165	77	26	133	94	19	192	80	32
21	Saichuan, Sichuan	1st	113	95	49	156	115	33	112	44	46	158	112	21	200	91	33
22	Changdu, Tibet	2nd	110	84	33	104	78	50	65	34	38	110	79	24	124	60	55
23	Gansu	2nd	128	109	45	153	151	112	134	67	37	145	95	24	196	99	43
24	Tibet	2nd	111	93	56	146	138	73	115	58	41	133	103	27	198	84	40
25	Beichuan, Sichuan	2nd	82	65	34	139	138	86	105	59	42	111	81	25	166	65	44
26	Liangshan, Sichuan	2nd	99	76	36	164	141	85	157	50	31	143	98	23	202	84	31
27	Guizhou	3rd	109	85	31	117	100	35	67	47	43	109	76	25	185	89	44
28	Yaan, Sichuan	2nd	123	91	26	166	164	135	154	62	33	151	110	22	198	74	36
29	Changdu, Tibet	2nd	93	72	35	140	110	46	107	49	38	125	88	19	182	79	48
30	Gansu	3rd	123	93	28	137	125	49	107	72	38	115	78	19	177	95	82
31	Qinghai	1st	121	82	22	128	111	39	96	53	42	120	87	24	158	70	51
32	Sichuan	2nd	141	102	25	146	122	48	115	45	36	141	100	20	192	81	40
33	Gansu	3rd	115	91	29	129	111	49	100	76	40	125	96	27	188	107	63
34	Qinghai	3rd	102	87	38	108	105	56	64	56	37	123	102	25	213	143	87
	R*		0.192	0.128	−0.020	0.014	−0.101	−0.004	0.056	−0.265	0.131	0.199	0.092	−0.181	−0.388	−0.460	−0.341

*The pearson's correlation coefficient between the color data (R, G or B values) and the total content of HAQs in the samples.

grading standards were saved in the network, and the BP neural network was able to produce a prediction. Although the determined sample grades are discrete numbers (1, 2, or 3) in the training process, the predicted values are continuous real numbers. The grade of an inputted sample could be designated based on the predicted value. For example, if the output value is in the range of (0.51–1.50], the sample should be designated as the grade 1 (Figure 4). Additionally, for the grade 2 and grade 3, the ranges are designated as (1.51–2.50] and (2.51–3.50], respectively. In the results predicted by the BP network, some output values were not in the range of (0.51–3.50]. These numbers were considered incorrect predictions.

The process can be summarized as follows:

(i) Input the quality evaluation parameters of the training samples into the network input nodes.

(ii) Create the BP neural network.

(iii) Select proper training functions and parameters.

(iv) Output the results from the prediction to the output nodes of the network.

(v) Input the three evaluation parameters for the samples.

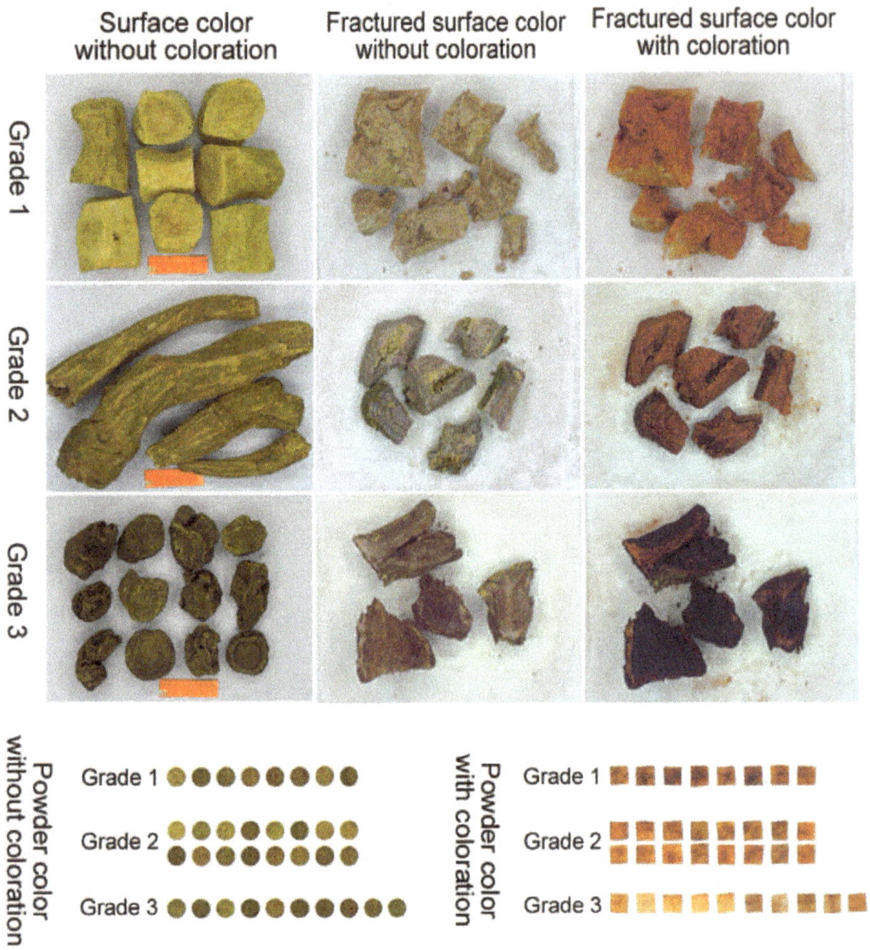

Figure 3. Representative images of rhubarb samples of different grades.

(vi) Proceed through the Matlab simulation.

```
[pn,meanp,stdp,tn,meant,stdt] = prestd(p,t); % normalizing
% establish neural network
net = newcf (minmax(ptr), [21 1], {'tansig' 'purelin'}, 'traingdx', 'learnsom');
% train the neural network
net.trainParam.epochs = 4500;
net.trainParam.goal = 0.000001;
net.trainParam.show = 40;
net.trainParam.lr = 0.05;
[net,tr] = train (net,ptr,ttr,[],[],val,test);
a = poststd(an,meant,stdt); % reverse normalization
% end
```

Color Conversion for Rhubarb Samples

Because the RGB color space consists of three dimensions, it is difficult to use RGB information to summarize the distribution of the rhubarb samples in each quality grade. To distinguish the lower and upper thresholds for grading different rhubarb samples, the RGB values were transformed into the CIE1931 XYZ color space, where the values can be normalized and plotted in a two-dimensional CIE1931xy chromaticity diagram. The formulas used to convert between the CIE XYZ and RGB color spaces are well documented [18,19]. The CIE XYZ color space is deliberately designed so that the Y parameter is a measure of the brightness or luminance of a color. The chromaticity of a color is then specified by the derived parameters x and y, two of the three normalized values which are functions of the three tristimulus values X, Y, and Z.

$$x = \frac{X}{X + Y + Z} \tag{1}$$

$$y = \frac{Y}{X + Y + Z} \tag{2}$$

$$z = \frac{Z}{X + Y + Z} = 1 - x - y \tag{3}$$

The derived color space specified by x and y can represent all of the chromaticities visible to the average person within a two-dimensional chromaticity diagram, which is a widely used tool to specify colors [18].

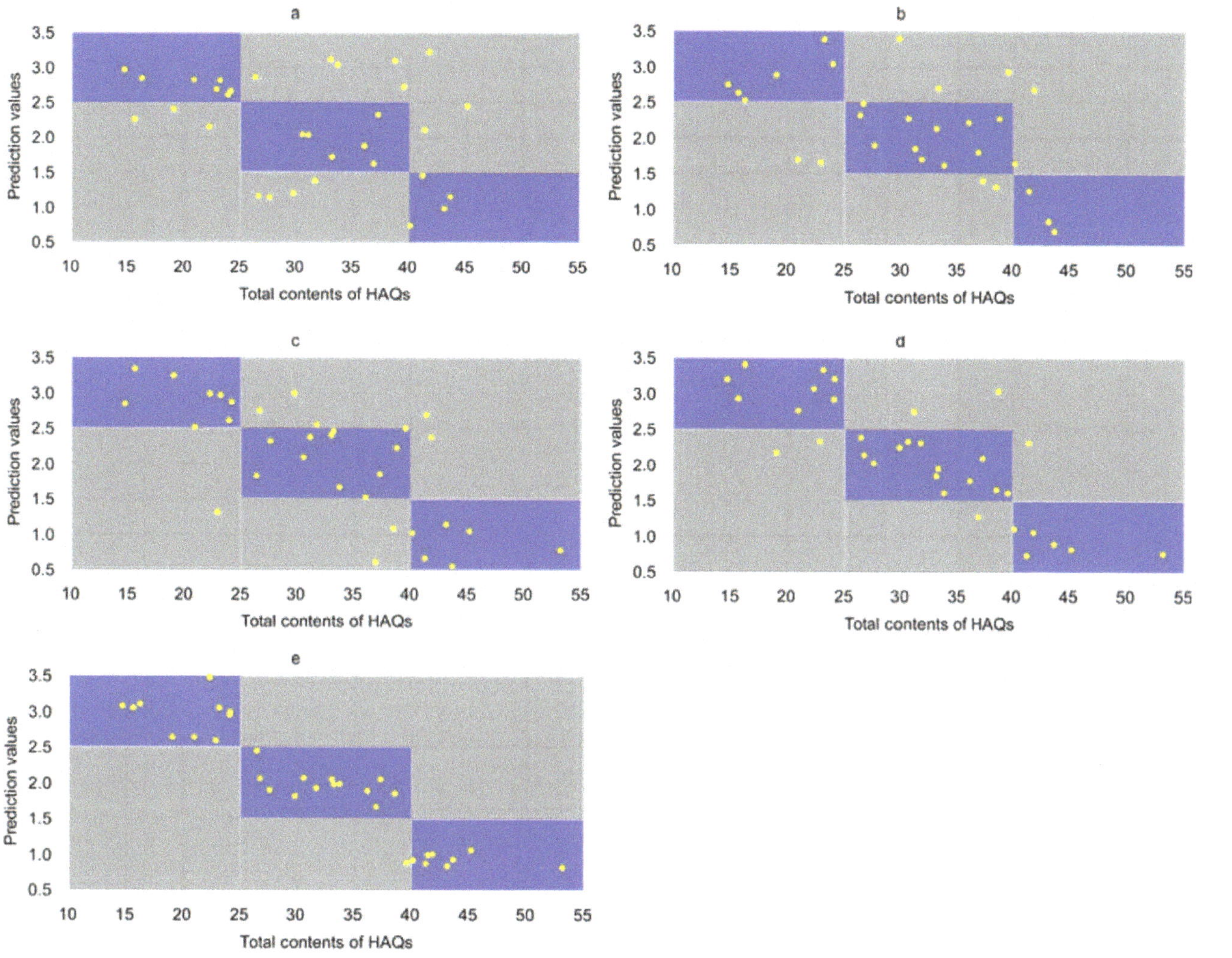

Figure 4. Color-based predictions of the grades of rhubarb samples from the BP network. All the thirty-four samples were counted here, including the training set and the test set. The blue areas indicate correct predictions, and the gray areas indicate incorrect predictions. a, Using the color from the surface of rhubarb without additional coloration as the input parameter, the percentage of correct predictions was 50.0% (17 correct predictions in 34 samples). b, When the colors of the fracture surfaces without development were input, the percent of correct predictions was 64.7% (22 correct predictions in 34 samples). c, When the color-enhanced fracture surfaces were analyzed, the percent of correct predictions was 73.5% (25 correct predictions in 34 samples). d, Using the powder without coloration as the input, the percent of correct predictions was 79.4% (27 correct predictions in 34 samples). e, Analysis of the powder after color development yielded predictions that were 91.2% accurate (31 correct predictions in 34 samples).

Design of the Colorimetric Grading Scale

To establish the color scale for colorimetric grading, we assumed that rhubarb samples of different quality would distribute randomly in a circle centered at the expected color values (points O_1, O_2 and O_3, shown in Figure 5a) for the samples. These values are typically within the radius of the maximum distance from the center in the chromaticity diagram. The centroid (point D) of the triangle that consists of the points O_1, O_2 and O_3 can be assigned as the division point that divides the samples into the different quality grades.

Results

Quality Grade Assignment for the Rhubarb Samples

Before the BP-ANN analysis, the rhubarb samples were divided into three grades according to the total content of the five HAQs (T_{HAQs}) based on the following definitions: grade 1, $T_{HAQs} \geq 40.00$ mg g^{-1}, grade 2, $25.00 < T_{HAQs} < 40.00$ mg g^{-1}, and grade 3, $T_{HAQs} \leq 25.00$ mg·g^{-1} (Table S1).

Color Quantization into RGB Values for the Rhubarb Samples

Images of a sample were captured in the standard lightbox and under natural light at different times (morning, noon, afternoon, evening) during the day using the optimized shooting conditions described above. Table 2 shows the relative standard deviations (RSD) of the R, G and B channels, which were 10.24%, 10.22% and 11.75%, respectively, when shooting under natural light at different time points. In contrast, the RSD for the R, G and B values were 0.94%, 1.13% and 1.81%, respectively, when shooting in the lightbox. The lighting conditions provided by the lightbox enable good reproducibility when acquiring images for color information. In this study, we acquired different colors of the herb, including the outside surface, a fracture surface, and a powder,

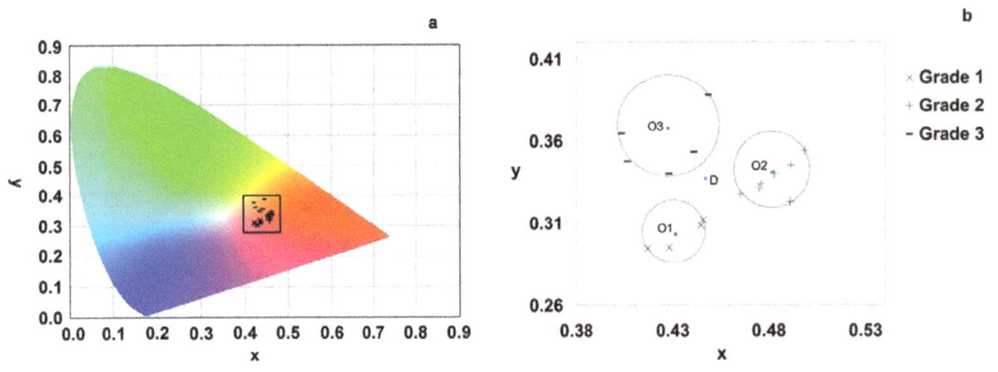

Figure 5. The distribution of the rhubarb samples in each grade in the CIE1931xy chromaticity diagram. a, The overall distribution of the samples in the two-dimensional coordinates overlaying on the CIE1931xy chromaticity diagram. The samples in the grade 1 mainly distribute in the lower left region favoring red-purple; the samples in the grade 2 distribute in the right region toward orange; and the samples in the grade 3 distribute in the upper left region tending toward yellow. b, Schematic diagram describing the geometric calculations for the segmentation points. The diagram represented the magnified region in the panel a.

with or without coloration by a developing reagent (Figure 3). The RGB values from the 34 rhubarb samples are shown in Table 1. The data of surface color with coloration were not listed and excluded from the research because the data varied greatly in different zones of the herb surface.

Neural Network Establishment and Prediction

The neural network was established firstly by processing the training set, and then the other samples were taken as the test set to assess the validity of the predictions and results from the network. We assumed the samples containing intermediate amount of HAQs in a certain quality grade are representative for the whole of the grade. So those samples of T_{HAQS} in the intermediate range (20% less than or greater than the upper or lower limit of each quality grade) were chosen as the training samples: The grade 1 consisted of samples 6, 7, 12, 15, 19, 20 and 21; the grade 2 contained samples 1, 2, 3, 4, 8, 11 and 17; and the grade 3 were samples 5, 9, 10, 14, 16, 27 and 30. After establishment of the BP network, the other thirteen samples out of the training set were input as test samples and predicted. The prediction accuracy by the BP network diversified depending on which form of color of the herb was examined. The prediction accuracy values of each kind of color were: 38.5% (5 correct predictions in 13 test samples) for the surface color, 92.3% (12 correct predictions in 13 test samples) for the powder color after coloration and 69.2% (9 correct predictions in 13 test samples) for the other three kinds of color. In addition, the predictions for the former training samples were also counted and combined with the results of the test samples. The prediction values were plotted with the contents of the five HAQs in Figure 4. It could be found that the color of the rhubarb powder after coloration attained the lowest wrong prediction of the quality grade for all the samples.

Table 2. The reproducibility of the RGB measurements.

Experiment	Under natural light			In standard lightbox		
	R	G	B	R	G	B
1	116	102	57	114	103	56
2	117	103	57	114	103	56
3	117	103	57	114	102	56
4	121	106	51	112	100	54
5	122	106	57	113	102	54
6	120	106	54	111	101	55
7	119	105	54	112	101	53
8	115	98	51	112	100	54
9	123	100	49	112	100	55
10	110	96	49	112	101	55
11	87	77	42	112	101	55
12	105	93	51	114	102	55
13	110	98	53	113	102	54
14	92	89	39	112	101	54
15	96	75	41	111	99	53
RSD (%)	10.24	10.22	11.75	0.94	1.13	1.81

Calculation of the Boundaries that Differentiate Grades of Rhubarb

The sixteen representative samples (sample 12, 15, 19 and 31 in the grade 1; sample 1, 3, 4, 24, 26, 28 and 32 in the grade 2; and sample 9, 10, 14, 33 and 34 in the grade 3) showing the least overlap in their distribution in the chromaticity diagram (i.e., distributed approximately 80% of the possible maximum distance from the center of each quality grade) were selected to determine the boundaries for differentiating the rhubarb grades. The acquired RGB values of the representative samples were converted to values within the CIE 1931xy color space and then plotted in the chromaticity diagram (Figure 5a). The distribution of the three grades of the rhubarb samples separated into distinct regions. According to the calculations described above, the mathematical expectation points (x, y) of each grade are O_1 (0.4315, 0.3031), O_2 (0.4819, 0.3408) and O_3 (0.4277, 0.3677). The division point D (x, y) is defined as the geometric center of the three mathematical expectation points calculated for the three grades and occurs at (0.4470, 0.3372). Figure 5b shows that the rhubarb samples in each grade distribute away from the division point (D) in three directions toward a different color category. The grade 1 tends toward the red-purple region; the grade 2 to the orange region; and the grade 3 to the yellow region. Thus, how the samples distribute can be used to determine the grade of an unknown rhubarb sample, specifically by comparing the color of the

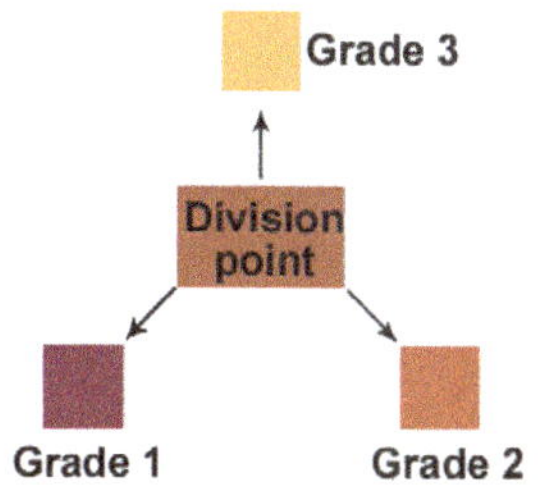

Figure 6. Differences between the color at the division point and the colors of the mathematical expectation points for each grade.

unknown with a colorimetric grading scale created based on the color of the division point (D). Corresponding ribbons was drawn using the software from the RGB values of the division point (D) and the mathematical expectation points (O_1, O_2, O_3) for each grade (Figure 6).

Discussion

Because of the convenience and speed of sensory evaluation compared with the laboratory analyses of chemical content, the desired color-based grading method would help in assessing the quality of rhubarb in the TCM marketplace. The approach for obtaining the color information is important for sensory evaluation. A colorimeter is a device that is commonly used to measure the color components of solid samples. In our preliminary experiment, we found that measuring the color of rhubarb by colorimeter was difficult because the plant's surface or fracture surface was not smooth and uniformly colored, which decreased the repeatability of the results. Unfortunately, most herbal medicines have various shapes that affect reproducibility. In this study, we used a digital camera to capture images of samples and extracted the color data from these images using Photoshop (Adobe Corporation, USA). Through this approach, the color data of the herbs are consistent with how colors are perceived by human vision. The RGB (red, green, blue) color model is one of the most widely used of the color systems. An additive model in which red, green, and blue light are summed to produce a broad array of colors, the model includes almost all of the colors that can be perceived by the human eye. In this study, the RGB values were used to represent color quantitatively. The RGB values could be converted into visual color, which made it possible to create a color scale that could be used as a reference for grading the quality of rhubarb.

Different concentrations of HAQs display different shades of yellow or red under a neutral or alkaline environment, respectively, which indicates a relationship between the color of the herb and its HAQ content. However, we found that the absolute values of Pearson's correlation coefficients between the contents of the five HAQs and the RGB values ranged from 0.004 to 0.460 (Table 1), showing non-significant linear correlation between the two variables. It could not be found a direct correlation between the color and quality of rhubarb because the RGB values are distributed in a non-linear space. So, we used artificial neural networks (ANNs), generally developed for non-linear mapping, generalization, self-organization and self-learning [20], to find relationships between the quality and the color of the samples. The most popular method used in ANN-based pattern recognition is the back-propagation (BP) trained, first-order neural network [21], which was used in this study. In Figure 4, it could be found that the outside surface color generated the lowest accuracy compared with the fracture surface color and the powder. After additional color development of the samples with a 0.5% NaOH aqueous solution, the rhubarb displayed a red to dark red color based on the Bornträger reaction of the base with the HAQs. Consequently, the coloration of the samples enhanced the accuracy of the network and increased the number of correct predictions for all sample types. The results suggested that measuring surface color of rhubarb is useless to some extent in assessment of its quality, because the color on the outside surface of the rhubarb can be more easily affected over the course of production and storage than the other sources of color data. The ununiformity was another defect of surface color in assessment of its quality. When the rhubarb is ground into powder form, the uniformity of color can be improved. In addition, developing the color of the HAQs has an advantage in reducing interference from other colored substances. Hence, the color-enhanced powder of rhubarb is preferred in color-based assessment of its quality.

The ANN results indicate that there is a positive but non-linear correlation between the quality of rhubarb and its color. However, the neural network is still a machine-based approach. To facilitate the quality assessment of rhubarb, we tried to establish a colorimetric grading scale to visually discriminate rhubarbs of varying quality. The boundaries of each quality grade of rhubarb were calculated according to their distribution in the chromaticity diagram (Figure 5b). The differences between the colors at the division point (D) and the colors of the calculated expected values for each grade can be distinguished with the naked eye, which enables the development of a color scale that can be printed on a card and used to grade rhubarb in the field [22]. For widespread use, the colorimetric grading scale could be printed on paper, similar to professional color cards such as Munsell color cards, to minimize the deviation between the theoretical and individually perceived colors.

In summary, the results of this study revealed that color or color parameters (RGB values) provided important information for the classification of quality of TCMs, such as rhubarb. However, the results varied depending on where the color was sampled: at the surface or fracture surface of the rhubarb, and with or without color development. The BP-ANN network achieved the highest percentage of correct predictions when analyzing powdered samples that were chemically processed to express color, which suggests that powders may be the best type of sample for the accurate grading of rhubarb. On the basis of the distribution of several rhubarb samples in the chromaticity diagram, we have designed a colorimetric grading scale to discriminate between rhubarbs of varying quality. By comparing the color of the sample with the colorimetric grading scale on the card, similar to determining pH using litmus paper, customers without experience in sensory evaluation could quickly assess the quality of rhubarb. This work illustrates the technical feasibility of color-based grading of rhubarb quality and provides useful references for the quantification and standardization of sensory evaluation-based quality control for TCMs, foods and other products.

Supporting Information

Table S1 Contents (mg g^{-1}) of the five HAQs in the rhubarb samples.
(DOC)

Text S1 Ultra Peformance liquid chromotography (UPLC) analysis.
(DOC)

Acknowledgments

The authors acknowledge Rui-xian Zhang, Wei Zhang and Su-min Hu for support in searching the ancient herbal books. The authors also acknowledge Ji Zhang for identifying the herb samples.

Author Contributions

Conceived and designed the experiments: XHX JBW. Performed the experiments: JBW LNZ QCZ XRZ. Analyzed the data: XHC LNZ QCZ JBW QFG BCL. Contributed reagents/materials/analysis tools: QFG BCL PZ YLZ. Wrote the paper: JBW QCZ LNZ YLZ.

References

1. Shahidi F, Rubin LJ, D'Souza LA, Teranishi R, Buttery RG (1986) Meat flavor volatiles: A review of the composition, techniques of analysis, and sensory evaluation. Crit Rev Food Sci 24(2): 141–243.
2. Evin F, Siekierski E (2002) Sensory evaluation of heating and air conditioning systems. Energ Buildings 34(6): 647–651.
3. Parpinello GP, Meluzzi A, Sirri F, Tallarico N, Versari A (2006) Sensory evaluation of egg products and eggs laid from hens fed diets with different fatty acid composition and supplemented with antioxidants. Food Res Int 39(1): 47–52.
4. Cunha CR, Dias AI, Viotto WH (2010) Microstructure, texture, colour and sensory evaluation of a spreadable processed cheese analogue made with vegetable fat. Food Res Int 43(3): 723–729.
5. Elortondo FJP, Ojeda M, Albisu M, Salmerón J, Etayo I, et al. (2007) Food quality certification: An approach for the development of accredited sensory evaluation methods. Food Qual Prefer 18(2): 425–439.
6. Parpinello GP, Versari A, Chinnici F, Galassi S (2009) Relationship among sensory descriptors, consumer preference and color parameters of Italian Novello red wines. Food Res Int 42(10): 1389–1395.
7. Zhu SH (2006) Modern commodity studies for traditional Chinese medicine. Beijing: People's Medical Publishing House. p.113.
8. Zhao ZZ, Liang ZT, Guo P (2011) Macroscopic identification of Chinese medicinal materials: Traditional experiences and modern understanding. J Ethnopharmcol 134(3): 556–564.
9. Wang JB, Zhang XR, Chu XH, Huang MJ, Jin C, et al. (2010) Delphi-based study on scientificity of organoleptic evaluation for rhubarb commercial specification. Chin J Chin Mat Med 35(20): 2657–2561.
10. Chu XH, Wang JB, Kong WJ, Zhao XJ, Liu FF, et al. (2011) Study on the reproducibility of organoleptic evaluation of commercial specification of *Rhizoma Coptidis* based on delphi method. World Sci Tech/Modern Tradit Chin Med Mat Med 13(2): 321–327.
11. Li ZL (2007) Origins of the Materia Medica (*Ben Cao Yuan Shi*). Beijing: People's Medical Publishing House.
12. Cuéllar MJ, Giner RM, Recio MC, Máñez S, Ríos JL (2001) Topical anti-inflammatory activity of some Asian medicinal plants used in dermatological disorders. Fitoterapia 72(3): 221–229.
13. Yokozawa T, Suzuki N, Okuda I, Oura H, Nishioka I (1985) Changes in the urinary constituents in rats with chronic renal failure during oral administration of rhubarb extract. Chem Pharm Bull 33, 4508–4514.
14. Wang JB, Zhao YL, Xiao XH, Li HF, Zhao HP, et al. (2009) Assessment of the renal protection and hepatotoxicity of rhubarb extract in rats. J Ethnopharmacol 124, 18–25.
15. Zhao YL, Wang JB, Zhou GD, Shan LM, Xiao XH (2009) Investigations of free anthraquinones from rhubarb against alpha-naphthylisothiocyanate- induced cholestatic liver injury in rats. Basic Clin Pharmacol 104(6), 463–469.
16. WHO Monographs on Selected Medicinal Plants (1999) Geneva: World Health Organization. p.231–240.
17. Pharmacopoeia of the People's Republic of China, First Div. (2010) Beijing: China Medical Science Press. p.22–23.
18. Rossel RAV, Minasny B, Roudier P, McBratney AB (2006) Colour space models for soil science. Geoderma 133(3–4): 320–333.
19. Mendoza F, Dejmek P, Aguilera JM (2006) Calibrated color measurements of agricultural foods using image analysis. Postharvest Biol Tec 41(3): 285–295.
20. Huang Y, Kangas LJ, Rasco BA (2007) Applications of artificial neural networks (ANNs) in food science. Crit Rev Food Sci 47(2): 113–26.
21. Agatonovic-Kustrin S, Beresford R (2000) Basic concepts of artificial neural network (ANN) modeling and its application in pharmaceutical research. J Pharmaceut Biomed 22(5): 717–727.
22. Xiao XH, Wang JB, Zhang XR, Chu XH (2011) The preparation method for the colorimetric grading scale card to discriminate the quality grade of Chinese materia medica. CN102042978A.

5

Chronic Administration of Anti-Stroke Herbal Medicine TongLuoJiuNao Reduces Amyloidogenic Processing of Amyloid Precursor Protein in a Mouse Model of Alzheimer's Disease

Ping He[1], Pengtao Li[2], Qian Hua[2], Yuan Liu[2], Matthias Staufenbiel[3], Rena Li[4], Yong Shen[1]*

1 Center for Advanced Therapeutic Strategies of Brain Disorders, Roskamp Institute, Sarasota, Florida, United States of America, **2** Department of Pathology, School of Preclinical Medicine, Beijing University of Chinese Medicine, Beijing, China, **3** Novartis Pharm Ltd., Nervous System Research, Basel, Switzerland, **4** Center for Hormone Advanced Science and Education, Roskamp Institute, Sarasota, Florida, United States of America

Abstract

Composed of Ginsenoside Rg1 and Geniposide, the herbal medicine TongLuoJiuNao (TLJN) injection liquid has anti-inflammatory properties and can improve learning and memory in mice. Recently, TLJN has been used to treat the patients with cerebral ischemic stroke and vascular dementia, which significantly increase the risk of developing Alzheimer's disease (AD) in the early human beings. Although beneficial effects of TLJN have been reported in the vascular-associated brain disorders, the roles of TLJN in AD brains are still not clear. In this study, we chronically administered TLJN in amyloid precursor protein (APP) Swedish mutant transgenic mice (APP23) from 6 months old of age, which is at the onset of Aβ plaques, to 12 months old. We found that TLJN significantly decreased Aβ production and deposition in the brain of APP23 mice. Furthermore, we observed that TLJN down-regulated the levels and activity of β-secretase 1 (BACE1) protein as well as the expression levels of γ-secretase complex components: PS1, nicastrin and anterior pharynx-defective 1 (APH1) but not presenilin enhancer 2 (PEN2). The results suggest an inhibitory effect of TLJN on amyloidogenic APP processing by down-regulating the cleavage enzymes BACE1 and γ-secretase.

Editor: Zhongcong Xie, Massachusetts General Hospital, United States of America

Funding: This work is supported by grants from NIH/NIA025888 (YS), NIH/NIAR01AG032441 (RL), Alzheimer Association: IIRG-09-61521 (YS) and IIRG-07-59510 (RL); AHAF: G2006-118 (RL) and A2008-642 (PH), The State Key Development Program for Basic Research of China: 2012CB518602 (PTL), Production of New Medicine Program of Ministry of Science and Technology of China: 2008ZX09101-027 (PTL) and National Natural Science Foundation of China: 81072901 (QH). The funders had no role in study design, data collection and analysis, decision to publish, or preparation of the manuscript.

Competing Interests: Matthias Staufenbiel is employed by Novartis Pharm Ltd. APP23 transgenic (20 males and 20 females in each age group) and non-transgenic wild type (20 males and 20 females in each age group) genotypes in our experiment are on the C57BL/6 background, which were provided by Novartis Institute for Biomedical Research. There is a patent of TongLuoJiuNao from Pengtao Li, Qian Hua and Yong Shen for Alzheimer's Disease treatment to declare. This does not alter the authors' adherence to all the PLOS ONE policies on sharing data and materials, as detailed online in the guide for authors.

* E-mail: yshen@rfdn.org

Introduction

TongLuoJiuNao (TLJN) injection liquid is an herbal medicine which is primarily composed of two active components: Ginsenoside Rg1 and Geniposide [1,2]. Nowadays, TLJN has been used in the treatment of patients with cerebral ischemic stroke and vascular dementia [3,4]. Ginsenosides belong to the class of steroid glycosides and triterpene saponins in the plant genus *Panax* (ginseng), which can suppress inflammation by nuclear factor κB (NF-κB) pathway [5,6] and tumor growth by inhibiting DNA polymerase activity [7,8]. Recent studies showed that Ginsenoside Rg1 could improve spatial learning and memory in rat models of Alzheimer's disease (AD) [9,10]. Another compound Geniposide in TLJN is an iridoid glycoside with a variety of biological activities including neuroprotection, anti-proliferation, and anti-oxidative stress [11,12]. Besides the beneficial roles of TLJN in acute ischemic stroke and vascular dementia [3,4], whether this anti-stroke herbal medicine could also be applied in the prevention and therapy of other neurological disorders such as AD is unknown.

AD is a neurodegenerative disease and pathologically characterized by excessive extracellular accumulation of amyloid β peptide (Aβ) in brains [13,14]. Aβ is generated from the cleavage of amyloid precursor protein (APP) by two enzymes: β-secretase 1 (BACE1) and γ-secretase [15,16]. Emerging evidence has shown that BACE1 expression levels and/or activities are increased in the brain of AD patients [17,18,19,20]. Herbal medicines have been introduced to alleviate demented symptoms of AD patients [21,22]. It has been suggested that Ginsenoside protects neurons against oxidative stress [23] and improves learning and memory functions [24,25]. Experimental studies showed that administration of Ginsenoside significantly reduced Aβ levels in brains of Tg2576 mice, an AD mouse model [26] and senescence-accerlerated mouse prone 8 (SAMP8) mice [10,27]. Furthermore, Ginsenoside is found to inhibit BACE1 activity by 80% in PC12 cells [28] and mouse neuroblastoma N2a cells expressing mutation human APP696 [29]. A recent report showed that TLJN increased the expression levels of IDE and NEP which both are involved in Aβ clearance [1].

In the present study, we intraperitoneally injected herbal medicine TLJN once a day in amyloid precursor protein (APP) Swedish double mutation transgenic mice (APP23) for 6 months (a critical period for Aβ deposition) [30]. We found that chronic administration of TLJN significantly reduced Aβ production and deposition and down-regulated BACE1 expression and activity as well as the expression of γ-secretase complex. However, Aβ degradation enzymes, neprilysin (NEP) and insulin degradation enzyme (IDE) were not affected in the animal model.

Materials and Methods

Component Analysis of Herbal Medicine TongLuaoJiuNao

TLJN was purchased from Kang Yuan Pharmaceutical Engineering Limited Company, Neimenggu, China (Catalog: 051125). In recent years, the active components in TLJN were identified and widely applied in clinic and experiments [1,2,31]. In brief, the components are extracted from *Panax notoginseng* and *Gardenia jasminoides*. The compounds were processed and purified in accordance with the protocol of the National Medical Dictionary of China. TLJN was obtained by high-performance liquid chromatography (HPLC). The results of HPLC were showed in **Fig. 1A** and the chemical structures of the two components in **Fig. 1B**. The chemical analysis revealed Ginsenoside Rg1 as $C_{42}H_{72}O_{14}$, molecular weight: 800 and Geniposide as $C_{17}H_{24}O_{10}$, molecular weight: 300 [1]. The final concentration of the compounds was measured by HPLC with Ginsenoside Rg1 (1.02 mg/ml) and Geniposide (4.95 mg/ml) [1,2,31].

Animals

All animal experiments were performed in compliance with a protocol approved by Roskamp Institute. APP23 transgenic genotypes (20 males in each group) in our experiments are on the C57BL/6 background, which are provided by Novartis Institute for Biomedical Research and the mice express mutated human βAPP (Swedish double mutation, KM670/671NL) under neuron-specific murine Thy-1 promoter element [32,33]. Non-transgenic wild type and APP23 mice were crossed and the progenies were genotyped and characterized as APP23 with PCR followed by Western blot for confirming brain holoAPP protein. The resulting littermates were used in experiments [30,34].

Herbal Medicine TLJN Administration

The concentration used for the experiments was based on the reference of daily dose given to patients in clinical practice [1,31]. For the observation of long-term effects on AD-like pathological changes, TLJN was administered from the age of 6th to 12th month (total six months). Mice were intraperitoneally injected once a day either with a dose of 300 μl herbal medicine TLJN solution per mouse (dilution of stock solution 1:2 distilled saline, n = 20) or with the same volume of distilled saline as vehicle groups (n = 20). This dose (0.1 mg of Genisenoside Rg1 and 0.5 mg of Geniposide) of TLJN per mouse here was demonstrated without potential side effects observed in long-term treatment [1,2,31].

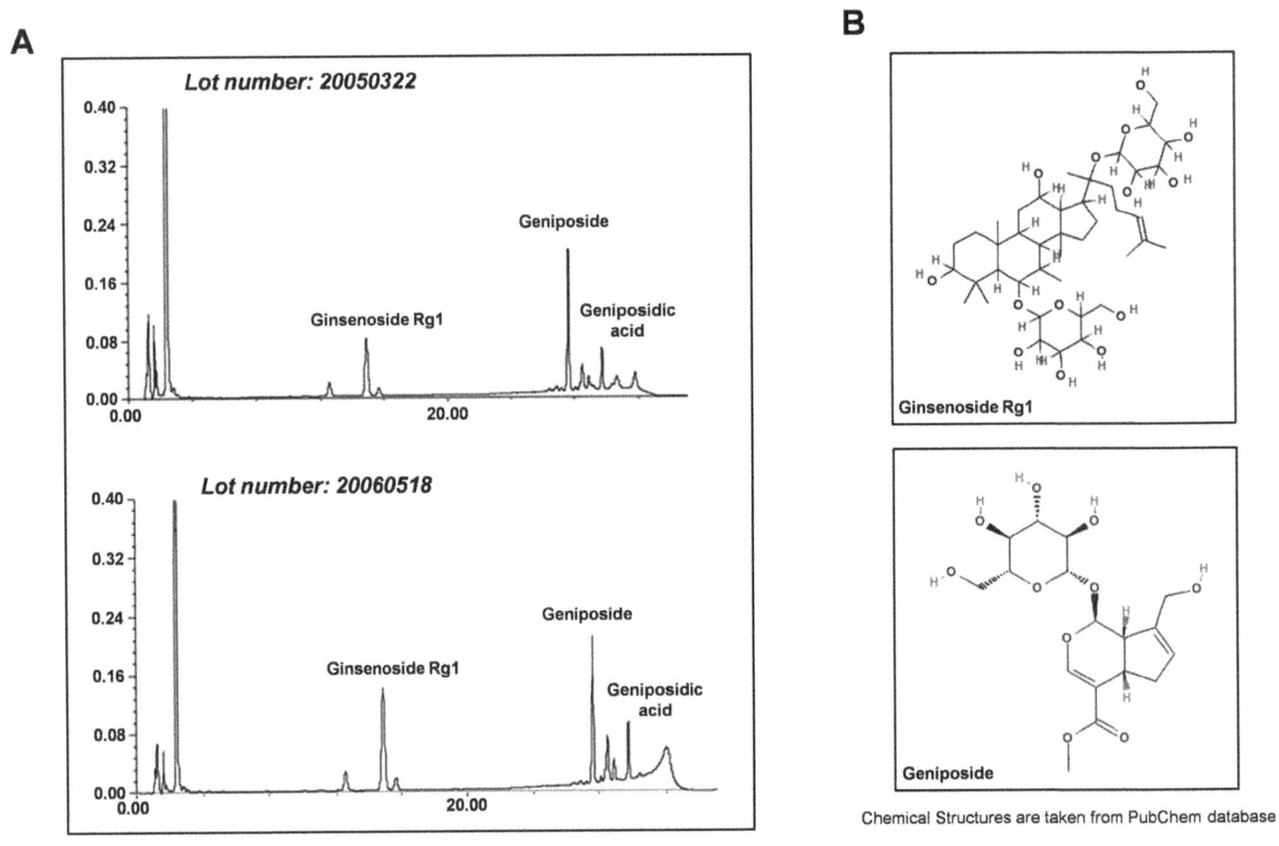

Figure 1. Chemical analysis of herbal medicine TongLuoJiuNao. (**A**) Ginsenoside and Geniposide in this study showed the same peak pattern. The figure was a representative of at least two separate experiments, each with triplicate samples. The chromatograms were scaled to the highest peak. (**B**) Chemical structure of Ginsenoside and Geniposide.

The treatment protocol for the herbal medicine is well tolerated by the animals. At the last day of the injection practice, mice were perfused with phosphate buffered saline (PBS) supplemented 10 U heparin. The brain tissues were dissected and the half of brain was post-fixed with 4% paraformaldehyde (PFA) for histological analysis and another half of the brain was stored in −80°C for biochemical analysis.

Aβ Enzyme-linked Immunosorbent Assay

Enzyme-linked immunosorbent assay (ELISA) quantification was performed as described previously [34,35,36]. The APP23 mice in the presence (n = 10) and absence of TLJN (n = 10) were used for the determination of Aβ40 and Aβ42 levels. The neocortex tissues were isolated and homogenized in M-PER mammalian protein extraction reagent (catalog: 78503, Thermo Fisher Scientific) and centrifuged at 14,000×g for 20 min at 4°C. Protein concentrations were measured by protein assays (Bio-Rad Laboratories, Hercules, CA) following manufacturer's instructions. The remaining pellet with insoluble Aβ was dissolved in 98% of formic acid and centrifuged at 4°C for 30 min. The supernatant from the pellet was collected for the assay of insoluble Aβ40 and Aβ42. The amount of Aβ40 and Aβ42 was measured with an Aβ40 and Aβ42 ELISA kit (KHB3481 and KHB3544, Invitrogen Life Technologies, Carlsbad, CA). The ELISA system has been extensively applied and there is no cross-reactivity between Aβ40 and Aβ42 protein. The quantitation of insoluble Aβ ELISA measurement was normalized to corresponding tissue protein concentration. Data were showed as Mean ± SD of four experiments.

BACE1 Activity Assay

An aliquot of neocortex tissue homogenates (n = 5 in each group) was further lysed with a lysis buffer described as previously [30,34]. Briefly, the supernatants were collected and BACE1 enzymatic activity was analyzed by using synthetic peptide substrates containing BACE1 cleavage site (HK(DABSYL)-SEVNLDAEFRQ(LY)) (BVI Substrate, a Lucifer Yellow labeled peptide, Catalog: #565781, Millipore Life Sciences Research, Billerica, MA). BACE1 substrate was dissolved in DMSO and mixed with HAc buffer (100 mM HAc and 100 mM NaCl, pH 4.5). An equal amount of protein was mixed with 100 μl of substrate. The fluorescence intensity was measured kinetically with a microplate reader for 2 hrs at 5 min reading intervals (Bio-Rad Laboratories) at an excitation wavelength of 430 nm and an emission wavelength of 520 nm. The average velocities were calculated and relative velocities compared to vehicle samples (100%) were plotted.

Western Blotting

Western blot was performed as described previously [34,37]. The neocortex from APP23 mice in the presence and absence of TLJN (n = 5 in each group) was homogenized in M-PER mammalian protein extraction reagent (catalog: 78503, Thermo Fisher Scientific) supplemented with Halt protease and phosphatase inhibitor single-use cocktail (Catalog: 78442, Thermo Fisher Scientific). Total proteins were separated by SDS-PAGE gel and then transferred to nitrocellulose membrane (Catalog: 162-0115, Bio-Rad Laboratories) using wet transfer equipment for overnight at 90 mA (Bio-Rad Laboratories). The blots were probed with antibodies as follows: mouse monoclonal antibody against APP (1:2000, clone: MABP21, catalog: #44–100, Invitrogen), mouse antibody against BACE1 ectodomain (1:2000, Clone: 137612, MAB931, R&D Systems), rabbit antibody against BACE1 N-terminal amino acids 46–62 (1:2000; MAB0681, Sigma-Aldrich, St. Louis, MO), mouse anti-soluble human APP β Swedish mutation (sAPPβ-sw, 1;1000, clone: 6A1, catalog: 10321, IBL-America, **Minneapolis, MN**), rabbit polyclonal NEP antibody (1:2000, sc-9149, Santa Cruz Biotechnology, Santa Cruz, CA), rabbit polyclonal IDE antibody (1:25000, PC730, Millipore), rabbit anti-anterior pharynx-defective 1 (APH1) polyclonal antibody (H2D, 1:5000, kind gift by Dr. Yueming Li, Memorial Sloan-Kettering Cancer Center, New York), rabbit polyclonal antibody against nicastrin (1:1000, PA1-758, Thermo Fisher Scientific), mouse antibody against presenilin 1 C-terminal loop (PS1, 1:1000, MAB5232, Millipore), rabbit polyclonal antibody against presenilin enhancer 2 (PEN2) (1:1000, clone: UD-1, PRB-560C, Covance), rat antibody against presenilin 1 N-terminal (1:1000, clone: hPS1-NT, MAB1563, Millipore), and mouse anti-β-actin antibody (1:5000, clone AC-15, A1978, Sigma-Aldrich). Secondary antibodies against mouse or rabbit IgG conjugated HRP were applied (SC-2004 and SC-2055; Santa Cruz Biotechnology). The membranes were developed with SuperSignal West Femto Maximum Sensitivity Substrate (Catalog: 34095, Thermo Fisher Scientific) and the chemiluminescent image signal was captured using ChemiDoc XRS (Bio-Rad Laboratories). Quantitatively, the densitometry of the protein amount was measured using Quantity One software (Version 4.6.0, Bio-Rad Laboratories). The ratio of targeting protein density versus corresponding β-actin signal was calculated and further compared to vehicle groups (as 100%). The final results were expressed as density folds of the experimental groups to that of vehicles, accordingly.

Histology and Immunostaining

Immunostaining was performed as described previously [30,34]. The treated mice (n = 6 in each group) were perfused using 0.1 M phosphate buffer. The half brain was post-fixed in 4% PFA. Brain sections were performed serially (30 μm). To observe the Aβ fibril aggregation, the sections were incubated in thioflavine S solution for 5 min (1:5000, T1892, Sigma-Aldrich). To test the Aβ accumulation, the sections were treated with 1% H_2O_2 for 10 min and blocked with 10% horse serum for 30 min. Monoclonal antibody against Aβ amino acid sequence 1–17 (1:2000, clone 6E10, MAB1560, Millipore) was incubated in 4°C overnight. Following the primary antibody, the biotinylated secondary antibody against mouse IgG was applied (1:1,000; Vector Labs, Burlingame, CA) for 30 min. Then VECTASTAIN Elite ABC kit (Vector Labs) was applied for 30 min and DAB (3,3′-diaminobenzidine) peroxidase substrate kit (Vector Labs) for 2 min. Counter staining was performed with Mayer's haematoxylin Solution (Sigma-Aldrich) for 1 min.

Quantification of Staining Structures

The sagittal sections per interval of 400 μm were chosen as histological and immunological staining. The counting of plaque number was carried out by an experimenter blind to the study [34]. A microscope (BX63; Olympus Corporation, Tokyo, Japan) with a 10x N PLAN, 20x and 40x PL FLUOTAR was used. Digitized images were captured with a DEI-470 digital camera (Optronics, Goleta, CA) on an Olympus microscope (Olympus). MagnaFire software (version 2.1C; Optronics) was applied. All of the immunopositive structures on each section were counted with same parameter. In general, 9–11 sections through the hippocampus formation per mouse were calculated (n = 6 mice in each group). The number of staining positive structures was totalized and expressed per section.

Statistical Analyses

Statistical analyses were performed as described previously [34,37]. Results were expressed as Mean ± SD and analyzed using a software program (SPSS version 11.5.1; SPSS). Student's *t* test was used as a comparison of two groups. The level of significance was $p \leq 0.05$.

Results

Herbal Medicine TLJN Reduces Aβ Levels and Deposition

Recent studies showed that Genisenosides could reduce Aβ42 levels in the brain of young Tg2576 mice [26]. At the age of 3–4 months old, there is not plaque formation yet in the brain of Tg2576 mice [38]. So, it is necessary to clarify whether Ginsenoside-induced reduction of Aβ levels is due to the decrease of insoluble Aβ aggregate in aged mice. To reveal the existence of plaques in the brain, the histological staining of thioflavine S, which binds to β sheet-rich fibril protein aggregates [39], was performed at the brain sections from the 12 months old APP23 mice in the presence and absence of TLJN (**Fig. 2A**). Results showed a significant reduction of thioflavine S positive deposits in TLJN-treated APP23 mice compared to vehicle groups (**Fig. 2B**, $*p<0.05$). A specific immunostaining identifying amyloid protein was also applied with antibody 6E10 recognizing Aβ1-17 fragment [40,41]. Representative images of Aβ-positive staining plaques were shown in **Fig. 2C.** The number of all immuno-positive plaques was counted per section and a significant decrease in the number of Aβ deposits was observed following chronic TLJN administration (**Fig. 2D**, $**p<0.05$). These data showed that TLJN could reduce amyloid protein aggregation.

To further confirm whether the decreased Aβ deposition induced by herbal medicine TLJN administration in APP23 mouse brains was due to insoluble Aβ reduction, we measured the levels of insoluble Aβ40 and Aβ42 by sandwich ELISAs (n = 10 each group) [34,36], which are primary Aβ species existing in amyloid plaques in AD brains [13,14,42], The pellets of detergent insoluble fractions from brain tissue homogenization were re-suspended with formic acid. Quantitative results showed that Aβ40 were significantly decreased by 34% in the subjects with TLJN chronic administration (2538±137 pg/mg) compared to the vehicle groups (3847±296 pg/mg) (Fig. 2E, $*p<0.05$). Insoluble Aβ42 levels were measured and observed a large decrease by 79% (893±32 pg/mg of in the presence of TLJN group vs 4192±381 pg/mg of the vehicle mice) (Fig. 2F, $**p<0.01$). These results suggest that TLJN could reduce Aβ levels, especially Aβ42 levels, consistent with previous report [26], and lead to the alleviation of Aβ pathology.

Herbal Medicine TLJN Down-regulates BACE1 Activity and Levels

BACE1 is an enzyme responsible for β-site APP cleavage to produce Aβ peptide [40,43,44,45,46]. We recently reported that BACE1 protein levels and activity are increased in sporadic AD brains [19,20]. Since Aβ level is reduced by TLJN application, we postulate that BACE1 might be one of the targets of TLJN. We detected BACE1 levels by Western blot (**Fig. 3A)** and found out a significant decrease of BACE1 protein levels in the TLJN application groups compared to vehicle groups (**Fig. 3A**).

It has been reported that Gensenoside Rg1 could inhibit BACE1 activity *in vitro* [28,29]. However, BACE1 activity has not been examined yet in the brain of APP transgenic mice treated with TLJN. Following the administration of TLJN for 6 months, the BACE1 activity was then examined. Quantification showed that BACE1 activity is significantly decreased in TLJN-treated groups compared to vehicles (**Fig. 3B**). These results suggest that in addition to reducing BACE1 protein levels, TLJN could also decrease BACE1 activity. Proteolytic enzyme BACE1 cleaves APP to produce a soluble N-terminal fragment APPβ (sAPPβ) [13,47]. To further verify the significant down-regulation of BACE1 by TLJN, Western blot were applied to test the secretion levels of sAPPβ fragments (**Fig. 3C**). We found a significant decrease of sAPPβ levels in the TLJN-treated APP23 mice (**Fig. 3C**, $*p<0.05$). To exclude the possibility that sAPPβ level decrease is due to the level reduction of substrate APP, APP was probed by Western blot. Results showed that there were no significant changes of APP protein levels in the groups between TLJN administration and vehicles (**Fig. 3D**), suggesting that TLJN down-regulates BACE1 but not APP expression in the brain of APP23 mice.

Herbal Medicine TLJN Reduces Expression Levels of γ-secretase Components

BACE1 cleavage generates a short C-terminal fragment (CTFβ) C99, which is then further processed by γ-secretase to produce Aβ peptide [16,48]. The γ-secretase is a complex composed of four components: PS1, nicastrin, APH1 and PEN2. It has not been reported that TLJN could modulate the components of γ-secretase. Here, using Western blot, we detected the expression levels of γ-secretase complex in the presence and absence of TLJN. We found that TLJN did not affect full length PS1 but lowered PS1 C-terminal fragment levels (**Fig. 4A**). TLJN also reduced the levels of both APH1 (**Fig. 4B**) and nicastrin (**Fig. 4C**). However, we did not find significant changes of the component PEN2 protein expression (**Fig. 4D**). These results suggest that TLJN reduces Aβ production through modulating the levels of γ-secretase components.

Herbal Medicine TLJN has Little Effect on Aβ Clearance Enzymes

In addition to BACE1 and γ-secretase which are responsible for Aβ production, there are two enzymes relevant to Aβ degradation and clearance: NEP and IDE [49], which contribute to the degradation of Aβ levels in brains. Recent data showed that TLJN increases NEP and IDE protein levels in a rat model of AD induced by $A\beta_{25-35}$ peptide intracerebral injection [1]. A recent report showed Geniposide could enhance IDE expression of cultured cortical neurons [50]. To examine the possibility that TLJN-induced Aβ reduction is also associated with Aβ degradation/or clearance in AD transgenic mice, we analyzed the levels of NEP and IDE in APP23 transgenic mouse brains with Western blotting. Unexpectedly, we did not find any significant elevation of either NEP (**Fig. 5A**) or IDE (**Fig. 5B**) levels following chronic TLJN administration in comparison to vehicle groups (n = 5 in each group).

Discussion

TLJN is a modern Chinese formula that has recently been applied in phase II clinical trial in patients with cerebral ischemic stroke and vascular dementia [3,4]. However, the roles of TLJN in AD still need to be tested in rigorous clinical trials. In the present study, we are the first to examine the effects of an anti-stroke herbal medicine TLJN on amyloid-related pathology in APP23 transgenic mice. Following TLJN chronic administration, we found in the brain tissues of APP23 mice that (1) Aβ levels and deposition were significantly decreased; (2) BACE1 protein levels as well as activity were significantly down-regulated; (3) the levels of γ-secretase components PS1, APH1 and nicastrin but not PEN2

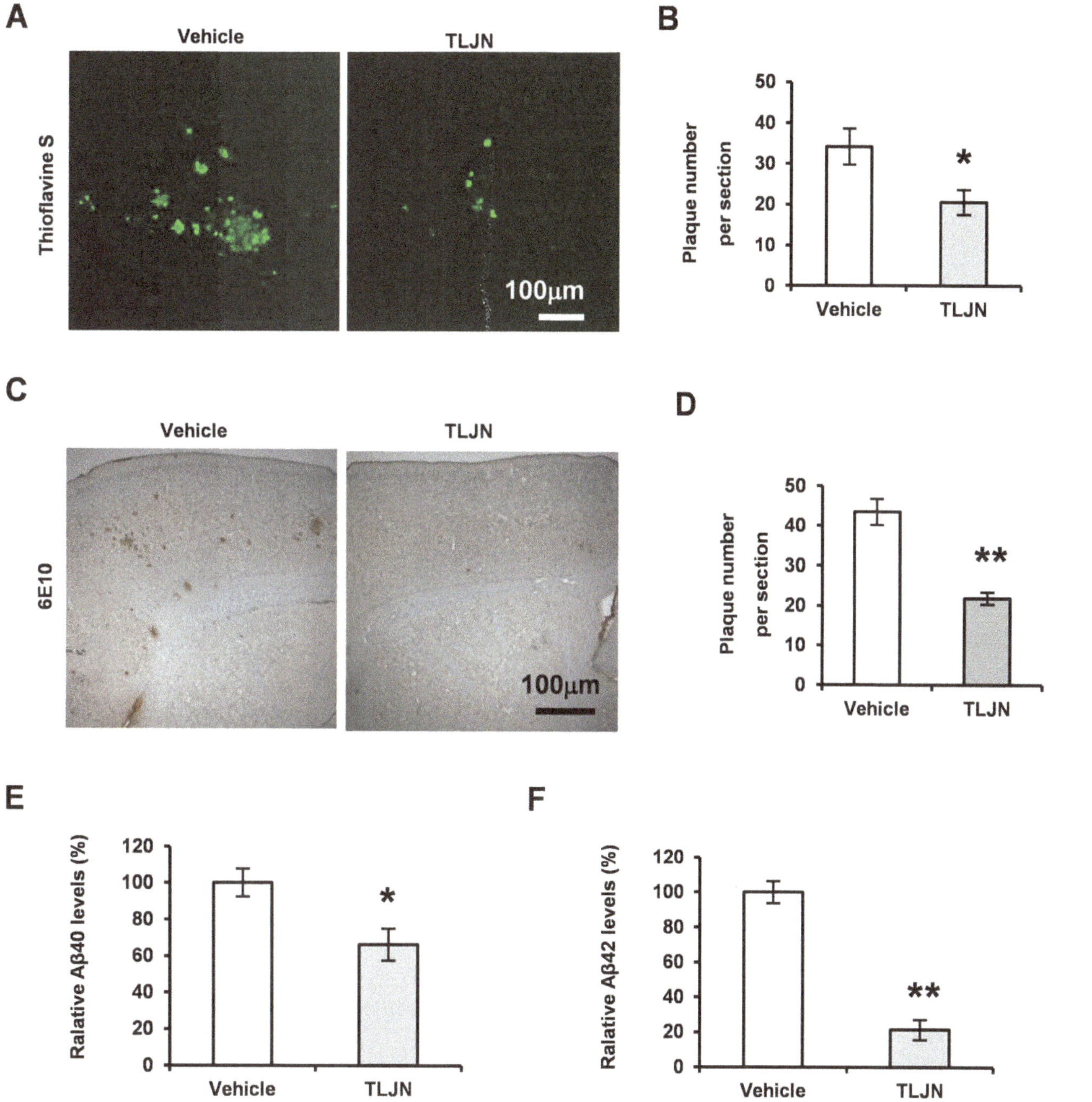

Figure 2. Herbal medicine TLJN reduces deposition and Aβ levels in APP23 mice. Representative images showed thioflavine S staining demonstrating insoluble Aβ deposition (**A**). The positive structures of thioflavine S histological staining were counted per section and statistical analysis showed a significant decrease in the number of plaques with TLJN treatment for 6 months (**B**, Mean ± SD, *$p<0.05$, Student *t*-test). Bar: 100 μm. Aβ accumulation was immunostained with 6E10 and microphotoimages were presented in (**C**). Similarly, 6E10-positive structures were counted and statistical analysis showed a significant decrease in the number of plaques in the brain treated with TLJN compared to vehicle groups (**D**, Mean ± SD, **$p<0.01$, Student *t*-test). Bar: 100 μm. ELISA was performed to measure insoluble Aβ40 and Aβ42 levels in the neocortex. Compared to vehicles, chronic treatment of TLJN significantly reduces Aβ40 (**E**) and Aβ42 levels (**F**) in the brain of APP23 mice (Mean ± SD, Student *t*-test, *$p<0.05$, **$p<0.01$).

were decreased; (4) there were not significant changes in the levels of the degrading enzymes NEP and IDE. Our finding of TLJN-decreased Aβ levels induced by TLJN is consistent with previous observations of Ginsenoside-induced Aβ level decrease [26,27,29,51]. Therefore, Ginsenoside in TLJN might be the main active ingredients responsible for decreasing Aβ levels. In addition to Aβ reduction, we also found a significant decrease in the number of insoluble Aβ plaques in the chronic presence of TLJN. The number decrease may be associated with total reduction of Aβ levels. Meanwhile, there is another possibility that Ginsenoside in TLJN inhibits transforming of soluble Aβ to insoluble or directly blocks the aggregation of insoluble Aβ.

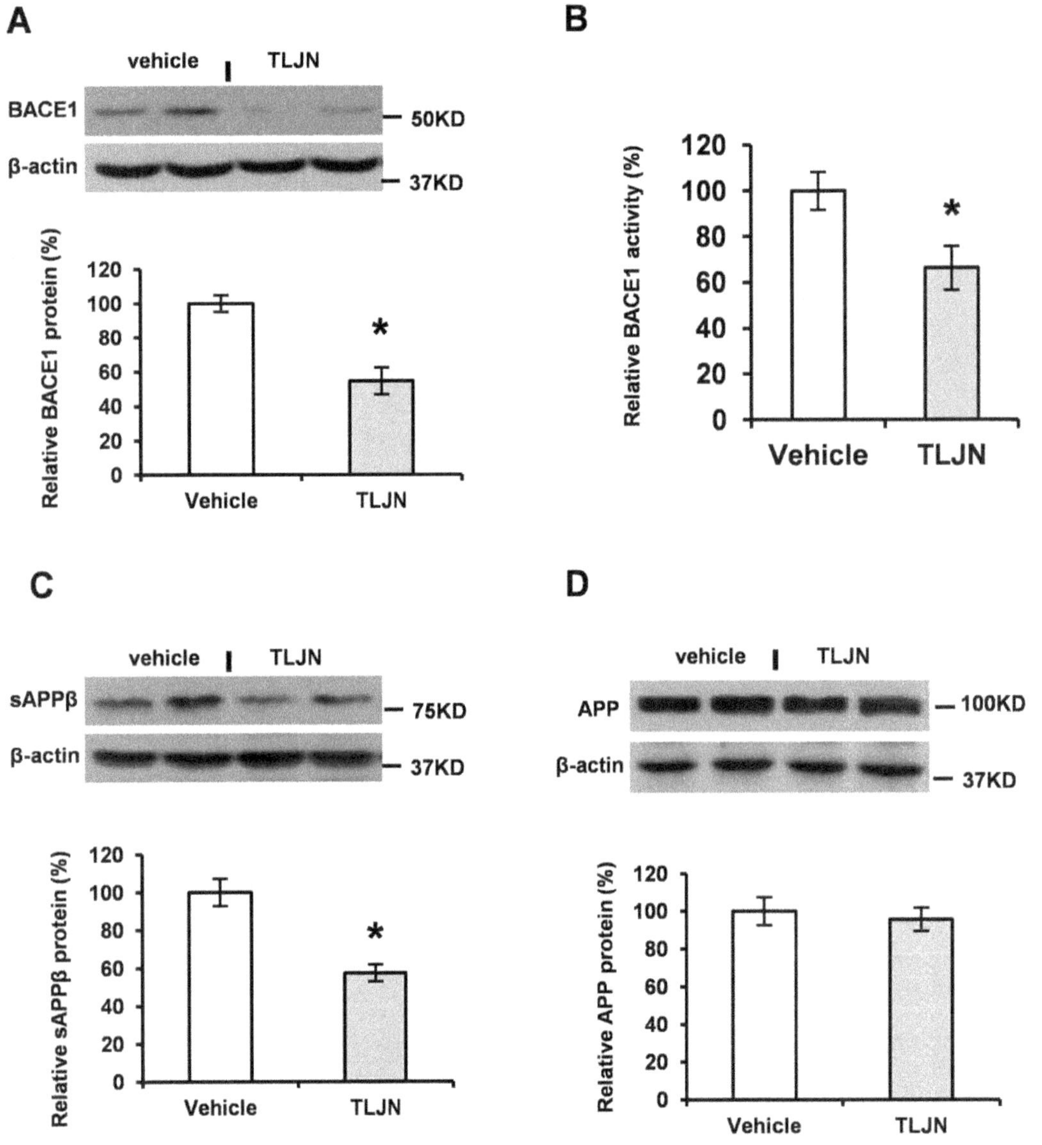

Figure 3. Herbal medicine TLJN down-regulates BACE1 levels and activity. BACE1 levels were probed by Western blot and its levels were normalized to β-actin level, accordingly (**A**). BACE1 activity was measured and relative activity levels were compared to vehicle controls (**B**, Mean ± SD, student t-test, *$p<0.05$). Soluble APP β fragment (sAPPβ) (**C**) and APP expression (**D**) were probed by Western blot and its levels were normalized to β-actin level, accordingly. Spot density analysis was performed and a significant decrease was observed in BACE1 (**A**), sAPPβ (**C**) but not APP levels (**D**) in TLJN-treated mice compared to vehicles. Statistical analysis was performed and significance was presented as *$p<0.05$ (Mean ± SD, Student *t*-test).

It has been reported that BACE1 is a stress-response protein [52], which means that its protein levels and/or activities might be modulated [53]. Here, we observed BACE1 level reduction in the brain treated with TLJN. In addition to TJLN-induced BACE1 protein level decrease, we also found that long-term TLJN treatment inhibited BACE1 activity in brains, consistent with the observation *in vitro* of BACE1 activity inhibition by the treatment of Ginsenoside Rg1 [28,29]. The mechanism involved in BACE1 down-regulation by TLJN remains to be confirmed. It has been found that glucose reduction could possibly be involved in the early events of AD pathogenesis [54,55]. It has been evidenced that glucose reduction as well as energy inhibition elevates BACE1 levels and activity in APP transgenic mice [54,56]. In contrast, Ginsenoside stimulates glucose uptake [23]. Therefore, the capability of Ginsenoside to improve glucose uptake could be a cause of the regulation of BACE1 level and activity by TLJN in the brain of APP23 mice. Ginsenoside has also been implicated in down-regulating NF-κB signaling, resulting in anti-inflammatory consequences [57,58,59]. Combining our previous finding that genetic inactivation of tumor necrosis factor receptor-mediated NF-κB signal transduction pathway results in the decrease of BACE1 levels, ultimately leads to Aβ reduction [34], hence we postulate that TLJN-containing Ginsenoside down-regulates NF-κB signaling, resulting BACE1 inhibition. Recently, Ginsenoside has been found to enhance the binding of peroxisome proliferator-activated receptor γ (PPARγ) to BACE1 promoter, which in turn inhibits the transcription and translation of BACE1 and thus suppress BACE1 activity [29].

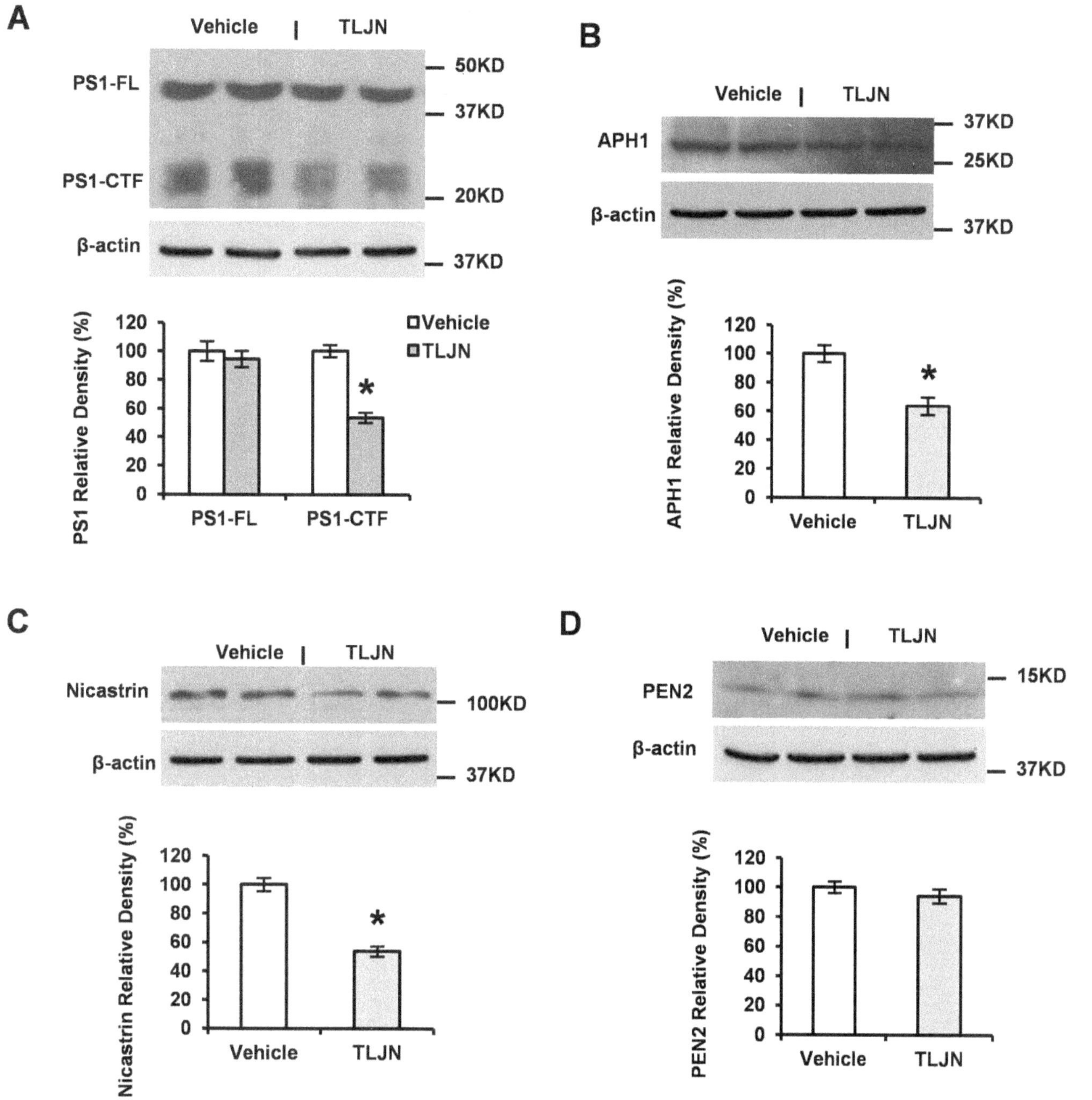

Figure 4. Herbal medicine TLJN reduces levels of γ-secretase components. APP23 mice were treated with TLJN for 6 months. Levels of γ-secretase components were analyzed by Western blotting. Representative images showed the bands of both PS1-CTF and PS1-FL (**A**), APH1 (**B**), nicastrin (**C**) and PEN2 (**D**). Then Spot density analysis was performed and a significant decrease was observed in PS1-CTF (**A**), APH1 (**B**) and nicastrin (**C**) but not in PS1-FL (**A**) and PEN2 (**D**). Significant differences were presented as *$p<0.05$ (Mean ± SD, Student *t*-test).

Another finding is that TLJN can partially decrease γ-secretase activity by reducing PS1, APH1 and nicastrin levels, which are components of γ-secretase enzyme complex. A number of small molecule γ-secretase inhibitors have been identified to block Aβ generation with high potency in cultured cells and in APP transgenic mouse models of AD [60,61,62]. However, It is noticed that γ-secretase also cleaves a number of additional substrates besides APP, such as Notch [48,63] and ErbB-4 [64], and thus γ-secretase inhibitors can suppress Notch processing [65,66]. Consequently, γ-secretase inhibition can result in serious adverse effects. Therefore, further elucidation of the mechanism of TLJN's action is highly desirable for pharmacological intervention in AD.

One recent report suggested that TLJN improves Aβ clearance enzyme IDE and NEP expression [1]. It has further been demonstrated that Geniposide has the capability to up-regulate IDE expression in cultured cortical neurons [50]. However, we did not find a significant elevation of either IDE or NEP levels in the brain chronically treated with TLJN. The previous observation of elevating IDE and NEP levels is based on a rat AD model induced by bilateral intra-hippocampal injection of Aβ peptide 25–35. The

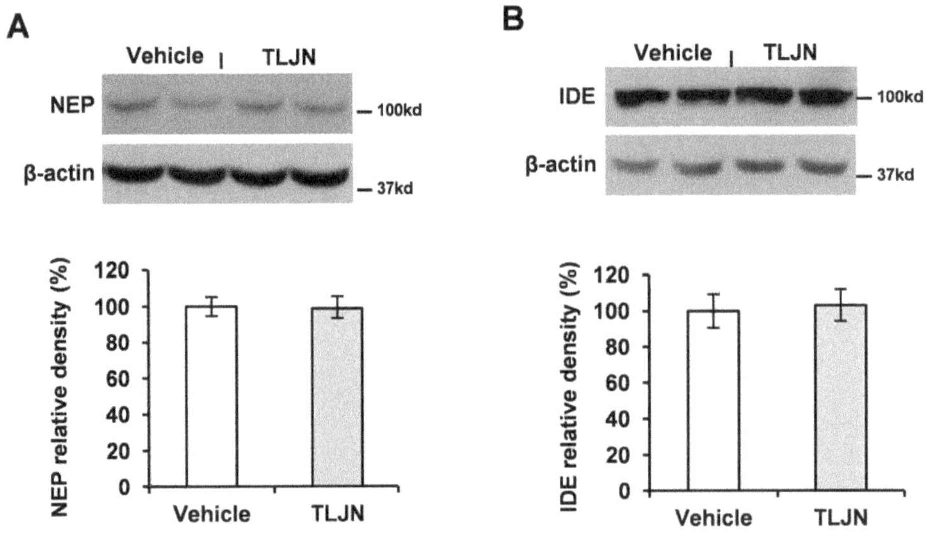

Figure 5. Herbal medicine TLJN has little effect on Aβ clearance enzyme expressions. APP23 were treated with TLJN for 6 months. Proteins from neocortex were loaded on an 8% Tris-Glycine gel. Membranes were blotted with rabbit polyclonal antibody against NEP (**A**) and antibody against IDE (**B**). Spot density analyses of NEP and IDE levels were performed and indicated as arbitrary units. No significant differences were presented as $p>0.05$ (Mean ± SD, Student *t*-test).

discrepancy of these results may be due to different AD models used.

Neuron injury and loss is an important cause of dementia in AD patients. Another compound in TLJN is Geniposide, which has biological activities of neuroprotection and anti-oxidative stress. Lines of evidence have shown that Geniposide promotes nuclear translocation of nuclear factor-E2-related factor 2 (Nrf2) [11]. Binding of Nrf2 to the antioxidant response element induces a battery of gene transcriptions that can coordinate a protective response against oxidative stressors [67]. Geniposide also up-regulates the expression of heme oxygenase-1 (HO-1) [68]. HO-1 is an enzyme which is responsible for degrading heme to carbon monoxide, free iron, and biliverdin and for the cell defense against oxidative stress [69]. There has been evidenced that Geniposide could enhance insulin secretion [70], which prevents oxidative stress-induced damage in AD [71]. Recently, it has been found that Geniposide could inhibit Aβ42-mediated cytotoxicity in neurons [50]. Therefore, the roles of Geniposide in neuroprotection might be one of the beneficial actions of TLJN.

In summary, besides the application in the patients with cerebral ischemic stroke [2,31,72], we have identified anti-stroke herbal medicine TLJN as a modulator of BACE1 and γ-secretase complex, which provides a mechanistic clue for the application in neurodegenerative diseases such as AD.

Author Contributions

Contributed reagents/materials/chemical analysis tools, including confirmation of chemical components of Ginsenoside and Geniposide in TLJN: PL QH YL MS. Wrote and revised the manuscript and addressed the questions from the reviewers: PH YS RL. Conceived and designed the experiments: YS PH PL QH RL. Performed the experiments: PH QH. Analyzed the data: PH RL YS.

References

1. Liu Y, Hua Q, Lei H, Li P (2011) Effect of Tong Luo Jiu Nao on Abeta-degrading enzymes in AD rat brains. J Ethnopharmacol 137: 1035–1046.
2. Li XJ, Hou JC, Sun P, Li PT, He RQ, et al. (2012) Neuroprotective effects of tongluojiunao in neurons exposed to oxygen and glucose deprivation. J Ethnopharmacol 141: 927–933.
3. Gu Z, Zhao J (2007) Clinical Trials of TongLuoJiuNao in Patients with Acute Brain Infarcts. Changchun Medical School of Chinese Medicine Bulletin.
4. Zhu W, Xiong J (2007) Clinical studies of TongLuoJiuNao in patients with acute infarcts. Hubei Med School of Chinese Medicine Bulletin 5: 4–39.
5. Kim BH, Lee YG, Park TY, Kim HB, Rhee MH, et al. (2009) Ginsenoside Rp1, a ginsenoside derivative, blocks lipopolysaccharide-induced interleukin-1beta production via suppression of the NF-kappaB pathway. Planta Med 75: 321–326.
6. Joo SS, Yoo YM, Ahn BW, Nam SY, Kim YB, et al. (2008) Prevention of inflammation-mediated neurotoxicity by Rg3 and its role in microglial activation. Biol Pharm Bull 31: 1392–1396.
7. Kim YJ, Kwon HC, Ko H, Park JH, Kim HY, et al. (2008) Anti-tumor activity of the ginsenoside Rk1 in human hepatocellular carcinoma cells through inhibition of telomerase activity and induction of apoptosis. Biol Pharm Bull 31: 826–830.
8. Lee SY, Kim GT, Roh SH, Song JS, Kim HJ, et al. (2009) Proteomic analysis of the anti-cancer effect of 20S-ginsenoside Rg3 in human colon cancer cell lines. Biosci Biotechnol Biochem 73: 811–816.
9. Zhang X, Wang J, Xing Y, Gong L, Li H, et al. (2012) Effects of ginsenoside Rg1 or 17beta-estradiol on a cognitively impaired, ovariectomized rat model of Alzheimer's disease. Neuroscience 220: 191–200.
10. Shi C, Zheng DD, Fang L, Wu F, Kwong WH, et al. (2012) Ginsenoside Rg1 promotes nonamyloidgenic cleavage of APP via estrogen receptor signaling to MAPK/ERK and PI3K/Akt. Biochim Biophys Acta 1820: 453–460.
11. Yin F, Liu J, Zheng X, Guo L, Xiao H (2010) Geniposide induces the expression of heme oxygenase-1 via PI3K/Nrf2-signaling to enhance the antioxidant capacity in primary hippocampal neurons. Biol Pharm Bull 33: 1841–1846.
12. Liu JH, Yin F, Guo LX, Deng XH, Hu YH (2009) Neuroprotection of geniposide against hydrogen peroxide induced PC12 cells injury: involvement of PI3 kinase signal pathway. Acta Pharmacol Sin 30: 159–165.
13. Bertram L, Tanzi RE (2008) Thirty years of Alzheimer's disease genetics: the implications of systematic meta-analyses. Nat Rev Neurosci 9: 768–778.
14. Hardy J, Selkoe DJ (2002) The amyloid hypothesis of Alzheimer's disease: progress and problems on the road to therapeutics. Science 297: 353–356.
15. Selkoe DJ (2003) Aging, amyloid, and Alzheimer's disease: a perspective in honor of Carl Cotman. Neurochem Res 28: 1705–1713.
16. Tanzi RE, Bertram L (2005) Twenty years of the Alzheimer's disease amyloid hypothesis: a genetic perspective. Cell 120: 545–555.
17. Fukumoto H, Cheung BS, Hyman BT, Irizarry MC (2002) Beta-secretase protein and activity are increased in the neocortex in Alzheimer disease. Arch Neurol 59: 1381–1389.
18. Holsinger RM, McLean CA, Beyreuther K, Masters CL, Evin G (2002) Increased expression of the amyloid precursor beta-secretase in Alzheimer's disease. Ann Neurol 51: 783–786.
19. Li R, Lindholm K, Yang LB, Yue X, Citron M, et al. (2004) Amyloid beta peptide load is correlated with increased beta-secretase activity in sporadic Alzheimer's disease patients. Proc Natl Acad Sci U S A 101: 3632–3637.

20. Yang LB, Lindholm K, Yan R, Citron M, Xia W, et al. (2003) Elevated beta-secretase expression and enzymatic activity detected in sporadic Alzheimer disease. Nat Med 9: 3–4.
21. Ji HF, Zhang HY (2008) Multipotent natural agents to combat Alzheimer's disease. Functional spectrum and structural features. Acta Pharmacol Sin 29: 143–151.
22. Williams P, Sorribas A, Howes MJ (2011) Natural products as a source of Alzheimer's drug leads. Nat Prod Rep 28: 48–77.
23. Bao HY, Zhang J, Yeo SJ, Myung CS, Kim HM, et al. (2005) Memory enhancing and neuroprotective effects of selected ginsenosides. Arch Pharm Res 28: 335–342.
24. Liu Y, Li X, Yuan HF (2006) [Progress of research on effects of ginsenoside Rg1 in promoting capability of learning and memory]. Zhongguo Zhong Xi Yi Jie He Za Zhi 26: 956–960.
25. Chang Y, Huang WJ, Tien LT, Wang SJ (2008) Ginsenosides Rg1 and Rb1 enhance glutamate release through activation of protein kinase A in rat cerebrocortical nerve terminals (synaptosomes). Eur J Pharmacol 578: 28–36.
26. Chen F, Eckman EA, Eckman CB (2006) Reductions in levels of the Alzheimer's amyloid beta peptide after oral administration of ginsenosides. FASEB J 20: 1269–1271.
27. Zhao H, Li Q, Zhang Z, Pei X, Wang J, et al. (2009) Long-term ginsenoside consumption prevents memory loss in aged SAMP8 mice by decreasing oxidative stress and up-regulating the plasticity-related proteins in hippocampus. Brain Res 1256: 111–122.
28. Wang YH, Du GH (2009) Ginsenoside Rg1 inhibits beta-secretase activity in vitro and protects against Abeta-induced cytotoxicity in PC12 cells. J Asian Nat Prod Res 11: 604–612.
29. Chen LM, Lin ZY, Zhu YG, Lin N, Zhang J, et al. (2012) Ginsenoside Rg1 attenuates beta-amyloid generation via suppressing PPARgamma-regulated BACE1 activity in N2a-APP695 cells. Eur J Pharmacol 675: 15–21.
30. He P, Cheng X, Staufenbiel M, Li R, Shen Y (2013) Long-term Treatment of Thalidomide Ameliorates Amyloid-like Pathology through Inhibition of β-Secretase in a Mouse Model of Alzheimer's Disease. PLoS One: Epub Feb 06.
31. Hua Q, Qing X, Li P, Li W, Hou J, et al. (2010) Brain microvascular endothelial cells mediate neuroprotective effects on ischemia/reperfusion neurons. J Ethnopharmacol 129: 306–313.
32. Sturchler-Pierrat C, Abramowski D, Duke M, Wiederhold KH, Mistl C, et al. (1997) Two amyloid precursor protein transgenic mouse models with Alzheimer disease-like pathology. Proc Natl Acad Sci U S A 94: 13287–13292.
33. Sommer B, Staufenbiel M (1998) A beta peptide deposition in the brains of transgenic mice: evidence for a key event in Alzheimer's disease pathogenesis. Mol Psychiatry 3: 284–286, 282–283.
34. He P, Zhong Z, Lindholm K, Berning L, Lee W, et al. (2007) Deletion of tumor necrosis factor death receptor inhibits amyloid beta generation and prevents learning and memory deficits in Alzheimer's mice. J Cell Biol 178: 829–841.
35. He P, Shen Y (2009) Interruption of beta-catenin signaling reduces neurogenesis in Alzheimer's disease. J Neurosci 29: 6545–6557.
36. Kuo YM, Beach TG, Sue LI, Scott S, Layne KJ, et al. (2001) The evolution of A beta peptide burden in the APP23 transgenic mice: implications for A beta deposition in Alzheimer disease. Mol Med 7: 609–618.
37. He P, Liu Q, Wu J, Shen Y (2012) Genetic deletion of TNF receptor suppresses excitatory synaptic transmission via reducing AMPA receptor synaptic localization in cortical neurons. FASEB J 26: 334–345.
38. Hsiao K, Chapman P, Nilsen S, Eckman C, Harigaya Y, et al. (1996) Correlative memory deficits, Abeta elevation, and amyloid plaques in transgenic mice. Science 274: 99–102.
39. LeVine H 3rd (1999) Quantification of beta-sheet amyloid fibril structures with thioflavin T. Methods Enzymol 309: 274–284.
40. Vassar R, Bennett BD, Babu-Khan S, Kahn S, Mendiaz EA, et al. (1999) Beta-secretase cleavage of Alzheimer's amyloid precursor protein by the transmembrane aspartic protease BACE. Science 286: 735–741.
41. Van Dooren T, Muyllaert D, Borghgraef P, Cresens A, Devijver H, et al. (2006) Neuronal or glial expression of human apolipoprotein e4 affects parenchymal and vascular amyloid pathology differentially in different brain regions of double- and triple-transgenic mice. Am J Pathol 168: 245–260.
42. Gandy S (2005) The role of cerebral amyloid beta accumulation in common forms of Alzheimer disease. J Clin Invest 115: 1121–1129.
43. Sinha S, Anderson JP, Barbour R, Basi GS, Caccavello R, et al. (1999) Purification and cloning of amyloid precursor protein beta-secretase from human brain. Nature 402: 537–540.
44. Hussain I, Powell D, Howlett DR, Tew DG, Meek TD, et al. (1999) Identification of a novel aspartic protease (Asp 2) as beta-secretase. Mol Cell Neurosci 14: 419–427.
45. Yan R, Bienkowski MJ, Shuck ME, Miao H, Tory MC, et al. (1999) Membrane-anchored aspartyl protease with Alzheimer's disease beta-secretase activity. Nature 402: 533–537.
46. Lin X, Koelsch G, Wu S, Downs D, Dashti A, et al. (2000) Human aspartic protease memapsin 2 cleaves the beta-secretase site of beta-amyloid precursor protein. Proc Natl Acad Sci U S A 97: 1456–1460.
47. Selkoe DJ (2011) Resolving controversies on the path to Alzheimer's therapeutics. Nat Med 17: 1060–1065.
48. Selkoe D, Kopan R (2003) Notch and Presenilin: regulated intramembrane proteolysis links development and degeneration. Annu Rev Neurosci 26: 565–597.
49. Farris W, Mansourian S, Chang Y, Lindsley L, Eckman EA, et al. (2003) Insulin-degrading enzyme regulates the levels of insulin, amyloid beta-protein, and the beta-amyloid precursor protein intracellular domain in vivo. Proc Natl Acad Sci U S A 100: 4162–4167.
50. Yin F, Zhang Y, Guo L, Kong S, Liu J (2012) Geniposide regulates insulin-degrading enzyme expression to inhibit the cytotoxicity of Abeta1–42 in cortical neurons. CNS Neurol Disord Drug Targets.
51. Shi YQ, Huang TW, Chen LM, Pan XD, Zhang J, et al. (2010) Ginsenoside Rg1 attenuates amyloid-beta content, regulates PKA/CREB activity, and improves cognitive performance in SAMP8 mice. J Alzheimers Dis 19: 977–989.
52. Cole SL, Vassar R (2008) The role of amyloid precursor protein processing by BACE1, the beta-secretase, in Alzheimer disease pathophysiology. J Biol Chem 283: 29621–29625.
53. Zhang C, Browne A, Divito JR, Stevenson JA, Romano D, et al. (2010) Amyloid-beta production via cleavage of amyloid-beta protein precursor is modulated by cell density. J Alzheimers Dis 22: 683–984.
54. Velliquette RA, O'Connor T, Vassar R (2005) Energy inhibition elevates beta-secretase levels and activity and is potentially amyloidogenic in APP transgenic mice: possible early events in Alzheimer's disease pathogenesis. J Neurosci 25: 10874–10883.
55. O'Connor T, Sadleir KR, Maus E, Velliquette RA, Zhao J, et al. (2008) Phosphorylation of the translation initiation factor eIF2alpha increases BACE1 levels and promotes amyloidogenesis. Neuron 60: 988–1009.
56. Vassar R (2007) Caspase-3 cleavage of GGA3 stabilizes BACE: implications for Alzheimer's disease. Neuron 54: 671–673.
57. Choi K, Kim M, Ryu J, Choi C (2007) Ginsenosides compound K and Rh(2) inhibit tumor necrosis factor-alpha-induced activation of the NF-kappaB and JNK pathways in human astroglial cells. Neurosci Lett 421: 37–41.
58. Choo MK, Sakurai H, Kim DH, Saiki I (2008) A ginseng saponin metabolite suppresses tumor necrosis factor-alpha-promoted metastasis by suppressing nuclear factor-kappaB signaling in murine colon cancer cells. Oncol Rep 19: 595–600.
59. Zhang Z, Li X, Lv W, Yang Y, Gao H, et al. (2008) Ginsenoside Re reduces insulin resistance through inhibition of c-Jun NH2-terminal kinase and nuclear factor-kappaB. Mol Endocrinol 22: 186–195.
60. Best JD, Jay MT, Otu F, Ma J, Nadin A, et al. (2005) Quantitative measurement of changes in amyloid-beta(40) in the rat brain and cerebrospinal fluid following treatment with the gamma-secretase inhibitor LY-411575 [N2-[(2S)-2-(3,5-difluorophenyl)-2-hydroxyethanoyl]-N1-[(7S)-5-methyl-6-oxo-6,7-d ihydro-5H-dibenzo[b,d]azepin-7-yl]-L-alaninamide]. J Pharmacol Exp Ther 313: 902–908.
61. Siemers ER, Dean RA, Friedrich S, Ferguson-Sells L, Gonzales C, et al. (2007) Safety, tolerability, and effects on plasma and cerebrospinal fluid amyloid-beta after inhibition of gamma-secretase. Clin Neuropharmacol 30: 317–325.
62. Siemers ER, Quinn JF, Kaye J, Farlow MR, Porsteinsson A, et al. (2006) Effects of a gamma-secretase inhibitor in a randomized study of patients with Alzheimer disease. Neurology 66: 602–604.
63. Schroeter EH, Kisslinger JA, Kopan R (1998) Notch-1 signalling requires ligand-induced proteolytic release of intracellular domain. Nature 393: 382–386.
64. Lee HJ, Jung KM, Huang YZ, Bennett LB, Lee JS, et al. (2002) Presenilin-dependent gamma-secretase-like intramembrane cleavage of ErbB4. J Biol Chem 277: 6318–6323.
65. Searfoss GH, Jordan WH, Calligaro DO, Galbreath EJ, Schirtzinger LM, et al. (2003) Adipsin, a biomarker of gastrointestinal toxicity mediated by a functional gamma-secretase inhibitor. J Biol Chem 278: 46107–46116.
66. Wong GT, Manfra D, Poulet FM, Zhang Q, Josien H, et al. (2004) Chronic treatment with the gamma-secretase inhibitor LY-411,575 inhibits beta-amyloid peptide production and alters lymphopoiesis and intestinal cell differentiation. J Biol Chem 279: 12876–12882.
67. Kraft AD, Johnson DA, Johnson JA (2004) Nuclear factor E2-related factor 2-dependent antioxidant response element activation by tert-butylhydroquinone and sulforaphane occurring preferentially in astrocytes conditions neurons against oxidative insult. J Neurosci 24: 1101–1112.
68. Yin F, Liu JH, Zheng XX, Guo LX (2010) GLP-1 receptor plays a critical role in geniposide-induced expression of heme oxygenase-1 in PC12 cells. Acta Pharmacol Sin 31: 540–545.
69. Jazwa A, Cuadrado A (2010) Targeting heme oxygenase-1 for neuroprotection and neuroinflammation in neurodegenerative diseases. Curr Drug Targets 11: 1517–1531.
70. Guo LX, Xia ZN, Gao X, Yin F, Liu JH (2012) Glucagon-like peptide 1 receptor plays a critical role in geniposide-regulated insulin secretion in INS-1 cells. Acta Pharmacol Sin 33: 237–241.
71. Duarte AI, Santos MS, Oliveira CR, Rego AC (2005) Insulin neuroprotection against oxidative stress in cortical neurons–involvement of uric acid and glutathione antioxidant defenses. Free Radic Biol Med 39: 876–889.
72. Hua Q, Zhu X, Li P, Tang H, Cai D, et al. (2008) Refined Qing Kai Ling, traditional Chinese medicinal preparation, reduces ischemic stroke-induced infarct size and neurological deficits and increases expression of endothelial nitric oxide synthase. Biol Pharm Bull 31: 633–637.

6

Hepatotoxicity or Hepatoprotection? Pattern Recognition for the Paradoxical Effect of the Chinese Herb *Rheum palmatum* L. in Treating Rat Liver Injury

Jia-bo Wang[1*⁹], Hai-ping Zhao[1,2⁹], Yan-ling Zhao[1], Cheng Jin[1], Dao-jian Liu[1], Wei-jun Kong[1,3], Fang Fang[1,3], Lin Zhang[1,3], Hong-juan Wang[1], Xiao-he Xiao[1]

1 Integrative Medicine Center, 302 Military Hospital, Beijing, People's Republic of China, **2** Key Laboratory of Modern Preparation of Traditional Chinese Medicine, Ministry of Education, Jiangxi University of Traditional Chinese Medicine, Nanchang, People's Republic of China, **3** Chengdu University of Traditional Chinese Medicine, Chengdu, People's Republic of China

Abstract

The hepatotoxicity of some Chinese herbs has been a cause for concern in recent years. However, some herbs, such as rhubarb, have been documented as having both therapeutic and toxic effects on the liver, leading to the complex problem of distinguishing the benefits from the risks of using this herb. To comparatively analyze the dose-response relationship between rhubarb and hepatic health, we administrated total rhubarb extract(RE) to normal and carbon tetrachloride(CCl_4)-treated rats for 12 weeks at 4 dosage levels(2.00, 5.40, 14.69 and 40.00 $g \cdot kg^{-1}$, measured as the quantity of crude material), followed by biochemical and histopathological tests of the rats' livers. A composite pattern was extracted by factor analysis, using all the biochemical indices as variables, into a visual representation of two mathematically obtained factors, which could be interpreted as the fibrosis factor and the cellular injury factor, according to the values of the variable loadings. The curative effect of administering the two lowest dosages of RE to CCl_4-treated rats was mainly expressed as a decrease in the extent of cellular injury. The hepatoprotective mechanism of RE might be related to its antioxidant effect, the antagonism of the free radical damage to hepatocytes caused by CCl_4. By contrast, the RE-induced liver damage was mainly expressed as a significant increase in the amount of fibrosis in both normal rats at all dosage levels and CCl_4-treated rats at the two highest dosage levels. Therefore, the hepatotoxic potential of RE could be attributable to the liver cell fibrosis induced by high doses of the herb. This study illustrates the bidirectional potential of rhubarb and demonstrates the feasibility of using factor analysis to study the dose-response relationships between herbal medicines and hepatotoxicity or the healing effects of these herbs by extracting the underlying interrelationships among a number of functional bio-indices in a holistic manner.

Editor: John E. Tavis, Saint Louis University, United States of America

Funding: This work was funded by the National Key Technologies R&D Program of China (No. 2009ZX09502-022) and by the National Natural Science Foundation of China (No. 30625042 and 30973947). The funders had no role in study design, data collection and analysis, decision to publish, or preparation of the manuscript.

Competing Interests: The authors have declared that no competing interests exist.

* E-mail: pharmacy302@126.com

⁹ These authors contributed equally to this work.

Introduction

Traditional Chinese herbal medicines are used worldwide, but there are a number of concerns regarding their use. Some researchers believe that herbal medicines are effective and safe, while others doubt their effectiveness and safety. The latter group has increased in number, especially after consecutive reports of adverse hepatotoxic effects of a number of phytomedicines, including *Polygonum multiflorum* [1], Shou-Wu Pian [2], Xiao-Chai-Hu-Tang (Syo-saiko-to), [3] and some herbs containing anthraquinones, such as *Sennae fructus angustifoliae* [4] and *Rheum palmatum* L. (rhubarb) [5]. Chitturi et al. believe that herbal hepatotoxicity is an expanding but poorly defined problem [6].

These herbal medicines, especially rhubarb and its constituent components, are frequently used as treatments for chronic liver diseases and as laxatives in Asian countries, and a number of cases have demonstrated their affirmative effectiveness and safety [7,8]. In addition to the clinical evidence of the effectiveness of rhubarb in treating chronic hepatic diseases, [9,10] many experiments at the animal, cellular and molecular levels have revealed that rhubarb and its anthraquinone constituents exert a protective effect against hepatic injury by inhibiting the carbon tetrachloride (CCl_4)-induced elevation of serum alanine aminotransferase (ALT), aspartate aminotransferase (AST), hyaluronic acid (HA) and laminin (LN) levels. [11,12]

In vitro and in vivo studies focusing on the anthraquinone constituents of rhubarb, however, have revealed conflicting results. A two-year National Toxicology Program (NTP) study, conducted by the U.S. Department of Health and Human Services (DHHS) on emodin, one of the main anthraquinone derivatives contained within rhubarb, demonstrated the hepatotoxic potential of emodin on normal rats and mice. The toxic effects included elevations of ALT levels, total bile acids (TBIL) levels and organ-weight-to-body-weight ratios (relative weights) of the liver, as well as decreases in alkaline phosphatase (AP) and total protein levels (TP). [13] Other investigators have reported that administration of rhubarb extracts (REs) led to elevations of serum ALT and TBIL levels in patients and experimental animals, leading to hepatitis and nephritis. [14–17]

The conflicting results of these reports might be due to the heterogeneity and complexity of herbal medicines with respect to their geographic origin, harvest season, and discrepancy of constituent components. Herbal medicines, which usually contain hundreds of chemical components with broad pharmacological targets and effects, present difficulties in describing overall biological profiles in a simple manner with a few essential factors that can be readily comprehended. Many phytopharmacologists have dedicated themselves to solving this provlem for decades. In recent years, pattern recognition, [18] a type of multivariate analysis approach, has become a promising method for identifying and interpreting meaningful regularities in noisy or complex systems, by analyzing data from different perspectives and summarizing them as useful information or by mining potential interrelationships. The factor analysis used in this study is a common pattern recognition method that reduces a large number of disease parameters to a relatively small number of independent factors, by describing the covariance structure of the observed data variables in terms of a few underlying and independent but non-measurable features called "factors". [19]

The aim of this study was to determine the paradoxical effects of liver protection and hepatotoxicity of rhubarb in the treatment of rat experimental hepatitis induced by carbon tetrachloride by categorizing a number of functional bio-indices into separate complementary domains (protection or toxicity) with no *a priori* assumptions. We believe that our data will provide useful information for the safe evaluation and proper application of rhubarb and, furthermore, will help increase our understanding of the rational use of phytomedicines.

Materials and Methods

Ethics Statement

This study was conducted in strict accordance with the recommendations of the Guidelines for the Care and Use of Laboratory Animals of the Ministry of Science and Technology of China. The animal protocol was approved by the Committee on the Ethics of Animal Experiments of the 302 Military Hospital (Approval ID: 09-056).

Animals and reagents

Male and female Sprague- Dawley rats, aged 6-8 weeks and weighing 180 ± 30 g, were obtained from the Laboratory Animal Center of the Academy of Military Medical Sciences (License No. SYXK 2007- 004). The animals were raised separately by gender and had unlimited access to food and water in an environmentally controlled breeding room (temperature 22±2°C, humidity 60–80%). The breeding room was illuminated by an artificial light cycle with 12 hours of light and 12 hours of darkness every day and was disinfected regularly.

Carbon tetrachloride (CCl_4) was purchased from Beijing Beihua Fine Chemicals Co. Ltd (Cat. #20060525), and olive oil was purchased from Sinopharm Chemical Reagent Beijing Co. Ltd (Cat. #F20080219). Both reagents were of AR grade.

Herb extraction and UPLC-MS/MS analysis

Rhubarb is the peeled and dried root of *Rheum palmatum* L., *R. tanguticum Maxim. ex* Balf. or *R. officinale* Baill. (Polygonaceae family), as stipulated in the Chinese Pharmacopoeia[20]. Rhubarb is also officially listed in European and Japanese pharmacopoeias. [21,22] *R. palmatum* was used in this study because it is described in all three pharmacopoeias and is more commonly used than the other species. The dried root and rhizome of *R. palmatum* L. were collected in Lixian County of the Gansu Province of China and were identified by Professor Xiao-he Xiao, a taxonomist at the Military Institute of Chinese Materia Medica. In total, 100 kg rhubarb was added to 600 L of 90% ethanol and then heated and extracted 3 times for 1 hour each time. The residual compounds after extraction were added to 1000 L of water and then heated and extracted for 1 hour. The filtrate was merged and sprayed dry, producing a yield of 29.3%. The samples were preserved for further experiments.

Rhubarb extract (RE) was analyzed for quality control by ultra-performance liquid chromatography coupled with an ultraviolet-visible detector and electrospray ionization tandem mass spectrometry (UPLC-UV-ESI-MS/MS). [23] The experimental conditions and data are provided in Text S1.

Animal model and study groups

In this study, a CCl_4-induced liver injury model was used because it has been well documented and demonstrated to have good repeatability and reliability. One experiment cycle continued for 16 weeks, and the following procedure was used immediately prior to the experiment, 180 rats were randomized into 10 groups of 18 animals each, with equal distributions by gender. The groups shown in Tables 1 and 2 were differentiated based on the treatment group and extract dosage. The rats in the five model groups (groups M and M_1-M_4) were injected intraperitoneally (i.p.) with CCl_4 oil (containing 1 portion CCl_4 and 9 portions olive oil, 5 ml/kg) 2 times per week for 12 weeks to induce chronic liver injury, and the rats in the other groups received normal saline (N.S.). The rats in all medication groups (groups N_1-N_4 and M_1-M_4) were administered RE intragastrically once per day from the 4th week until the end of the 16th week. Rats in the control (group N) and model (group M) groups were administered normal saline intragastrically. The RE dosages were 2.00, 5.40, 14.69 and 40.00 g/kg (measured as the quantity of crude material) per kg of body weight once per day and were equivalent to between 4 and 80 times the human upper dosage limit stipulated in the Chinese Pharmacopoeia (0.5 g/kg). Food and water were available *ad libitum* for all rats throughout the experiment.

Histopathologic examination and biochemical analysis

Necropsies were performed on all the animals at the end of the experiment. Tissues for histopathologic examination were fixed and preserved in 10% neutral buffered formalin, processed and trimmed, embedded in paraffin, sectioned to a thickness of approximately 5μm, and stained with hematoxylin and eosin (HE).

Biochemical analyses were performed on all animals. The biochemical parameters of serum ALT, AST, AP, urea nitrogen (SUN), creatinine (CREA), TP, albumin (ALB), globulin (GLO), calcium, inorganic phosphate, total cholesterol (CHOL) and TBIL levels were measured by the Clinical Laboratory of 302 Military Hospital of China. The levels of HA, LN and transforming growth factor β_1 (TGF-β_1) in rat serum were quantitated by chemiluminescence using assay kits from Beijing Deyuan Biomedical Engineering Corporation, China.

Statistical analysis

The experimental values were expressed as means ± standard deviation (means ± SD). All data were analyzed using the Statistical Package for the Social Sciences for Windows, version 13.0 (SPSS Inc, Chicago, IL, USA). The groups were compared

Table 1. Liver toxicity induced by rhubarb extract in normal rats with regard to survival and biochemical indices.

Groups	N	ND_1	ND_2	ND_3	ND_4
Dosage (g/kg)	0	2	5.4	14.69	40
Survival[a]	18	18	17	15	14
ALT (U/L)	73.00±17.70	104.86±10.17	119.43±31.36$^{\triangle}$	125.43±19.86$^{\triangle}$	175.86±22.75$^{\triangle}$
AST (U/L)	149.57±27.78	187.00±37.46	207.86±71.81	268.00±57.83$^{\triangle}$	261.00±48.55$^{\triangle}$
AP (U/L)	53.71±21.26	73.00±28.14	89.29±18.31	97.29±21.48$^{\triangle}$	116.43±19.7$^{\triangle}$
TBIL (μmol/L)	1.09±0.32	1.01±0.59	1.24±0.30	1.50±0.53	1.66±0.75$^{\triangle}$
TP (g/L)	69.71±12.31	74.14±13.56	76.29±11.34	84.43±10.72	87.71±8.12$^{\triangle}$
GLO (g/L)	27.57±7.50	34.43±6.48	35.71±5.77	46.29±9.72	51.43±7.57$^{\triangle}$
HA (ng/L)	203.30±71.98	220.4±73.97	277.79±23.17$^{\triangle}$	281.46±44.08$^{\triangle}$	350.13±47.98$^{\triangle}$
LN (ng/L)	31.53±5.05	36.76±10.47	38.01±8.43	48.47±10.22$^{\triangle}$	54.19±9.78$^{\triangle}$
TGF-β_1 (pg/L)	18.23±1.42	20.87±1.95	19.09±3.38	29.82±6.27	39.19±7.76$^{\triangle}$

N, normal rat group without treatment; ND_1-ND_4, normal rat groups treated with rhubarb extract at dosages of 2.00, 5.40, 14.69 and 40.00 g kg^{-1}, respectively. ALT, serum alanine aminotransferase; AST, serum aspartate aminotransferase; AP, alkaline phosphatase; TBIL, total bile acids; TP, total protein; GLO, globulin; HA, hyaluronic acid; LN, laminin; TGF-β_1, transforming growth factor β_1.
[a] The initial number of animals in each group of the study was 18.
$^{\triangle}$ *P<0.05* compared to the N group.

using ANOVA and multivariate statistical analysis, and the significance probability was set at $P=0.05$.

The factor analysis model was as follows:

$$y_c = l_{c1}F_1 + l_{c2}F_2 + l_{c3}F_3 + ... + l_{cn}F_n + \varepsilon_c$$

where y_c is the cth original variable, $c=1, \ldots, p$, p is the number of original variables, $l_{c1}, l_{c2}, l_{c3}, \ldots, l_{cn}$ are the factor loadings, $F_1, F_2, F_3, \ldots, F_n$ are the (new) factors, n is the number of factors, and ε_c the error term related to y_c. [24] The correlation coefficients were analyzed by principal component analysis and subsequent rotation according to the standard varimax criterion. The correlation between parameters was attributed to their common dependence on independent entities called "factors." The coefficients that linked the parameters to factors were named "factor loadings".

Results

Study design

This study included two parts. First, a comparative experiment was designed to investigate the dose-responses of RE to normal and CCl_4-treated rats. Standard blood chemistry analyses were used to evaluate liver damage and histological changes were assessed. All doses were set at high levels to uncover potential toxicities to rigorously investigate the hepatic risks of RE.

Table 2. Protective effect of rhubarb extract against CCl_4-induced liver injury with regard to the survival and biochemical indices in the model groups.

Groups	M	MD_1	MD_2	MD_3	MD_4
Dosage (g/kg)	0	2	5.4	14.69	40
Survival[a]	16	18	15	13	11
ALT (U/L)	519.14±64.46$^{\triangle}$	261.14±46.52*	213.43±33.16*	183.14±33.26*	253.43±55.24*
AST (U/L)	775.14±119.95$^{\triangle}$	421.00±35.13*	234.71±43.18*	268.57±77.34*	367.57±104.59*
AP (U/L)	140.57±58.8$^{\triangle}$	58.86±15.55*	63.57±20.56*	83.00±18.35	103.57±27.67
TBIL (μmol/L)	2.34±0.24$^{\triangle}$	1.49±0.71*	1.24±0.72*	1.64±1.07	2.89±0.72*
TP (g/L)	92.43±14.12$^{\triangle}$	71.00±10.85*	71.00±6.68*	75.71±9.41	87.14±7.99
GLO (g/L)	58.43±9.36$^{\triangle}$	29.86±10.93*	33.00±3.51*	38.14±8.28	49.71±6.70
HA (ng/L)	362.17±36.88$^{\triangle}$	284.23±38.73*	310.29±70.63*	436.37±61.71*	508.10±62.38*
LN (ng/L)	53.31±23.25$^{\triangle}$	36.59±10.25	38.64±7.85	52.49±6.93	91.96±19.21*
TGF-β_1 (pg/L)	33.07±11.06$^{\triangle}$	30.69±6.75	32.48±5.73	34.08±6.71	53.77±10.45*

M, model rat group without treatment; MD_1-MD_4, model rat groups treated with rhubarb extract at dosages of 2.00, 5.40, 14.69 and 40.00 g kg^{-1}, respectively. ALT, serum alanine aminotransferase; AST, serum aspartate aminotransferase; AP, alkaline phosphatase; TBIL, total bile acids; TP, total protein; GLO, globulin; HA, hyaluronic acid; LN, laminin; TGF-β_1, transforming growth factor β_1.
[a] The initial number of animals in each group of the study was 18.
$^{\triangle}$ *P<0.05* compared to the N group.
**P<0.05*, compared to the M group.

Second, a factor analysis approach was utilized to mathematically illustrate the bidirectional effect of liver protection and hepatotoxicity of RE on subjects under different physiological conditions. The mathematical modeling process used a dimension reduction effect to convert the original dataset of numerous disease variables into a relatively small number of independent "factors" that are not measurable but are easy to comprehend, including the protection factor and the lesion factor.

Identification of the chemical constituents in rhubarb extract (RE)

In a previous study, it was demonstrated that the major components contained in RE are anthraquinone derivatives and tannin-related compounds. [25] Using liquid chromatography coupled with tandem mass spectrometry, seventeen compounds were identified in this study, and their structures were tentatively assigned as twelve anthraquinone derivatives and five tannin-related compounds. The identified chemical constituents (Table S1) and the contents of the index compounds in the RE (Table S2) are summarized in the supplementary materials to illustrate the chemical basis of the RE utilized in this study. The chemical structures of the identified constituents in RE are depicted in Figures S1 and S2. The chromatographic profile is depicted in Fig. 1.

Common changes

All the RE-treated rats had a dose-related fur color change patterns, ranging from yellow to red, that appeared early in the study with exposure to increasing concentrations of RE. Red-to-brown urine and reddish-brown staining of the anal area were also noted for all rats that were treated with RE. Marked and chronic diarrhea accompanied by emaciation and inactivity were observed in all model and normal rats that were treated with 40 g/kg, but not the lower doses, of RE. During RE administration, the rats in the CCl_4-treated groups had lower increases in weight than those in the normal groups at the same dosage. Rats in all the RE-administered groups had negative dose-related body weight changes, and the rats in the highest dosage group had the lowest increase in weight until cessation of RE administration.

Histopathology

Dosage-dependent vacuolar degeneration of the hepatic portal area and/or hyperplasia of interstitial fibrous tissue were observed in over 67% of animals in the ND_1-ND_4 groups.

In the control group (group N), all rats exhibited normal histology. By contrast, 16 out of 18 animals in the model group (group M) exhibited vacuolar degeneration, which was characterized by small or medium vacuole formation in hepatocytes accompanied by nuclear loss or dislocation to the margins of the vacuoles. Hepatocytes with large nuclei were occasionally observed. Small focal lymphocytic infiltration of the stroma and/or portal area was also observed in 12 out of 18 animals in group M. Moreover, an obviously thickened envelope and fibrosis of the portal area and/or stroma were observed in 11 out of 18 animals in group M. The animals in groups MD_1-MD_4 showed decreases in vacuolar degeneration and lymphocytic infiltration in hepatocytes with increasing RE dosages. Over 67% of the animals in both groups MD_1 and MD_2 exhibited notably alleviated fibrosis of the liver envelope, portal area, and/or stroma, whereas 67% of the animals in the MD_3 group and 88% of the animals in the MD_4 group exhibited obvious aggravation of fibrosis. Typical histopathologic changes are depicted in Fig. 2.

Biochemical indices

The biochemical indices that changed significantly in the study groups are shown in Tables 1 and 2.

In the control group (N) and RE-treated normal rat groups (ND_1-ND_4), the indices exhibited overall dose-dependent increasing trends (Table 1). Compared to the group N, serum ALT and HA values increased significantly in the ND_2, ND_3 and ND_4 groups ($P<0.05$) and AST, LN and TGF-β_1 values increased significantly in the ND_3 and ND_4 groups ($P<0.05$), whereas TBIL values increased significantly in the ND_4 group only ($P<0.05$).

The serum ALT and AST values of all RE-treated model groups (MD_1-MD_4) were significantly lower than those of group M without treatment ($P<0.05$). However, these two indices stopped declining and started to increase when the dosage increased from the second dosage (MD_2, 5.40 g/kg) to the third (MD_3, 14.69 g/kg). Regarding the TBIL, HA, LN and TGF-β_1 levels, the values

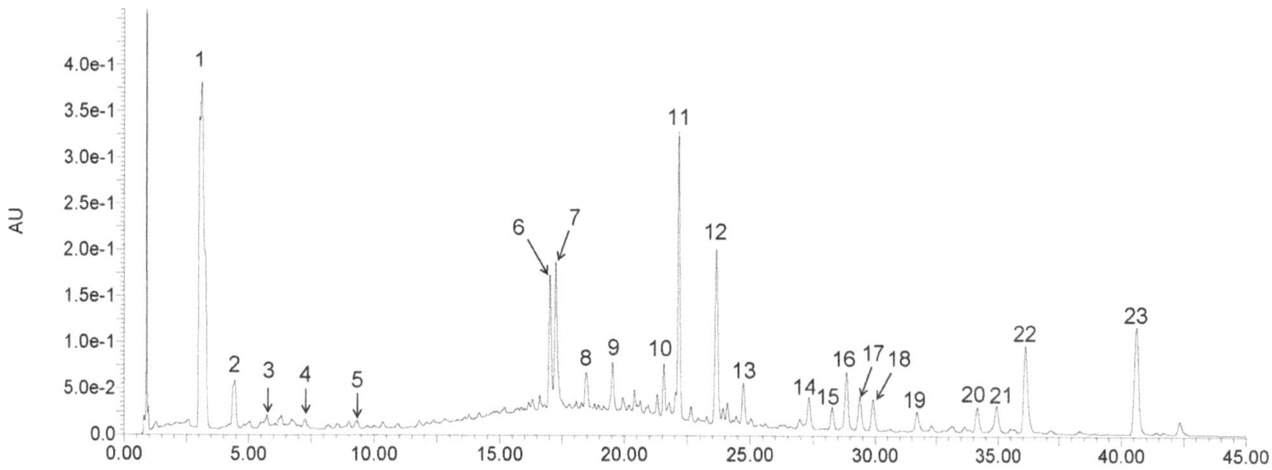

Figure 1. UPLC/UV chromatogram at 280 nm of the extract of *Rheum palmatum* L. Seventeen compounds were identified by electrospray ionization tandem mass spectrometry: galloyl glucose (1), glucopyranosyl-galloyl-glucose (3), catechin glucopyranoside (4), isomer of catechin glucopyranoside (5), aloe emodin *O*-glucoside (9), rhein *O*-glucoside (10), cinnamoyl-*O*-galloyl-glucose (11), laccaic acid D *O*-glucoside (13), dehydroxylaccaic acid D *O*-glucoside (14), chrysophanol *O*-glucoside (15), isomer of chrysophanol *O*-glucoside (16), emodin *O*-glucoside (17), laccaic acid D (19), physcion *O*-glucoside (20), emodin (21), acetyl- chrysophanol (22) and physcion (23). The other six chromatographic peaks (2, 6-8, 12 and 18) are unknown compounds.

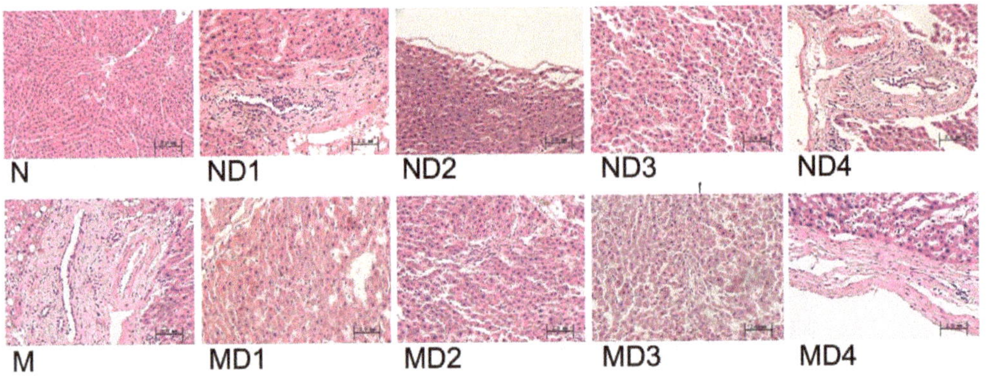

Figure 2. Typical histopathologic section photographs of rats in different groups (HE stained, 200× magnification). Dose-dependent vacuolar degeneration of the portal area and/or hyperplasia of the interstitial fibrous tissue were observed in the normal groups ND_1–ND_4. Obviously thickened envelopes and fibrosis of the portal area and/or stroma was observed in the animals of group M. This toxic degeneration caused by CCl_4 was improved after treatment with rhubarb extract in groups MD_1–MD_4. Notably, alleviation of fibrosis of the liver envelope, portal area, and/or stroma was observed in the animals in the MD_1 and MD_2 groups, whereas aggravation of fibrosis was found in over 67% of animals in the MD_3 and MD_4 groups. N, normal rat group without treatment; ND_1-ND_4, normal rat groups treated with rhubarb extract at dosages of 2.00, 5.40, 14.69 and 40.00 g kg^{-1}, respectively. M, model rat group without treatment; MD_1-MD_4, model rats groups treated with rhubarb extract at dosages of 2.00, 5.40, 14.69 and 40.00 g kg^{-1}, respectively.

of the maximum dosage group (MD_4 group) were even higher than those of group M without treatment ($P<0.05$) (Table 2).

Factor analysis using biochemical indices as variables

Bartlett's test of sphericity indicated a correlation between the currently used variables because the correlation matrix was significantly different from the identity matrix ($P<0.01$). The KMO measure of sampling adequacy was 0.789, which was higher than the acceptable criterion of 0.5. [26] The eigenvalues of the 9 factors are depicted in a scree plot in Fig. 3. Several methods were used to determine the number of meaningful factors that should be extracted. As a general rule, factors with an eigenvalue greater than 1.0 are retained. [27] The rationale for this rule is that the amount of variance accounted for by each factor should be at least equal to the variance of one variable. [24] This criterion indicated that two factors should be extracted in the present study. The first

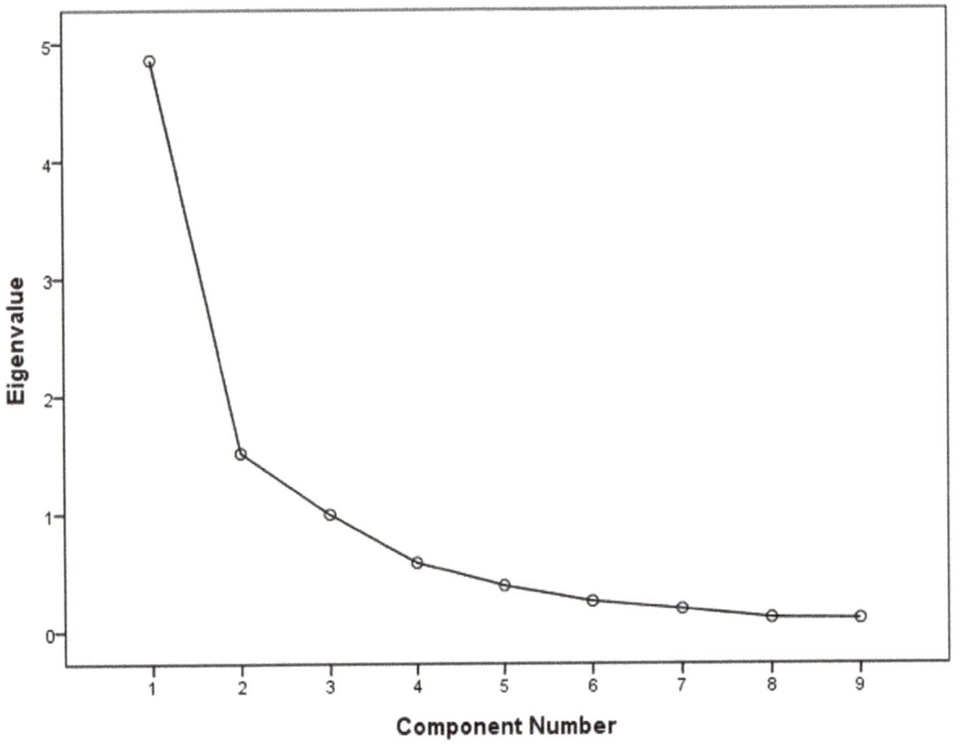

Figure 3. Scree plot depicting the eigenvalues of the factors extracted by factor analysis using biochemical indices as variables. The two factors with eigenvalue greater than 1.0 were retained in subsequent analyses.

and second factors accounted for 53.985% and 16.856% of the total variability, respectively. These two primary factors could explain 70.840% of the total variability in the dataset. The results of the factor analysis and a suggested interpretation are shown in Table 3. In interpreting the retained factors, we only selected variables with loadings above 0.5 or below -0.5 (i.e., variables with high influence).[28] According to this criterion, factor 1 could be labeled as "fibrosis" because the selected biochemical variables including HA, LN and TGF-β_1 (all loadings >0.85) are related to the fibrotic course[29-31] and factor 2 could be labeled as "cellular injury" because it was mainly affected by ALT and AST (both loadings >0.90), which were altered when the hepatocellular membrane was damaged.

The graphical representation of the dose-response relationship of RE, using these two statistically obtained factors as the axes to show the distribution pattern of different study groups in the plot, is depicted in Fig. 4. In the graphical representation, the toxicity- and pharmacologically induced variation patterns of the biochemical indices could be deduced from the ordered distribution of the studied groups. The untreated N group and the untreated M group are represented at the left lower side and upper right side of the diagram, respectively. The distance of group M away from group N illustrated certain hepatotoxic effects of both enzyme variations and fibrosis in rats with CCl_4-induced hepatitis compared to normal animals. The values of the fibrosis factor of the normal rat groups increased in all dosage groups (ND_1-ND_4, dosages from 2.00 to 40 g/kg), whereas their values of the cellular injury factor did not significantly increase. In the model rat groups, the values of the cellular injury factor of the first (MD_1, 2.00 g/kg) and second (MD_2, 5.40 g/kg) dosage groups decreased compared to the value of the untreated model group (M), whereas the values decreased by a smaller degree when the dosage was further increased. Although the values of the fibrosis factor of the MD_1 and MD_2 groups decreased slightly compared to the value of the M group, the values of the MD_3 (14.69 g/kg) and MD_4 (40.00 g/kg) groups shifted to an increasing trend with increasing dosage.

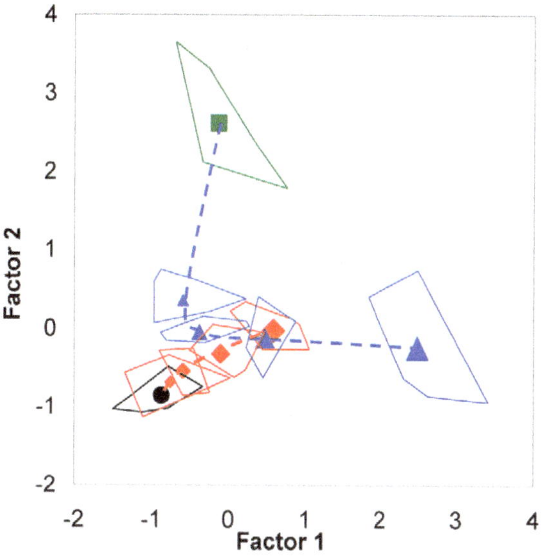

Figure 4. Dose-response relationships of rhubarb extract to both normal and model rats, as represented by a factor plot. The alteration pattern of the dose-response relationship between rhubarb extract and hepatic health in normal rats showed an almost linear variation: factor 1, considered in relation to fibrosis and called the "fibrosis factor", showed a notable increasing trend with increasing of dosage levels (ND_1-ND_4, dosages of 2.00, 5.40, 14.69 and 40.00 g kg^{-1}, respectively), whereas factor 2, considered in relation to cell membrane integrality and called the "cellular injury factor", revealed a nonsignificant increase. By contrast, the alteration pattern in the model rat groups assumed a parabolic shape with increasing dosages. The factor 1 values decreased in the MD_1 and MD_2 groups but decreased to a small degree when the dosage was further increased. The factor 2 values decreased slightly in the MD_1 and MD_2 groups and then shifted to a significant increasing trend with increasing dosages in the MD_3 and MD_4 groups. The center points of the different groups are labeled as follows: untreated normal rats group (N, ■ green square); normal rat groups treated with rhubarb extract at different dosages (ND_1-ND_4, ◆) (symbol size indicates dosage); untreated model rat group (M, ●); and model rat groups treated with rhubarb extract at different dosages (MD_1-MD_4, ▲ blue triangle) (symbol size indicates dosage). The border lines around the center points are presented for the range of original data points of the studied groups.

Table 3. Results of factor analysis after a varimax rotation[a].

Variable	Factor 1	Factor 2
AST	0.068	**0.910**
ALT	0.090	**0.901**
ALP	0.348	**0.620**
TP	0.448	**0.514**
GLO	**0.526**	**0.675**
TBIL	**0.685**	0.434
HA	**0.856**	0.264
TGF-β_1	**0.856**	0.121
LN	**0.896**	0.103
Eigenvalue	4.859	1.517
Cumulative proportion [b]	53.985	70.840
Suggested interpretation	Fibrosis	Cellular injury

ALT, serum alanine aminotransferase; AST, serum aspartate aminotransferase; AP, alkaline phosphatase; TBIL, total bile acids; TP, total protein; GLO, globulin; HA, hyaluronic acid; LN, laminin; TGF-β_1, transforming growth factor β_1.

[a] The loadings, eigenvalues, cumulative proportion of the total variance and a suggested interpretation are provided for the two factors. Only variables with loadings above 0.5 or below -0.5 were used in the interpretation (displayed in bold).

[b] The cumulative proportion is the cumulative proportion of the total variance in the data. Because the variables are standardized to a variance of 1, the total eigenvalue is equal to 9 (number of variables).

Discussion

It has been previously reported that the protective effect of rhubarb against CCl_4-induced liver lesions was largely attributed to the inhibition of the generation of free radicals and antioxidant activity. [32,33] The mechanism of CCl_4-induced liver injury is generally interpreted as follows: the compound is bioactivated by cytochrome P450 2E1 to the trichloromethyl free radical (•CCl_3) and then further converted to a peroxy radical (CCl_3O_2•), which leads to a chain reaction auto-oxidation of the fatty acids in the cytoplasmic membrane phospholipids causing functional and morphological changes to the cell membrane. [34] As a consequence, the cell membranes of hepatocytes become more permeable, and enzymes such as ALT and AST can leak out into the bloodstream, leading to increased levels of these enzymes in the blood. These increases reflect the degree of hepatocyte damage and necrosis [35] and vice versa. Therefore, it could be inferred that the pharmacological activity of rhubarb in treating liver injury is strongly related to its antioxidant effects via the protection of hepatic cells against free radical damage. This outcome manifested as a decrease in the cellular injury factor, (shown in Fig. 4), which was closely correlated with biomarkers such as ALT and AST (shown in Table 2).

The anti-oxidative effects [36] of rhubarb anthraquinone derivatives, along with their hepatoprotective effects, [11] have been reported. In addition, a series of tannin-related compounds with strong antioxidant effects have been identified in RE (see Supplementary Materials). In a previous report, the antioxidant activities of rhubarb tannins were verified. [37] Therefore, we believe that rhubarb tannins and anthraquinone derivatives may all contribute to the hepatoprotective effects of rhubarb against CCl_4-induced liver damage.

The hepatoprotective effect of rhubarb and its components has also been documented as antagonizing α-naphthylisothiocyanate (ANIT)-[38] and concanavalin A [39]- induced experimental liver injury. In a previous study, we found that free anthraquinones extracted from rhubarb, such as rhein and emodin, exhibited protective activity against ANIT-induced cholestatic liver injury by reducing the serum levels of glutamate-pyruvate transaminase, glutamic oxaloacetic transaminase and the serum total bilirubin, direct bilirubin, alkaline phosphatase, γ-glutamyltransferase and total bile acids. These effects were markedly different from the effects on CCl_4-induced liver injury. The morphological alterations induced by ANIT in rats, including the necrosis of hepatocytes and biliary epithelial cells, as well as neutrophil infiltration and sinusoid congestion, were also alleviated by concurrent intragastric administration of these free anthraquinones. [8] Some clinical evidence has also revealed a hepatoprotective effect of rhubarb against infantile cholestatic hepatitis[40] and acute icteric hepatitis [41]. The protective effect against CCl_4-induced liver damage reported in this study demonstrated only one aspect of the pharmacological potential of rhubarb to protect the liver. Although there is some evidence of the protective potential of this herb against liver injury due to multiple causes, the molecular mechanisms of this protection remain unclear. Rigorous clinical studies and in-depth experimental studies are needed to demonstrate rhubarb's hepatoprotective effects and mechanisms of action.

In our study, dose-dependent alterations of liver fibrosis associated with increases in the fibrosis factor were clearly observed in the rats in the normal groups (Figs 2 and 4). Although the occurrence of fibrosis of the liver tissues of normal rats that were treated with rhubarb has been reported infrequently, this phenomenon warrants further consideration. Elevation of TBIL, TP and GLO levels in serum have also been found in normal rat groups. These alterations usually occur along with hepatic impairment, indicating functional deterioration of the liver. Although the hepatoprotective effects of anthraquinone derivatives are well documented, it has also been reported that the total anthraquinone derivatives isolated from rhubarb show some hepatotoxic potential in rats in a six month-long experiment. [14] Therefore, the dose-response relationship between rhubarb anthraquinones and liver health warrants further investigation.

The alteration pattern of the fibrosis factor in the model rat groups assumed a parabolic shape with increasing dosages of RE (shown in Fig. 4). At lower dosages (MD_1, 2.00 g/kg and MD_2, 5.40 g/kg), rhubarb demonstrated some ameliorative effects on liver injury by decreasing the fibrosis caused by CCl_4; however, the fibrosis was aggravated rather than alleviated when the dosage was increased further (MD_3, 14.69 g/kg and MD_4, 40.00 g/kg). Therefore, we believe that the hepatotoxic potential of rhubarb is strongly related to liver fibrosis, although this effect is undetectable when the normal dosage recommended in the Chinese Pharmacopoeia (0.5 g/kg) is administered. [20]

The results of the factor analysis of biochemical indices indicated that the parallel histopathological changes arose coincidently. The vacuolar degeneration, and lymphocyte infiltration and fibrosis observed in the hepatocytes of CCl_4-treated rats were alleviated after treatment with RE, demonstrating the herb's effectiveness in protecting hepatocytes from the toxicant. However, the anti-fibrotic effect of RE that was observed in the lower dosage groups was reversed with further increases in the RE dosage. The dose-dependent hyperplasia of interstitial fibrous tissue was also observed in liver tissue sections from normal rats that were treated with RE, which was in accordance with the variations in the fibrosis factor.

A classical description of the understanding of such bidirectional effects of rhubarb and other herbal medicines, *You Gu Wu Yun*, was recorded in the Chinese Medical Treatise *Su Wen* (translated as *Plain Questions*, part of *The Yellow Emperor's Classic of Internal Medicine*), which was written 2,500 years ago.[42] The archaic and recondite wording of *You Gu Wu Yun* can be explained as follows. A drug will reveal its therapeutic effect when it is prescribed to patients with the correct indications; however, it may produce deleterious effects in both sick and healthy people as a result of incorrect indications. Another translation of the wording implies that the dosage of the drug is critical to its rational application in the clinic to balance the benefits and risks. Ancient Traditional Chinese Medicine (TCM) has effectively relied on the theory of *You Gu Wu Yun* as an important set of guidelines in the treatment of diseases and disorders. The dose-related bidirectional effect of TCM illustrated in this study supports the aforementioned theory. The pattern recognition approach proposed in this report opens an avenue to decode the ancient TCM theory and to elucidate its medical implications with the use of modern biochemical tools.

In conclusion, the findings of this study illustrate the bidirectional potential, both liver protection and hepatotoxicity, of rhubarb on CCl_4-treated and normal rats and demonstrate the feasibility of using a multivariate analysis approach factor analysis, to study the dose-response (therapeutic efficacy versus toxicity) relationships of traditional herbal medicines by revealing the underlying interrelationships within a number of functional bio-indices in a holistic manner. This study provides a paradigm for a better understanding and scientific assessment of the benefits and risks of herbal medicines to facilitate the rational clinical administration of these medicines.

Supporting Information

Figure S1 Chemical structures of the free anthraquinones in the rhubarb extract.
(TIF)

Figure S2 Chemical structures of the tannin-related compounds in the rhubarb extract.
(TIF)

Table S1 Identification of the chemical constituents in the rhubarb extract.
(DOC)

Table S2 The contents (%) of anthraquinones and tannins in the rhubarb extract.
(DOC)

Text S1 UPLC- ESI-MS/MS analysis.
(DOC)

Acknowledgments

We gratefully acknowledge Yuan-li Mao and her colleagues for performing biochemical analysis.

Author Contributions

Conceived and designed the experiments: XHX JBW. Performed the experiments: JBW HPZ WJK FF HJW. Analyzed the data: CJ JBW HPZ WJK YLZ LZ. Contributed reagents/materials/analysis tools: YLZ CJ. Wrote the paper: JBW YLZ HPZ DJL.

References

1. Medicines And Healthcare Products Regulatory Agency. *Polygonum multiflorum* and liver reactions. Available: http://www.mhra.gov.uk/Howweregulate/Medicines/Herbalmedicines/HerbalSafetyNews/Currentsafetyissues/CON2023590.
2. Mazzanti G, Battinelli L, Daniele C, Mastroianni CM, Lichtner M, et al. (2004) New case of acute hepatitis following the consumption of Shou Wu Pian, a Chinese Herbal product derived from *Polygonum multiflorum*. Ann Intern Med 140: W30.
3. Itoh S, Marutani K, Nishijima T, Matsuo S, Itabashi M (1995) Liver injuries induced by herbal medicine, Syo-saiko-to (xiao-chai-hu-tang). Digest Dis Sci 40: 1845–1848.
4. Vanderperren B, Rizzo M, Angenot L, Haufroid V, Jadoul M, et al. (2005) Acute liver failure with renal impairment related to the abuse of senna anthraquinone glycosides. Ann Pharmacother 39: 1353–1357.
5. Yuen MF, Tam S, Fung J, Wong DK, Wong BC, et al. (2006) Traditional Chinese medicine causing hepatotoxicity in patients with chronic hepatitis B infection: a 1-year prospective study. Aliment Pharmacol Ther 24: 1179–1186.
6. Chitturi S, Farrell GC (2000) Herbal hepatotoxicity: An expanding but poorly defined problem. J Gastroen Hepatol 15: 1093–1099.
7. World Health Organization (1999) WHO Monographs on Selected Medicinal Plants. Geneva: World Health Organization. pp 231–240.
8. Zhao YL, Wang JB, Zhou GD, Shan LM, Xiao XH (2009) Investigations of free anthraquinones from rhubarb against α- naphthylisothiocyanate- induced cholestatic liver injury in rats. Basic Clin Pharmacol Toxicol 104: 463–469.
9. Huang ZH, Dong YS, Ye WY (1997) Clinical observation on treatment of infantile cholestatic hepatitis syndrome by rhubarb. Chin J Integr Trad West Med 17: 459–461.
10. Wang GS (1985) Clinical and experimental study on the treatment of severe subacute hepatitis with traditional Chinese medicinal compounds. Chin J Integr Trad West Med 5: 329–331, 322.
11. Arosio B, Gagliano N, Fusaro LM, Parmeggiani L, Tagliabue J, et al. (2000) Aloe-Emodin quinone pretreatment reduces acute liver injury induced by carbon tetrachloride. Pharmacol Toxicol 87: 229–233.
12. Jin H, Sakaida I, Tsuchiya M, Okita K (2005) Herbal medicine Rhei rhizome prevents liver fibrosis in rat liver cirrhosis induced by a choline- deficient L-amino acid- defined diet. Life Sci 76: 2805–2816.
13. National Toxicology Program (2001) Technical report on the toxicology and carcinogenesis studies of emodin in F344/N rats and B6C3F1 mice. Series No. 493. NIH Publication No. 01-3952. U.S. Department of Health and Human Services, Public Health Service, National Institutes of Health, Research Triangle Park, NC.
14. Zhang LY, Jiang ZZ, Pu CH, Yan M (2004) Six- month oral toxicity study of total anthraquinone in radix et rhizoma rhei in SD rats. Chin J Biochem Pharm 25: 206–209.
15. Xu Y (2005) Clinical analysis of 30 cases of drug-induced liver injury by Chinese medicine. Modern J Integr Trad Chin West Med 14: 600–601.
16. Tian Y, Yang J, Lu JY (2008) Toxic effect of rhubarb overdose on mouse hepatocytes. Chin J Histochem Cytochem 17: 303–307.
17. Wang JB, Zhao YL, Xiao XH, Li HF, Zhao HP, et al. (2009) Assessment of the renal protection and hepatotoxicity of rhubarb extract in rats. J Ethnopharmacol 124: 18–25.
18. Wael ED (1997) Pattern recognition approaches in biomedical and clinical magnetic resonance spectroscopy: a review. NMR Biomed 10: 99–124.
19. Tafeit E, Möller R, Sudi K, Reibnegger G (2000) Artificial neural networks compared to factor analysis for low- dimensional classification of high-dimensional body fat topography data of healthy and diabetic subjects. Comput Biomed Res 33: 365–374.
20. (2005) Pharmacopoeia of the People's Republic of China, First Div. Beijing: China Chemical Industry Press. pp 17–18.
21. (2001) European Pharmacopoeia, 4th ed. Strasbourg: European Directorate for the Quality of Medicines, Council of Europe. 1858 p.
22. Japanese Pharmacopoeia, 15th ed (2006) Tokyo: Pharmaceutical and Food Safety Bureau, Ministry of Health, Labour and Welfare. 1344 p.
23. Ye M, Han J, Chen H, Zheng J, Guo D (2007) Analysis of phenolic compounds in rhubarbs using liquid chromatography coupled with electrospray ionization mass spectrometry. J Am Soc Mass Spectrom 18: 82–91.
24. Sharma S (1996) Applied Multivariate Techniques. New York: Wiley Press. pp 90–143.
25. Qin Y, Wang JB, Kong WJ, Zhao YL, Yang HY, et al. (2011) The diarrheogenic and antidiarrhoeal bidirectional effects of rhubarb and its potential mechanism. J Ethnopharmacol 133(3): 1096–1102.
26. Leung TF, Wong GW, Ko FW, Lam CW, Fok TF (2005) Clinical and atopic parameters and airway inflammatory markers in childhood asthma: a factor analysis. Thorax 60: 822–826.
27. Cattell RB (1966) The Scree test for the number of factors. Multivariate Behav Res 1: 245–276.
28. Thoefner MB, Ersbøll AK, Jensen AL, Hesselholt M (2001) Factor analysis of the interrelationships between clinical variables in horses with colic. Prev Vet Med 48: 201–214.
29. Tong Z, Chen R, Alt DS, Kemper S, Perbal B, et al. (2009) Susceptibility to liver fibrosis in mice expressing a connective tissue growth factor transgene in hepatocytes. Hepatology 50: 939–947.
30. Miele L, Forgione A, La Torre G, Vero V, Cefalo C, et al. (2009) Serum levels of hyaluronic acid and tissue metalloproteinase inhibitor-1 combined with age predict the presence of nonalcoholic steatohepatitis in a pilot cohort of subjects with nonalcoholic fatty liver disease. Transl Res 154: 194–201.
31. Attallah AM, Toson EA, Shiha GE, Omran MM, Abdel-Aziz MM, et al. (2007) Evaluation of serum procollagen aminoterminal propeptide III, laminin, and hydroxyproline as predictors of severe fibrosis in patients with chronic hepatitis C. J Immunoassay Immunochem 28: 199–211.
32. Liu L, Mei QB, Li BL, Zhou SY, Cao ZX (2001) Antioxidation of *Tanguficum* Maxim polysaccharide on acute liver injury mice. J Fourth Mil Med Univ 22: 530–533.
33. Wan SH, Ding YQ, Pu XH, Guo L, Kang TG (2006) Protective effect of hydroxy- anthroquinones from *Rheum Palmatum* L. on acute liver injure of rats induced by CCl_4. Chinese Pharmacological Bulletin 22: 1405–1406.
34. Jeong HG (1999) Inhibition of cytochrome P450 2E1 expression by oleanolic acid: hepatoprotective effects against carbon tetrachloride- induced hepatic injury. Toxicol Lett 105: 215–222.
35. Napoli J, Prentice D, Niinami C, Bishop GA, Desmond P, et al. (1997) Sequential increases in the intrahepatic expression of epidermal growth factor, basic fibroblast growth factor, and transforming growth factor beta in a bile duct ligated rat model of cirrhosis. Hepatology 26: 624–633.
36. Luo ZY, Huang X, Bao GR (2007) ESR study on the scavenging effects of the main ingredients in *Rheum palmatum* L. on superoxide anion radical. Chin Arch Tradit Chin Med 25: 612–614.
37. Iizuka A, Iijima OT, Kondo K, Itakura H, Yoshie F, et al. (2004) Evaluation of Rhubarb using antioxidative activity as an index of pharmacological usefulness. J Ethnopharmacol 91: 89–94.
38. Ding Y, Zhao L, Mei H, Zhang SL, Huang ZH, et al. (2008) Exploration of Emodin to treat alpha-naphthylisothiocyanate-induced cholestatic hepatitis via anti-inflammatory pathway. Eur J Pharmacol 590(1-3): 377–386.
39. Mase A, Makino B, Tsuchiya N, Yamamoto M, Kase Y, et al. (2010) Active ingredients of traditional Japanese (kampo) medicine, inchinkoto, in murine concanavalin A-induced hepatitis. J Ethnopharmacol 127(3): 742–749.
40. Huang ZH, Dong YS, Ye WY (1997) Clinical observation on treatment of infantile cholestatic hepatitis syndrome by rhubarb. Zhongguo Zhong Xi Yi Jie He Za Zhi 17(8): 459–461.
41. Wu CX (1984) A preliminary study on the effect of a single Rheum officinale in heavy doses in the treatment of acute icteric hepatitis. Zhong Xi Yi Jie He Za Zhi 4(2): 88–89.
42. Ni M (1995) The Yellow Emperor's Classic of Medicine: A New Translation of the Neijing Suwen with Commentary. Boston: Shambhala.

7

A Review of Potential Harmful Interactions between Anticoagulant/Antiplatelet Agents and Chinese Herbal Medicines

Hsin-Hui Tsai[1,2], Hsiang-Wen Lin[1,2,3]*, Ying-Hung Lu[1], Yi-Ling Chen[1], Gail B. Mahady[4]

1 School of Pharmacy and Graduate Institute, College of Pharmacy, China Medical University, Taichung, Taiwan, **2** Department of Pharmacy, China Medical University Hospital, Taichung, Taiwan, **3** Department of Pharmacy Administration, College of Pharmacy, University of Illinois at Chicago, Chicago, Illinois, United States of America, **4** Department of Pharmacy Practice, College of Pharmacy, PAHO/WHO Collaborating Centre for Traditional Medicine, University of Illinois at Chicago, Chicago, Illinois, United States of America

Abstract

Background: The risks attributed to drug-herb interactions, even when known, are often ignored or underestimated, especially for those involving anti-clotting drugs and Chinese medicines. The aim of this study was to structurally search and evaluate the existing evidence-based data associated with potential drug interactions between anticoagulant/antiplatelet drugs and Chinese herbal medicines (CHMs) and evaluate the documented mechanisms, consequences, and/or severity of interactions.

Methodology and Findings: Information related to anticoagulant/antiplatelet drug-CHM interactions was retrieved from eight interaction-based textbooks, four web resources and available primary biomedical literature. The primary literature searches were conducted in English and/or Chinese from January 2000 through December 2011 using the secondary databases (e.g., PubMed, Airiti Library, China Journal full-text database). The search terms included the corresponding medical subject headings and key words. Herbs or natural products not used as a single entity CHM or in Chinese Medicinal Prescriptions were excluded from further review. The corresponding mechanisms and severity ratings of interactions were retrieved using *MicroMedex®*, *Lexicomp®* and *Natural Medicines Comprehensive Database®*. Finally, we found 90 single entity CHMs contributed to 306 documented drug-CHM interactions. A total of 194 (63.4%) interactions were verified for its evidence describing possible mechanisms and severity. Of them, 155 interactions (79.9%) were attributable to pharmacodynamic interactions, and almost all were rated as moderate to severe interactions. The major consequences of these interactions were increased bleeding risks due to the additive anticoagulant or antiplatelet effects of the CHMs, specifically danshen, dong quai, ginger, ginkgo, licorice, and turmeric.

Conclusions/Significance: Conventional anticoagulants and antiplatelet drugs were documented to have harmful interactions with some commonly used single entity CHMs. For those patients who are taking conventional anti-clotting medications with CHMs for cardiovascular or cerebrovascular diseases, the potential risks of increased bleeding due to drug-CHM interactions should not be ignored.

Editor: Dermot Cox, Royal College of Surgeons, Ireland

Funding: This study was fully supported by the Committee on Chinese medicine and Pharmacy, Department of Health, Executive Yuan, Taiwan, R.O.C. (grant number: CCMP99-RD-016) and partially supported by National Science Council (grant number: NSC 99-2320-B-039 -031 -MY3). Those founders have no role in study design, data collection, and analysis, decision to publish, or preparation of the manuscript.

Competing Interests: The authors have declared that no competing interests exist.

* E-mail: hsiangwl@mail.cmu.edu.tw

Introduction

Ischemic heart disease and stroke are the two primary causes of death worldwide, accounting for 24% of all deaths reported in 2008 [1]. Anticoagulants and antiplatelet drugs are important standard therapies used to prevent clot formation in the treatment and prevention of cardiovascular and cerebrovascular diseases [2]. However, most anticoagulant and antiplatelet agents have drug interactions with a variety of other medications, foods, and dietary supplements [3,4]. A systematic review published in 2008 reported that medications with anticoagulant or antiplatelet activity are most likely to have interactions with herbal medicines [5]. Specifically, those patients given anticoagulant agents are at a higher risk of suffering from potentially harmful drug interactions, compared to other cardiovascular drugs, when co-administered with herbal medicines [6].

The use of complementary and alternative medicine (CAM), including herbal medicines, is widespread and has increased worldwide over the last decade [7,8]. A systematic review of CAM found that the prevalence of CAM use varied widely from 9% to 65% [9]. Nearly 40% of patients with cardiovascular disease or stroke had used CAM therapies concomitantly with their prescribed medications [10,11]. Traditional Chinese Medicine (TCM) is one of the dominant forms of CAM for many Asian populations [7,12,13], including those who migrated to western countries. A substantial percentage of Asian patients were likely to use TCM in combination with the conventional medicines [14–17]. For instance, 13% of patients using anticoagulant or antiplatelet agents were also prescribed concentrated CHMs concomitantly in a Taiwanese population-based study [17].

To date, there is very limited documented information about potential prescription drug interactions with CHMs. Considerable proportions of clinical practitioners or patients underreport their use of natural health products, including CHMs [18]. The majority of physicians and professional trainees have limited training on herbal adverse events, toxicities, and drug interactions [19]. The lack of training and education may be associated with a reduced recognition of potential drug-herb interactions, specifically their occurrence and associated adverse events. While patients taking anticoagulant/antiplatelet drugs are more likely to be exposed to potential drug-herb interactions (i.e., increased risks of bleeding [20]), the aim of this study was to systematically review the available published evidence-based data and biomedical reports associated with drug interactions between anticoagulant/antiplatelet drugs and CHMs, and further to evaluate the documented mechanisms, consequences, and/or severity of interactions.

Materials and Methods

Evidence retrieval and literature search

The evidence regarding "harmful" interactions between anticoagulant/antiplatelet drugs and herbal medications used in TCM (in terms of Chinese herbal medicine [CHM]) was the main focus and extracted from eight interaction-based textbooks [21–28], four web resources [29–32], and available primary biomedical literature sources. In this review, we defined CHM as the same definition derived from the web site of National Center for Complementary and Alternative Medicine and originally cited from Chinese Materia Medica [33]. The search of primary articles was conducted in four English and three Chinese secondary databases, including MEDLINE, PubMed, EMBASE, Cochrane Library, Airiti Library, Index to Taiwan Periodical Literature System, and the China Journal full-text database. The search terms in these databases included the corresponding medical subject headings (MeSH terms) and key words as follows: 'herb drug interactions'; 'anticoagulants' OR 'antiplatelet drugs' OR 'warfarin' OR 'heparin' OR 'aspirin' OR 'clopidogrel' OR 'dipyridamole' OR 'ticlopidine' AND 'Traditional Chinese Medicine' OR 'Chinese medication' OR 'herbal medicine' OR 'phytotherapy' AND 'interaction.' The searches were restricted to either the English or Chinese language during 2000 to 2011 (from January 2000 through December 2011). The articles were selected based on the title and abstract. The selected articles were retrieved independently by two authors (YLC, YHL), and then validated by the other two authors (HHT, HWL). Specifically, all retrieved literature were selected regardless of types of study, i.e., animal studies, clinical trials, observational studies, or review articles. Those in vitro studies or literature without interaction reports, or corresponding studies about pure compounds (but not for single entity CHMs), were excluded.

Evidence extraction and review

Initially, any level of evidence-based interactions, as long as it was retrieved from the aforementioned books, web sites, or primary literature, between the anticoagulant/antiplatelet agents and any natural products or herbs (i.e., either being classified as CHMs or not) was first extracted and documented. However, animal-derived medications used in TCM were not included. Then, we used a standardized data abstraction checklist on *Excel*® spreadsheet to extract all relevant data, including common name, scientific name and/or binomial source, plant parts, dose, route of administration, drug name, consequence of interactions, and evidence resources, etc, if they were available. Data for all anticoagulant/antiplatelet agents was extracted regardless of belonging to a drug class or an individual drug. The anticoagulants were composed of heparin and warfarin while antiplatelet agents included aspirin, clopidogrel, dipyridamole and ticlopidine. All relevant data in the literature was extracted and compiled by two of the authors (YLC, YHL), and then validated by the other two authors (HHT, HWL). To cross-validate the retrieved and reviewed information, we conducted the focus group review and discussions. A focus group included five experienced pharmacists practicing in either Western medicine or Chinese medicine on a daily basis in Taiwanese hospitals. Any disagreements about classifications and information conflict were resolved by consensus. Specifically, all of the members in the focus group were trained in both Western and Chinese medicines in a School of Pharmacy and/or their master graduate programs. They all have more than 15 years of experience practicing in TCM pharmacy or clinical pharmacy services in hospitals that provide medical services with both Western and TCM medicines. None of these members were authors.

Data management and analysis

Next, the following review and analysis particularly focused on those single entity CHMs commonly listed in Chinese Medicine books, including the Taiwan Herbal Pharmacopoeia (THP) [34], Chinese Medicinal Herbs Preparation [35], and Chinese Materia Medica [36]. Thus, those natural products or herbs that were not documented in the aforementioned books and/or any combination of Chinese Medicinal Prescriptions, which were listed in some ancient TCM books, were excluded for further analyses. Moreover, those single entity CHMs included for further review were verified by two experienced pharmacists who were members of the focus group.

To obtain proof about clinical significance of interactions, we identified and verified the severity ratings and possible mechanisms of each interaction using three well-known interactions databases (*MicroMedex*® [37], Lexi-Interact in *Lexicomp*® [38], or "Natural Product/Drug Interaction Checker" in *Natural Medicines Comprehensive Database*® *(NMCD*®) [39]). Because of the various definitions of severity ratings among these three databases, we compiled the rating schemes and categorized the severity of each interaction into six types in this review: "contraindicated," "major," "moderate," "minor," "no interaction," and "no available information for the item." The comparisons of severity rating definitions in different databases with this review were listed in Table 1. Accordingly, the mechanisms for interactions were also categorized into pharmacokinetics, pharmacodynamics, pharmacokinetics plus pharmacodynamics, and unknown based upon the records from these three databases. All of the related data was compiled and managed using the *Excel*® spreadsheets. Last, the descriptive analyses were performed to explore the frequency and proportion of the retrieved evidence associated with the interaction numbers, the corresponding types of retrieved mechanisms and severity ratings of interactions.

Result

Literature search and evidence retrieval

A total of 154 articles were selected from the initial 550 retrieved literature reports based on their relevance to the purpose

Table 1. The comparisons of severity rating definitions in different databases with current review.

	MicroMedex®	Lexicomp®	NMCD®	Current review
Contraindicated	Do not use combination; contraindicated.	-	-	Interactions with severity rated as "contraindicated" according to MicroMedex®.
Major	Combination may cause life-threatening damage and/or need medical intervention to prevent severe adverse effect.	Effects may result in death, hospitalization, permanent injury, or therapeutic failure.	Do not use combination; contraindicated; strongly discourage patients from using this combination; a serious adverse outcome could occur.	Interactions with severity rated as "major" in any of the three databases.
Moderate	Combination may cause worsen the patient's condition and/or need to change the therapy.	Medical intervention needed to treat effects; effects do not meet criteria for Major.	Use cautiously or avoid combination; warn patients that a significant interaction or adverse outcome could occur.	Interactions rated as "moderate" and without "major" score in any of these databases.
Minor	Do not need to change the therapy.	Effects would be considered tolerable in most cases; no need for medical intervention.	Be aware that there is a chance of an interaction; advise patients to watch for warning signs of a potential interaction.	Interactions rated as "minor" and without "moderate" or "major" score in any of these databases.
No interaction	-	-	-	There was no documented interaction between the medication and the single entity CHM
No available documented information for the item	-	-	-	There was no available information about the single entity CHM in these databases.

NMCD: Natural Medicines Comprehensive Database.

of review. After thorough evaluation and analysis, 98 articles with full text (75 review articles [5,6,40–112], and 23 primary studies, i.e., 4 animal studies [113–116], 4 clinical trials [117–120], and 15 observational studies [20,121–134]) were included for further evaluation (Figure 1). The summaries of retrieved primary literature are listed in Table 2, while the summaries of retrieved review articles are listed in Appendix S1. The retrieved data missing information concerning the common name, scientific name, plant source, plant parts, and dose for the natural products/herbs or CHM were excluded from Table 2 and Appendix S1, but may be accessed upon specific request to the authors.

Initially, there were 417 interactions in total obtained from the aforementioned evidence-based resources. Of them, 235 interactions between anticoagulant/antiplatelet agents and specific single CHMs were extracted for further evaluation. After expanding the interactions to individual medications from the different drug classes, a total of 306 interactions between distinct anticoagulant/antiplatelet agents and single entity CHMs were identified. Warfarin and aspirin accounted for the majority of documented, evidenced-based interactions with single entity CHMs (Figure 2). Overall, 90 distinct single entity CHMs contributed to the 306 documented interactions.

Severity rating and mechanisms upon availability in three databases

Of the 306 interactions between distinct anticoagulant/antiplatelet agents and single entity CHMs, 203 (66.3%), 292 (95.4%), and 99 (32.3%) drug-CHM interactions were retrieved with some relevant information about interactions from *MicroMedex®*, *NMCD®*, and *Lexicomp®*, respectively. However, only 62 (20.2%), 172 (56.2%), and 83 (27.1%) of these interactions in *MicroMedex®*, *NMCD®*, and *Lexicomp®*, respectively, contained identifiable severity ratings and interaction mechanisms (Figure 3). Overall, a total of 194 (63.4%) interactions were found to have severity ratings and mechanisms in at least one of these databases. While 50 interactions with information in *MicroMedex®* (80.6%) were categorized as the moderate interactions, 132 interactions documented in *NMCD®* (76.7%) were classified as moderate. However, all of the 83 documented interactions in *Lexicomp®* were found to have major drug-CHM interactions (Figure 3). Consequently, of all 194 interactions being identified with the severity rating in any of the three databases, only 29 (15.0%) were found in all of the three databases, 65 (33.5%) could be identified in two databases, while more than half (100, 51.5%) were documented in only one database.

Of those identifiable mechanisms for interactions, the majority (155, 79.9%) were attributable to pharmacodynamic-related mechanisms. 8.3% were attributed to pharmacokinetic-related mechanisms and 11.3% were the results of both pharmacodynamic and pharmacokinetic mechanisms. Most of the pharmacodynamic-related interactions were due to the additive anticoagulant/antiplatelet effect of the single entity CHM. For example, some CHMs, i.e., clove (*Eugenia caryophyllata*), cat's claw (*Uncaria tomentosa*), and ginger (*Zingiber officinale*), were reported to inhibit cyclooxygenase activity, platelet aggregation, and thromboxane synthetase activity, respectively [37,39]. Most of these potential interactions have not been documented in clinical practice. In contrast, a few documented single entity CHMs with pharmacodynamic-related interactions causing decreased anticoagulant effects were reported in the literature. For example, alfalfa (*Medicago sativa*) and green tea (*Camellia sinensis*) may antagonize the anticoagulant effects of warfarin due to the presence of vitamin K in these products [37,39]. As for the documented pharmacokinetic-related interactions, the majority were due to the inhibition

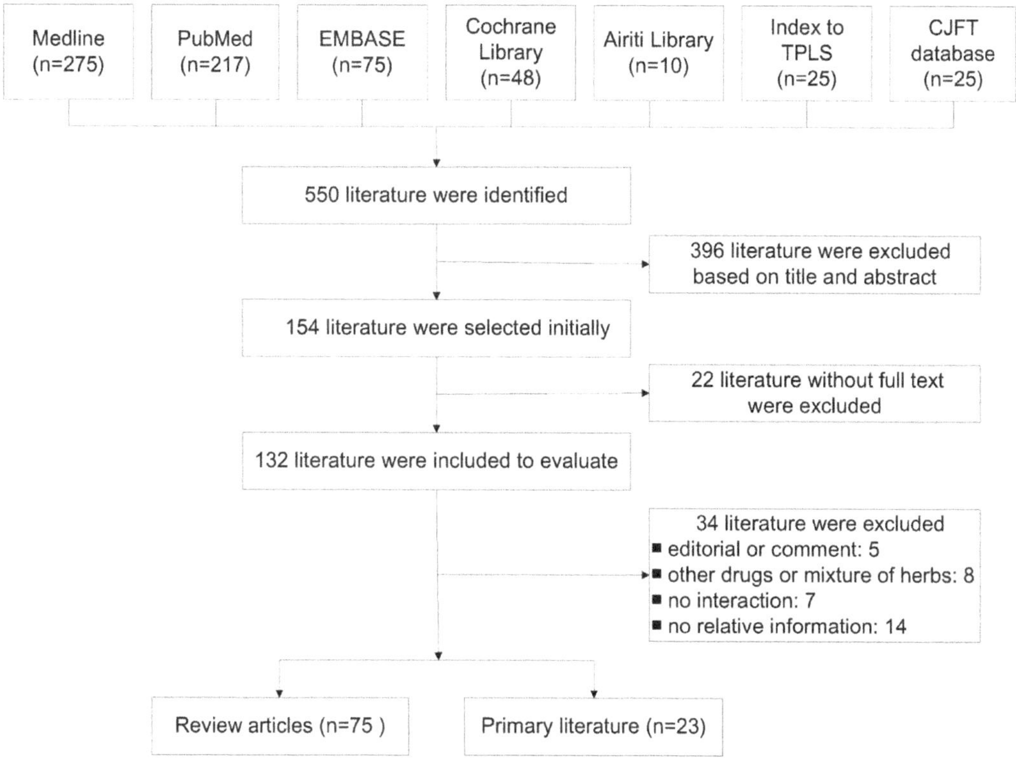

Figure 1. Flow chart of primary literature search. TPLS: Taiwan Periodical Literature System; CJFT: China Journals Full-text.

of warfarin or clopidogrel metabolism *via* the Cytochrome P450 (CYP) pathway, including CYP 1A2, 3A4, and 2C9. For example, dandelion (*Taraxacum officinale*), bitter orange (*Citrus aurantium*), and milk thistle (*Silybum marianum*) were reported to inhibit CYP1A2, 3A4, and 2C9, respectively. Therefore, these herbal products may inhibit warfarin or clopidogrel catabolism, and result in an increase in their anticoagulation/antiplatelet activities [39]. Similarly, ginkgo (*Ginkgo biloba*), red clover (*Trifolium pratense*), and Siberian ginseng (*Eleutherococcus senticosus*) were documented to inhibit all of these three CYP enzymes, thus similar effects on the anticoagulation action of warfarin or clopidogrel may be expected [37,39].

Consequences of drug–CHM Interactions

Of the 90 interactions that involve a single entity CHM, the majority would result in an increased risk of bleeding when used in combination with anticoagulants or antiplatelet agents (Table 3). For instance, commonly used CHMs including danshen (*Salvia miltiorrhiza*), dong quai (*Angelica sinensis*), ginger (*Zingiber officinale*), and licorice (*Glycyrrhizae uralensis*) were documented to have major interactions with anticoagulants or antiplatelet drugs. The combinations causing major interactions may cause life-threatening damage and/or severe adverse events. Thus, we strongly discourage patients and clinicians from using these combinations [37–39]. Specifically, celery, a functional food and classified as a CHM in the Chinese Materia Medica, is reported to increase bleeding in Philp's book and a few review articles and was then verified in the *Lexicomp*® record [26,81,82,85,94]. There were no published primary data that describe the rationale or potential mechanism of this interaction. Therefore, interpretation of the data related to celery should be cautious.

Furthermore, a few reports showed that single entity CHMs may decrease the effectiveness of anticoagulant/antiplatelet agents. Agrimony (*Agrimonia eupatoria*), myrrh (*Commiphora myrrha*), and St. John's wort (*Hypericum perforatum*) were documented to result in a decreased effectiveness of warfarin [21,22,24,25,72,135], while pepper (*Piper nigrum*) and cannabis (*Cannabis sativa*) were reported to reduce the antiplatelet efficacy of aspirin [28]. Nevertheless, we also noted the conflicting consequences of interactions reported in the different evidence resources. Some evidence suggested that alfalfa, Asian ginseng (*Panax ginseng*), green tea, and Siberian ginseng may reduce the anticoagulant effects of anticoagulant/antiplatelet agents [5,37,73,74], while some published data suggested that these single entity CHMs might increase the risk of bleeding episodes if they were used concurrently with anticoagulants and antiplatelet drugs [38,39,73].

Discussion

In this review, the potential interactions between anticoagulant/antiplatelet drugs and single entity CHMs were analyzed and evaluated based on retrievable and published evidence. We found 90 commonly used single entity CHMs (such as danshen, dong quai, ginger, and licorice) were involved in 306 evidence-based drug interactions with anticoagulant and/or antiplatelet drugs. Warfarin and aspirin were the two drugs reported to have the largest numbers of documented interactions with the greatest number of single entity CHMs. Most of these interactions were moderate to severe and attributable to pharmacodynamic mechanisms. The majority of these interactions were found to increase the risks of bleeding.

In the United States and Singapore, 10–20% of patients used herbal therapies or CHMs when using prescribed anticoagulant or

Table 2. Summary of the included primary literature and the retrieved relevant information about natural products or herbs (including CHMs).

Clinical trials

Reference	Natural products/ herbs (including CHMs)	Dose schedule of Natural products/herbs (including CHMs)	Medication	Study design	Observed/measured outcomes
Abdul 2010 [117]	Commercial products of echinacea (oral)	14 days	Warfarin (oral)	Open-label, randomized, three-treatment, cross-over study	INR, platelet activity, Warfarin concentration
Jiang 2006 [118]	Commercial products of St John's wort, Asian ginseng, ginkgo, or ginger (oral)	7 or 14 days	Warfarin (oral)	Two randomized, open-label, controlled, crossover studies	INR, Warfarin concentration
Jiang 2004 [119	Commercial products of St John's wort, ginseng (oral)	7 days or 14 days	Warfarin (oral)	Open-label, three-way crossover randomized study	Platelet aggregation, INR, Warfarin protein binding, Warfarin concentration
Yuan 2004 [120]	Root of American ginseng (oral)	3 weeks	Warfarin (oral)	Randomized, double-blind, placebo-controlled trial.	INR, Warfarin concentration

Animal studies

Reference	Natural products/ herbs (including CHMs)	Preparation of Natural products/herbs (including CHMs)	Medication	Animal model	Observed/measured outcomes
Kuo 2006 [113]	Dried roots of danshen	Ethyl acetate extracts	7-Hydroxywarfarin	Mice	The effect on CYP
Li 2010 [114]	Dried fruits of danggui and honghua	Aqueous extracts	Clopidogrel	Rat	Bleeding time and hematology parameters
Makino 2002 [115]	Commercial product of Kangen-Karyu	Aqueous extracts	Warfarin	Rat	Plasma concentration, prothrombin time, bleeding time
Wu 2010 [116]	Commercial product of danshen	Ethyl acetate extracts	Warfarin	Rat	Pharmacokinetics parameters

Observational studies

Reference	Natural products/herbs (including CHMs)	Medication	Study design	Population (number of participants)	Observed/measured outcomes
Blalock 2009 [121]	Herbs and natural products	Conventional medication	Population-based epidemiological study	Data from Johnston County Osteoarthritis Project (n = 2523)	Prevalence of exposure to potential interactions
Bush 2007 [122]	Herbal and dietary substances	General	Survey	Outpatients from clinics (n = 804)	The rate of potential and observed adverse herb-drug interactions
Canter 2004 [123]	Herbal and nutritional supplements	General	Self-completed survey	Elderly outpatients (n = 271)	Associated risks of negative interactions with prescription drugs
Chan 2011 [124]	Ginkgo biloba	Antiplatelet or anticoagulant agents	Retrospective population based study	Combination users of ginkgo and antiplatelet or anticoagulant agents (n = 3579 or 15397)	The prevalence and frequency of co-prescription, the relative risk of hemorrhage associated with combination
Chan 2011 [125]	Herbs	Warfarin	Survey	Patients with nonvalvular atrial fibrillation (n = 250)	Effect of concomitant herbal intake on anticoagulation control
Charrois 2007 [126]	Natural health products	General	Survey	Community pharmacists (n = 132)	Community pharmacists' knowledge of interactions
Clauson 2008 [127]	St. John's wort	General	Evaluation of label	-	Identification of labeling of 8 clinically relevant safety issues
Dergal 2002 [128]	Herbal medicines	Prescription and over-the-counter drugs	Survey	Older adults (≥65 years) attending a memory clinic (n = 195)	The frequency of potential interactions between herbal medicines and conventional drug therapies.
Goldman 2008 [129]	Natural health products	General	Survey	Parents and patients 0 to 18 years at a large pediatric emergency department (n = 1804)	The frequency of concurrent use and potential interactions

Table 2. Cont.

Observational studies

Reference	Natural products/herbs (including CHMs)	Medication	Study design	Population (number of participants)	Observed/measured outcomes
Rogers 2001 [130]	Herbs	General	Survey	Emergency department patients with heart disease, diabetes, psychiatric disorders, and/or hypertension (n = 944)	Prevalence and occurrence of sever herb-drug interactions.
Saw 2006 [20]	Herbs	Antiplatelet/anti coagulant drugs	Cross-sectional survey	Patients from cardiology, neurology, infectious and nephrology wards (n = 250)	Assessing the use of herbal medicines in medical patients that may interact with antiplatelet or anticoagulant therapy
Segal 2006 [131]	Matricaria chamomilla	Warfarin	Case report	70-year-old woman	-
Shalansky 2007 [132]	Complementary and alternative medicine	Warfarin	Prospective, longitudinal study	Adults prescribed warfarin for an expected duration of at least 4 months (n = 171)	Risk factors for bleeding events and supratherapeutic INR
Su 2010 [133]	Shengmai-yin	Warfarin	Case report	A 71-year-old man	-
Lai 2010 [134]	Chinese herbal medicines	Warfarin	Case-crossover study	Warfarin users from database (n = 4211)	Causal inference of potential interactions

CYP: cytochrome P450; VKORC1: vitamin K epoxide reductase complex subunit 1; INR: international normalized ratio.

antiplatelet medications for cardiovascular diseases or stroke [10,11]. A survey also showed that one in five patients in Malaysia who took anticoagulant or antiplatelet drugs, also concurrently used herbal therapies [20]. While the use of TCM is prevalent among Asian populations [12,13], there is also an increasing trend of using TCM in Western countries. Thus, it is necessary that clinicians be aware of these drug-CHMs interactions in order to effectively manage those patients who are using anticoagulant/antiplatelet drugs with the listed CHMs.

In this review, the majority of documented interactions were rated as "major or severe" in scale. However, the actual consequences of concurrent use might be changed depending on the used medications, dose levels, binomial source, plant parts, and/or route of administration of CHMs, in addition to the patients' characteristics (such as genetic differences and dietary habits), their use patterns, and combinations of single CHMs and/or Chinese Medicinal Prescriptions (based on TCM theory). As for the safety and effectiveness of using anticoagulants and antiplatelets, health care providers need to be more judicious in counseling their patients regarding the possibility of interactions between these drugs and herbal remedies or CHMs. If concurrent use is unavoidable, then health care providers should closely monitor patients for potential adverse events associated with these possible interactions (e.g., increased international normalized ratio, bleeding).

In fact, the interactions between herbal remedies or CHMs and drugs are often more complex due to the multiple ingredients found in all single entity CHMs [87,94] and their binomial source, plant parts, dose, quality, preparation and/or route of administration [54]. Again, the likelihood of drug-CHM interactions may be different when using combinations of several single entity CHMs or those Chinese Medicinal Prescriptions. In particular, Chinese Medicinal Prescriptions (combined TCM medicines based on the theory of TCM) are sometimes the first line of therapy in Asian countries [136,137]. For instance, Jia Wei Hiaxo Yao San is commonly used for anxiety, irritability, and depression, and is one of the most frequently used Chinese Medicinal Prescriptions in Taiwan. This well known ancient Chinese herbal formula is generally used for liver Qi stagnation but contains at least ten distinct entity of CHMs [137], including dong quai, ginger, and licorice, which are documented to have major interactions with anticoagulant or antiplatelet drugs [37–39]. Therefore, those patients using Jia Wei Hiaxo Yao San might encounter higher bleeding risks due to the occurrence of significant major interactions. In this case, health care professionals could more aggressively take appropriate actions to prevent them from causing serious life threatening adverse events in their patients if they were aware of such potential risks.

In this review, we also found that the major documented mechanisms of interactions between anticoagulant/antiplatelet drugs and CHMs were attributable to their pharmacodynamic interactions, especially due to additive anticoagulant or antiplatelet effects. Many of the commonly used CHMs such as clove, danshen, ginger, and licorice are documented to have intrinsic anticoagulant or antiplatelet properties [85,138]. However, these blood-activating or stasis-resolving CHMs (e.g., danshen, and dong quai) are widely used in TCM for the treatment of cardiovascular or cerebrovascular diseases. Although some clinical studies have been conducted to investigate the effects of these CHMs on stroke or coronary diseases [139,140], further large scale, rigorous clinical trials are needed to confirm the benefits and risks of using these CHMs. With limited robust evidence and clinical trials supporting the use of CHMs, it is crucial for physicians and pharmacy practitioners to educate their patients on why they need to disclose their concurrent use of conventional medications and CAM, including CHMs, especially for those patients who are taking anticoagulant or antiplatelet drugs.

Currently, there is no single comprehensive database to identify the facts of drug-CHM interactions, levels of evidence sufficiency, corresponding mechanism, and/or clinical significance. Instead, we utilized three commonly used natural products or drug interaction-related databases to identify and verify the information

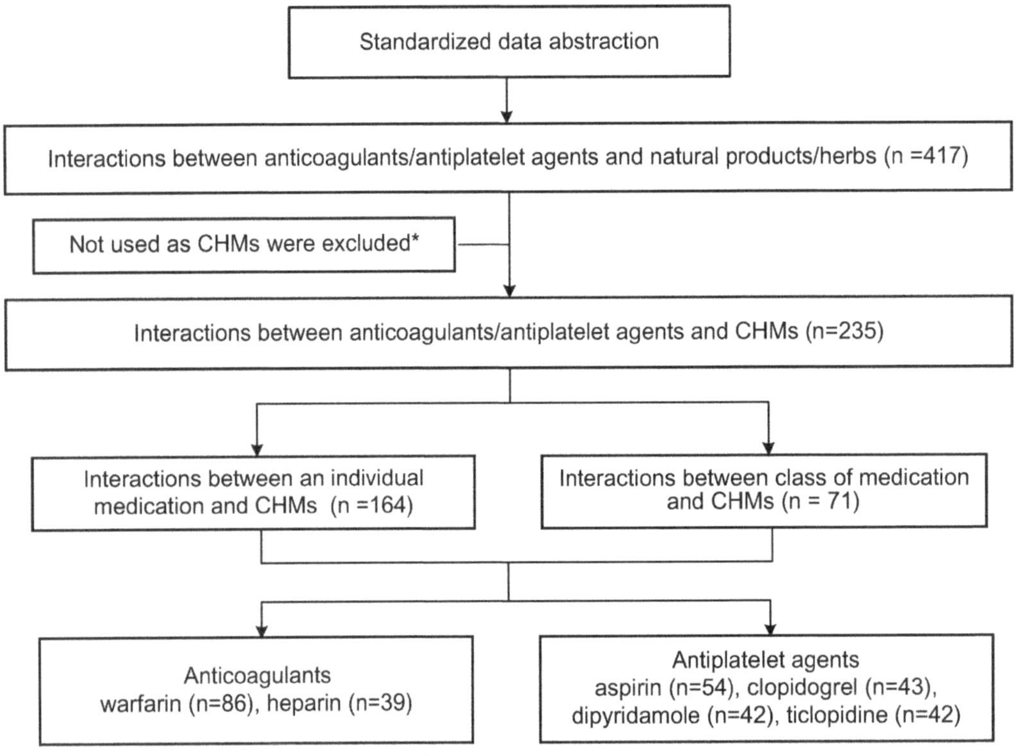

Figure 2. Retrieved findings of interactions between anticoagulant/antiplatelet agents and single Chinese herbal medicines. * Natural products or herbs which were not identified in the Taiwan Herbal Pharmacopoeia, Chinese Medicinal Herbs Preparation, or Chinese Materia Medica were excluded. CHMs: Chinese herbal medicines.

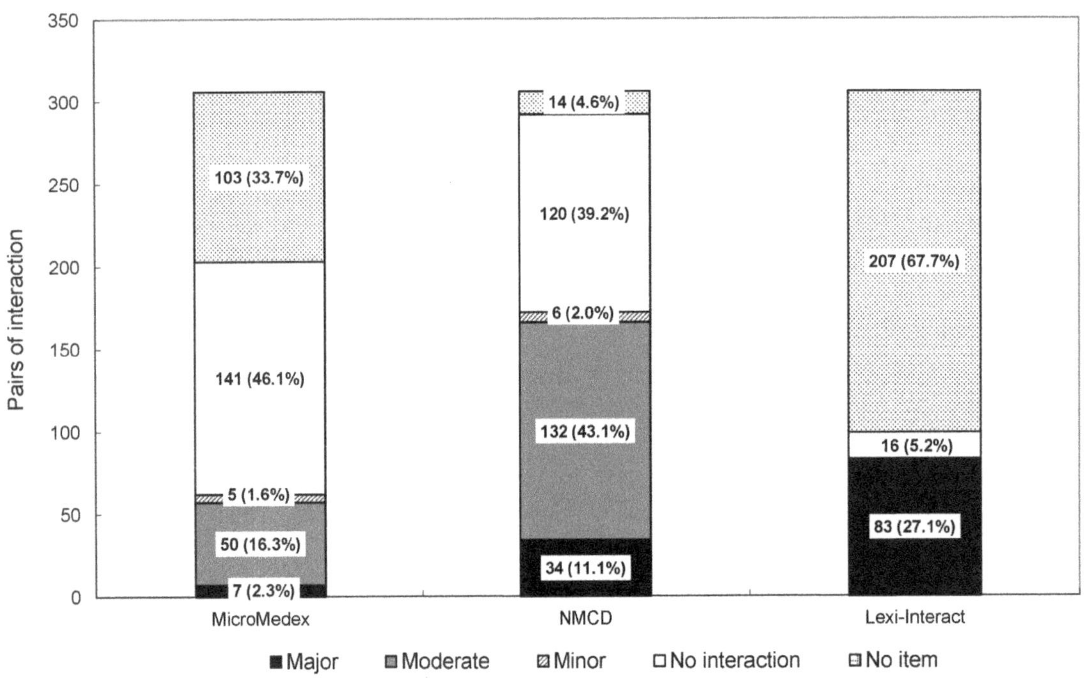

Figure 3. Documented severity ratings of interactions between distinct anticoagulant/antiplatelet agents and single Chinese herbal medicines. The total interactions between distinct anticoagulant/antiplatelet agents and single CHMs were 306. The classification of "No interaction" meant that there is no interaction between the medication and the single CHMs, while "No item" meant that there was no available information about the single CHMs in the database. NMCD: Natural Medicines Comprehensive Database.

Table 3. Documented interactions between anticoagulant/antiplatelet drugs and Chinese herbal medicine, [a] which might increase the risks of bleeding.

Severity rating [b]	CHM documented to increase bleeding risks of the six anticoagulant/antiplatelet drugs	CHM documented to increase bleeding risks of at least one of the six anticoagulant/antiplatelet drugs
Major	Celery, Chamomile, Danshen, Dong quai, Evening primrose, Fenugreek, Garlic, Ginger, Ginkgo, Horse chestnut, Licorice, Red clover, Reishi,[c] Turmeric, Willow	Cat's claw
Moderate	Andrographis, Bogbean, Cayenne, Clove, Flaxseed, Kudzu, Onion, Saw palmetto	Aloe vera, Asafetida, Bitter orange, Blackcurrant seed, Burdock, Cassia, Cinchona, Coltsfoot, Da huang, Eucalyptus, Lycium, Milk thistle, Nutmeg, Peony, Royal jelly, Safflower, Soybean, Valerian, Yarrow
No available information for the item	Artichoke, Astragalus, Dandelion,[d] Glehnia, Kelp, Lavender, Meadowsweet,[e] Red yeast rice,[f] Skullcap	American ginseng, Angelica,[f] Artemesia, Black cohosh,[f] Chrysanthemum flower, Corydalis yanhuso, Dang shen, Erigeron, Geum japonicum, Hawthorn,[e] Horseradish, Jamaica quassia, Japanese brome, Lovage, Magnolia bark, Motherwort, Plantain, Pubescent angelica, Rue, Shiitake, Sweet melilot, Tamarind,[e] Wood ear mushrooms

[a]Chinese herbal medicine were identified according to Taiwan Herbal Pharmacopoeia,[34] Chinese Medicinal Herbs Preparation,[35] or Chinese Materia Medica.[36].
[b] The severity rating was categorized according to *MicroMedex®*, *Lexicomp®* and *Natural Medicines Comprehensive Database®*. Interactions with severity rated as major in any of the three databases were included in the "major" type, while interactions rated as moderate and without major score in any database were included in the "moderate" type. "No available documented information for the item" meant that there was no available information about the single CHM in these databases.
[c] Interaction with heparin is lack of information about severity rating.
[d] Interaction with clopidogrel or warfarin is moderate. [e] Interaction with aspirin is moderate. [f] Interaction with warfarin is moderate.

needed and retrieved this information regarding their mechanism and severity rating. The results of this review show that more than half of documented drug interactions retrieved from books, web sites, or primary literature could be identified in *NMCD®*, and less of them could be retrieved in *MicroMedex® or Lexicomp®*. This finding is consistent with the results of a previous study which was conducted in 2008 to evaluate the commonly used dietary supplement databases [141]. Of these databases, *NMCD®* had been recognized as the most appropriate database used to answer questions (including drug interactions) about dietary supplements [141]. In addition, we also found that only a few interactions could be identified in all of the tertiary literature (*MicroMedex®*, Drug interaction facts) and there existed variations in the severity rating of interactions [142]. This finding is also in agreement with Abarca's evaluation, which concluded that only a few major drug-drug interactions were listed in the four available interaction compendium and with very little agreement among them [142]. Thus, further rigorous qualitative studies that include opinions from a variety of experts on CHMs and drug interactions are needed to provide more consistent and robust information about the levels of clinical significance and mechanisms and combinations to be avoided to prevent drug-CHM interactions from occurring.

Nevertheless, our review has a number of limitations. First, there exists discordance in the nomenclature of Chinese medicine and herbs, as well as in both of the English and Chinese resources that need to be addressed. In particular, some evidence was retrieved from the English resources showing that an inconsistency of homonyms, synonyms, or translation may exist. Furthermore, only a small portion of the literature listed the common names of the natural products or herbal remedies, and the majority of them lacked any information on the scientific names and/or binomial source. Therefore, we need to be cautious when interpreting the findings on the natural products, herbs and CHMs per se. Second, the majority of literature reports did not specify which parts of natural products/herbs and CHMs (e.g., roots, leaves, seeds, or flowers) were used, on what doses, or which routes of administration were taken. In fact, the active ingredients and doses of CHMs may vary by situation and person based on TCM theory. Usually, the kinds and parts of CHMs and their preparation procedures are chosen based upon the stages of patients' disease status or condition. Lastly, only those interactions with evidence-based data retrieved from *MicroMedex®*, *NMCD®*, or *Lexicomp®*, were further reviewed for the corresponding mechanisms and rating of severity in this study. Thus, the interpretations might be subjective to information obtained from the retrieved database(s), and validated by the reviewers and members in the focus group. However, we have tried our best to screen and highlight the interactions using the best available evidence and consistent approach, although not all reports or studies were published or relevant documented interactions analyzed.

Conclusions

Conventional anticoagulants and antiplatelet drugs were documented to have harmful interactions with some commonly used single entity CHMs. Concurrent use of some herbal remedies may increase or reduce the pharmacologic effects of anticoagulant and antiplatelet drugs with moderate or severe consequences. For those patients who are taking conventional anti-clotting medications with CHMs for cardiovascular or cerebrovascular diseases, the potential risks of increased bleeding due to drug-CHM interactions should not be ignored. This review provides some guidance to health care professionals as to how to recognize the potential risks of interactions between anticoagulants/antiplatelets and single entity CHMs. Moreover, it is critical for all health care professionals to be able to initiate and effectively communicate and discuss the proper use of CHM-related products with conventional medications (i.e., anticoagulant or antiplatelet agents for cardiovascular or cerebrovascular diseases) because many patients may not voluntarily disclose their CHM-related use to their physicians.

Supporting Information

Appendix S1 Summary of review articles to retrieve relevant information about interactions between antico-

agulants/antiplatelet drugs and natural products/herbs (including CMHs).
(DOCX)

Appendix S2 PRISMA checklist.
(DOCX)

Acknowledgments

The authors would like to express their gratitude to Chiu-Lin Tsai for his insights and comments initially on the identification of CHMs, Po-Ming Huang and Shan-Chieh Wu for their assistance with the review and manuscript, Jun-Fon Wang and Po-Ming Huang for their help on data management, the other reviewers for their insights of drug-CHM interaction information, as well as Dan Lu, Matthias C. Lu and Jenna Beall for their comments on the manuscript.

Author Contributions

Conceived and designed the experiments: HHT HWL. Performed the experiments: YHL YLC HHT HWL. Analyzed the data: HHT. Wrote the paper: HHT HWL. Reviewed and revised the manuscript: GBM.

References

1. World Health Organization (WHO) (2008). The 10 leading causes of death by broad income group. http://www.who.int/mediacentre/factsheets/fs310/en/. Accessed May 25, 2012.
2. Furie KL, Kasner SE, Adams RJ, Albers GW, Bush RL, et al. (2011) Guidelines for the prevention of stroke in patients with stroke or transient ischemic attack: a guideline for healthcare professionals from the american heart association/american stroke association. Stroke 42: 227–276.
3. Holbrook AM, Pereira JA, Labiris R, McDonald H, Douketis JD, et al. (2005) Systematic overview of warfarin and its drug and food interactions. Arch Intern Med 165: 1095–1106.
4. Dunn SP, Macaulay TE (2011) Drug-Drug Interactions Associated with Antiplatelet Therapy. Cardiovasc Hematol Agents Med Chem 9: 231.
5. Ulbricht C, Chao W, Costa D, Rusie-Seamon E, Weissner W, et al. (2008) Clinical evidence of herb-drug interactions: a systematic review by the natural standard research collaboration. Curr Drug Metab 9: 1063–1120.
6. Izzo AA, Di Carlo G, Borrelli F, Ernst E (2005) Cardiovascular pharmacotherapy and herbal medicines: the risk of drug interaction. Int J Cardiol 98: 1–14.
7. Su D, Li L (2011) Trends in the use of complementary and alternative medicine in the United States: 2002–2007. J Health Care Poor Underserved 22: 296–310.
8. Rossler W, Lauber C, Angst J, Haker H, Gamma A, et al. (2007) The use of complementary and alternative medicine in the general population: Results from a longitudinal community study. Psychol Med 37: 73–84.
9. Ernst E (2000) Prevalence of use of complementary/alternative medicine: a systematic review. Bull World Health Organ 78: 252–257.
10. Yeh GY, Davis RB, Phillips RS (2006) Use of complementary therapies in patients with cardiovascular disease. Am J Cardiol 98: 673–680.
11. Lee GBW, Charn TC, Chew ZH, Ng TP (2004) Complementary and alternative medicine use in patients with chronic diseases in primary care is associated with perceived quality of care and cultural beliefs. Fam Pract 21: 654–660.
12. Chang LC, Huang N, Chou YJ, Lee CH, Kao FY, et al. (2008) Utilization patterns of Chinese medicine and Western medicine under the National Health Insurance Program in Taiwan, a population-based study from 1997 to 2003. BMC Health Serv Res 8: 170.
13. Lim MK, Sadarangani P, Chan HL, Heng JY (2005) Complementary and alternative medicine use in multiracial Singapore. Complement Ther Med 13: 16–24.
14. Lai D, Chappell N (2007) Use of Traditional Chinese Medicine by older Chinese immigrants in Canada. Fam Pract 24: 56–64.
15. Chen FN, Lee CPD, Hsieh CL, Lin CC, Chiang HM, et al. (2008) Survey on Adult Behavior and Medication of Chinese and Western Medicine-Based on the Outpatients of a Medical Center in Mid-Taiwan. J Int Chin West Med 10: 25–34.
16. Rochelle TL, Marks DF (2010) Medical pluralism of the Chinese in London: an exploratory study. Br J Health Psychol 15: 715–728.
17. Tsai HH, Lin HW, Chien CR, Li TC (2012) Concurrent use of antiplatelets, anticoagulants, or digoxin with Chinese medications: a population-based cohort study. Eur J Clin Pharmacol DOI 10.1007/s00228-012-1359-6.
18. Alherbish A, Charrois TL, Ackman ML, Tsuyuki RT, Ezekowitz JA (2011) The prevalence of natural health product use in patients with acute cardiovascular disease. PLoS One 6: e19623.
19. Suchard JR, Suchard MA, Steinfeldt JL (2004) Physician knowledge of herbal toxicities and adverse herb-drug interactions. Eur J Emerg Med 11: 193–197.
20. Saw JT, Bahari MB, Ang HH, Lim YH (2006) Potential drug-herb interaction with antiplatelet/anticoagulant drugs. Complement Ther Clin Pract 12: 236–241.
21. Mahady GB (2001) Botanical dietary supplements: Quality, safety and efficacy. Lisse, The Netherlands: Swets & Zeitlinger Publishers.
22. Cassileth BC, Yeung KS (2003) Herb-drug interactions in oncology. Hamilton: London BC Decker Inc.
23. Ulbricht CE (2005) Natural standard herbs & supplement reference: Evidence-based clinical review. St. Louis, Mo.: Mosby/Elsevier.
24. Tatro DS (2011) Drug interaction facts. Saint Louis: Wolters Kluwer Health/Facts & Comparisons.
25. Stargrove MB, Treasure J, McKee DL (2008) Herb, nutrient, and drug interactions: Clinical implications and therapeutic strategies. St. Louis: Mosby Elsevier.
26. Philp RB (2004) Herbal-drug interactions and adverse effects: An evidence-based quick reference guide. USA: McGraw-Hill Professional.
27. Jennes F, Flaws B (2007) Herb toxicities & drug interactions: A formula approach. Boulder: Blue Poppy Press.
28. Williamson E, Driver S, Baxter K (2009) Stockley's herbal medicines interactions. London: Pharmaceutical Press.
29. Committee on Chinese Medicine and Pharmacy, Department of Health, Executive Yuan. Abstract of yearbook. http://www.ccmp.gov.tw/en/research/result.asp?relno = 51&level = C. Accessed March 10, 2012.
30. Department of Health, Executive Yuan, R.O.C. (TAIWAN). Government research bulletin. http://grbsearch.stpi.narl.org.tw/GRB/. Accessed March 15, 2012.
31. Office of Dietary Supplements. *Dietary Supplement Fact Sheets*. http://ods.od.nih.gov/factsheets/list-all/. Accessed March 19, 2012.
32. National Center for Complementary and Alternative Medicine. *Herbs at a Glance*. http://nccam.nih.gov/health/herbsataglance.htm. Accessed March 20, 2012.
33. National Center for Complementary and Alternative Medicine (2010) *Traditional Chinese Medicine*: An Introduction. http://nccam.nih.gov/health/whatiscam/chinesemed.htm. Accessed March 1, 2012.
34. Committee on Chinese Medicine and Pharmacy (2004) Taiwan Herbal Pharmacopoeia. Taipei: Department of Health, Executive Yuan.
35. Chang HC, Tsai KU (2003) Chinese Medicinal Herbs Preparation. Taichung: China Medical University.
36. State Administration of Traditional Chinese Medicine (1999) Chinese Materia Medica. Shanghai: Shanghai scientific and Technical Publishers.
37. MICROMEDEX® 1.0 (Healthcare Series). Interaction Database. http://www.thomsonhc.com/hcs/librarian/ND_T/HCS/ND_PR/Main/CS/A304ED/DUPLICATIONSHIELDSYNC/95C0EB/ND_PG/PRIH/ND_B/HCS/ND_P/Main/PFActionId/hcs.Interactions.FindDrugInteractions. Accessed April 15, 2012.
38. Lexicomp. Lexi-Interact Online (2012). http://www.uptodate.com/crlsql/interact/frameset.jsp.Accessed April 18, 2012.
39. Natural Medicines Comprehensive Database. *Natural Product/Drug Interaction Checker*. http://naturaldatabase.therapeuticresearch.com/nd/Search.aspx?s = ND&cs = &pt = 7&rli = 1&sh = . Accessed April 20, 2012.
40. Awang DV, Fugh-Berman A (2002) Herbal interactions with cardiovascular drugs. J Cardiovasc Nurs 16: 64–70.
41. Bone KM (2008) Potential interaction of Ginkgo biloba leaf with antiplatelet or anticoagulant drugs: what is the evidence? Mol Nutr Food Res 52: 764–771.
42. Borrelli F, Izzo AA (2009) Herb-drug interactions with St John's wort (Hypericum perforatum): an update on clinical observations. AAPS J 11: 710–727.
43. Brazier NC, Levine MA (2003) Drug-herb interaction among commonly used conventional medicines: a compendium for health care professionals. Am J Ther 10: 163–169.
44. Bressler R (2005) Herb-drug interactions. Interactions between saw palmetto and prescription medications. Geriatrics 60: 32.
45. Bressler R (2005) Herb-drug interactions: interactions between ginseng and prescription medications. Geriatrics 60: 16–17.
46. Bressler R (2005) Herb-drug interactions. St. John's wort and prescription medications. Geriatrics 60: 21–23.
47. Bressler R (2005) Herb-drug interactions: interactions between Ginkgo biloba and prescription medications. Geriatrics 60: 30–33
48. Butterweck V, Derendorf H (2008) Potential of pharmacokinetic profiling for detecting herbal interactions with drugs. Clin Pharmacokinet 47: 383–397.
49. Chan E, Tan M, Xin J, Sudarsanam S, Johnson DE (2010) Interactions between traditional Chinese medicines and Western therapeutics. Curr Opin Drug Discov Devel 13: 50–65.
50. Chavez ML, Jordan MA, Chavez PI (2006) Evidence-based drug-herbal interactions. Life Sci 78: 2146–2157.
51. Choi YH, Chin YW, Kim YG (2011) Herb-drug interactions: focus on metabolic enzymes and transporters. Arch Pharm Res 34: 1843–1863.
52. Cohen PA, Ernst E (2010) Safety of herbal supplements: a guide for cardiologists. Cardiovasc Ther 28: 246–253.

53. Colalto C (2010) Herbal interactions on absorption of drugs: Mechanisms of action and clinical risk assessment. Pharmacol Res 62: 207–227.
54. Coxeter PD, McLachlan AJ, Duke CC, Roufogalis BD (2004) Herb-drug interactions: an evidence based approach. Curr Med Chem 11: 1513–1525.
55. De Smet PAGM, Floor-Schreudering A, Bouvy ML, Wensing M (2008) Clinical risk management of interactions between natural products and drugs. Curr Drug Metab 9: 1055–1062.
56. Di Carlo G, Borrelli F, Ernst E, Izzo AA (2001) St John's wort: Prozac from the plant kingdom. Trends Pharmacol Sci 22: 292–297.
57. Di YM, Li CG, Xue CC, Zhou S-F (2008) Clinical drugs that interact with St. John's wort and implication in drug development. Curr Pharm Des 14: 1723–1742.
58. Ernst E (2000) Herb-drug interactions: potentially important but woefully under-researched. Eur J Clin Pharmacol 56: 523–524.
59. Ernst E (2004) Risks of herbal medicinal products. Pharmacoepidemiol Drug Saf 13: 767–771.
60. Fugh-Berman A (2000) Herb-drug interactions. Lancet 355: 134–138.
61. Fugh-Berman A, Ernst E (2001) Herb-drug interactions: review and assessment of report reliability. Br J Clin Pharmacol 52: 587–595.
62. Gardiner P, Phillips R, Shaughnessy AF (2008) Herbal and dietary supplement – drug interactions in patients with chronic illnesses. Am Fam Physician 77: 73–78.
63. Greenblatt DJ, von Moltke LL (2005) Interaction of warfarin with drugs, natural substances, and foods. J Clin Pharmacol 45: 127–132.
64. Greeson JM, Sanford B, Monti DA (2001) St. John's wort (Hypericum perforatum): a review of the current pharmacological, toxicological, and clinical literature. Psychopharmacology (Berl) 153: 402–414.
65. Haller CA (2006) Clinical approach to adverse events and interactions related to herbal and dietary supplements. Clin Toxicol (Phila) 44: 605–610.
66. Holcomb SS (2009) Common herb-drug interactions: what you should know. Nurse Pract 34: 21–29.
67. Hu Z, Yang X, Ho PCL, Chan SY, Heng PWS, et al. (2005) Herb-drug interactions: a literature review. Drugs 65: 1239–1282.
68. Huang S-M, Lesko LJ (2004) Drug-drug, drug-dietary supplement, and drug-citrus fruit and other food interactions: what have we learned? J Clin Pharmacol 44: 559–569.
69. Izzo AA (2005) Herb-drug interactions: an overview of the clinical evidence. Fundam Clin Pharmacol 19: 1–16.
70. Izzo AA, Ernst E (2001) Interactions between herbal medicines and prescribed drugs: a systematic review. Drugs 61: 2163–2175.
71. Izzo AA, Ernst E (2009) Interactions between herbal medicines and prescribed drugs: an updated systematic review. Drugs 69: 1777–1798.
72. Javed F, Golagani A, Sharp H (2008) Potential effects of herbal medicines and nutritional supplements on coagulation in ENT practice. J Laryngol Otol 122: 116–119.
73. Ko RJ (2004) A U.S. perspective on the adverse reactions from traditional Chinese medicines. J Chin Med Assoc 67: 109–116.
74. Kuhn MA (2002) Herbal remedies: drug-herb interactions. Crit Care Nurse 22: 22–28, 30, 32.
75. Madabushi R, Frank B, Drewelow B, Derendorf H, Butterweck V (2006) Hyperforin in St. John's wort drug interactions. Eur J Clin Pharmacol 62: 225–233.
76. Markowitz JS, DeVane CL (2001) The emerging recognition of herb-drug interactions with a focus on St. John's wort (Hypericum perforatum). Psychopharmacol Bull 35: 53–64.
77. McFadden R, Peterson N (2011) Interactions between drugs and four common medicinal herbs. Nurs Stand 25: 65–68.
78. Mills E, Wu P, Johnston BC, Gallicano K, Clarke M, et al. (2005) Natural health product-drug interactions: a systematic review of clinical trials. Ther Drug Monit 27: 549–557.
79. Norred CL, Brinker F (2001) Potential coagulation effects of preoperative complementary and alternative medicines. Altern Ther Health Med 7: 58–67.
80. Nutescu E, Chuatrisorn I, Hellenbart E (2011) Drug and dietary interactions of warfarin and novel oral anticoagulants: An update. J Thromb Thrombolysis 31: 326–343.
81. Nutescu EA, Shapiro NL, Ibrahim S, West P (2006) Warfarin and its interactions with foods, herbs and other dietary supplements. Expert Opin Drug Saf 5: 433–451.
82. Ohnishi N, Yokoyama T (2004) Interactions between medicines and functional foods or dietary supplements. Keio J Med 53: 137–150.
83. Pal D, Mitra AK (2006) MDR- and CYP3A4-mediated drug-herbal interactions. Life Sci 78: 2131–2145.
84. Poppenga RH (2002) Herbal medicine: potential for intoxication and interactions with conventional drugs. Clin Tech Small Anim Pract 17: 6–18.
85. Samuels N (2005) Herbal remedies and anticoagulant therapy. Thromb Haemost 93: 3–7.
86. Singh YN (2005) Potential for interaction of kava and St. John's wort with drugs. J Ethnopharmacol 100: 108–113.
87. Skalli S, Zaid A, Soulaymani R (2007) Drug interactions with herbal medicines. Ther Drug Monit 29: 679–686.
88. Tachjian A, Maria V, Jahangir A (2010) Use of herbal products and potential interactions in patients with cardiovascular diseases. J Am Coll Cardiol 55: 515–525.
89. Tirona RG, Bailey DG (2006) Herbal product-drug interactions mediated by induction. Br J Clin Pharmacol 61: 677–681.
90. Tomlinson B, Hu M, Lee VWY (2008) In vivo assessment of herb-drug interactions: possible utility of a pharmacogenetic approach? Mol Nutr Food Res 52: 799–809.
91. Ueng YF, Chen RM (2004) The role of cytochrome P450 in herb-drug interactions. Curr Pharmacogenomics Person Med 2: 209–218.
92. Venkataramanan R, Komoroski B, Strom S (2006) In vitro and in vivo assessment of herb drug interactions. Life Sci 78: 2105–2115.
93. Whitten DL, Myers SP, Hawrelak JA, Wohlmuth H (2006) The effect of St John's wort extracts on CYP3A: a systematic review of prospective clinical trials. Br J Clin Pharmacol 62: 512–526.
94. Williamson EM (2003) Drug interactions between herbal and prescription medicines. Drug Saf 26: 1075–1092.
95. Williamson EM (2005) Interactions between herbal and conventional medicines. Expert Opin Drug Saf 4: 355–378.
96. Wittkowsky AK (2008) Dietary supplements, herbs and oral anticoagulants: the nature of the evidence. J Thromb Thrombolysis 25: 72–77.
97. Woodward KN (2005) The potential impact of the use of homeopathic and herbal remedies on monitoring the safety of prescription products. Hum Exp Toxicol 24: 219–233.
98. Yang XX, Hu ZP, Duan W, Zhu YZ, Zhou SF (2006) Drug-herb interactions: Eliminating toxicity with hard drug design. Curr Pharm Des 12: 4649–4664.
99. Zhou L, Zuo Z, Chow MS (2005) Danshen: an overview of its chemistry, pharmacology, pharmacokinetics, and clinical use. J Clin Pharmacol 45: 1345–1359.
100. Zhou S, Chan E, Pan S-Q, Huang M, Lee EJD (2004) Pharmacokinetic interactions of drugs with St John's wort. J Psychopharmacol 18: 262–276.
101. Zhou S, Gao Y, Jiang W, Huang M, Xu A, et al. (2003) Interactions of herbs with cytochrome P450. Drug Metab Rev 35: 35–98.
102. Zhou S-F, Zhou Z-W, Li C-G, Chen X, Yu X, et al. (2007) Identification of drugs that interact with herbs in drug development. Drug Discov Today 12: 664–673.
103. Mao XQ, Xie HT, Zhou HH (2007) MDR-and CYP3A4-mediated drug-herbal Interactions. Chinese Journal of Clinical Pharmacology and Therapeutics 12: 728–734.
104. Wang TY (2011) Outcomes Influenced by Drug Interactions. The Journal of Long Term Care 15: 24–32.
105. Wang YY (2003) Interactions between warfarin and other anticoagulant agents or herbal medicine. The Journal of Taiwan Pharmacy 19: 5–10.
106. Li JY, Shih HJ, Tsai ML (2008) Interactions between warfarin and chinese herbal medicine. The Journal of Taiwan Pharmacy 24: 135–142.
107. Lin JJ (2003) Interactions between Herbal and Conventional Therapies: Focus on Ginseng and Ginkgo Biloba. Show Chwan Medical Journal 4: 1–4.
108. Chen FP, Zhong MX, Huang XZ (2011) The whole aspects of interaction between traditional Chinese medicine and western medicine. Family Medicine & Primary Medical Care 26: 168–176.
109. Chen JF, Hu YJ, Miao CY (2007) Advancement of pharmacokinetic studies on Chinese herbal medicine-synthetic drug interactions. Clin J Clin Pharmacol Ther 12: 1348–1353.
110. Peng B, Li JR, He R (2010) The research status of herb-drug interactions. World Science and Technology-Modernization of Traditional Chinese Medicine. doi: 10.3969/j.issn.1674–3849.2010.02.024.
111. Tsai CH, Lu CY (2009) Analysis on the interaction of warfarinand ginseng. Taipei Journal of Chinese Medicine 15: 98–109.
112. Lai YC, Chen YL, Lai JS (2007) Toxicity of Chinese Herbal Medicine and drug-herb Interactions. The Chung Shan Medical Journal 18: 343–357.
113. Kuo YH, Lin YL, Don MJ, Chen RM, Ueng YF (2006) Induction of cytochrome P450-dependent monooxygenase by extracts of the medicinal herb Salvia miltiorrhiza. J Pharm Pharmacol 58: 521–527.
114. Li Y, Wang N (2010) Antithrombotic effects of Danggui, Honghua and potential drug interaction with clopidogrel. J Ethnopharmacol 128: 623–628.
115. Makino T, Wakushima H, Okamoto T, Okukubo Y, Deguchi Y, et al. (2002) Pharmacokinetic interactions between warfarin and kangen-karyu, a Chinese traditional herbal medicine, and their synergistic action. J Ethnopharmacol 82: 35–40.
116. Wu WWP, Yeung JHK (2010) Inhibition of warfarin hydroxylation by major tanshinones of Danshen (Salvia miltiorrhiza) in the rat in vitro and in vivo. Phytomedicine 17: 219–226.
117. Abdul MI, Jiang X, Williams KM, Day RO, Roufogalis BD, et al. (2010) Pharmacokinetic and pharmacodynamic interactions of echinacea and policosanol with warfarin in healthy subjects. Br J Clin Pharmacol 69: 508–515.
118. Jiang X, Blair EYL, McLachlan AJ (2006) Investigation of the effects of herbal medicines on warfarin response in healthy subjects: a population pharmacokinetic-pharmacodynamic modeling approach. J Clin Pharmacol 46: 1370–1378.
119. Jiang X, Williams KM, Liauw WS, Ammit AJ, Roufogalis BD, et al. (2004) Effect of St John's wort and ginseng on the pharmacokinetics and pharmacodynamics of warfarin in healthy subjects. Br J Clin Pharmacol 57: 592–599.
120. Yuan CS, Wei G, Dey L, Karrison T, Nahlik L, et al. (2004) Brief communication: American ginseng reduces warfarin's effect in healthy patients: a randomized, controlled Trial. Ann Intern Med 141: 23–27.

121. Blalock SJ, Gregory PJ, Patel RA, Norton LL, Callahan LF, et al. (2009) Factors associated with potential medication-herb/natural product interactions in a rural community. Altern Ther Health Med 15: 26–34.
122. Bush TM, Rayburn KS, Holloway SW, Sanchez-Yamamoto DS, Allen BL, et al. (2007) Adverse interactions between herbal and dietary substances and prescription medications: a clinical survey. Altern Ther Health Med 13: 30–35.
123. Canter PH, Ernst E (2004) Herbal supplement use by persons aged over 50 years in Britain: frequently used herbs, concomitant use of herbs, nutritional supplements and prescription drugs, rate of informing doctors and potential for negative interactions. Drugs Aging 21: 597–605.
124. Chan ALF, Leung HWC, Wu J-W, Chien T-W (2011) Risk of hemorrhage associated with co-prescriptions for Ginkgo biloba and antiplatelet or anticoagulant drugs. J Altern Complement Med 17: 513–517.
125. Chan H-T, So L-T, Li S-W, Siu C-W, Lau C-P, et al. (2011) Effect of herbal consumption on time in therapeutic range of warfarin therapy in patients with atrial fibrillation. J Cardiovasc Pharmacol 58: 87–90.
126. Charrois TL, Hill RL, Vu D, Foster BC, Boon HS, et al. (2007) Community identification of natural health product-drug interactions. Ann Pharmacother 41: 1124–1129.
127. Clauson KA, Santamarina ML, Rutledge JC (2008) Clinically relevant safety issues associated with St. John's wort product labels. BMC Complement Altern Med 8: 42.
128. Dergal JM, Gold JL, Laxer DA, Lee MSW, Binns MA, et al. (2002) Potential interactions between herbal medicines and conventional drug therapies used by older adults attending a memory clinic. Drugs Aging 19: 879–886.
129. Goldman RD, Rogovik AL, Lai D, Vohra S (2008) Potential interactions of drug-natural health products and natural health products-natural health products among children. J Pediatr 152: 521–526.
130. Rogers EA, Gough JE, Brewer KL (2001) Are emergency department patients at risk for herb-drug interactions? Acad Emerg Med 8: 932–934.
131. Segal R, Pilote L (2006) Warfarin interaction with Matricaria chamomilla. CMAJ 174: 1281–1282.
132. Shalansky S, Lynd L, Richardson K, Ingaszewski A, Kerr C (2007) Risk of warfarin-related bleeding events and supratherapeutic international normalized ratios associated with complementary and alternative medicine: a longitudinal analysis. Pharmacotherapy 27: 1237–1247.
133. Su Q, Li Y (2010) Interaction between warfarin and the herbal product shengmai-yin: A case report of intracerebral hematoma. Yonsei Med J 51: 793–796.
134. Lai JN (2010) Causal inference of bleeding complications in patients with warfarin treatment in Taiwan – a eleven year follow up study. Yearbook of Chinese Medicine and Pharmacy 28: 291–388.
135. Al Faraj S (2005) Antagonism of the anticoagulant effect of warfarin caused by the use of Commiphora molmol as a herbal medication: a case report. Ann Trop Med Parasitol 99: 219–220.
136. Yamashita H, Tsukayama H, Sugishita C (2002) Popularity of complementary and alternative medicine in Japan: a telephone survey. Complement Ther Med 10: 84–93.
137. Hsieh SC, Lai JN, Lee CF, Hu FC, Tseng WL, et al. (2008) The prescribing of Chinese herbal products in Taiwan: a cross-sectional analysis of the national health insurance reimbursement database. Pharmacoepidemiol Drug Saf 17: 609–619.
138. Mousa SA (2010) Antithrombotic effects of naturally derived products on coagulation and platelet function. Methods Mol Biol 663: 229–240.
139. Xu G, Zhao W, Zhou Z, Zhang R, Zhu W, et al. (2009) Danshen extracts decrease blood C reactive protein and prevent ischemic stroke recurrence: A controlled pilot study. Phytother Res 23: 1721–1725.
140. Zhu YF, Luo HM, Deng ZL, Fu DY, Yao W, et al. (2012) Effects of the Chinese patent medicine, Honghua injection, on platelet glycoprotein Tib/Ufa receptors in patients with acute coronary syndrome: A randomized controlled trial. Zhong Xi Yi Jie He Xue Bao 10: 318–323.
141. Clauson KA, Peak AS, Marsh WA, DiScala S, Bellinger RR (2008) Clinical decision support tools: focus on dietary supplement databases. Altern Ther Health Med 14: 36–40.
142. Abarca J, Malone DC, Armstrong EP, Grizzle AJ, Hansten PD, et al. (2004) Concordance of severity ratings provided in four drug interaction compendia. J Am Pharm Assoc 44: 136–141.

8

The Efficacy of Chinese Herbal Medicine as an Adjunctive Therapy for Advanced Non-small Cell Lung Cancer

Shi Guang Li[1,2], Hai Yong Chen[3], Chen Sheng Ou-Yang[1,2], Xi-Xin Wang[4], Zhen-Jiang Yang[1,2], Yao Tong[3]*, William C.S. Cho[5]*

1 Graduate School, Guangzhou University of Chinese Medicine, Guangzhou, China, **2** Department of Oncology and Hematology, Shenzhen Hospital of Traditional Chinese Medicine, Shenzhen, Guangdong Province, China, **3** School of Chinese Medicine, Li Ka Shing Faculty of Medicine, The University of Hong Kong, Hong Kong SAR, China, **4** Shanxi Province Hospital of Traditional Chinese Medicine, Taiyuan, Shanxi Province, China, **5** Department of Clinical Oncology, Queen Elizabeth Hospital, Hong Kong SAR, China

Abstract

Many published studies reflect the growing application of complementary and alternative medicine, particularly Chinese herbal medicine (CHM) use in combination with conventional cancer therapy for advanced non-small cell lung cancer (NSCLC), but its efficacy remains largely unexplored. The purpose of this study is to evaluate the efficacy of CHM combined with conventional chemotherapy (CT) in the treatment of advanced NSCLC. Publications in 11 electronic databases were extensively searched, and 24 trials were included for analysis. A sum of 2,109 patients was enrolled in these studies, at which 1,064 patients participated in CT combined CHM and 1,039 in CT (six patients dropped out and were not reported the group enrolled). Compared to using CT alone, CHM combined with CT significantly increase one-year survival rate (RR = 1.36, 95% CI = 1.15–1.60, p = 0.0003). Besides, the combined therapy significantly increased immediate tumor response (RR = 1.36, 95% CI = 1.19–1.56, p<1.0E−5) and improved Karnofsky performance score (KPS) (RR = 2.90, 95% CI = 1.62–5.18, p = 0.0003). Combined therapy remarkably reduced the nausea and vomiting at toxicity grade of III–IV (RR = 0.24, 95% CI = 0.12–0.50, p = 0.0001) and prevented the decline of hemoglobin and platelet in patients under CT at toxicity grade of I–IV (RR = 0.64, 95% CI = 0.51–0.80, p<0.0001). Moreover, the herbs that are frequently used in NSCLC patients were identified. This systematic review suggests that CHM as an adjuvant therapy can reduce CT toxicity, prolong survival rate, enhance immediate tumor response, and improve KPS in advanced NSCLC patients. However, due to the lack of large-scale randomized clinical trials in the included studies, further larger scale trials are needed.

Editor: John D. Minna, Univesity of Texas Southwestern Medical Center at Dallas, United States of America

Funding: These authors have no support or funding to report.

Competing Interests: The authors have read the journal's policy and have the following conflicts: William Cho is a PLOS ONE Editorial Board member. This does not alter the authors' adherence to all the PLOS ONE policies on sharing data and materials.

* E-mail: a94720348@gmail.com (YT); williamcscho@gmail.com (WCSC)

These authors contributed equally to this work.

Introduction

Lung cancer is the most common malignancy worldwide and a leading cause of cancer-related deaths. In 2012, it is estimated that 160,300 deaths (87,700 in men, 72,600 in women) from lung cancer would occur in the United States [1].

The non-small cell lung cancer (NSCLC) is the most common form of lung cancer, which accounts for approximately 85% of all lung cancer cases. Nowadays the standard treatment for patient with advanced NSCLC who has a good performance status, platinum-based chemotherapy (CT) is the first-line regimen [2,3]. However, platinum-based CT has the potential for severe adverse events, and the International Adjuvant Lung Cancer Trial suggests that more deaths in the CT group and the benefit of CT decreased over time [4,5]. In spite of the development of new CT regimens use in the treatment of NSCLC, the prognosis of the patients remains poor. Its five-year survival rate is as low as 15.9% [6,7]. Thus, there is an increasing awareness to maximize tumor control, prolong overall survival, minimize CT side-effects and improve quality of life (QoL).

In complementary and alternative medicine (CAM), Chinese herbal medicine (CHM) has become increasingly popular for the patients with advanced NSCLC. Recent studies have reported some CHMs in associated with platinum-based CT have definite superiority in relieving the symptoms of lung cancer patients, reducing the severe adverse effects (AEs) of standard cancer therapy, enhancing short-term efficacy and improving patients QoL [8]. There are a variety of herbs being used in different combinations and forms, such as oral administration and intravenous injection, to treat advanced NSCLC combined with platinum-based CT. However, albeit a number of studies being published in Chinese, the evidence on efficacy of CHM as adjuvant therapy to conventional CT is not well demonstrated in the Western world. Thus, the aim of this study is to carry out a comprehensive systematic review about the efficacy of CHM as an adjunctive therapy for advanced NSCLC.

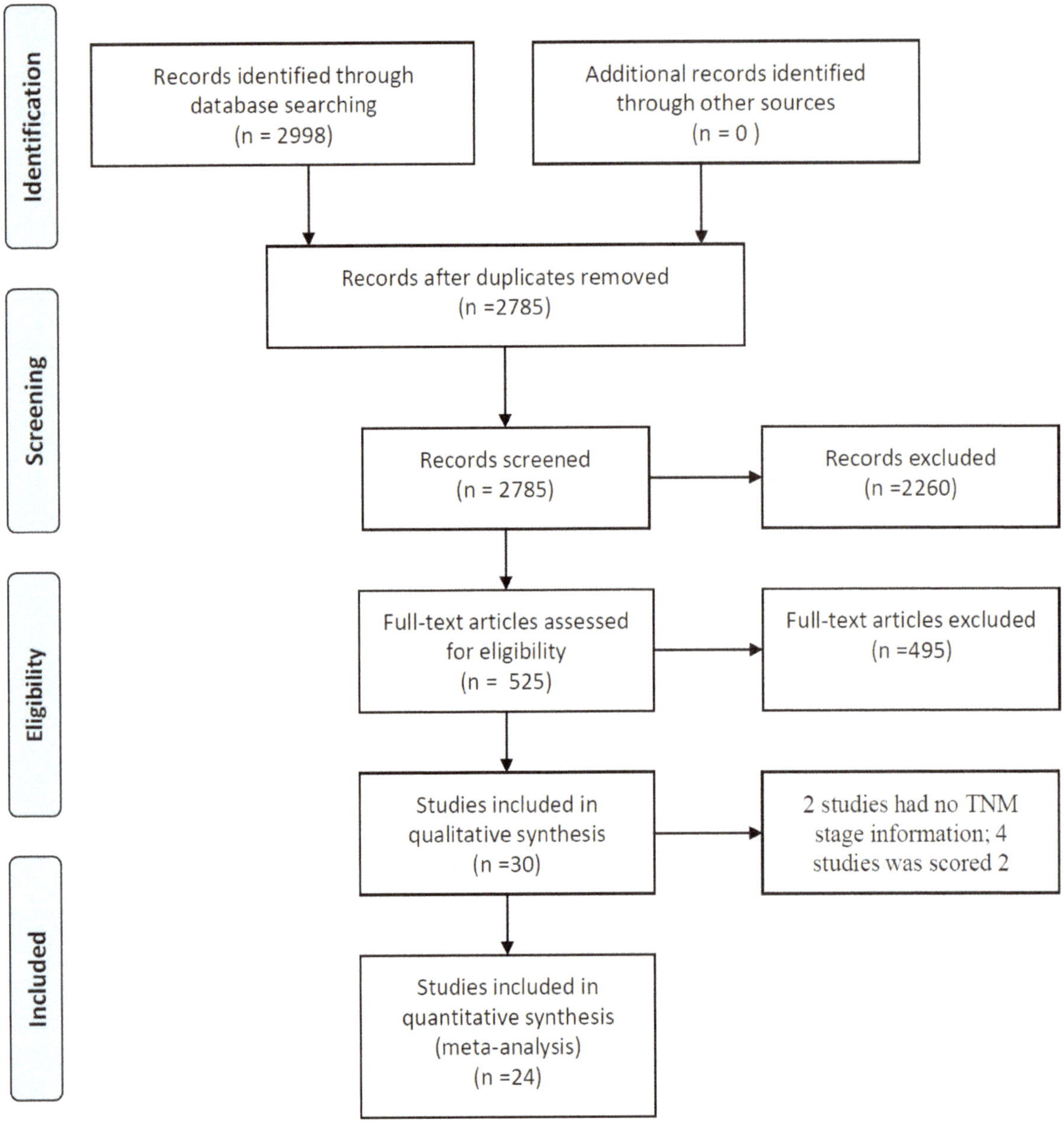

Figure 1. Flow chart of study selection.

Study or Subgroup	Experimental Events	Experimental Total	Control Events	Control Total	Weight	Risk Ratio M-H, Fixed, 95% CI
Chen et al 2008	27	51	23	49	18.9%	1.13 [0.76, 1.67]
Chen et al 2011	26	40	14	37	11.7%	1.72 [1.07, 2.75]
Li et al 2003	17	40	8	40	6.5%	2.13 [1.04, 4.35]
Lu and Wei 2009	20	30	14	30	11.3%	1.43 [0.90, 2.26]
Yang 2007	14	32	13	34	10.2%	1.14 [0.64, 2.04]
Zhang et al 2008	23	51	18	55	14.0%	1.38 [0.85, 2.24]
Zhang et al 2012	44	63	32	56	27.4%	1.22 [0.92, 1.62]
Total (95% CI)		**307**		**301**	**100.0%**	**1.36 [1.15, 1.60]**
Total events	171		122			

Heterogeneity: $Chi^2 = 4.24$, df = 6 (P = 0.64); $I^2 = 0\%$

Test for overall effect: Z = 3.61 (P = 0.0003)

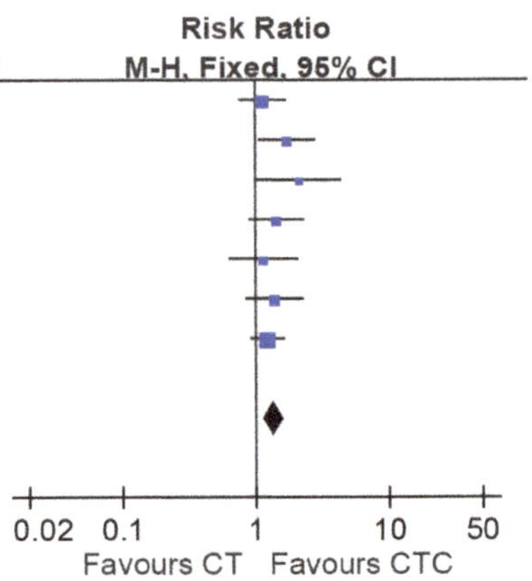

Figure 2. Number of patients with survival >one-year. Overall survivals estimated from meta-analysis of pairwise comparisons in the patients with chemotherapy combined Chinese herbal medicine (CTC, treatment group) versus patients in chemotherapy (CT, control group).

Study or Subgroup	Experimental Events	Experimental Total	Control Events	Control Total	Weight	Risk Ratio M-H, Fixed, 95% CI
Chen et al 2008	24	51	16	49	7.2%	1.44 [0.88, 2.37]
Deng et al 2012	10	28	7	30	3.0%	1.53 [0.68, 3.47]
Huang et al 2011	8	29	5	28	2.2%	1.54 [0.57, 4.15]
Huang et al 2012	6	29	8	28	3.6%	0.72 [0.29, 1.82]
Li et al 2003	7	40	5	40	2.2%	1.40 [0.48, 4.04]
Li et al 2009	26	42	16	41	7.1%	1.59 [1.01, 2.49]
Lin 2008	42	58	28	57	12.4%	1.47 [1.08, 2.01]
Lin and Zheng 2011	7	30	5	30	2.2%	1.40 [0.50, 3.92]
Lu and Wei 2009	16	30	13	30	5.7%	1.23 [0.73, 2.09]
Sun 2011	13	30	10	29	4.5%	1.26 [0.66, 2.40]
Xu et al 2007	17	60	11	56	5.0%	1.44 [0.74, 2.81]
Yang 2007	9	32	9	34	3.8%	1.06 [0.48, 2.34]
Zhang et al 2008	23	51	19	55	8.0%	1.31 [0.81, 2.10]
Zhang et al 2012	20	63	11	56	5.1%	1.62 [0.85, 3.07]
Zheng et al 2010	15	30	14	30	6.1%	1.07 [0.63, 1.81]
Zhou et al 2005	27	103	13	92	6.0%	1.86 [1.02, 3.38]
Zhou et al 2012	4	25	1	25	0.4%	4.00 [0.48, 33.33]
Zhu and Guo 2011	41	92	35	90	15.5%	1.15 [0.81, 1.62]
Total (95% CI)		**823**		**800**	**100.0%**	**1.36 [1.19, 1.56]**
Total events	315		226			

Heterogeneity: Chi² = 7.39, df = 17 (P = 0.98); I² = 0%
Test for overall effect: Z = 4.50 (P < 0.00001)

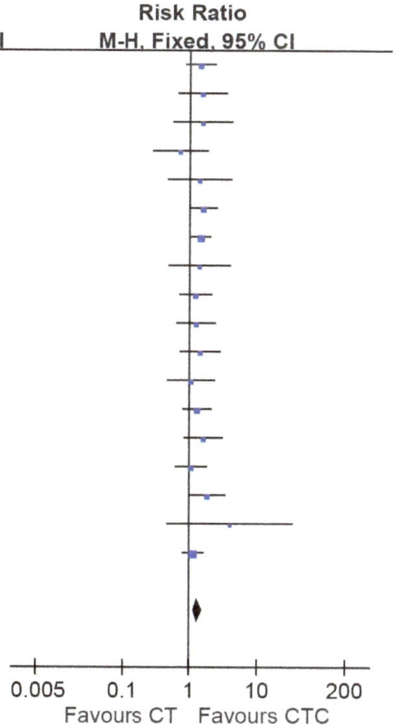

Figure 3. Immediate tumor responses. Immediate tumor responses estimated from meta-analysis of pairwise comparisons in patients with chemotherapy combined Chinese herbal medicine (CTC, treatment group) versus patients in chemotherapy (CT, control group).

Methods

Clinical trials were retrieved from 11 databases as well as from conference papers and theses. The studies were reviewed independently by SGL and HYC. The data from included studies were extracted by the first reviewer and verified by the second reviewer. Discrepancies were rectified referring to the original articles. Only the studies which satisfied the criteria were included in the meta-analysis.

Search Strategy

The terms retrieved in databases were as the following: (non-small-cell lung cancer OR non-small-cell lung carcinoma OR NSCLC OR squamous cell lung carcinoma large cell lung carcinoma OR lung adenocarcinoma) AND (Chinese medicine OR traditional Chinese medicine OR Chinese herbal medicine OR Chinese herbal drug OR traditional herbal medicine OR herbal medicine OR traditional Japanese medicine OR traditional medicine OR ethnomedicine OR folk medicine OR folk remedies OR home remedies OR indigenous medicine OR primitive medicine OR materia medica OR homeopathic remedies OR nosodes OR traditional East Asian medicine OR traditional Far Eastern medicine OR Far East medicine OR Oriental medicine OR Korean medicine OR Tibetan medicine OR herb OR herbaceous agent OR medicinal plant OR medicinal herbs OR medicinal plant product OR plant extract OR plant preparation OR herbal preparation OR botanic OR botany OR Kampo OR Kanpo OR traditional Mongolian medicine OR Mongolian folk

Study or Subgroup	Experimental Events	Experimental Total	Control Events	Control Total	Weight	Risk Ratio M-H, Fixed, 95% CI
Li et al 2009	26	42	7	41	24.7%	3.63 [1.77, 7.41]
Sun 2011	5	30	4	29	14.2%	1.21 [0.36, 4.06]
Xu et al 2007	13	60	5	56	18.0%	2.43 [0.92, 6.37]
Yao et al 2011	29	43	3	43	10.4%	9.67 [3.18, 29.36]
Zhang et al 2012	9	63	6	56	22.1%	1.33 [0.51, 3.51]
Zhu et al 2011	13	32	3	31	10.6%	4.20 [1.32, 13.31]
Total (95% CI)		**270**		**256**	**100.0%**	**3.25 [2.22, 4.77]**
Total events	95		28			

Heterogeneity: Chi² = 10.15, df = 5 (P = 0.07); I² = 51%
Test for overall effect: Z = 6.04 (P < 0.00001)

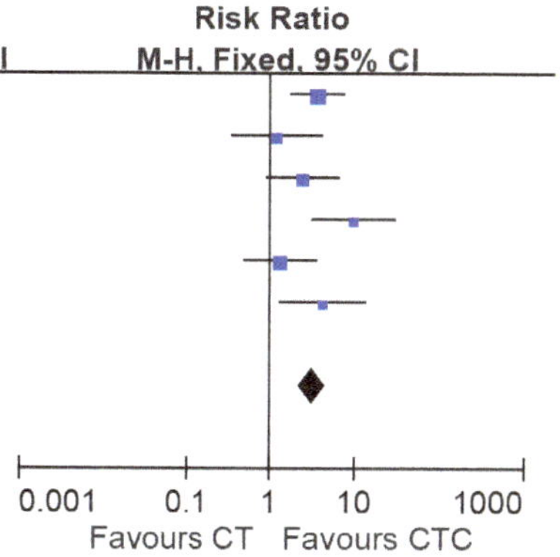

Figure 4. Quality of life. The quality of life changes on Karnofsky performance scale (KPS) were estimated from meta-analysis of pairwise comparisons in patients with Chinese herbal medicine (CTC, treatment group) versus patients in chemotherapy (CT, control group). KPS improvement (the increase of KPS ≥10).

A. Nausea and vomiting at toxicity grade of III~IV

	Experimental		Control			Risk Ratio
Study or Subgroup	**Events**	**Total**	**Events**	**Total**	**Weight**	**M-H, Fixed, 95% CI**
Huang et al 2011	0	29	0	28		Not estimable
Huang et al 2012	3	28	7	29	20.9%	0.44 [0.13, 1.55]
Lu and Wei 2009	2	30	6	30	18.2%	0.33 [0.07, 1.52]
Xu et al 2007	1	60	3	56	9.4%	0.31 [0.03, 2.90]
Zheng et al 2010	2	30	17	30	51.5%	0.12 [0.03, 0.47]
Total (95% CI)		**177**		**173**	**100.0%**	**0.24 [0.12, 0.50]**
Total events	8		33			

Heterogeneity: Chi² = 2.18, df = 3 (P = 0.54); I² = 0%

Test for overall effect: Z = 3.81 (P = 0.0001)

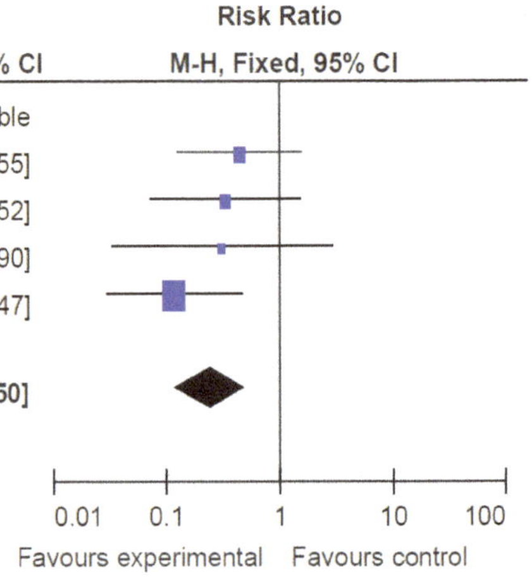

B. Hemoglobin decline at the toxicity grade of I~IV

	Experimental		Control			Risk Ratio
Study or Subgroup	**Events**	**Total**	**Events**	**Total**	**Weight**	**M-H, Fixed, 95% CI**
Huang et al 2011	11	29	13	28	11.5%	0.82 [0.44, 1.51]
Li and Li et al 2012	16	40	20	39	17.6%	0.78 [0.48, 1.27]
Lu and Wei 2009	5	30	9	30	7.8%	0.56 [0.21, 1.46]
Sun 2011	4	30	16	29	14.1%	0.24 [0.09, 0.64]
Xu et al 2007	31	60	39	56	35.0%	0.74 [0.55, 1.00]
Zhu and Guo 2011	8	92	16	90	14.0%	0.49 [0.22, 1.09]
Total (95% CI)		**281**		**272**	**100.0%**	**0.64 [0.51, 0.80]**
Total events	75		113			

Heterogeneity: Chi² = 6.64, df = 5 (P = 0.25); I² = 25%

Test for overall effect: Z = 3.96 (P < 0.0001)

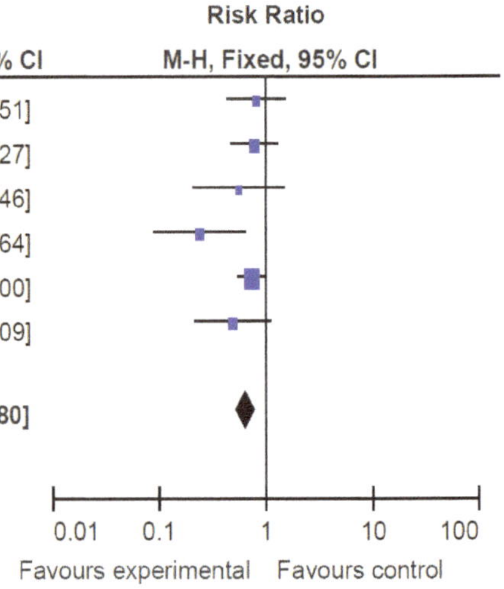

C. Hemoglobin decline at the toxicity grade of III~IV

	Experimental		Control			Risk Ratio
Study or Subgroup	**Events**	**Total**	**Events**	**Total**	**Weight**	**M-H, Fixed, 95% CI**
Huang et al 2011	1	29	2	28	13.3%	0.48 [0.05, 5.03]
Li and Li et al 2012	2	40	5	39	33.2%	0.39 [0.08, 1.89]
Lu and Wei 2009	0	30	0	30		Not estimable
Sun 2011	0	30	2	29	16.7%	0.19 [0.01, 3.87]
Xu et al 2007	4	60	2	56	13.6%	1.87 [0.36, 9.80]
Zhu and Guo 2011	1	92	1	90	6.6%	0.98 [0.06, 15.40]
Zhu et al 2011	0	32	2	31	16.6%	0.19 [0.01, 3.88]
Total (95% CI)		**313**		**303**	**100.0%**	**0.58 [0.26, 1.29]**
Total events	8		14			

Heterogeneity: Chi² = 3.35, df = 5 (P = 0.65); I² = 0%

Test for overall effect: Z = 1.33 (P = 0.18)

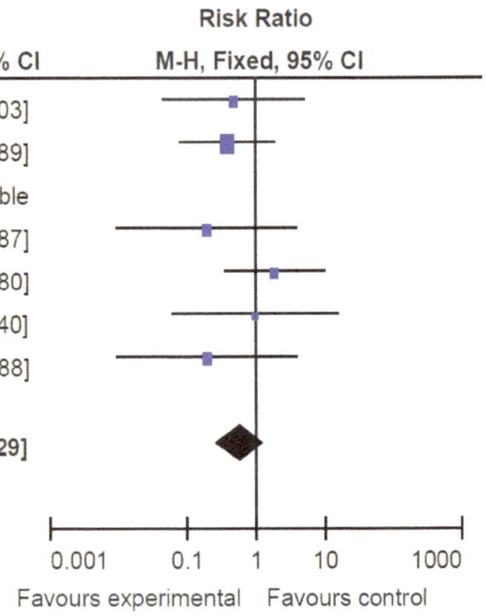

Figure 5. Reduction of adverse effects. Reduction of adverse effects estimated from meta-analysis of pairwise comparisons in patients with Chinese herbal medicine (CHM, treatment group) versus patients without CHM (control group). (**A**) Number of patients with nausea and vomiting at toxicity grade of III-IV. (**B**) Number of patients with hemoglobin decline at the toxicity grade of I-IV with CTC therapy. (**C**) Number of patients with hemoglobin decline at the toxicity grade III–IV with CTC therapy.

medicine OR Mongolian medicine OR phytotherapy OR herb therapy OR herbal therapy OR ethnopharmacology OR ethnobotany OR phytogenic OR alternative medicine OR alternative therapy OR complementary therapy OR complementary medicine OR TCM OR CHM OR Zhong Yi Xue) AND (clinical trial OR randomized controlled trial OR controlled clinical trial OR multicenter study OR phase 1 clinical trial OR phase 2 clinical trial OR phase 3 clinical trial OR phase 4 clinical trial). The terms in Chinese adopted from the above terms were retrieved in Chinese databases.

Databases

The databases in English language included EMBASE (1974 to September 2012), MEDLINE (1946 to September 2012), AMED (from 1985 to September 2012), EBM Reviews included Cochrane Database of Systematic Reviews (2005 to September 2012), ACP Journal Club (1991 to September 2012), Database of Abstracts of Reviews of Effects (September 2012), Cochrane Central Register of Controlled Trials (September 2012), Cochrane Methodology Register (September 2012), Health Technology Assessment (September 2012), NHS Economic Evaluation Database (September 2012). The databases in Chinese included CNKI (China Knowledge Resource Integrated Database, China academic journals, conference proceedings and theses; 1979 to September 2012).

Inclusion Criteria

Studies included in the meta-analysis had to meet all of the following criteria: (1) Participants: NSCLC patients had to be diagnosed by pathological sections and were treated by the CT. (2) Type of studies: only clinical randomized controlled trials (RCTs) were eligible. (3) Type of intervention: studies reported CT combined with or without CHM. For studies using other agents as the third arm, only the two arms using CHM and/or CT will be included for analysis. (4) Type of outcome measurements: overall survival rate and tumor response were the main outcome measurements; other outcome measurement included reduction in AEs of CT, improvement in clinical symptoms and blood disorders were also considered.

Exclusion Criteria

Clinical trials were excluded if they did not meet the above criteria. In addition, studies with the followings were also excluded: (1) CHM were used in both of the intervention group and control group; (2) Non-original research (e.g. review article, letter to the editor); (3) Duplicated publications.

Outcome Measures

Survival rate, tumor response of CHM on the number of patients with complete response (CR) or partial response (PR), as well as those with progressive disease (PD) based on the WHO scale were examined. The improved or stable performance status of patients were investigated based on the Karnofsky performance score (KPS), in which 100 refers to a normal subject with no complaints, 70 refers to a patient unable to carry on normal activity, 50 refers to a patient who requires considerable assistance, 40 refers to a disabled patient and 30 refers to a hospitalization-recommended patient. The efficacy of CHM on relieving the AEs of CT including nausea and vomiting, hemoglobin (HB), platelet (PLT) were studied by grading the acute and subacute AEs of cancer treatment.

Quality Assessment

Methodological quality of RCTs was assessed using the five-point Jadad scale [9]. All trials were reviewed by at least two reviewers and any disagreement was resolved by third reviewer consensus. In addition, the risk of bias for the included studies was also assessed.

Data Analysis

The Review Manager 5.1 software (Nordic Cochrane Centre, Copenhagen, Denmark) was employed for data analysis. The effect data is expressed as relative risk (RR) with 95% confidence interval (CI). If the heterogeneity exists in pooled studies (I^2>50%), a random model was applied, otherwise the fix model was applied. Statistic significant difference was considered as $p<0.05$.

Results

Characteristics of the Included Studies

In the study, 2,998 articles were retrieved. 30 studies were finally included. Among these studies, six studies were not pooled for analysis as four studies had Jadad score 2 [10–13], and other two studies did not report tumor-node-metastasis (TNM) staging information [14,15]. Therefore, 24 eligible studies were included for meta-analysis. The study selection process details were described in Figure 1. A sum of 2,109 patients was enrolled in these studies, at which 1,064 patients participated in CT combined CHM (CTC) and 1,039 in CT (six patients dropped out and were not reported the group enrolled). A total 78 patients withdraw or dropped out, 36 patients in CTC, 36 in CT and six patients in groups not specified.

All the patients recruited in the 24 studies were at stage III to IV of NSCLC TNM, and all of the studies were graded at least Jadad score 3. The risk of bias of all studies was shown in Table S1. The course of treatment varied from 4 to 16 weeks in the included studies. A list of therapeutic approaches and outcome assessment in each study, and the quality of studies assessed by five-point Jadad scale was listed in Table 1. All studies had claimed the baseline were comparable except one study [32] including age, gender, histopathology or TNM stage as shown in Table S2.

Survival

One-year survival was analyzed as shown in Figure 2. One-year survival in pooled studies showed a significant rise in CTC compared to CT alone (RR = 1.36, 95% CI = 1.15–1.60, p = 0.0003, seven studies, 608 patients), with low heterogeneity (I^2 = 0%) [16–22]. A half-year survival also demonstrated a favor of CTC compared to CT alone (RR = 1.18, 95% CI = 1.04–1.33, p = 0.008, two studies, 157 patients) as shown in Figure S1.

Immediate Tumor Response

As shown in Figure 3, CTC therapy was associated with a significant increase in the number of patients who reported complete or partial response (RR = 1.36, 95% CI = 1.19–1.56,

Table 1. Characteristics of the included studies.

Study	No. of participants/dropout or withdrawal	TNM stage	Control group intervention	CHM formula	Assessment of outcome	Duration (week)	Jadad scale
Chen et al. 2008 [16]	106/6 dropout patients	IIIB–IV	NP	Shengmai injection Gujin grand decoction	Tumor response, survival rate, chemotoxicity	12	3
Chen et al. 2011 [17]	77/0	IIIB–IV	NP/TP	Feiji recipe	Tumor response, survival rate, CD62P	8	3
Deng et al. 2012 [23]	60/drop out: 2 patients in CTC and 3 patients in CT	IIIB–IV	TP/DP	Feitai capsule	Tumor response, CT completion rate, CT delay rate	12	4
Huang et al. 2011 [24]	60/3 withdrawals	IIIB–IV	GP	Yinqi Yangyin decoction	Tumor response, survival rate, chemotoxicity, KPS	8	3
Huang et al. 2012 [25]	60/3 withdrawals	IIIB–IV	GP	Ziyin Qinre Jiedu decoction	Tumor response, chemotoxicity, KPS	11.4	3
Li and Li 2012 [39]	80/1 withdrawal	III–IV	TP	Jianpi Yangxue decoction	Chemotoxicity	3	3
Li et al. 2003 [18]	80/drop out: 7 patients in CTC and 5 patients in CT	III–IV	CAP/EP/CT combined with radiotherapy	Intravenous injection of Xiaoji decoction based on syndrome differentiation	Tumor response, survival rate, chemotoxicity, KPS, CD4, CD8	8	4
Li et al. 2009 [26]	83/0	IIIB–IV	MVP	Haishensu	Tumor response, survival rate, chemotoxicity, KPS, body weight	4	4
Lin 2008 [27]	129/drop out: 5 patients in CTC and 4 patients in CT; withdraw: 2 patients in CTC and 3 patients in CT	IIIB–IV	MVP combined with radiotherapy	Fuzheng Kangai decoction	Tumor response, chemotoxicity, KPS	12	3
Lin and Zheng 2011 [28]	64/drop out: 2 patients in CTC and 2 patients in CT	III–IV	NVB/+DDP	Hechan Pian plus CHMs based on syndrome differentiation	Tumor response, chemotoxicity, body weight	12	3
Lu and Wei 2009 [19]	60/0	III–IV	NP combined with radiotherapy	Shenmai injection	Tumor response, chemotoxicity, survival rate	8	3
Shan et al. 2011 [38]	60/0	III–IV	NP/NC/TP/GP	CHM decoction and intravenous dripping of patent Chinese medicine Yanshu injection	EORTC QLQ-LC43	8	3
Sun 2011 [29]	60/withdraw:1 patient in CT	IIIB–IV	NP	Fuzheng Jiedu decoction	Tumor response, chemotoxicity, KPS, NK cells	9	3
Xu et al. 2007 [30]	120/drop out: 4 patients in CT	III–IV	NP/GP/MVP	Kangliu Zengxiao decoction, Feiyan Ning decoction	Survival rate, KPS, main clinical symptoms, chemotoxicity	12–16	4
Yang 2007 [20]	77/drop out: 4 patients in CTC and 3 patients in CT; withdraw: 2 patients in CTC and 2 patients in CT	III–IV	NP	Shengmai injection and Meihua Dianshe pill	Cost-tumor control rate ratio and cost-one year survival rate ratio	8–16	4
Yao et al. 2011 [35]	86/0	III–IV	NP/CE/TP	Yangyin Ruanjian decoction	Quality of life, size of tumor, body weight, survival rate	12	3
Zhang et al. 2008 [22]	120/drop out: 9 patients in CTC and 5 patients in CT	III–IV	NP	Artesunate	Tumor response, survival rate, chemotoxicity, mean survival time, time to progression	8	4
Zhang et al. 2012 [21]	135/16 dropouts	IIIB–IV	NP/TP/GP	Feiliuping extract	Therapeutic effect, immune function, KPS, median life span, survival rate of one year	6	4

Table 1. Cont.

Study	No. of participants/dropout or withdrawal	TNM stage	Control group intervention	CHM formula	Assessment of outcome	Duration (week)	Jadad scale
Zheng et al. 2007 [37]	40/drop out: 2 patients in CTC and 1 patient in CT	III–IV	NP/CE/TP	Feiliuping decoction	NK cytoactivity, CD3, CD4, CD4/CD8, KPS, MDC	8	3
Zheng et al. 2010 [31]	60/0	IIIB–IV	DP	Shenmai injection	Tumor response, chemotoxicity	8	3
Zhou et?al. 2005 [32]	324/30 drop out and withdrawals; CTC and CT were analyzed only. (CTC:103;CT:92; CM:99)	III–IV	NP	Hechan Pian/Shenyi Jiaonang based on syndrome differentiation	Overall response rate, median survival time, cost-effect	12	4
Zhou et al. 2012 [33]	52/2 withdrawals	III–IV	TP/NP/DP/GP	Yiqi Yangyin Huatan decoction based on syndrome differentiation	RECIST evaluation, cost/therapeutic effect ratio	8	3
Zhu and Guo 2011 [34]	182/0	III–IV	TP/NP/GP	Yanshu injection	Tumor response, median survival time, serum tumor markers, chemotoxicity, CD3, CD4, CD4/CD8	16	3
Zhu et al. 2011 [36]	127/3 withdrawals; CTC and CT were analyzed only (CTC: 32; CT:31; other two group: 30, 31 respectively)	III–IV	NP/GP	Kangliu Zengxiao decoction	Clinical symptoms, adverse effect, KPS, NK cytoactivity, CD3, CD4, CD4/CD8	8	4

Abbreviations: CAP = cyclophosphamide+adriamycin+cisplatinum, CHM = Chinese herbal medicine, CT = chemotherapy, CTC = chemotherapy combined with Chinese herb medicine, DDP = cisplatinum, DP = docetaxel+cisplatinum, EP = VP-16+ cisplatinum, GP = gemcitabine+cisplatinum, KPS = Karnofsky performance score, MDC = macrophage-derived chemokine, MVP = mitomycin+vindesine+cisplatinum, NC = vinorelbine+cisplatinum, NP = vinorelbine+cisplatinum, NVB = vinorelbine, RECIST = Response Evaluation Criteria in Solid Tumors, TP = paclitaxel+cisplatinum.

p<1.0E−5, 18 studies, 1,623 patients) [16,18–34]. In addition, the advantage of CTC therapy was found in the number of patients who reported complete, partial and stable response (RR = 1.14, 95% CI = 1.08–1.19, p<1.0E-5, 19 studies, 1,697 patients, figure not showed).

Performance Status

Two types of KPS data were reported in the studies, the improvement of KPS (ten-point cutoff) and the value of KPS in pre- and post-treatment. Six studies of the 24 studies, with evaluation of 526 patients were being analyzed. 35.1% and 10.9% of patients reported improved (the increase of KPS≥10) in CTC (n = 270) and in CT (n = 256), respectively. Significant findings with improvement were shown in the CTC (RR = 2.90, 95% CI = 1.62–5.18, p = 0.0003, six studies, 526 patients) (Figure 4) [21,26,29,30,35,36]. There was no significant heterogeneity among these studies ($I^2 = 51\%$). Dropping one of any studies did not alter the result that favor of CTC. The value of KPS was reported with pre-treatment in seven studies [19,24–26,30,34,37] and post-treatment in four studies [24,25,34,37]. The pooled studies showed that the KPS of pre-treatment had no significant difference in CTC and CT (SMD = −0.04, 95% CI = −0.20-0.12, p = 0.64, $I^2 = 0\%$). However, the pooled studies indicated the heterogeneity in the four studies of post-treatment (SMD = 1.03, 95% CI = −0.09–2.14, p = 0.07, $I^2 = 95\%$). Interestingly, these four studies all claimed significant improvement in CTC compared to CT.

Reduction in CT Toxicity

Nausea and vomiting are common AEs of CT. A significant reduction of nausea and vomiting at toxicity grade of III–IV in CTC compared to CT therapy was found (RR = 0.24, 95% CI = 0.12–0.50, p = 1.0E−4, five studies, 350 patients) [19,24,25,30,31] (Figure 5A). However, there was significant heterogeneity in the studies with reduction of nausea and vomiting at toxicity grade of I–IV (data not shown). One study reported a significant reduction of nausea and vomiting in CTC compared to CT at the 10th day of second treatment, based on the questionnaire EORTC QLQ-LC43 (combination of EORTC QLQ-C30 and QLQ-LC13) [38]. The study was not pooled due to the different data types.

The decrease of HB at the toxicity grade of I–IV in patients with CTC therapy was significant reduced (RR = 0.64, 95% CI = 0.51–0.80, p<1.0E−4, six studies, 553 patients, Figure 5B) [19,24,29,30,34,39]; yet CTC therapy did not show a significant difference in the decline of HB at the toxicity grade of III–IV (RR = 0.58, 95% CI = 0.26–1.29, p = 0.18, seven studies, 616 patients) compared to CT alone (Figure 5C) [19,24,29,30,34,36,39].

The inhibition of white blood cells (WBCs) at the toxicity grade of III–IV or I–IV in patients with CTC therapy was significant reduced (RR = 0.36, 95% CI = 0.26–0.52, p<1.0E−5, nine studies, 666 patients; RR = 0.75, 95% CI = 0.67–0.84, p<1.0E−5, eight studies, 603 patients, respectively) (Figure 6A and Figure 6B) [19,24,25,27,29–31,36,39].

The decrease of PLTs in numbers at the toxicity grade of III–IV was significant prevented in patients with CTC therapy (RR = 0.34, 95% CI = 0.17–0.68, p = 0.002, seven studies, 557 patients) [19,24,25,29,34,36,39]. The decrease of PLTs in numbers at the toxicity grade of III–IV was significant dismissed in patients with CTC therapy (RR = 0.43, 95% CI = 0.31–0.60, p<1E−5, six studies, 494 patients) [19,24,25,29,34,39]. In addition, our study showed CTC therapy significantly prevented

A. WBC reduction at the toxicity grade of III~IV

Study or Subgroup	Experimental Events	Experimental Total	Control Events	Control Total	Weight	Risk Ratio M-H, Fixed, 95% CI
Huang et al 2011	2	29	3	28	3.2%	0.64 [0.12, 3.57]
Huang et al 2012	2	28	3	29	3.1%	0.69 [0.12, 3.83]
Li and Li et al 2012	6	40	12	39	12.9%	0.49 [0.20, 1.17]
Lin 2008	7	58	20	57	21.4%	0.34 [0.16, 0.75]
Lu and Wei 2009	3	30	6	30	6.4%	0.50 [0.14, 1.82]
Sun 2011	0	30	1	29	1.6%	0.32 [0.01, 7.61]
Xu et al 2007	12	60	23	56	25.2%	0.49 [0.27, 0.88]
Zheng et al 2010	2	30	8	30	8.5%	0.25 [0.06, 1.08]
Zhu et al 2011	0	32	16	31	17.7%	0.03 [0.00, 0.47]
Total (95% CI)		**337**		**329**	**100.0%**	**0.36 [0.26, 0.52]**
Total events	34		92			

Heterogeneity: Chi² = 5.97, df = 8 (P = 0.65); I² = 0%

Test for overall effect: Z = 5.58 (P < 0.00001)

Risk Ratio M-H, Fixed, 95% CI

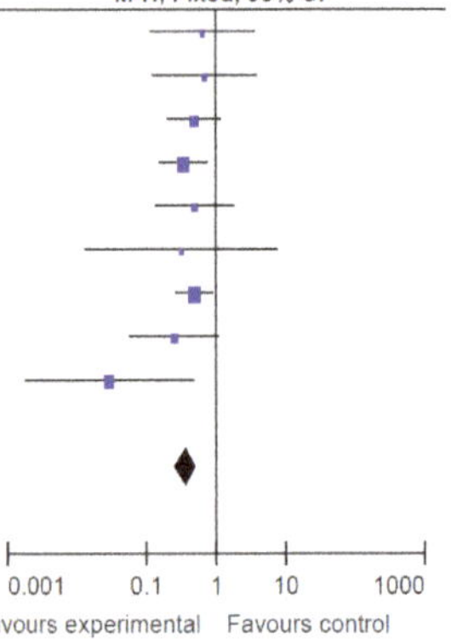

B. WBC reduction at the toxicity grade of I~IV

Study or Subgroup	Experimental Events	Experimental Total	Control Events	Control Total	Weight	Risk Ratio M-H, Fixed, 95% CI
Huang et al 2011	9	29	12	28	5.7%	0.72 [0.36, 1.44]
Huang et al 2012	5	28	12	29	5.5%	0.43 [0.17, 1.07]
Li and Li et al 2012	25	40	31	39	14.6%	0.79 [0.59, 1.05]
Lin 2008	37	58	50	57	23.4%	0.73 [0.59, 0.90]
Lu and Wei 2009	17	30	24	30	11.1%	0.71 [0.49, 1.02]
Sun 2011	5	30	13	29	6.1%	0.37 [0.15, 0.91]
Xu et al 2007	42	60	42	56	20.2%	0.93 [0.75, 1.17]
Zheng et al 2010	24	30	29	30	13.5%	0.83 [0.68, 1.00]
Total (95% CI)		**305**		**298**	**100.0%**	**0.75 [0.67, 0.84]**
Total events	164		213			

Heterogeneity: Chi² = 8.72, df = 7 (P = 0.27); I² = 20%

Test for overall effect: Z = 4.84 (P < 0.00001)

Risk Ratio M-H, Fixed, 95% CI

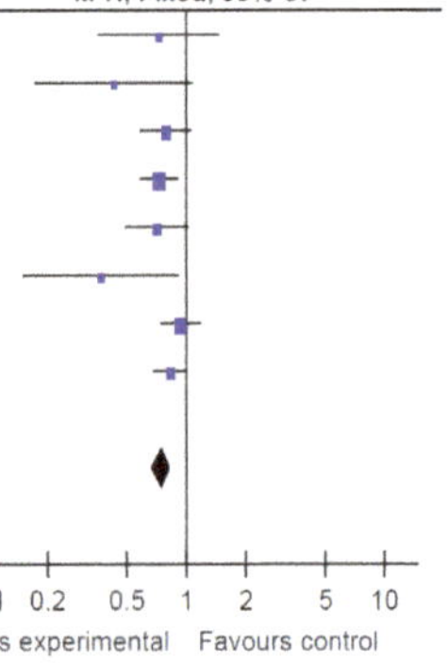

C. Platelet reduction at the toxicity grade of III~IV

Study or Subgroup	Experimental Events	Experimental Total	Control Events	Control Total	Weight	Risk Ratio M-H, Fixed, 95% CI
Huang et al 2011	2	29	4	28	13.9%	0.48 [0.10, 2.43]
Huang et al 2012	2	28	4	29	13.4%	0.52 [0.10, 2.61]
Li and Li et al 2012	1	40	3	39	10.4%	0.33 [0.04, 2.99]
Lu and Wei 2009	0	30	0	30		Not estimable
Sun 2011	0	30	1	29	5.2%	0.32 [0.01, 7.61]
Zhu and Guo 2011	4	92	14	90	48.4%	0.28 [0.10, 0.82]
Zhu et al 2011	0	32	2	31	8.7%	0.19 [0.01, 3.88]
Total (95% CI)		**281**		**276**	**100.0%**	**0.34 [0.17, 0.68]**
Total events	9		28			

Heterogeneity: Chi² = 0.71, df = 5 (P = 0.98); I² = 0%

Test for overall effect: Z = 3.05 (P = 0.002)

Risk Ratio M-H, Fixed, 95% CI

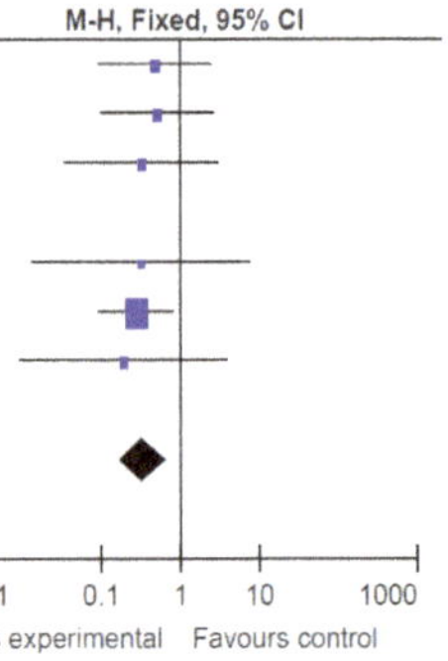

D. Platelet reduction at the toxicity grade of I~IV

Study or Subgroup	Experimental Events	Experimental Total	Control Events	Control Total	Weight	Risk Ratio M-H, Fixed, 95% CI
Huang et al 2011	7	29	14	28	15.9%	0.48 [0.23, 1.02]
Huang et al 2012	7	28	15	29	16.5%	0.48 [0.23, 1.00]
Li and Li et al 2012	8	40	12	39	13.6%	0.65 [0.30, 1.42]
Lu and Wei 2009	6	30	13	30	14.5%	0.46 [0.20, 1.05]
Sun 2011	2	30	6	29	6.8%	0.32 [0.07, 1.47]
Zhu and Guo 2011	9	92	29	90	32.7%	0.30 [0.15, 0.60]
Total (95% CI)		**249**		**245**	**100.0%**	**0.43 [0.31, 0.60]**
Total events	39		89			

Heterogeneity: Chi² = 2.40, df = 5 (P = 0.79); I² = 0%

Test for overall effect: Z = 5.01 (P < 0.00001)

Risk Ratio M-H, Fixed, 95% CI

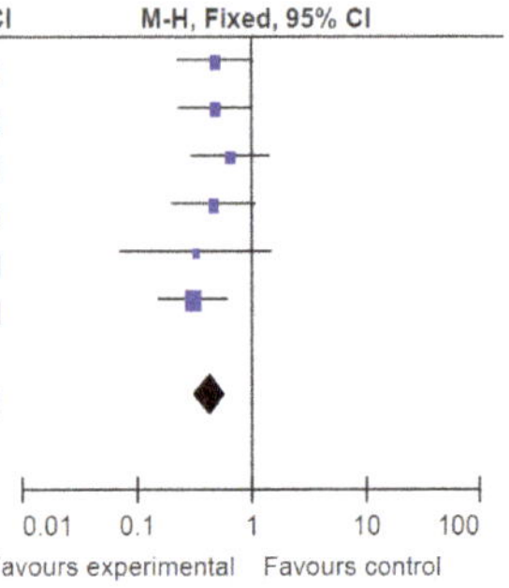

Figure 6. Reduction of adverse effects. Reduction of adverse effects estimated from meta-analysis of pairwise comparisons in patients with Chinese herbal medicine (CHM, treatment group) versus patients without CHM (control group). (**A**) The inhibition of white blood cells (WBCs) at the toxicity grade of III–IV. (**B**) The inhibition of WBCs at the toxicity grade of I–IV. (**C**) The decrease of platelets in numbers at the toxicity grade of III–IV. (**D**) The decrease of platelets in numbers at the toxicity grade of I–IV.

the decline of PLTs at the toxicity grade of III–IV and I–IV when dropped any one study.

Herbs Frequently used in NSCLC

19 studies have reported herbs and decoctions. Among them, *Radix Astragalus*, *Radix Adenophorae* and *Radix Ophiopogonis* are the most commonly used herbs for NSCLC (Table 2).

Discussion

Recent studies showed that the use of CAM has increasingly gained recognition and usage in cancer patients [40,41]. CHM is especially popular among the CAM usage as palliative care for cancer patients, but the efficacy of the combined use of CAM and CT on advanced NSCLC cancer remains under explored due to language barrier of many studies reported in Chinese language [42]. Meta-analysis is a powerful statistical analysis of results from individual studies, which increases the precision of a treatment effect and settles controversies studies [43]. In the present study, the pooled data with advanced NSCLC has shown that combined therapy significantly improved the survival rates, immediate tumor response and performance status of advanced NSCLC patients. We also found that, when compared with CT alone, the CTC therapy significantly reduce AEs associated with chemotherapeutic interventions, including nausea and vomiting, decrease in the peripheral blood leukocytes and HB (Figure 5 and Figure 6).

In contrast to most of the previous meta-analyses in this area, our systematic review set the inclusion criteria with Jadad score ≥3 to increase the study quality and included studies with stage III–IV of TNM to minimize the heterogeneity among the studies. It is also encouraging to see that the adjunctive use of CHM with CT may prolong survival in advanced stage NSCLC patients, and CT-related side effects appear to be less frequent and milder in the use of concomitant CAM treatment, which suggest CAM may enhance the compliance to CT and eventually result in improving KPS of patients. The efficacy of CHM as an adjuvant therapy for NSCLC is in line with our previous findings in colorectal cancer, hepatocellular carcinoma and nasopharyngeal carcinoma [44–46].

Table 2. Herbs frequently used for non-small cell lung cancer.

Chinese herbal medicine	Frequency	
	Count	%
Radix Astragalus	10	52.6
Radix Adenophorae	8	42.1
Radix Ophiopogonis	7	36.8
Radix Glycyrrhizae	5	26.3
Poria	5	26.3
Herba Oldenlandia Diffusa	5	26.3
Radix Asparagi	4	21.1
Semen Persicae	4	21.1
Radix Notoginseng	4	21.1

According to Chinese medicine theory, illness is caused by the disharmony of yin and yang, and Chinese medicine aims to restore the balance of yin and yang to alleviate the disease symptoms. CHMs have been commonly used in Asia for thousands of years. Interestingly, it is reported that 61 out of 74 lung cancer patients recruited by 17 Community Clinical Oncology Program (CCOP) affiliates throughout the United States have used CAM while undergoing CT or radiation therapy [47]. However, the potential for integrating CAM into conventional CT treatment remains to be evaluated [48]. *Radix Astragalus, Radix Adenophorae, Radix Ophiopogonis, Radix Glycyrrhizae, Poria and Oldenlandia diffusa* identified in the study have the function of tonifying qi, nourishing yin and removing blood stasis, which are in accordance to the commonest symptoms in NSCLC patients undergoing CT (i.e. blood stasis, vital energy and yin deficiency). It is in line with other findings that *Radix Astragalus, Radix Ophiopogonis and Oldenlandia diffusa* are commonly used for NSCLC [49]. Besides, it has also been reported that there was a significant effectiveness of adding astragalus-based herbal treatment to standard CT regimens [50]. Several experimental researches have revealed that *Adenophora Polysaccharides* and *Oldenlandia diffusa* extract could effectively inhibited the growth of cancer cell lines and induced significant increase of apoptosis. Furthermore, there was a significant inhibition of lung metastases in animal model with no noticeable AEs [51,52]. *Radix Adenophorae* and *Radix Ophiopogonis* were also shown to have anti-inflammation and immunomodulating effects [53,54]. Our previous studies have demonstrated that *Radix Astragalus*, the dried root of *Astragalus membranaceus*, has anti-tumor, immunomodulating and immunorestorative effects *in vivo* and *in vitro* [55,56]. It is in accordance with other findings that *Radix Astragulus* has immunologic benefits by stimulating macrophage, natural killer cell activity but inhibiting T-helper cell type 2 cytokines [57]. In addition, the combination of *Radix Astragulus* and *Radix Angelicae* increased WBC, HB and PLT in cyclophosphamide-induced anemic rat [58]. This study also indicated that these two herbs are associated with enhancing erythropoietin expression [58]. Erythropoietin is also able to prevent against cisplatin cytotoxicity in cells via several mechanisms [59,60]. These findings may give some insights on the mechanism of how CHM improved the hematological parameters in this systematic review. Furthermore, *Radix Astragalus* also reduced toxicity induced by cyclophosphamide [61]. Though the molecular mechanism is not fully understood, the immunostimulating effects and the reduction of chemotherapy-induced toxicity may be the two major advantages for CHM as adjuvant therapy in NSCLC treatment.

Survival rate, immediate tumor response and chemo-toxicity are three major outcomes in the studies. However, not all the studies simultaneously reported the three outcomes. For example, Zhang et al. [21] reported all three outcomes while Li and Li [39] reported the reduction of chemo-toxicity only. Nevertheless, we analyzed all available data in these reports without any subjective selection. KPS is a scale for the evaluation of cancer patients. In this study, we analyzed continuous data (average of KPS scores) and discontinuous data (patient number with an increase of KPS≥10). There is significant heterogeneity when we pooled studies with continuous data, although the baseline has no heterogeneity in the meta-analysis. The variation of KPS value in the studies may be due to the differences in treatment duration, treatment methods and the herb prescriptions in different studies. Therefore, the change of KPS in patients is more accurate to indicate the efficacy of treatments in pooled studies. The interval of ten in KPS normally shows a significant change of performance status as described by previous publications [26,57,62,63]. Hence, we adopted a ten-point increase as the cutoff for improved performance status. The findings showed a significant improvement in KPS with CTC treatment.

In conclusion, the evidence from the meta-analysis of the included studies shows that CHM as adjuvant therapy has advantages in NSCLC patients. However, due to the complex nature of CHM interventions, particular attention should be paid to apply appropriate and rigorous research methodologies to investigate CHM as a holistic system [64]. Therefore a large scale RCT integrated the Chinese Medicine methodology of pattern diagnosis and treatment is warranted for further study.

Supporting Information

Figure S1 Number of patients with survival >half-year. Overall survivals estimated from meta-analysis of pairwise comparisons in the patients with chemotherapy combined Chinese herbal medicine (CTC, treatment group) versus patients in chemotherapy (CT, control group).
(TIF)

Table S1 The risk of bias of the included studies.
(DOC)

Table S2 Age, gender and baseline of studies.
(DOC)

Author Contributions

Interpretation of data and manuscript revision: SGL HYC CSOY XXW ZJY YT WCC. Conceived and designed the experiments: WCC YT. Analyzed the data: SGL HYC. Wrote the paper: SGL HYC.

References

1. Siegel R, Naishadham D, Jemal A (2012) Cancer statistics, 2012. CA Cancer J Clin 62: 10–29.
2. Pfister DG, Johnson DH, Azzoli CG, Sause W, Smith TJ, et al. (2004) American Society of Clinical Oncology treatment of unresectable non-small-cell lung cancer guideline: update 2003. J Clin Oncol 22: 330–353.
3. Azzoli CG, Temin S, Aliff T, Baker S Jr, Brahmer J, et al. (2011) 2011 Focused update of 2009 American Society of Clinical Oncology Clinical practice guideline update on chemotherapy for stage IV non-small-cell lung cancer. J Clin Oncol 29: 3825–3831.
4. Arriagada R, Dunant A, Pignon JP, Bergman B, Chabowski M, et al. (2010) Long-term results of the international adjuvant lung cancer trial evaluating adjuvant cisplatin-based chemotherapy in resected lung cancer. J Clin Oncol 28: 35–42.
5. Kato H, Tsuboi M, Kato Y, Ikeda N, Okunaka T, et al. (2005) Postoperative adjuvant therapy for completely resected early-stage non-small cell lung cancer. Int J Clin Oncol 10: 157–164.
6. Gkiozos I, Charpidou A, Syrigos K (2007) Developments in the treatment of non-small cell lung cancer. Anticancer Res 27: 2823–2827.
7. Baggstrom MQ, Stinchcombe TE, Fried DB, Poole C, Hensing TA, et al. (2007) Third-generation chemotherapy agents in the treatment of advanced non-small cell lung cancer: a meta-analysis. J Thorac Oncol 2: 845–853.
8. Chen YZ, Li ZD, Gao F, Zhang Y, Sun H, et al. (2009) Effects of combined Chinese drugs and chemotherapy in treating advanced non-small cell lung cancer. Chin J Integr Med 15: 415–419.
9. Jadad AR, Moore RA, Carroll D, Jenkinson C, Reynolds DJ, et al. (1996) Assessing the quality of reports of randomized clinical trials: is blinding necessary? Control Clin Trials 17: 1–12.
10. Huang C, Liao TH (2008) Effect of combination of Chenxialiujun decoction and chemotherapy on non-small lung cell cancer. Hebei J Tradit Chin Med 30: 1287–1288.
11. Liang QL, Zhang Y, Xie JR, Li SJ, Luo HQ, et al. (2007) Clillical study on effcacy of compound Dashen droplet pill with chemotherapy in treating advanced non-small cell lung cancer. Shanghai J Tradit Chin Med 41: 22–24.
12. Qi YF, Li XR, Li HJ (2011) Clinical study on lung cancer treated by Dahuang Zhechong Wan. Chin J Inf Tradit Chin Med 18: 15–17.
13. Yan GY, Xu ZY, Deng HB, Wan ZY, Zhang L, et al. (2011) Effect s of chemotherapy combined with Chinese herbal medicine Kangliu Zengxiao decoction on tumor markers of patient s with advanced non-small cell lung cancer: a randomized, controlled trial. J Chin Integr Med 9: 525–530.
14. Yang PY, Jia YJ, Chen J, Li XJ, Sun YY, et al. (2011) A clinical study of Xiaoyan decoction combined with chemotherapy on the immune function of the NSCLC patients with "Qi deficiency and blood statsis". J New Chin Med 43: 64–65.
15. Wang YC, Zhang RH (2009) Clinical effect of non-small cell lung cancer treated by combined chemotherapy with Zhongliuan capsule. Chin Tradit Patent Med 31: 669–673.
16. Chen Y, Di L, Zhang S, Chen M, Sun H, et al. (2008) The randomized, multicenter, controlled clinic trail for treating advanced non-small cell lung cancer with combined traditional chinese medicine and vinorelbine (Navelbine, NVB) plus cisplatin (DDP) chemotherapy. Zhongguo Fei Ai Za Zhi 11: 441–444.
17. Chen XZ, Huang ZQ, Yang YL, Qian HQ, Liang GW, et al. (2011) The intervention effect of Feiji recipe on CD62P of non-small cell lung cancer patients. Chin Med Mod Distance Ed China 9: 93–95.
18. Li LN, Liu WS, Xu K, Wu WY, Liu YL, et al. (2003) The prognosis factors of comprehensive treatment with traditional Chinese medicine to non-small cell lung cancer. Shanxi Cancer Med 11: 44–47.
19. Lu XA, Wei YR (2009) Therapeutic effect of combination of Shenmai injection and radio-chemotherapy on advanced non-small cell lung cancer. Hebei J Tradit Chin Med 31: 597–599.
20. Yang HL (2007) Cost-effect analysis of integrated Chinese and Western medical treatment for advanced non-small cell lung cancer. J Tradit Chin Med 48: 232–234.
21. Zhang PT, Lin HS, Yu MW, Yang ZY, Dong HT, et al. (2012) Application of traditional Chinese medicine and Western medical therapeutic evaluation methodologies for the combination treatment with Feiliuping extract and chemotherapy in advanced non-small cell lung cancer. J Tradit Chin Med 53: 403–406.
22. Zhang Z, Yu SQ, Miao L, Huang XY, Zhang XP, et al. (2008) Artesunate combined with vinorelbline plus cisplatin in treatment of advanced non-small cell lung cancer: a randomized controlled trial. Zhong Xi Yi Jie He Xue Bao 6: 134–138.
23. Deng S, Ouyang X, Yu Z, Dai X, Chen X, et al. (2012) Influence of Chinese herbal medicine Feitai capsule on completion or delay of chemotherapy in patients with stage IIIB/IV non-small cell lung cancer: a randomized controlled trial. Zhong Xi Yi Jie He Xue Bao 10: 635–640.
24. Huang YL, Hou AJ, Hu Y, Zhou L, Gao HF (2011) The clinical effect of Yi Qi Yang Yin Chinese medicine combined with GP chemotherapy to the advanced non-small cell lung cancer patients. J New Chin Med 43: 47–49.
25. Huang YL, Hou AJ, Zhou L, Hu Y, Shen XY (2012) Clinical study on non-small cell lung cancer treated by Zi Yin Qin Re herbs combined with chemotherapy. Liaoning Tradit Chin Med J 2: 53.
26. Li GY, Yu XM, Zhang HW, Zhang B, Wang CB, et al. (2009) Haishengsu as an adjunct therapy to conventional chemotherapy in patients with non-small cell lung cancer: a pilot randomized and placebo-controlled clinical trial. Complement Ther Med 17: 51–55.
27. Lin J (2008) Clinical study on the combined Chinese and Western medicine in treating 58 cases of non-small cell lung cancer. Henan J Tradit Chin Med 28: 29–31.
28. Lin LZ, Zheng XT (2011) Clinical observation of the therapeutic effect of traditional Chinese medicine in the treatment of elderly non-small cell lung cancer. Tradit Chin Drug Res Clin Pharmacol 22: 120–122.
29. Sun QS (2011) Clinical observation of the therapeutic effect of chemotherapy plus traditional Chinese medicine in the treatment of advanced non-small cell lung cancer. Hainan Med J 22: 31–33.
30. Xu ZY, Jin CJ, Shen DY, Li M, Zhou WD, et al. (2007) Clinical study on treatment of advanced non-small cell lung cancer with Chinese herbal medicine in different stages combined with chemotherapy. Zhongguo Zhong Xi Yi Jie He Za Zhi 27: 874–878.
31. Zheng QH, Liao XF, Wang Y (2010) Thirty cases of docetaxel plus cisplatin with Shenmai injection in treatment of advanced non-small cell lung cancer. Jiangxi J Tradit Chin Med 57–58.
32. Zhou DH, Lin LZ, Zhou YQ, Luo RC, LIu KF, et al. (2005) Cost-effectiveness analysis of three therapeutic regimens for advanced non-small cell lung cancer. Chin J Clin Oncol 32: 1081–1084.
33. Zhou L, Liu JX, Li HG, Zhao LH, Liu LS, et al. (2012) Comparative study on treatment of advance non-small cell lung cancer by two methods. Shanghai J Tradit Chin Med 5: 8.
34. Zhu LM, Guo JF (2011) Clinical study of Yanshu injection on treating advanced non-small cell lung cancer. Chin J Clin Oncol Rehabil 18: 380–384.
35. Yao QB, Wang LX, Ni W, Shen YL, Zhu Y, et al. (2011) Clinical observation of "Yang Yin Ruan Jian" on non-small cell lung cancer. J Zhejiang Chin Med Uni 35: 501–503.

36. Zhu LM, Zhang H, Zhou H, Pan CF, Shen KP, et al. (2011) Time-effect relationship of Kangliu Zengxiao decoction in reducing chemotherapy associated adverse reactions in patients with advanced non-small cell lung cancer. J Shanghai Jiaotong Uni (Med Sci) 31: 797–801.
37. Zheng HG, Pu BK, Lin HS, Xiong L, Hua BJ, et al. (2007) The efficacy of Feiliuping decoction on dendritic cell subtypes and immune function in patients with non-small cell lung carcinoma. Beijing J Tradit Chin Med 26: 214–217.
38. Shan M, Han B, You J (2011) Assessment of therapeutic efficacy on treating advanced non-small cell lung cancer in the aged by Chinese medicine adopting the international questionnaire of quality of life. Zhongguo Zhong Xi Yi Jie He Za Zhi 31: 873–879.
39. Li Y, Li C (2012) Clinical study of treatment of cancer chemotherapy by Jianpi Yangxue Tang. Guangming J Chin Med 27: 108–109.
40. Hyodo I, Amano N, Eguchi K, Narabayashi M, Imanishi J, et al. (2005) Nationwide survey on complementary and alternative medicine in cancer patients in Japan. J Clin Oncol 23: 2645–2654.
41. Chang KH, Brodie R, Choong MA, Sweeney KJ, Kerin MJ (2011) Complementary and alternative medicine use in oncology: a questionnaire survey of patients and health care professionals. BMC Cancer 11: 196.
42. Li JH (1996) A study on treatment of lung cancer by combined therapy of traditional Chinese medicine and chemotherapy. Zhongguo Zhong Xi Yi Jie He Za Zhi 16: 136–138.
43. Bent S (2008) Herbal medicine in the United States: review of efficacy, safety, and regulation: grand rounds at University of California, San Francisco Medical Center. J Gen Intern Med 23: 854–859.
44. Cho WC, Chen HY (2009) Transcatheter arterial chemoembolization combined with or without Chinese herbal therapy for hepatocellular carcinoma: meta-analysis. Expert Opin Investig Drugs 18: 617–635.
45. Cho WC, Chen HY (2009) Clinical efficacy of traditional Chinese medicine as a concomitant therapy for nasopharyngeal carcinoma: a systematic review and meta-analysis. Cancer Invest 27: 334–344.
46. Zhong LL, Chen HY, Cho WC, Meng X, Tong Y (2012) The efficacy of Chinese herbal medicine as an adjunctive therapy for colorectal cancer: a systematic review and meta-analysis. Complementary therapies in medicine. Complement Ther Med 20: 240–252.
47. Yates JS, Mustian KM, Morrow GR, Gillies LJ, Padmanaban D, et al. (2005) Prevalence of complementary and alternative medicine use in cancer patients during treatment. Supportive Care Cancer 13: 806–811.
48. Brake MK, Bartlett C, Hart RD, Trites JR, Taylor SM (2011) Complementary and alternative medicine use in the thyroid patients of a head and neck practice. Otolaryngol Head Neck Surg 145: 208–212.
49. Chen S, Flower A, Ritchie A, Liu J, Molassiotis A, et al. (2010) Oral Chinese herbal medicine (CHM) as an adjuvant treatment during chemotherapy for non-small cell lung cancer: a systematic review. Lung Cancer 68: 137–145.
50. Dugoua JJ, Wu P, Seely D, Eyawo O, Mills E (2010) Astragalus-containing Chinese herbal combinations for advanced non-small-cell lung cancer: a meta-analysis of 65 clinical trials enrolling 4751 patients. Lung Cancer 1: 85–100.
51. Li Y, Li C-H, Tang F-T, Li X-F (2004) Pharmacological action of adenophora polysaccharides. Chin J Integr Med 10: 78–80.
52. Gupta S, Zhang D, Yi J, Shao J (2004) Anticancer activities of Oldenlandia diffusa. J Herb Pharmacother 4: 21–33.
53. Wu X, Dai H, Huang L, Gao X, Tsim KW, et al. (2006) A fructan, from Radix Ophiopogonis, stimulates the proliferation of cultured lymphocytes: structural and functional analyses. J Nat Products 69: 1257–1260.
54. Roh SS, Kim SH, Lee YC, Seo YB (2008) Effects of Radix Adenophorae and cyclosporine A on an OVA-induced murine model of asthma by suppressing to T cells activity, eosinophilia, and bronchial hyperresponsiveness. Mediators Inflamm 2008: 781425.
55. Cho WC, Leung KN (2007) In vitro and in vivo immunomodulating and immune restorative effects of Astragalus membranaceus. J Ethnopharmacol 113: 132–141.
56. Cho WC, Leung KN (2007) In vitro and in vivo anti-tumor effects of Astragalus membranaceus. Cancer Lett 252: 43–54.
57. McCulloch M, See C, Shu XJ, Broffman M, Kramer A, et al. (2006) Astragalus-based Chinese herbs and platinum-based chemotherapy for advanced non-small-cell lung cancer: meta-analysis of randomized trials. J Clin Oncol 24: 419–430.
58. Chang MS, Kim do R, Ko EB, Choi BJ, Park SY, et al. (2009) Treatment with Astragali radix and Angelicae radix enhances erythropoietin gene expression in the cyclophosphamide-induced anemic rat. J Med Food 12: 637–642.
59. Rjiba-Touati K, Ayed-Boussema I, Belarbia A, Azzebi A, Achour A, et al. (2013) Protective effect of recombinant human erythropoeitin against cisplatin cytotoxicity and genotoxicity in cultured Vero cells. Exp Toxicol Pathol 65: 181–187.
60. Li J, Vesey DA, Johnson DW, Gobe G (2007) Erythropoietin reduces cisplatin-induced apoptosis in renal carcinoma cells via a PKC dependent pathway. Cancer Biol Ther 6: 1944–1950.
61. Kim W, Kim SH, Park SK, Chang MS (2012) Astragalus membranaceus ameliorates reproductive toxicity induced by cyclophosphamide in male mice. Phytother Res 26: 1418–1421.
62. Yates JW, Chalmer B, McKegney FP (1980) Evaluation of patients with advanced cancer using the Karnofsky performance status. Cancer 45: 2220–2224.
63. Glare P (2005) Clinical predictors of survival in advanced cancer. J Support Oncol 3: 331–339.
64. Flower A, Witt C, Liu JP, Ulrich-Merzenich G, Yu H, et al. (2012) Guidelines for randomised controlled trials investigating Chinese herbal medicine. J Ethnopharmacol 140: 550–554.

9

The Root Extract of the Medicinal Plant *Pelargonium sidoides* Is a Potent HIV-1 Attachment Inhibitor

Markus Helfer[1], Herwig Koppensteiner[1], Martha Schneider[1], Stephanie Rebensburg[1], Sara Forcisi[2], Constanze Müller[2], Philippe Schmitt-Kopplin[2], Michael Schindler[1], Ruth Brack-Werner[1]*

1 Institute of Virology, Helmholtz Zentrum München - German Research Center for Environmental Health, Neuherberg, Germany, **2** Research Unit Analytical BioGeoChemistry, Helmholtz Zentrum München - German Research Center for Environmental Health, Neuherberg, Germany

Abstract

Global HIV-1 treatment would benefit greatly from safe herbal medicines with scientifically validated novel anti-HIV-1 activities. The root extract from the medicinal plant *Pelargonium sidoides* (PS) is licensed in Germany as the herbal medicine EPs®7630, with numerous clinical trials supporting its safety in humans. Here we provide evidence from multiple cell culture experiments that PS extract displays potent anti-HIV-1 activity. We show that PS extract protects peripheral blood mononuclear cells and macrophages from infection with various X4 and R5 tropic HIV-1 strains, including clinical isolates. Functional studies revealed that the extract from PS has a novel mode-of-action. It interferes directly with viral infectivity and blocks the attachment of HIV-1 particles to target cells, protecting them from virus entry. Analysis of the chemical footprint of anti-HIV activity indicates that HIV-1 inhibition is mediated by multiple polyphenolic compounds with low cytotoxicity and can be separated from other extract components with higher cytotoxicity. Based on our data and its excellent safety profile, we propose that PS extract represents a lead candidate for the development of a scientifically validated herbal medicine for anti-HIV-1 therapy with a mode-of-action different from and complementary to current single-molecule drugs.

Editor: Paul Zhou, Pasteur Institute of Shanghai, Chinese Academy of Science, China

Funding: Financial support for this study was provided by intramural funding of the Helmholtz Zentrum München. The funders had no role in study design, data collection and analysis, decision to publish, or preparation of the manuscript.

Competing Interests: Co-author Michael Schindler is a PLOS ONE editorial board member. This does not alter the authors' adherence to all the PLOS ONE policies on sharing data and materials.

* E-mail: brack@helmholtz-muenchen.de

Introduction

As of August 2012, 23 single-molecule drugs were approved for anti-HIV-1 therapy in the USA by the FDA [1]. The continuous need for the development of new therapeutic anti-HIV-1 agents arises from the rapid emergence of viruses resistant to these drugs (reviewed in [2], [3]), the necessity for continuous life-long treatment [4], the challenges of providing antiretroviral treatment in resource-limited settings [5] and the need for novel drugs with fewer adverse effects [6].

Natural products and herbal medicines are a promising source of new therapeutic agents and for the development of complementary and alternative medicines to conventional drug regimens [7]. While medicinal plants have been reported to display anti-HIV-1 activity (reviewed in [8,9]), herbal preparations are currently not part of conventional therapeutic regimens. Antiviral potencies and modes-of-actions of medicinal plants are poorly understood. Therefore they have been considered mainly as sources for the isolation of single anti-HIV-1 hit molecules by conventional drug-discovery approaches [9,10]. However, herbal preparations may also contain unique mixtures of molecules that act in concert to display novel bioactivities [11]. Herbal preparations have many potential benefits for anti-HIV therapy, including the complementation of existing drug therapies, improvement of anti-HIV treatment in resource-limited settings and reduction of the risk of emergence of viral resistance. Furthermore, they may display novel modes-of-action, which are different from current single-molecule drugs. Thus it is worthwhile to perform detailed and rigorous experimental investigations to evaluate anti-HIV-1 activities of herbal extracts.

Pelargonium sidoides (PS) is an indigenous medicinal plant of South Africa which has been used as a traditional medicine for the treatment of various ailments for over a century [12]. A proprietary extract from PS roots known as EPs®7630 or Umckaloabo® has been evaluated in numerous clinical trials for safety and alleviation of symptoms associated with acute bronchitis and is licensed in Germany as herbal medicine for the treatment of upper respiratory tract infections. PS extract contains numerous different metabolites [13] and has been shown to inhibit viruses associated with respiratory diseases like influenza viruses [14,15] and herpes virus [16].

The proven safety profile, richness in metabolites and demonstrated activities against various viruses led us to evaluate PS extract for anti-HIV-1 activity. We demonstrate that PS extract potently inhibits infection by HIV-1 strains with different tropisms. Anti-HIV-1 activity of PS extract is based on a new mode-of-action that diminishes infectivity of virus particles and prevents their attachment to host cells. Chemical analysis indicated that anti-HIV activity is mediated by multiple polyphenolic compounds. These results support PS extract as a lead candidate for the development into an herbal medicine with a novel mode of anti-HIV-1 activity.

Materials and Methods

Virus production

Virus stocks were produced by HEK293T cells transfected with proviral plasmids and analyzed for infectivity, signal induction, absence of cell toxicity and p24 quantity as described in [17].

The X4- tropic strain HIV-1_{LAI} [18] was produced by transfection with the proviral plasmid pLAI.2, the R5-tropic strain HIV-$1_{AD8(R5)}$ [19] with pNL(AD8), the R5-tropic GFP reporter virus HIV-1 NL4-3 Gag-iGFP [20] with pBR-NL4-3 V92th014.12-IRES-eGFP, the R5-tropic HIV-1ΔEnv$_{JRFL(R5)}$ [21] by co-transfecting pNL4.3ΔEnv and pSVIIIenvJRFL. HIV-1 particles pseudotyped with the VSV-G envelope protein were produced by co-transfecting pSG3ΔEnv and pM2.G (Addgene, MA). Clinical isolates CH077 and STCOr1 were produced by transfection with the appropriate proviral plasmids [22]. P-891 was isolated from serum of an HIV-1 infected individual as described [17]. Non-commercial providers of plasmids are listed in the "Acknowledgements".

Cells and cell culture

LC5-CD4 is a HeLa subline engineered for cell-surface expression of CD4 [17]. The HIV-1 reporter cell line LC5-RIC contains a reporter gene for Rev- and Tat-dependent expression of a red fluorescent protein [17]. LC5-RIC-R5 cells were generated by stable transfection of LC5-RIC cells with plasmids containing human CCR5 cDNA in the pMSCVPuro backbone [23]. LC5-RIC, LC5-RIC-R5 and HEK293T (ATCC®-Number CRL-11268) cells were cultured as described [17]. Human peripheral blood mononuclear cells (PBMCs) were isolated from buffy coats by Ficoll (Biochrom AG) gradient centrifugation as described in [24]. Cells were washed and treated with ammonium chloride potassium (ACK) buffer (Gibco), to remove residual platelets and erythrocytes, respectively. PBMCs were stored at -80°C in batches of 1×10^7 cells pooled from 4 donors in 1 ml VLE-RPMI 1640 medium (Biochrom AG, Berlin) with 20% FCS (Gibco) and 10% DMSO (Sigma Aldrich). Primary human macrophages were isolated from PBMCs as described in [20].

Reference HIV-1 inhibitors

AZT was purchased from Sigma Aldrich and His-Griffithsin from Biomol GmbH. The following reagents were obtained through the NIH AIDS Research and Reference Reagent Program, Division of AIDS, NIAID, NIH: bicyclam JM-2987 (hydrobromide salt of AMD-3100) [25,26]; T-20, Fusion Inhibitor from Roche; Efavirenz; His-Griffithsin from Drs. Barry O'Keefe and James McMahon [27].

Generation of crude PS extracts and isolation of polyphenols

Crude *PS* extract was generated from dried plant roots obtained from Amarelo (www.amarelo24.de). Roots were ground with a ball mill (Minimill Pulverisette 23; Fritsch, Idar-Oberstein). 10 g powdered roots were stirred in 50 ml water (dd$H_2$0) for ~2h at room temperature (RT). Boiling, while not necessary, did not affect anti-HIV activity. The extract was cleared by centrifugation (4000 g). Aliquots of the extract were evaporated in an Eppendorf Vacuum Concentrator, the dry mass weighed and dd$H_2$0 added to generate extract stock solutions with 10 mg dry mass per ml. All PS extract stock solutions were sterilized by filtration (0.45 µM syringe-filter; Merck Millipore Ltd) and stored at -20°C until use.

Enrichment of *PS*-derived polyphenols (PSPP). 2.5 g of polyvinylpyrrolidone (PVPP; Sigma-Aldrich) was added to 50 ml of PS extract stock solution (10 mg/ml), vortexed, and polyphenols allowed to adsorb to PVPP at RT for 15 min before centrifugation at 4000 g. The supernatant represented the polyphenol-depleted fraction and the pellet the polyphenol-enriched fraction. The pellet was washed 3 times with 25 ml dd$H_2$0 and polyphenols eluted by washing 3 times with 25 ml 0.5 N NaOH. The pooled eluates were adjusted to pH 7 with 2 N HCl. The polyphenol-depleted and polyphenol-enriched fractions were purified by solid phase extraction (SPE) (Agilent Bond Elut C18). SPE-purified eluates were evaporated and dissolved in dd$H_2$0 to generate stock solutions with 10 mg per ml.

Assays

Assays for inhibition of HIV-1 infection of LC5-RIC cells and primary human cells are described in Materials and Methods S1.

HIV-1-cell attachment assays were performed with the HIV-1 NL4-3 Gag-iGFP reporter virus and LC5-RIC-R5 cells in the presence of the HIV-1 fusion inhibitor T-20 (50 nM). LC5-RIC-R5 cells (2×10^5) were seeded onto 24×24 mm cover slips placed in 6-well plates. 24 hours later, the culture medium was replaced by fresh medium containing inhibitor compounds (100 µg/ml PS-extract or polyphenol enriched PS-extract, or 5 nM Griffithsin reference compound) and virus inoculum (8.5 pg p24/cell). After 4 h incubation at 37°C, the cells were washed once with PBS and cell membranes stained with DiD (Invitrogen) according to the manufacturer's protocol. Cells were then fixed in 2% paraformaldehyde (PFA) in PBS at room-temperature for 10 minutes and treated with DAPI-staining solution for 5 minutes at room temperature for staining of cellular DNA. The cells were washed, coverslips fixed onto glass-slides with Moviol and dried in the dark overnight. Samples were analyzed by fluorescence microscopy (Nikon TiE equipped with Perkin Elmer UltraView Vox System). Exposure-times: GFP: 100 ms, DAPI: various, DiD: various, Brightfield: various. Counting of virus particles (GFP spots defined as all pixels within a radius of 1 µm around the brightest spot, intensity threshold 755) was performed using Volocity 6.2.1-software (Perkin Elmer). DiD/DAPI-positive cells were counted manually.

Cell viability was analyzed by MTT (3-(4,5-Dimethylthiazol-2-yl)-2,5-diphenyltetrazolium bromide) assay as described in [17].

Quantification of HIV-1 DNA and RNA levels

HIV-1 DNA copy numbers and viral RNA were determined by quantitative PCR as described in Materials and Methods S1.

Chromatographic Separation of PS Extract was performed by UPLC (Ultra Performance Liquid Chromatography) of PS extract purified by solid phase extraction (for details see Materials and Methods S1).

Ultrahigh Resolution Mass Spectrometry was performed by ICR/FTMS (Ion Cyclotron Resonance/Fourier Transformation Mass Spectrometry). Details, including description of methods for evaluation of complex mass data, are provided in Materials and Methods S1.

Statistical Analysis

EC_{50}/CC_{50} values were calculated with GraphPad Prism v5, using the equation for sigmoidal dose-response with variable slope. Statistical significances were determined by one-way Anova with Bonferroni post-hoc test. **** $p<0.0001$.

Results

Anti-HIV-1 activity of PS root extract

Initial testing of PS-root extract for anti-HIV-1 activity with EASY-HIT technology [17] revealed dose-dependent inhibition of HIV-1 infection for all extract preparations examined, including the commercial herbal medicine EPs®7630 (Figure S1). The EASY-HIT assay gauges antiviral effects by measuring infection parameters associated with two temporally distinct steps of the HIV-1 replication cycle (i.e. expression of early viral proteins Tat and Rev = step 1 and release of infectious virions = step 2, resp.) with an HIV-1 reporter cell line [17]. Multiple tests showed that PS extract was similarly effective at reducing infection parameters at both steps, with half-maximal inhibition (EC_{50}) at 8.13 µg/ml (±4.82; n = 19) for step 1 and 8.00 µg/ml (±2.26; n = 2) for step 2 (Figure 1). This indicates that PS extract interferes with HIV-1 replication at an early step of the HIV-1 replication cycle [17].

To determine anti-HIV activity of PS extract with primary HIV-1 target cells, we used *ex vivo* cultures of human peripheral blood mononuclear cells (PBMC) and monocyte-derived macrophages (MDM). Both primary HIV-1 target cell types yielded EC_{50} values comparable to those measured for the reporter cells in the EASY-HIT system (Figure 1). Inhibition of infection of PBMCs by PS extract was determined by measuring infectious virus titers of supernatants of cultures exposed to HIV-1_{LAI} and different concentrations of PS extract (EC_{50} = 5.70±2.7 µg/ml; n = 4). PS-mediated inhibition of infection of MDMs was analyzed with an R5 reporter virus that coexpresses Nef and EGFP from a bicistronic mRNA (R5 HIV-1NL4-3 IRES-eGFP [20]) and analyzing proportions of EGFP-positive cells by flow cytometry (EC_{50} = 8.27±2.75 µg/ml; n = 3).

We also investigated whether PS extracts can inhibit infection by clinical HIV-1 isolates. Clinical isolates were derived from serum of a chronically infected individual (P-891; [17]) and from blood of acutely (CH077) or chronically (STCOr1) infected individuals [22]. As shown in Figure 1*E*, PS extract was active against all clinical isolates investigated, yielding EC_{50} values below 6 µg/ml.

In all assays evaluating PS-mediated inhibition of HIV-1 infection, viability of cells exceeded 80%, confirming that inhibition of infection was not caused by PS-induced cytotoxicity.

Together, these results demonstrate that PS extract inhibits HIV-1 infection of various HIV-1 target cell types, including primary cells, and acts against various HIV-1 isolates, including clinical HIV-1 isolates.

PS extract interferes with HIV-1 entry into the host cell.

To narrow down the stage of the HIV-1 replication cycle at which PS extract inhibits HIV-1 replication, we first performed time-of-addition (TOA) assays with PS extract [17,28]. The HIV-1 entry inhibitors Griffithsin [27] and T-20 [29] and the reverse transcription inhibitor AZT [30] were used as reference compounds. The TOA profiles indicate that PS extract acts at a very early stage of HIV-1 replication which precedes reverse transcription (Figure 2*A*). For further confirmation, we investigated whether treatment with PS extract reduced levels of input viral RNA. Experiments were performed in the presence of reverse transcriptase inhibitor (Efavirenz) to maximize accumulation of input viral RNA. RNA was isolated from cells exposed to the virus +/- PS extract for 4 hours and levels of input RNA quantified by RT-PCR using HIV-1 specific primers. As shown in Figure 2*B*, PS treatment led to a strong reduction of input viral RNA levels in virus-exposed cells, compared to levels of HIV-1 RNA in cells exposed to the virus without PS treatment. As expected, PS treatment also strongly diminished levels of HIV-1 DNA in cells exposed to the virus without Efavirenz (Figure 2*C*). Together, the facts that PS extract behaves like validated entry inhibitors in TOA experiments and the dramatic reduction of levels of input HIV-1 RNA and HIV-1 DNA in virus-exposed cells caused by treatment with PS extract indicate that PS blocks HIV-1 entry into host cells.

Entry is mediated by the HIV-1 envelope protein. Therefore we investigated the influence of viral envelope proteins on the antiviral activity of PS by comparing inhibitory effects of PS extract on infection by HIV-1 particles pseudotyped with different envelope proteins. Virions carrying the vesicular stomatitis virus G-envelope protein on their surface were on average 10-fold less sensitive to inhibition by PS extract than HIV-1 with native envelope proteins (Figure 2*D*). In contrast, PS extract was similarly efficient at inhibiting infection of virus particles with different HIV-1 envelope proteins (i.e. X4 (LAI) and R5 (AD8 and JRFL)). These results demonstrate that PS extract inhibits HIV-1 entry by interfering with the function of the envelope proteins independent of their coreceptor tropism.

Since PS extract perturbs functionality of the HIV-1 envelope, we investigated whether PS extract interferes with infectivity of HIV-1 particles. Virus preparations were pre-incubated with PS extract without target cells prior to assaying their infectivity. Pre-incubation assays were also performed with the reference compounds Griffithsin, the CXCR4 antagonist AMD3100 [31], the fusion inhibitor T-20 and the reverse transcriptase inhibitor Efavirenz [32]. As shown in Figure 3, virus pre-incubation with PS extract resulted in stronger inhibition of infection (PS panel, green curve, EC_{50} 3.9±0.3 µg/ml) than simultaneous addition of virus and PS extract to LC5-RIC cells (PS panel, blue curve, EC_{50} 14.3±1.1 µg/ml). Virus pre-incubation also enhanced the inhibitory activity of Griffithsin, but not of the other reference compounds (other panels, green and blue curves).

Next we tested whether anti-HIV-1 activity of PS extract involves association of extract ingredients with target cells LC5-RIC target cells were pre-incubated with PS extract or the reference inhibitors for 4 hours, and subsequently exposed to HIV-1_{LAI} virus in the absence of inhibitor. While PS extract displayed no antiviral activity under these conditions (Figure 3, PS panel, black curve), all reference inhibitors showed measurable anti-HIV-1 activities (other panels, black curves), although the compounds were removed and cells were washed after the 4-hour pre-incubation period.

Together these results show that PS extract is an HIV-1 entry inhibitor that directly diminishes the infectivity of viral particles.

PS extract inhibits attachment of HIV-1 to host cells.

PS extract might target a pre- or post binding step to diminish HIV-1 infectivity and inhibit entry. We thus investigated whether PS extract affects the attachment of HIV-1 to target cells. Assays were performed with GFP-labeled infectious R5 virus particles (R5 HIV-1 NL4-3 Gag-iGFP; [20]) and LC5-RIC-R5 cells. Spinning disc confocal fluorescence microscopy was used to visualize and quantify GFP-labeled HIV-1 particles associated with target cells. All assays were performed in the presence of the fusion inhibitor T-20 to promote accumulation of cell surface bound HIV-1. Tests were performed with HIV-1 inhibitor solutions validated for anti-HIV-1 activity (EC_{50} PS: 7.9±0.8 µg/ml; GRFT: 0.34±0.04 nM). The results are shown in Figure 4. As expected, GFP-labeled HIV-1 particles efficiently attached to the cells in the absence of inhibitor (attachment control, 25.1±5.6 GFP-spots per cell). In contrast, PS extract completely blocked cellular HIV-1 attachment, yielding similarly low numbers of GFP signals per cell

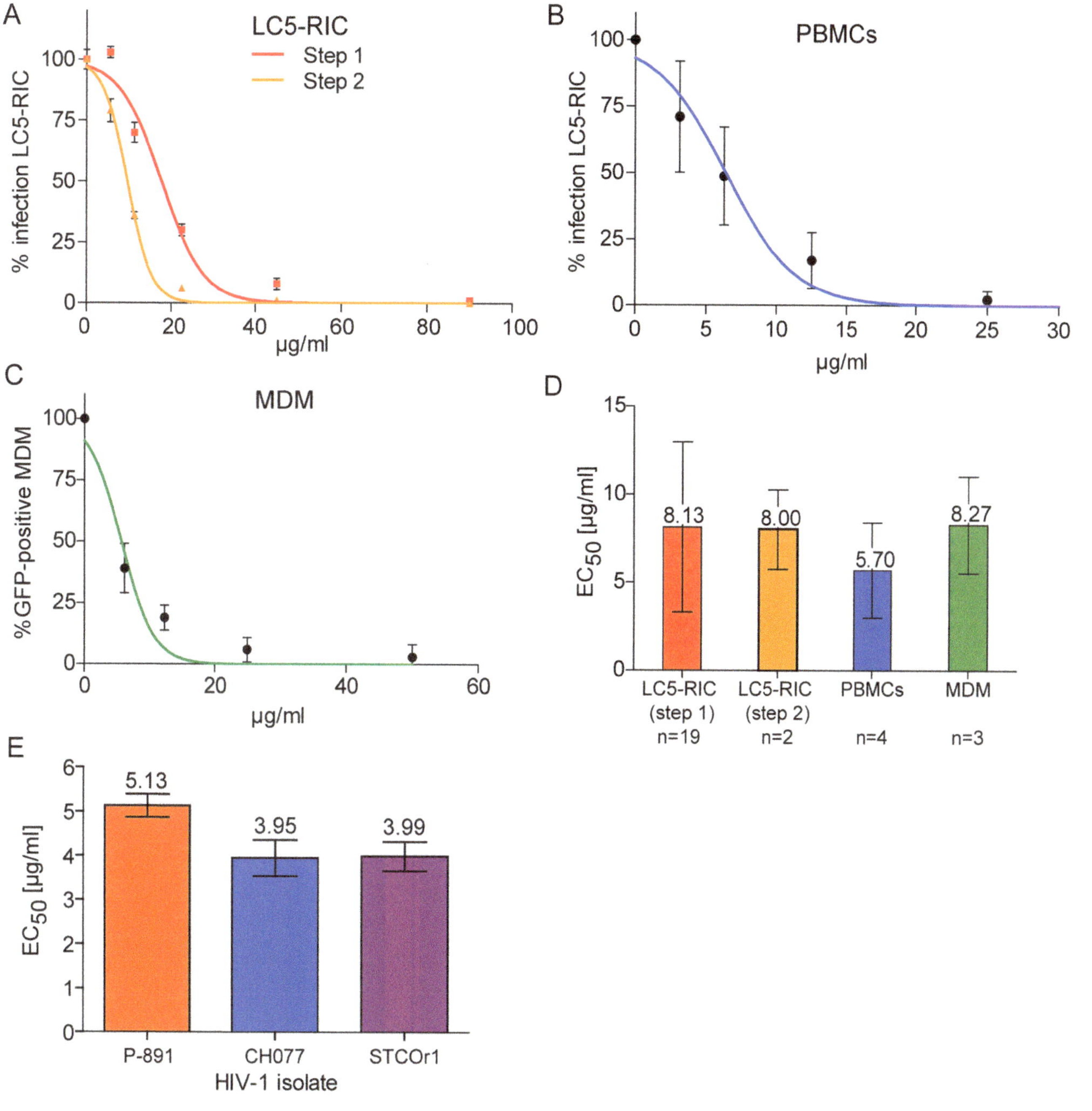

Figure 1. Evaluation of anti-HIV-1 activity of *Pelargonium sidoides* (PS) aqueous root extract with various HIV-1 target cells and HIV-1 isolates. Panels A-C show representative results for dose-dependent inhibition of HIV-1 infection of LC5-RIC indicator cells, human peripheral blood mononuclear cells (PBMC) and human monocyte-derived macrophages (MDM) by PS extract. Data for infection of PS-treated cultures are expressed in percentage of values measured for untreated cultures (=100% infection). The graph in D shows the EC_{50} values calculated from multiple independent infection experiments (n = number of independent infection experiments) for each cell type. Panel E shows HIV-1 inhibitory activity (EC_{50}) of PS extract against clinical HIV-1 isolates. *A*, HIV-1 reporter cells (LC5-RIC) were exposed to HIV-1_{LAI} and serial dilutions of PS extract and infection assayed by measuring reporter gene expression (step 1) and production of infectious virus (step 2). Mean values and standard deviation of the mean are indicated for each extract dilution. *B*, IL-2 stimulated PBMCs were exposed to HIV-1_{LAI} and different concentrations of PS extract and levels of infectious virus in culture supernatants of PBMCs assayed with LC5-RIC cells. Results are shown for 4 independent infection experiments using PBMCs that were pooled from 4 different donors, with each extract concentration assayed in triplicate in each experiment. *C*, MDMs were exposed to the HIV-1 reporter virus R5 HIV-1NL4-3 IRES-eGFP that coexpresses Nef and EGFP from a bicistronic mRNA via an IRES element. Three days later, proportions (%) of GFP positive cells were determined by flow cytometry. Data were normalized to values for untreated cells. Results are shown for three independent infection experiments with MDMs from different donors. *D*, The graph shows EC_{50} values (effective concentration for half-maximal inhibition) for each cell type, calculated from the compiled results of multiple independent infection experiments. n = number of independent infection experiments with triplicate analysis of each extract concentration. Mean values and standard deviations of the mean are indicated for each cell type. *E*, HIV-1 reporter cells (LC5-RIC-R5) were exposed to the indicated clinical HIV-1 isolates and serial dilutions of PS extract in triplicate wells and reporter gene expression was measured 5 days post infection. Mean values and standard deviations of the mean are indicated for each HIV-1 isolate.

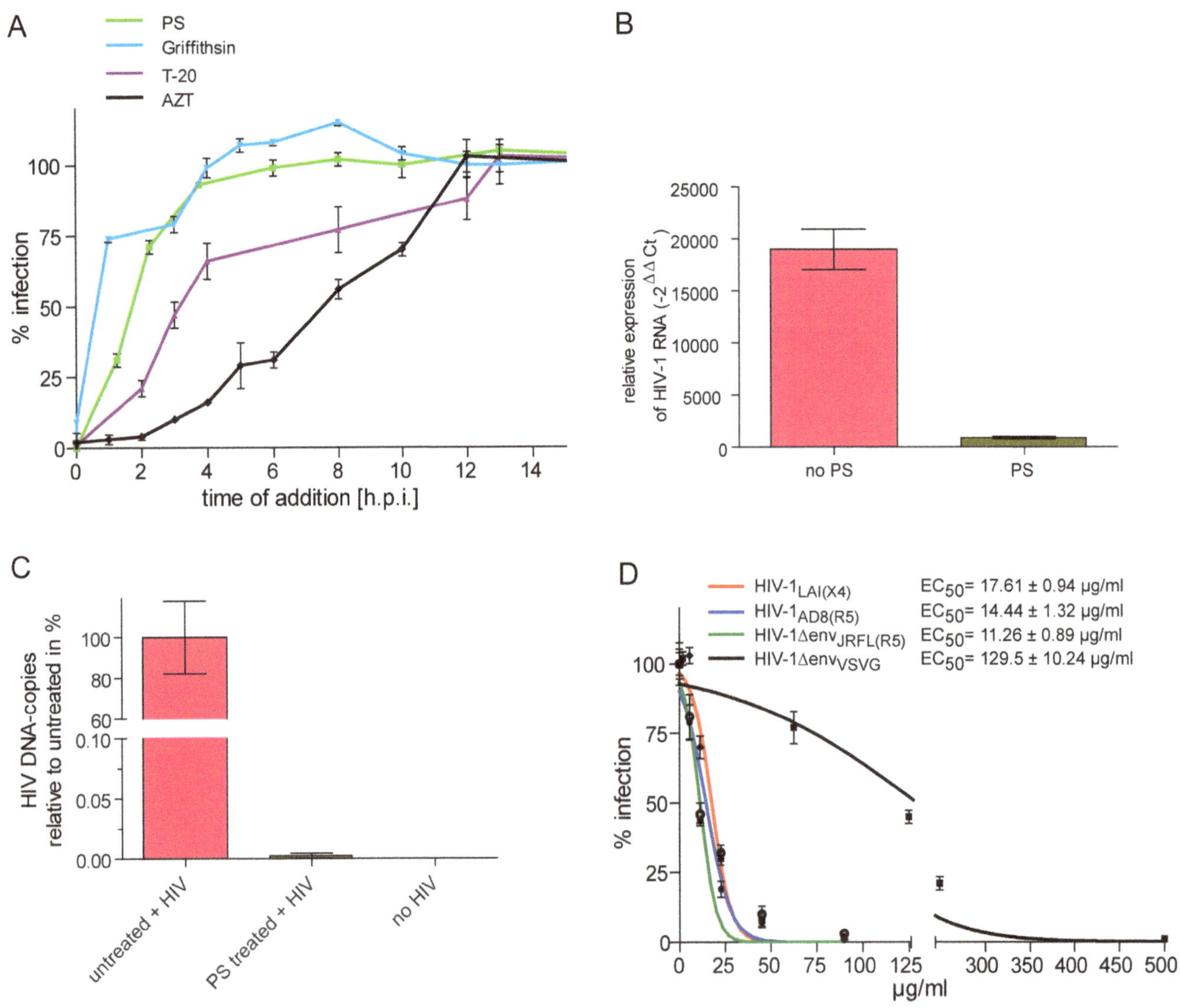

Figure 2. PS extracts inhibit entry of HIV-1 into the host cell. *A*, Comparison of time-of-addition (TOA) profiles of PS extract and reference compounds that inhibit HIV-1 entry (i.e. Griffithsin and T-20) and reverse transcription (AZT), respectively. For TOA assays, virus preparations (HIV-1_{LAI}) were added to LC5-RIC cells and HIV-1 inhibitors added either simultaneously with the virus (time point 0) or at later time points (h.p.i. = hours post infection) at concentrations yielding maximum inhibition (i.e. $>5\times EC_{50}$). Cultures were assayed for reporter expression 48 hours after virus addition and fluorescent signal intensities normalized to those of cultures exposed to virus in the absence of inhibitors. Each time point was measured in triplicate. Mean values and standard deviation of the mean are indicated for each time point. *B*, Reduction of input HIV-1 viral RNA levels by treatment with PS-extract. LC5-CD4 cells were exposed to HIV-1_{LA1} and Efavirenz in the presence or absence of PS extract (50 µg/ml) in triplicate samples. After 4 hours exposure time, RNA was isolated from each sample, cDNA prepared and real-time PCR performed with HIV-1 specific primers to quantify viral RNA levels. HIV-1 transcript levels were normalized to RPII. Relative expression was calculated by the $-2^{-\Delta\Delta CT}$ method. The data is expressed as fold expression of HIV-1 RNA in HIV-1 exposed/treated samples compared to unexposed/untreated samples. Columns indicate mean values and error bars the standard deviations of the means. *C*, Reduction of HIV-1 DNA loads in HIV-1-exposed PBMCs by treatment with PS extract. HIV-1 DNA levels were determined by real-time PCR in peripheral blood derived mononuclear cells treated with PS extract during exposure to HIV-1 and in untreated infected cells (analysed in triplicate samples). Columns indicate mean values and error bars the standard deviations of the means. *D*, Influence of envelope proteins on the inhibition of virus infection by PS extract. LC5-RIC cells were exposed to HIV-1 variants with different HIV-1 envelope proteins representing different virus tropisms (HIV-1_{LAI}: X4-tropic; HIV-1-AD-8 and HIV-1$\Delta Env_{JRFL(R5)}$: R5-tropic) or HIV-1 based virus particles pseudotyped with an envelope protein (G-protein) from a heterologous virus (*Vesicular Stomatitis Virus*; HIV-1ΔEnv_{VSVG}) in the presence of different concentrations of PS extract. Cultures were assayed for reporter expression 48 hours after virus addition and fluorescent signal intensities normalized to those of cultures exposed to virus without inhibitors. Mean values of triplicate wells and standard deviation of the mean are indicated for each extract concentration.

as the background control (PS, 1.1±0.4; background, 0.5±0.7). Treatment with Griffithsin resulted in a small although significant increase in the number of cell-associated virus particles (36±4.2 GFP-spots per cell), which is in line with previous evidence for the enhancement of virus binding to the CD4 receptor by Griffithsin [33]. Thus, PS extract prevents HIV-1 attachment to target cells, which is a novel mode of entry inhibition.

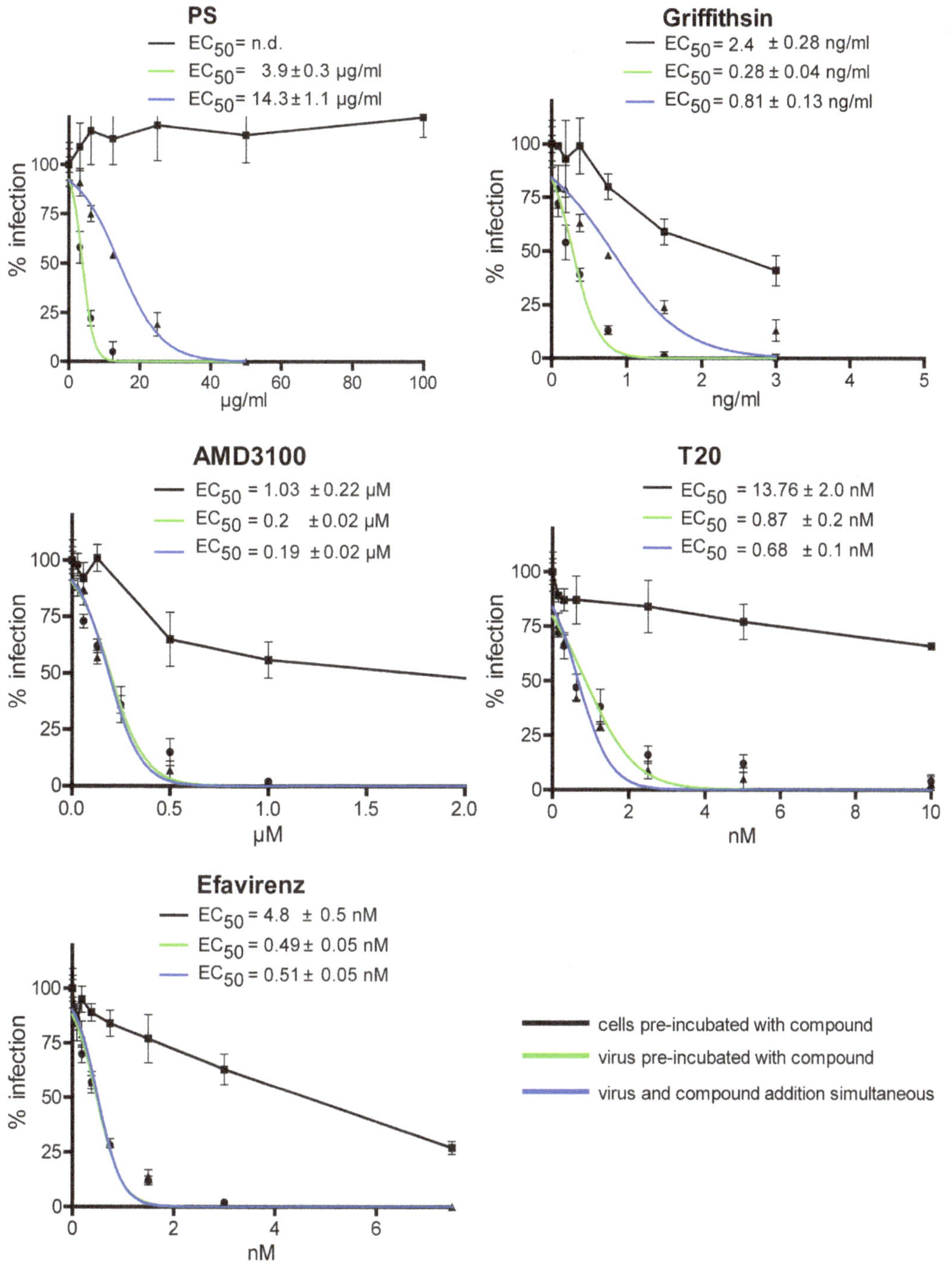

Figure 3. Effects of pre-incubation of virus preparations or target cells with PS extracts or reference compounds on inhibition of HIV-1 infection. Inhibition of HIV-1 infection by PS extract was enhanced by pre-incubation of virus preparations with PS extract, compared to inhibition of infection without virus pre-incubation. HIV-1 target cells pre-incubated with PS extract prior to infection did not retain HIV-1 inhibitory activity. Virus pre-incubation (green curves): Inhibitory activity of PS extract was assayed with HIV-1_{LAI} virus preparations pre-incubated with different concentrations of PS extract for 4 hours before adding to LC5-RIC cells. Target cell pre-incubation (black curves): LC5-RIC cells were incubated with different concentrations of inhibitors and subsequently exposed to HIV-1_{LAI} in fresh medium in the absence of inhibitors. No pre-incubation (blue curves): Virus and inhibitors were added simultaneously to LC5-RIC cells. The entry inhibitors Griffithsin, AMD3100 and T20 and the reverse transcriptase inhibitor Efavirenz were analyzed as reference compounds. Mean values of triplicate wells and standard deviation of the mean are indicated for each extract concentration.

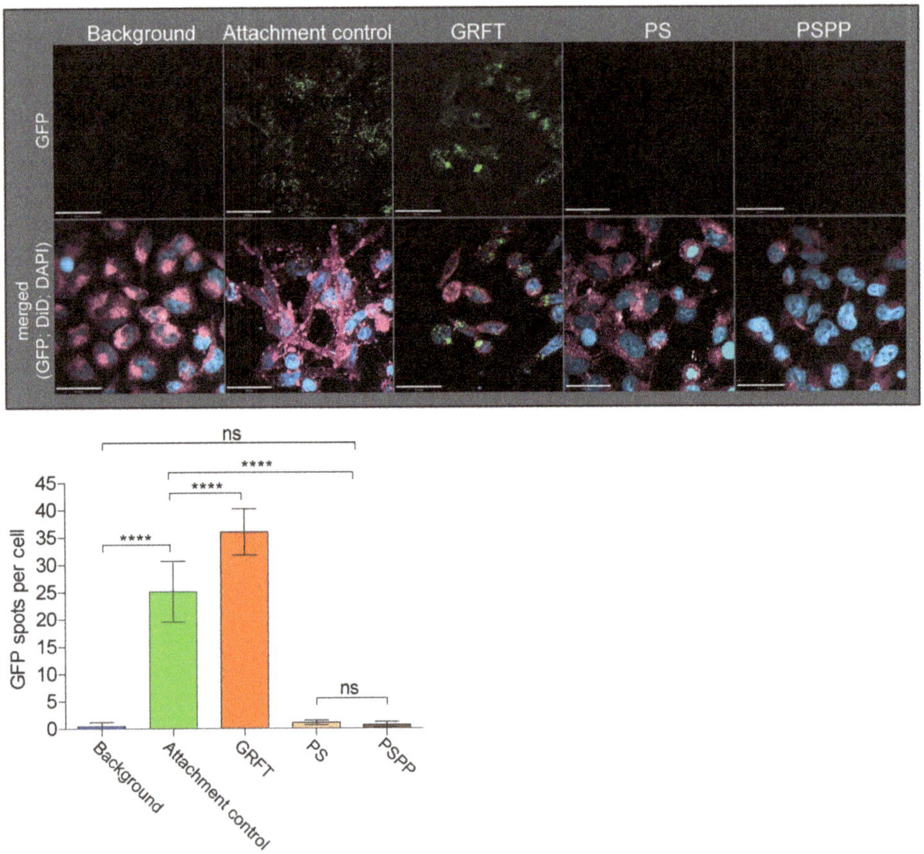

Figure 4. PS extracts inhibit attachment of virus particles to host cells. The effects of PS extract (PS), polyphenols enriched from PS extract (PSPP) by adsorption to polyvinylpolypyrrolidone and the reference compound Griffithsin (GRFT) on virus attachment were determined by fluorescent imaging of virus particles associated with host cells. Controls consisted of cells without virus inoculum (background) and cells exposed to virus particles in the absence of inhibitory compounds (attachment control). LC5-RIC-R5 cells were exposed to fluorescently tagged R5 virus particles (R5 HIV-1 NL4-3 Gag-iGFP) in the presence of the fusion inhibitor T20. Cells were stained with DiD (membrane stain; pink) and DAPI (DNA stain; blue). *A*, Representative images are shown for each sample. Scale bars: 35 µm. *B*, Quantitative analysis of cell-associated fluorescent signals. Quantification of cell-associated GFP signals was performed with Volocity 6.2.1 imaging software. Cells were identified manually. 160-180 cells from at least 5 images were analyzed for each sample. Mean values and standard deviations are shown. Statistical significances were determined by one-way Anova with Bonferroni post-hoc test. **** $p<0.0001$.

Anti-HIV-1 activity of PS extract is mediated by polyphenol compounds.

The high complexity and diversity of the metabolic pool of the PS plant [13] raises the possibility that anti-HIV-1 activity of PS extract may be exerted by multiple compounds. For chemical characterization of anti-HIV-1 activity, PS extract was separated by UPLC-chromatography and anti-HIV-1 activity of fractions determined with the EASY-HIT system. Chemical structures within the fractions were identified by ICR/FTMS (Ion Cyclotron Resonance/Fourier Transformation Mass Spectrometry). This technology allows to distinguish between several thousands of ions with extremely high mass accuracy [34] and enables prediction of the molecular formula of detected compounds and their putative annotation [35].

Several fractions dispersed throughout the chromatogram displayed anti-HIV-1 activity (Figure 5*A*). This indicates that multiple chemical compounds in the PS extract have anti-HIV-1 activity. ICR/FTMS analysis combined with structural data-mining, statistical analysis and mass network analysis revealed that fractions with anti-HIV-1 activity were selectively enriched for various aromatic and oxygen rich compounds (Figure 5*B*). These were annotated as polyphenolic compounds, mainly belonging to the classes of flavonoids and leuco-anthocyanidins.

To investigate involvement of polyphenols in anti-HIV activity of PS extract, we used adsorption of polyphenols to polyvinylpolypyrrolidone [36] to produce a PS-derived polyphenol fraction (PSPP). Specific enrichment of polyphenols in this fraction was confirmed by ICR/FTMS (Figure S2).

Analysis of anti-HIV-1 activity of the PSPP fraction showed that it also inhibited HIV-1 infection (Figure 6*A*, *B*). Anti-HIV-1 activity of the PSPP extract was confirmed with primary target cells (PBMCs) and HIV-1 reporter cells (LC5-RIC) and for different HIV-1 isolates, including clinical isolates. The EC_{50} values for PSPP-mediated HIV-1 inhibition were <7 µg/ml, and were comparable to the EC_{50} values measured for the crude PS extract (Figure 1). In contrast, anti-HIV-1 activity of the polyphenol-depleted fraction was severely diminished (EC_{50} ~200 µg/ml; not shown). Strikingly, the PSPP fraction was much less cytotoxic for PBMC [50% cytotoxic concentration (CC_{50})≥1200 µg/ml] than the crude PS extract (CC_{50}≤250 µg/ml) (Figure 6*A*). This resulted in a strongly improved therapeutic index (CC_{50}/EC_{50}) for PSPP (324), which is about 9-fold higher than for crude PS extract (~35). PSPP treatment also inhibited

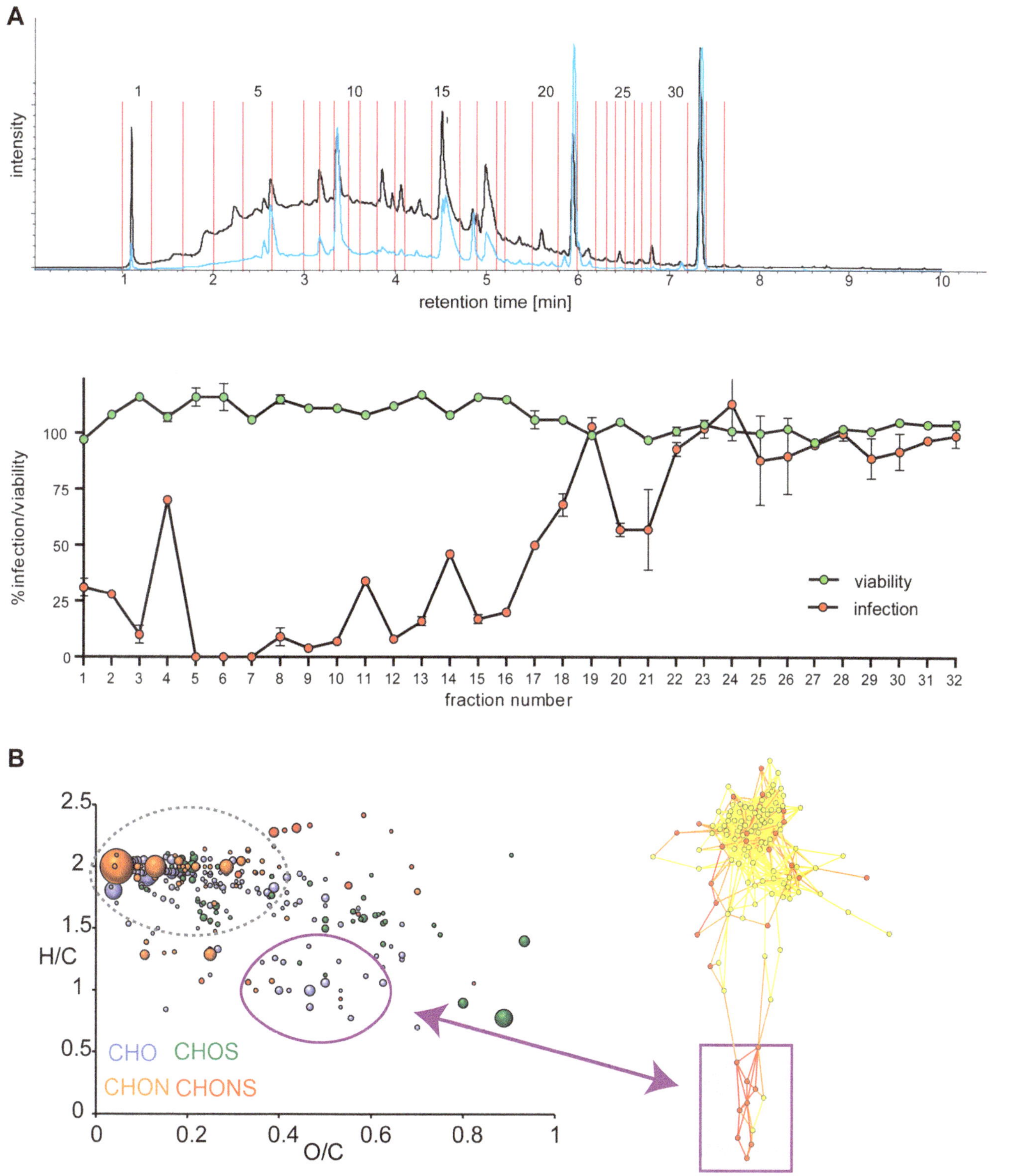

Figure 5. Chemical analysis of anti-HIV activity of PS extract. PS extract was purified by solid phase extraction and separated by UPLC-chromatography. Fractions were analyzed for anti-HIV activity with the EASY-HIT assay and for effects on cell viability by MTT assay. Chemical structures in fractions were analyzed by a combination of ICR/FTMS (Ion Cyclotron Resonance/Fourier Transformation Mass Spectrometry), structural data-mining, statistical analysis and mass network analysis. *A*, Profiling of anti-HIV activity shows inhibitory activity in multiple UPLC-fractions. The UV-chromatogram (top) displays the signal intensities at 289 (black graph) and 330 (blue graph) nm used for peak-oriented identification of PS fractions. The profile below the UV-chromatogram shows a plot of the anti-HIV-1-activity (red data points) and cell viability (green data points) of the corresponding UPLC fractions. *B*, Chemical diversity of anti-HIV activity. The van Krevelen diagram at the left shows the chemical diversity of compounds discriminating fractions with strong anti-HIV-1 activity (3, 5-10, 12) from non-active fractions (19, 22-32). Discriminatory compounds included groups of polyphenolic compounds like flavonoids and leuco-anthocyanidins (encircled in violet) as well as aliphatic oxygen poor, hydrogen

rich lipid compounds (encircled in grey). The graph at the right shows mass networks in highly active fractions (i.e. fractions 5-10, 12, 13, 15, 16; red) versus poorly active fractions (1, 2, 4, 11, 14, 17, 19-21, yellow). The networks include a cluster of masses predominantly associated with high anti-HIV activity (framed in violet) that map to the group of polyphenolic compounds in the van Krevelen diagram (violet arrow).

attachment of virus particles to cells (Figure 4) and dramatically reduced input viral RNA levels (Figure 6*C*) indicating that PSPP inhibits HIV-1 by the same mechanism of action as crude PS extract.

In sum, the antiviral activity of PS extract can be attributed to polyphenolic secondary metabolites belonging to the classes of flavonoids and leuco-anthocyanidins. The potent anti-HIV-1 activity and reduced cytotoxicity of the PSPP fraction indicate that enrichment of polyphenols from PS root extracts eliminates cytotoxic molecules, while retaining HIV-1 inhibitors.

Discussion

This study demonstrates that PS root extract, including the commercial herbal medicine EPs®7630, is a highly reliable source of robust anti-HIV-1 activity. PS extract prevents attachment of virus particles to host cells and hence HIV-1 entry. Our results suggest that HIV-1 inhibitory molecules in PS extracts target HIV-1 envelope proteins, since virus particles bearing the heterologous VSV-G protein instead of HIV-1 proteins in their envelopes are much less sensitive to inhibition by PS extract. The mode-of-action of PS extract exhibits a combination of features that set it apart from approved anti-HIV-1 drugs and from investigational entry inhibitors including lectins [37,38], polyanionic compounds [39,40] and synthetic anti-lipopolysaccharide peptides (SALPs) [41], of which several are under development as microbicides and drug candidates. For one, PS extract prevents attachment of virus particles to host cells. In contrast, the lectin Griffithsin, which was assayed as reference compound, did not inhibit HIV-1 attachment and therefore blocks entry at a later stage. Other plant derived

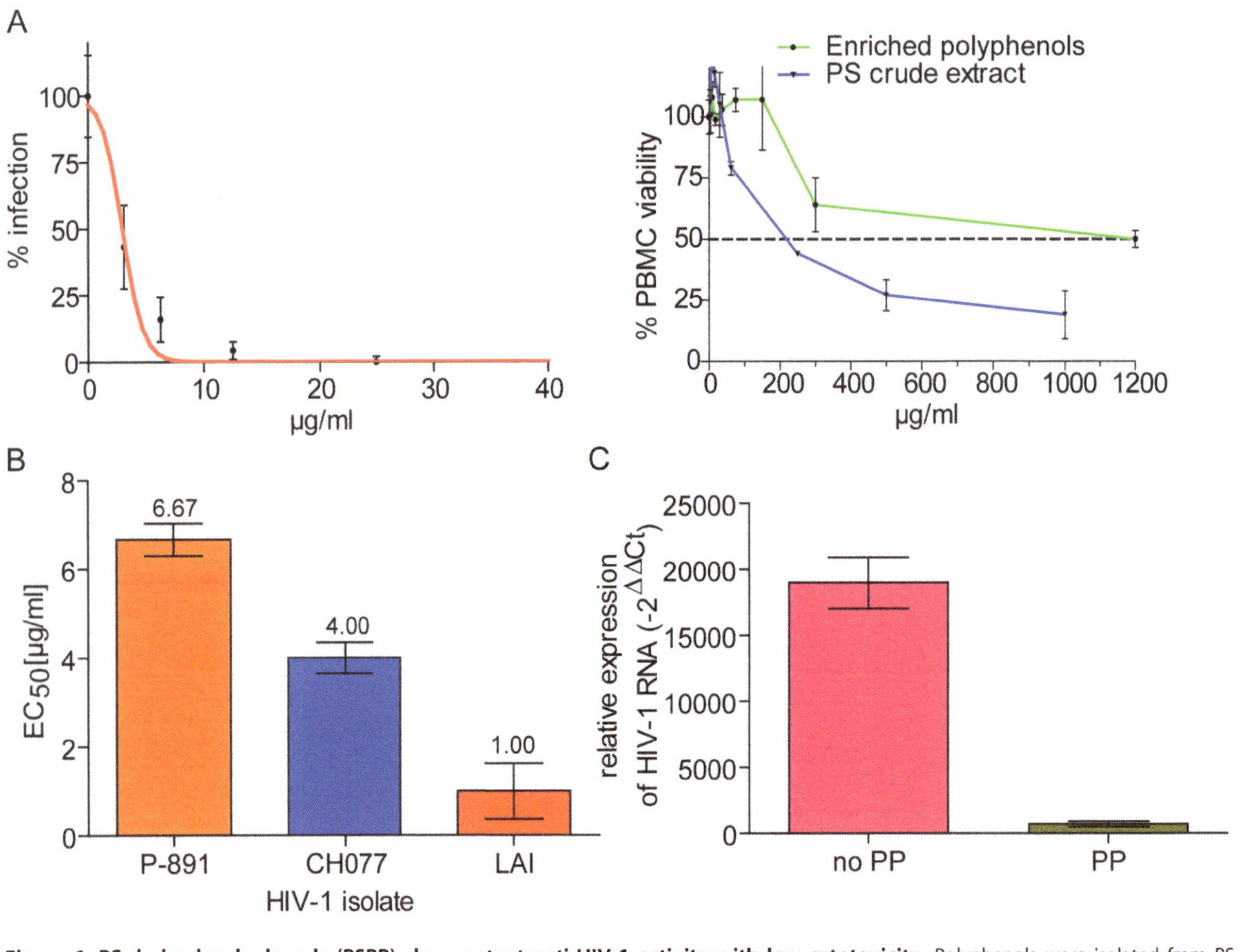

Figure 6. PS-derived polyphenols (PSPP) show potent anti-HIV-1 activity with low cytotoxicity. Polyphenols were isolated from PS extract by adsorption to polyvinylpolypyrrolidone. *A*, Effects of PSPP treatment on HIV-1 infection and viability of PBMCs. The left panel shows dose-dependent inhibition of infection of PBMCs with HIV-1_{LAI}. The data represents results from 3 independent infection experiments in which quadruplicate wells were assayed for each extract concentration. Mean values and standard deviations of the means are indicated. The EC_{50} value calculated from these data is 2.98±0.2. The right panel shows the effects of enriched polyphenols and the crude PS extract on the viability of PBMCs. PBMCs were exposed to different concentrations of PSPP or the crude PS extract and effects on cell viability measured by MTT assay. Mean values and standard deviations of the means are indicated for each concentration (triplicate samples). *B*, Anti-HIV-1 activity of PSPP against different HIV-1 isolates. For further details see legend to Fig. 1E. *C*, Reduction of input viral RNA levels by PSPP treatment. For details see legend to Figure 2*B*.

HIV-1 entry inhibitors epigallocatechin gallate (EGCg) and theaflavin also act after attachment [42,43,44] and in this respect are similar to Griffithsin but different from PS extract. Second, PS exerts potent anti-HIV-1 activity independent of the viral coreceptor tropism. This is in contrast to polyanions that mainly target CXCR4-using HIV-1 strains [45], and to compounds that act by blocking single HIV-1 cell surface co-receptors (e.g. AMD3100 [31]) or CCR5 (e.g. Maraviroc; [46]). Third, PS extract directly interferes with the infectivity of HIV-1 particles before they interact with the host cell and thus has virucidal activity. This is in contrast to entry inhibitors that bind to molecules on the surface of host cells (e.g. SALPs, Maraviroc and Griffithsin [47]) or that interfere with entry processes that take place after the virus has bound to the host cell (T20).

Interestingly, PS extract was also reported to display virucidal activity against herpesvirus [16], but not against influenza virus [15]. This indicates that PS inhibits HIV-1 and herpesviruses by mechanisms different from those involved in inhibition of influenzavirus and suggests that PS extract contains multiple antiviral compounds with different activities.

In addition to the novel mode-of-action, PS extract has several other characteristics that highlight it as an attractive candidate for HIV-1 preventive and therapeutic strategies. We demonstrate that anti-HIV activity of PS extract is exerted by the concerted action of a unique combination of polyphenolic antiviral ingredients. Conceivably, this may reduce the risk of the emergence of drug-resistant viruses, compared to treatment with single-molecule drugs.

Furthermore, safety of PS extract was demonstrated in at least 18 clinical trials, involving treatment of children and adults with upper respiratory tract diseases with EPs®7630 over several weeks [12,48]. We show that enrichment of polyphenols by adsorption to polyvinylpyrrolidone further reduces cytotoxicity for PBMCs, improving the therapeutic index of PS-mediated antiviral activity. Clinical safety of PS extracts and the compelling evidence for *in vitro* anti-HIV-1 activity presented in our study encourages future testing of PS extract and PS-derived polyphenol-enriched formulations in HIV-1 infected individuals.

Because PS extract inhibits HIV-1 entry by a novel mode-of-action, it may complement the activity of current microbicide candidates and thus improve prevention of HIV-1 transmission. For anti-HIV-1 therapy, PS extract may supplement first-line treatment regimens, which so far do not include entry inhibitors. Furthermore, PS extract may help decrease virus burden during interruption of conventional drug treatment. Another remarkable feature of the anti-HIV-1 activity of PS extract is its robustness against boiling, drying and extreme pH conditions. Thus we show that PS-extract can be easily produced from PS roots and is amenable to long-term storage at room temperature without loss of anti-HIV-1 activity. This indicates the possibility to use PS-polyphenolic drugs as anti-HIV-1 therapy in resource limited settings. Of note, PS is a medicinal plant habituated in South Africa. Hence, it is highly likely that there will be a high level of compliance towards a PS-based antiviral therapeutic regimen in this region, which is strongly affected by the AIDS pandemic.

Conclusions

Here we demonstrate that an aqueous extract from roots of *Pelargonium sidoides* plants contains robust and potent anti-HIV-1 activity. PS extract prevents HIV-1 particles from attaching to host cells and displays a novel mode-of-action different from other HIV-1 entry inhibitors. Chemical analysis indicates that anti-HIV-1 activity is mediated by the concerted action of multiple polyphenolic compounds which can be separated from components of the extract with higher cytotoxicity by adsorption to polyvinylpyrrolidone.

Based on its potent anti-HIV activity and its extensively studied safety profile, we conclude that PS extract represents a promising lead candidate for the development of a herbal medicine for HIV-1 treatment. The novel mode of anti-HIV activity suggests that PS extract may be useful for complementation of other anti-HIV-1 agents in the therapy of HIV-infected individuals and in protection against HIV-1 infection. Finally, our study demonstrates the amenability of PS extract for experimental analyses, suggesting the use of PS extract as a research tool to advance the development of new anti-HIV agents that protect potential HIV-1 target cells from virus exposure in humans.

Supporting Information

Materials and Methods S1 Assays for testing of inhibition of HIV-1 infection. Quantification of HIV-1 DNA- and RNA-levels. Chromatographic separation of PS extracts. Ultrahigh resolution mass spectrometry.
(DOCX)

Figure S1 Inhibition of HIV-1 infection by different preparations of PS root extracts, including the commercial herbal medicine EPs® 7630. PS extract from plants were prepared from dry or fresh PS roots as described in the main text (Materials and Methods). For analysis of anti-HIV activity of the commercial herbal medicine Umckaloabo/EPs®7630 (purchased from a local pharmacist), aqueous samples were prepared by removing ethanol in the commercial formulation by evaporation in an Eppendorf Vacuum Concentrator and restoration of the original sample volume with ddH_20. Anti-HIV-1 activity was evaluated in LC5-RIC cultures exposed to $HIV1_{LAI}$. Each extract concentration was tested in triplicate. Fluorescent signal intensities of treated cultures were normalized to those of untreated cultures assayed in the same plate (100% infection). Mean values (columns) and standard deviation of the mean are indicated for each extract dilution.
(DOCX)

Figure S2 ICR/FT-MS analysis of crude PS extract and a PS-derived polyphenolic (PSPP) fraction with polyvinylpyrrolidone-adsorbing compounds confirms enrichment of polyphenols in the PSPP fraction. 12 Tesla ICR/FT-MS (Ion Cyclotron Resonance/Fourier Transformation -Mass Spectrometry) measurements in negative electrospray ionization mode were conducted of crude PS extract (A) and PSPP (B) to describe their compositional space. Hundreds of assigned elemental formulas are projected in the van Krevelen diagrams (A, B, C). High H/C ratio indicates relative high aliphaticity and low aromaticity, whereas high O/C ratio relates to oxygenated compounds; the bubble size is proportional to the signal intensities in (A) PS extract, (B) the PSPP fraction and (C) to the signal increase in PVPP relative to PS extracts (ratio of intensities PSPP/PS). Crude Pelargonium extracts possesses a high diversity of small molecule components (<1kDa) within a wide domain of polarity and structural characteristics. The PSPP fraction showed an enrichment of polyphenolic compounds in the domain (H/C 0.5-1; O/C 0.4-0.6, violet circle) (B and C); most aliphatic lipid structures (H/C 1.5-2 O/C 0-0.4) are eliminated in PSPP fraction.
(DOCX)

Acknowledgments

We thank Ben Berkhout (University of Amsterdam, The Netherlands) for providing the plasmid pLAI.2, Paul Clapham (University of Massachusetts

Medical School, Worcester, MA, USA) for the plasmids pNL4.3ΔEnv and pSVIIIenvJRFL and Dr. Olaf Kutsch (University of Alabama, Birmingham, Ala, USA) for the CCR5-expression plasmid in the pMSCVpuro backbone. We thank Beatrice Hahn, University of Pennsylvania School of Medicine for permission to use infectious molecular clones of CH077 and STC0r1 clinical isolates and Frank Kirchhoff, University of Ulm, for providing the appropriate plasmids. pNL(AD8) and pSG3ΔEnv were obtained through the NIH AIDS Reagent Program, Division of AIDS, NIAID, NIH from Dr. Eric O. Freed and Drs. John C. Kappes and Xiaoyun Wu, respectively. We thank Ulrike Protzer for continuous support and encouragement and Ingrid Huelsmeier and Ute Finkel for expert technical assistance.

Author Contributions

Conceived and designed the experiments: MH RBW M. Schneider M. Schindler PSK HK. Performed the experiments: MH HK M. Schneider SR SF CM. Analyzed the data: MH HK M. Schneider M. Schindler SR SF CM RBW PSK. Wrote the paper: MH HK M. Schneider M. Schindler SR SF CM RBW PSK.

References

1. AIDSinfo USDoHaHSH (2012) HIV and Its Treatment – FDA-Approved Anti-HIV Medications.
2. Tang MW, Shafer RW (2012) HIV-1 Antiretroviral resistance: Scientific principles and clinical applications. Drugs 72: e1–e25.
3. Stadeli KM, Richman DD (2012) Rates of emergence of HIV drug resistance in resource-limited settings: a systematic review. Antiviral therapy.
4. Marcus KA, Sorbello A, Truffa M, Williams J, Raine JM, et al. (2012) Current advances in pharmacovigilance in the USA and Europe: meeting the challenges of safety monitoring in HIV. Current Opinion in HIV and AIDS 7: 292–298.
5. Vella S, Schwartländer B, Sow SP, Eholie SP, Murphy RL (2012) The history of antiretroviral therapy and of its implementation in resource-limited areas of the world. AIDS 26: 1231–1241.
6. Hawkins T (2010) Understanding and managing the adverse effects of antiretroviral therapy. Antiviral research 85: 201–209.
7. Cordell GA, Colvard MD (2012) Natural products and traditional medicine: turning on a paradigm. Journal of natural products 75: 514–525.
8. Mukhtar M, Arshad M, Ahmad M, Pomerantz RJ, Wigdahl B, et al. (2008) Antiviral potentials of medicinal plants. Virus research 131: 111–120.
9. Singh IP, Bodiwala HS (2010) Recent advances in anti-HIV natural products. Natural product reports 27: 1781–1800.
10. Cos P, Maes L, Vlietinck A, Pieters L (2008) Plant-derived leading compounds for chemotherapy of human immunodeficiency virus (HIV) infection-an update (1998–2007). Planta Med 74: 1323–1337.
11. Gertsch J (2011) Botanical drugs, synergy, and network pharmacology: forth and back to intelligent mixtures. Planta Medica-Natural Products and Medicinal-Plant Research 77: 1086.
12. Brendler T, Van Wyk B-E (2008) A historical, scientific and commercial perspective on the medicinal use of *Pelargonium sidoides* (Geraniaceae). Journal of ethnopharmacology 119: 420–433.
13. Kolodziej H (2007) Fascinating metabolic pools of *Pelargonium sidoides* and *Pelargonium reniforme*, traditional and phytomedicinal sources of the herbal medicine Umckaloabo ® Phytomedicine 14: 9–17.
14. Michaelis M, Doerr HW, Cinatl J (2011) Investigation of the influence of EPs ® 7630, a herbal drug preparation from *Pelargonium sidoides*, on replication of a broad panel of respiratory viruses. Phytomedicine 18: 384–386.
15. Theisen LL, Muller CP (2012) EPs® 7630 (Umckaloabo®), an extract from *Pelargonium sidoides* roots, exerts anti-influenza virus activity in vitro and in vivo. Antiviral research.
16. Schnitzler P, Schneider S, Stintzing F, Carle R, Reichling J (2008) Efficacy of an aqueous *Pelargonium sidoides* extract against herpesvirus. Phytomedicine: international journal of phytotherapy and phytopharmacology 15: 1108.
17. Kremb S, Helfer M, Heller W, Hoffmann D, Wolff H, et al. (2010) EASY-HIT: HIV full-replication technology for broad discovery of multiple classes of HIV inhibitors. Antimicrobial agents and chemotherapy 54: 5257–5268.
18. Peden K, Emerman M, Montagnier L (1991) Changes in growth properties on passage in tissue culture of viruses derived from infectious molecular clones of HIV-1_{LAI}, HIV-1_{MAL}, and HIV-1_{ELI}. Virology 185: 661–672.
19. Freed EO, Englund G, Martin MA (1995) Role of the basic domain of human immunodeficiency virus type 1 matrix in macrophage infection. Journal of virology 69: 3949–3954.
20. Koppensteiner H, Banning C, Schneider C, Hohenberg H, Schindler M (2012) Macrophage internal HIV-1 is protected from neutralizing antibodies. Journal of virology 86: 2826–2836.
21. Peters PJ, Bhattacharya J, Hibbitts S, Dittmar MT, Simmons G, et al. (2004) Biological analysis of human immunodeficiency virus type 1 R5 envelopes amplified from brain and lymph node tissues of AIDS patients with neuropathology reveals two distinct tropism phenotypes and identifies envelopes in the brain that confer an enhanced tropism and fusigenicity for macrophages. Journal of virology 78: 6915–6926.
22. Parrish NF, Gao F, Li H, Giorgi EE, Barbian HJ, et al. (2013) Phenotypic properties of transmitted founder HIV-1. Proceedings of the National Academy of Sciences 110: 6626–6633.
23. Jones J, Whitford W, Wagner F, Kutsch O (2007) Optimization of HIV-1 infectivity assays. BioTechniques 43: 589.
24. Fuss IJ, Kanof ME, Smith PD, Zola H (2009) Isolation of whole mononuclear cells from peripheral blood and cord blood. Current Protocols in Immunology7.11–7.1. 8.
25. De Clercq E, Yamamoto N, Pauwels R, Balzarini J, Witvrouw M, et al. (1994) Highly potent and selective inhibition of human immunodeficiency virus by the bicyclam derivative JM3100. Antimicrobial agents and chemotherapy 38: 668–674.
26. Hendrix CW, Flexner C, MacFarland RT, Giandomenico C, Fuchs EJ, et al. (2000) Pharmacokinetics and safety of AMD-3100, a novel antagonist of the CXCR-4 chemokine receptor, in human volunteers. Antimicrobial agents and chemotherapy 44: 1667–1673.
27. Mori T, O'Keefe BR, Sowder II RC, Bringans S, Gardella R, et al. (2005) Isolation and characterization of griffithsin, a novel HIV-inactivating protein, from the red alga Griffithsia sp. Journal of Biological Chemistry 280: 9345–9353.
28. Daelemans D, Pauwels R, De Clercq E, Pannecouque C (2011) A time-of-drug addition approach to target identification of antiviral compounds. Nature Protocols 6: 925–933.
29. Kilby JM, Hopkins S, Venetta TM, DiMassimo B, Cloud GA, et al. (1998) Potent suppression of HIV-1 replication in humans by T-20, a peptide inhibitor of gp41-mediated virus entry. Nature medicine 4: 1302–1307.
30. De Clercq E (2009) The history of antiretrovirals: key discoveries over the past 25 years. Reviews in medical virology 19: 287–299.
31. Hendrix CW, Collier AC, Lederman MM, Schols D, Pollard RB, et al. (2004) Safety, pharmacokinetics, and antiviral activity of AMD3100, a selective CXCR4 receptor inhibitor, in HIV-1 infection. JAIDS Journal of Acquired Immune Deficiency Syndromes 37: 1253–1262.
32. Sluis-Cremer N, Tachedjian G (2008) Mechanisms of inhibition of HIV replication by nonnucleoside reverse transcriptase inhibitors. Virus research 134: 147.
33. Alexandre KB, Gray ES, Pantophlet R, Moore PL, McMahon JB, et al. (2011) Binding of the mannose-specific lectin, griffithsin, to HIV-1 gp120 exposes the CD4-binding site. Journal of virology 85: 9039–9050.
34. Forcisi S, Moritz F, Kanawati B, Tziotis D, Lehmann R, et al. (2013) Liquid chromatography–mass spectrometry in metabolomics research: Mass analyzers in ultra high pressure liquid chromatography coupling. Journal of Chromatography A 1292: 51–65.
35. Overy DP, Enot DP, Tailliart K, Jenkins H, Parker D, et al. (2008) Explanatory signal interpretation and metabolite identification strategies for nominal mass FIE-MS metabolite fingerprints. Nature Protocols 3: 471–485.
36. Magalhães PJ, Vieira JS, Gonçalves LM, Pacheco JG, Guido LF, et al. (2010) Isolation of phenolic compounds from hop extracts using polyvinylpolypyrrolidone: characterization by high-performance liquid chromatography-diode array detection-electrospray tandem mass spectrometry. Journal of chromatography 1217: 3258–3268.
37. François K, Balzarini J (2010) Potential of carbohydrate-binding agents as therapeutics against enveloped viruses. Medicinal Research Reviews 32: 349–387.
38. Huskens D, Schols D (2012) Algal lectins as potential HIV microbicide candidates. Marine drugs 10: 1476-1497.
39. Hertje M, Zhou M, Dietrich U (2010) Inhibition of HIV-1 Entry: Multiple Keys to Close the Door. ChemMedChem 5: 1825–1835.
40. Gibson R, Arts E (2012) Past, Present, and Future of Entry Inhibitors as HIV Microbicides. Current HIV research 10: 19.
41. Krepstakies M, Lucifora J, Nagel C-H, Zeisel MB, Holstermann B, et al. (2012) A new class of synthetic peptide inhibitors blocks attachment and entry of human pathogenic viruses. Journal of Infectious Diseases 205: 1654–1664.
42. Yamaguchi K, Honda M, Ikigai H, Hara Y, Shimamura T (2002) Inhibitory effects of (–)-epigallocatechin gallate on the life cycle of human immunodeficiency virus type 1 (HIV-1). Antiviral research 53: 19–34.
43. Hamza A, Zhan C-G (2006) How can (-)-epigallocatechin gallate from green tea prevent HIV-1 infection? Mechanistic insights from computational modeling and the implication for rational design of anti-HIV-1 entry inhibitors. The Journal of Physical Chemistry B 110: 2910–2917.
44. Yang J, Li L, Tan S, Jin H, Qiu J, et al. (2011) A natural theaflavins preparation inhibits HIV-1 infection by targeting the entry step: Potential applications for preventing HIV-1 infection. Fitoterapia.
45. Moulard M, Lortat-Jacob H, Mondor I, Roca G, Wyatt R, et al. (2000) Selective interactions of polyanions with basic surfaces on human immunodeficiency virus type 1 gp120. Journal of virology 74: 1948–1960.
46. Dorr P, Westby M, Dobbs S, Griffin P, Irvine B, et al. (2005) Maraviroc (UK-427,857), a potent, orally bioavailable, and selective small-molecule inhibitor of chemokine receptor CCR5 with broad-spectrum anti-human immunodeficiency virus type 1 activity. Antimicrobial agents and chemotherapy 49: 4721–4732.

47. Kouokam JC, Huskens D, Schols D, Johannemann A, Riedell SK, et al. (2011) Investigation of griffithsin's interactions with human cells confirms its outstanding safety and efficacy profile as a microbicide candidate. Plos one 6: e22635.

48. Timmer A, Günther J, Rücker G, Motschall E, Antes G, et al. (2008) *Pelargonium sidoides* extract for acute respiratory tract infections. Cochrane Database Syst Rev 3.

Traditional Herbal Medicine Use Associated with Liver Fibrosis in Rural Rakai, Uganda

Brandon J. Auerbach[1,2]*, Steven J. Reynolds[3,4], Mohammed Lamorde[1,5], Concepta Merry[1,5,6], Collins Kukunda-Byobona[8], Ponsiano Ocama[2,7], Aggrey S. Semeere[1,7], Anthony Ndyanabo[9], Iga Boaz[9], Valerian Kiggundu[9], Fred Nalugoda[9], Ron H. Gray[9,10], Maria J. Wawer[9,10], David L. Thomas[4], Gregory D. Kirk[11], Thomas C. Quinn[3,4], Lara Stabinski[3,11], on behalf of the Rakai Health Sciences Program

1 Infectious Diseases Institute, College of Health Sciences, Makerere University, Kampala, Uganda, **2** Harvard Medical School, Boston, Massachusetts, United States of America, **3** Division of Intramural Research, National Institute of Allergy and Infectious Diseases, National Institutes of Health, Bethesda, Maryland, United States of America, **4** Division of Infectious Diseases, Department of Medicine, School of Medicine, Johns Hopkins University, Baltimore, Maryland, United States of America, **5** Department of Pharmacology and Therapeutics, School of Medicine, University of Dublin, Trinity College, Dublin, Ireland, **6** St James's Hospital, Dublin, Ireland, **7** Department of Medicine, College of Health Sciences, Makerere University, Kampala, Uganda, **8** Department of Botany, Makerere University, Kampala, Uganda, **9** Rakai Health Sciences Program, Entebbe, Uganda, **10** Department of Population, Family, and Reproductive Health, Bloomberg School of Public Health, Johns Hopkins University, Baltimore, Maryland, United States of America, **11** Department of Epidemiology, Bloomberg School of Public Health, Johns Hopkins University, Baltimore, Maryland, United States of America

Abstract

Background: Traditional herbal medicines are commonly used in sub-Saharan Africa and some herbs are known to be hepatotoxic. However little is known about the effect of herbal medicines on liver disease in sub-Saharan Africa.

Methods: 500 HIV-infected participants in a rural HIV care program in Rakai, Uganda, were frequency matched to 500 HIV-uninfected participants. Participants were asked about traditional herbal medicine use and assessed for other potential risk factors for liver disease. All participants underwent transient elastography (FibroScan®) to quantify liver fibrosis. The association between herb use and significant liver fibrosis was measured with adjusted prevalence risk ratios (adjPRR) and 95% confidence intervals (CI) using modified Poisson multivariable logistic regression.

Results: 19 unique herbs from 13 plant families were used by 42/1000 of all participants, including 9/500 HIV-infected participants. The three most-used plant families were Asteraceae, Fabaceae, and Lamiaceae. Among all participants, use of any herb (adjPRR = 2.2, 95% CI 1.3–3.5, p = 0.002), herbs from the Asteraceae family (adjPRR = 5.0, 95% CI 2.9–8.7, p<0.001), and herbs from the Lamiaceae family (adjPRR = 3.4, 95% CI 1.2–9.2, p = 0.017) were associated with significant liver fibrosis. Among HIV infected participants, use of any herb (adjPRR = 2.3, 95% CI 1.0–5.0, p = 0.044) and use of herbs from the Asteraceae family (adjPRR = 5.0, 95% CI 1.7–14.7, p = 0.004) were associated with increased liver fibrosis.

Conclusions: Traditional herbal medicine use was independently associated with a substantial increase in significant liver fibrosis in both HIV-infected and HIV-uninfected study participants. Pharmacokinetic and prospective clinical studies are needed to inform herb safety recommendations in sub-Saharan Africa. Counseling about herb use should be part of routine health counseling and counseling of HIV-infected persons in Uganda.

Editor: John E. Tavis, Saint Louis University, United States of America

Funding: The study was primarily funded by the United States National Institutes of Health (NIH) Bench to Bedside Program. Additional support was provided by the Division of Intramural Research, National Institutes of Allergy and Infectious Diseases, National Institutes of Health. Support was also provided by the National Institute on Drug Abuse (PI: DLT, R01-AI-16078) and the American Cancer Society (PI: GDK, MRSG-07-284-01-CCE). The study was jointly conducted and benefited from close collaboration of researchers from the intramural NIH Laboratory of Immunoregulation, Johns Hopkins University, the Infectious Diseases Institute of Makerere University, and the Rakai Health Sciences Program. Support for the RHSP HIV Care Program was provided by the President's Emergency Fund for AIDS Relief (PEPFAR) and support for the Rakai Community Cohort Study was provided by the Department of the Army, United States Army Medical Research and Material Command Cooperative Agreement DAMD17-98-2-8007; grants R01 A134826 and R01 A134265 from the National Institute of Allergy and Infectious Diseases; grant R01 016078 (DLT) from the National Institute on Drug Abuse; and grant 5P30HD06826 from the National Institute of Child and Health Development. BJA and ASS were funded by the Fogarty International Clinical Research Scholars (FICRS) program of the NIH, administered by the Vanderbilt University Institute for Global Health (R24 TW007988). The funders had no role in study design, data collection and analysis, decision to publish, or preparation of the manuscript.

Competing Interests: The authors have declared that no competing interests exist.

* E-mail: brandon_auerbach@hms.harvard.edu

Introduction

Traditional herbal medicines are commonly used for HIV/AIDS and other health conditions in Uganda and sub-Saharan Africa, often in parallel with programs that provide antiretroviral therapy (ART). In the 1990's an estimated 80% of Ugandans living in rural villages used traditional healers for primary health care [1]. A study of 137 HIV-infected Ugandans receiving ART found that 60% used herbs concurrently with ART [2].

In Uganda traditional herbal medicines are usually boiled extracts of herbs taken orally [3]. Some potentially hepatotoxic traditional herbal medicines used in Uganda and sub-Saharan Africa include *Hoodia gordoni* [4], kava [5], *Phytolacca dioica* [6], and herbs from the Asteraceae family [7]. Little is known about the hepatotoxicity of other commonly used herbs or the contribution of herbs to the burden of liver fibrosis and hepatocellular carcinoma in sub- Saharan Africa, including when used concomitantly with ART. Data on the specific types of herbs taken by HIV-infected persons in Uganda is limited, as is information about their components, side effects, toxicities, and ART interactions [8].

In Rakai, Uganda, liver toxicity associated with herbal medicine may be of particular concern given the high prevalence of significant liver disease (17%) among HIV-infected persons in Rakai recently identified by transient elastography (FibroScan®, Echosense, Paris, France) [9]. In the aforementioned study, reported herbal medicine use was associated with a two-fold increased risk of significant liver disease, defined as a transient elastography score equivalent to METAVIR liver fibrosis stage 2 (portal fibrosis with few septa) or greater [9]. The study presented here follows up on this prior investigation with an in-depth analysis of the herbs used by study participants and their relation to liver fibrosis.

Methods

This cross-sectional study enrolled 500 HIV-infected participants receiving care at five HIV care clinics within the Rakai Health Sciences Program (RHSP) HIV Care Program. 500 HIV-uninfected participants from the Rakai Community Cohort Study (RCCS) were frequency- matched to these participants by age, gender, and community. Begun in 1994 in one of Uganda's hardest-hit regions by the HIV epidemic, the RCCS conducts annual surveys in a population of 10,000–15,000 people aged 15–49 years, and is described in detail elsewhere [10]. Participants underwent a detailed liver-disease focused risk factor questionnaire which included an assessment of herbal drug use, venous blood collection, and transient elastography (FibroScan®, Echosense, Paris, France) to quantify liver fibrosis.

Ethics Statement

Written informed consent was obtained from all participants. Institutional Review Boards of theNational Institute of Allergy and Infectious Diseases, the Johns Hopkins Medical Institutions, the Scientific and Ethics Committee of the Uganda Virus Research Institute, and the Uganda National Council for Science and Technology approved this study. The study protocol conforms to the ethical guidelines of the 1975 Declaration of Helsinki, and is registered on clinicaltrials.gov (#NCT00782158).

Herb Use Assessment

Participants were asked about any current herb use and then to name the two herbs they used most often. Scientific names were assigned to local herb names in consultation with local traditional medicine practitioners and a member of Makerere University Botany Department (CKB). The Makerere University Herbarium database was also used to validate herb identities. Some participants reported non-plant substances such as clay and spiritual charms as herb use. Participants reporting use of non-plant based entities were reclassified as non-herb users in this analysis.

Laboratory Assays

HIV-1 serology was determined by two HIV-1 enzyme immuno-assays: Vironostika HIV-1 (OrganonTeknika, Charlotte, North Carolina, USA) and Cambridge Biotech (Worcester, Massachusetts, USA). Participants with discrepant HIV-1 enzyme immune assay results were tested with western blot (HIV-1 Western Blot; Bio-Merieux-Vitek, St. Louis, Missouri, USA). For HIV-infected participants, current CD4 count (within 12 months) and CD4 count nadir were abstracted from the RHSP HIV Care Program database. CD4 counts were measured by FACSCalibur flow cytometer (software version 1.4, Becton Dickinson, San Jose, California, USA). Hepatitis B virus surface antigen (HBsAg) was determined using ELISA (ETI-MAK-2 Plus, Diasorin, Vercelli, Italy). Alanine aminotransferase (ALT) was tested using standard methods (COBAS CII; Roche, Basel, Switzerland), and hepatotoxicity was defined by ALT elevations and classified according to AIDS Clinical Trial Group criteria [11]. The upper limit of normal for ALT was defined as 19 IU/L in women and 39 IU/L in men [12,13].

Transient Elastography

Transient elastography or FibroScan® is a novel, validated, noninvasive technology for the evaluation of fibrosis in chronic liver disease [14]. A FibroScan® is approximately the size of an ultrasound unit. A probe placed over a patient's abdomen produces vibration and the speed of the responding elastic wave is detected by ultrasound. The propagation of these waves through the liver is directly correlated to the degree of liver stiffness. The results are instantaneously received as a single, quantitative parameter of liver stiffness measurement (LSM, reported in kPa). Each transient elastography scan takes ten liver stiffness measurements in rapid succession over several seconds. The median of the ten measurements is reported as the final liver stiffness measurement. The procedure is non-invasive, painless, has no side effects, and requires only a few minutes to perform. The device requires minimal training and does not need to be performed by advanced medical personnel.

In this study a conservative liver stiffness measurement cutoff of ≥9.3 kPa, from a validation study in persons of predominantly African descent, was used to define significant fibrosis equivalent to METAVIR fibrosis stage 2 (portal fibrosis with few septa) or greater [15]. Two study nurses at the Rakai Health Science Program study site conducted all transient elastography scans after receiving certification from the manufacturer. According to manufacturer recommendations, scans with high variability—defined as an interquartile range greater than 30% of the median LSM value from an individual examination—were not considered valid and were excluded from the analysis. Participants with invalid scans on an initial attempt were repositioned and rescanned up to 4 times to achieve a valid scan.

Statistics

Baseline demographic, behavioral and clinical characteristics were compared by HIV status. Differences in continuous variables were assessed using t-tests and Wilcoxon-Mann-Whitney tests. Categorical variables were compared using Pearson's chi squared test.

Table 1. Baseline characteristics of study participants.

	HIV-infected pts (n = 500)	HIV-uninfected pts (n = 500)	
	n (% or IQR)	n (% or IQR)	p value
Characteristic			
Median Age, years	38 (IQR 31–44)	37 (IQR 32–44)	0.025
Female	312 (67%)	333 (67%)	0.89
Heavy Liquor use (>1.25 L/week)	11 (2%)	9 (2%)	0.65
Lifetime occupational fishing	5 (1%)	1 (0.2%)	0.65
HBsAg positive	23 (5%)	14 (3%)	0.10
Valid TE scan	468 (94%)	494 (99%)	<0.001
Herb Use			
Current herb use	8 (2%)	33 (7%)	0.0001
Known herbs	5 (0.9%)	16 (3%)	0.015
Unknown herbs	4 (0.9%)	17 (3%)	0.004
Asteraceae family	2 (0.4%)	6 (1%)	0.16
Fabaceae family	0 (0%)	6 (1%)	0.014
Lamiaceae family	1 (0.2%)	4 (0.8%)	0.18
ACTG Heptatotoxicty Criteria			
Median ALT (U/L)	22 (IQR 16–31)	19 (IQR 15–25)	<0.001
Grade 0 (<1.25×ULN) by ALT	354 (71%)	414 (83%)	
Grade 1 (1.25–2.5×ULN) by ALT	122 (24%)	77 (15%)	
Grade 2 (2.6–5×ULN) by ALT	19 (4%)	9 (2%)	
Grade 3 (5.1–10×ULN) by ALT	5 (1%)	0 (0%)	
Grade 4 (>10×ULN) by ALT	0 (0%)	0 (0%)	
CD4 and ART Characteristics			
Current CD4 count (cells/uL)	449 (IQR 320–642)		
Nadir CD4 count (cells/uL)	214 (IQR 130–350)		
Nadir CD4 count <100 cells/uL	95 (19%)		
On ART	302 (60%)		
ART duration (months)	19 (IQR 9–38)		

HIV (Human Immunodeficiency Virus), IQR (Interquartile Range), HBsAg (Hepatitis B Surface Antigen), ACTG (AIDS Clinical Trials Group), CD4 (Cluster of Differentiation 4 positive Helper T cells), ART (Antiretroviral Therapy).

The primary outcome measure was liver fibrosis. Because odds ratios may overestimate the magnitude of association between variables if the outcome of interest is common, adjusted prevalence risk ratios (adjPRR) with 95% confidence intervals (95% CI) were estimated using modified Poisson regression [16]. The multivariable models adjusted for HIV, gender, occupation in the fishing industry, chronic hepatitis B infection (positive hepatitis B surface antigen), and drinking ≥1.25 liters per week of liquor, as these risk factors were associated with liver disease in previous analysis of this study population [9]. Age was included in all models and nadir CD4 cell count and ART status were included in models restricted to HIV- infected participants for reasons of biologic plausibility. STATA version 11.0 (STATA Corp, College Station, TX) was used for statistical analysis.

Results

Baseline Characteristics

The HIV-infected and uninfected groups each had 67% females (see table 1). The median age of 38 years in the HIV-infected group was close to the median age of 37 years in the HIV-uninfected group ($p = 0.025$). Only 2% of both HIV-infected and uninfected participants were heavy liquor drinkers ($p = 0.65$). The prevalence of chronic HBV infection was similar in both groups, 5% in HIV-infected participants and 3% in HIV-uninfected participants ($p = 0.010$). 29% of HIV-infected participants and 17% of HIV-uninfected participants had any grade 1 or higher hepatotoxicity by AIDS Clinical Trial Group (ACTG) criteria ($p < 0.001$). No participants demonstrated grade 4 hepatotoxicity.

At the time of enrolment HIV-infected participants had a median CD4 count of 449 cells/μL (IQR 320–642) and 60% were receiving ART with a median duration of 19 months (IQR 9–38). Demographics of the HIV-infected group were also similar to participants in the Rakai Health Sciences HIV Care Program, in which 65% of participants are female, 64% are on ART, and the median CD4 count is 480 cells/μL.

468/500 (94%) of HIV-infected participants and 494/500 (99%) of HIV-uninfected participants had valid elastography scans. Those with valid scans were included in the assessment of liver fibrosis and were included in the regression models.

Table 2. Characteristics of participants reporting current herb use.

	Using Herbs (n = 42)	Not Using Herbs (n = 958)	
Characteristic	**n (% or IQR)**	**n (% or IQR)**	**p value**
Median Age, years	39 (32–44 IQR)	38 (31–44 IQR)	0.61
Female	27 (64%)	643 (67%)	0.15
Heavy Liquor use (>1.25 L/week)	3 (7%)	17 (2%)	0.015
Lifetime occupational fishing	1 (2%)	5 (0.5%)	0.13
HBsAg positive	2 (5%)	35 (4%)	0.73
HIV infected	9 (20%)	491 (50%)	0.0001

L (Liters), HBsAg (Hepatitis B Surface Antigen), HIV (Human Immunodeficiency Virus).

Characteristics of Herb Users

42/1000 (4%) of all participants reported current use of traditional herbal medicines, including 9/500 (2%) of HIV-infected participants and 33/500 (7%) HIV-uninfected participants (table 1). 21/42 (50%) of participants could name at least one herb they were taking. 4/46 (9%) of participants reporting

Table 3. Characteristics of known herbs in the Asteraceae, Fabaceae, and Lamiaceae families.

Family (n taking)	Scientific Name	Local Names (n taking)	English Name	Taken in Rakai for:	Known Pharmacology	Known Liver Toxicity and/or ART Interaction
Asteraceae (8)	*Vernonia amygdalina*	Mululuza (4)	Bitter leaf	Fever, fever with jaundice	Contains alkaloids, saponins, tannins, flavonoids, steroid glycosides, sesquiterpine lactone [32]	Hepatotoxic at high doses (750 mg/kg) [24]. One herb from the Veronia genus (V. lasiopus) was hepatotoxic in an in-vitro rat precision cut liver slice model [33]. Many herbs in the Asteraceae family contain pyrrolizidine alkaloids, which are associated with veno-occlusive liver disease [17]
	Vernonia genus	Kiluluuza (2)				
	Microglossa densiflora	Kafugankande, Akafugankande (1)		Fever, indigestion, loose stools, parasites	Microglossa family contains clerodane diterpenoids [34]	A similar herb from the Microglossa family (M. *pyrifolia*) was hepatotoxic in an *in-vitro* rat precision cut liver slice model [33]. Many herbs in the Asteraceae family contain pyrrolizidine alkaloids, which are associated with veno-occlusive liver disease [17]
	Aspilia africana	Makaayi (1)	Wild sunflower	Fever with jaundice	Contains saponins, tannins, terpenoids, Sesquiterpenes, monoterpenes [35,36]	No hepatoxicity in rat in vivo model [38]. Many herbs in the Asteraceae family contain pyrrolizidine alkaloids, which are associated with veno-occlusive liver disease [17]
Fabaceae (6)	*Pseudarthria hookeri*	Bikakala, Kikakala, Omukakala, Mukakala (4)		Fever, fever with jaundice, allergy, cough, wounds	May have estrogenic activity [37]	Many herbs in the Fabaceae family contain pyrrolizidine alkaloids, which are associated with veno-occlusive liver disease [17]
	Indigofera congesta	Namasumi (2)	Indigo	Fever with jaundice, antenatal health	Indigofera family members contain flavonoids, saponins, quinones, sterols/ triterpenes, tannins, gallic acid, caffeic acid, rutin and myricetin [38]	Many herbs in the Fabaceae family contain pyrrolizidine alkaloids, which are associated with veno-occlusive liver disease [17]
Lamiaceae (5*)	*Ocimum gratissimum*	Mujaaja, Omujaaja (3)	African basil	Epigastric pain	Contains tannin phlobaphenes, flavones, flavonols, xanthones, chalcones, aurones, terpenes, flavononols, leucoanthocyanidins, catechins [39]	Herb from Ocimum genus (O. *lamiifolium*) was hepatotoxic in an *in-vitro* rat precision cut liver slice model [33], Ocimum *gratissimum* caused hepatoxicity *in-vivo* rabbit liver model [25]
	Hoslundia opposita	Kamunye (3)		To replace blood, postnatal health, vomiting during fever and jaundice	Contains sesquiterpenes and sesquiterpene alcohols [40]	

*one patient took both Ocimum gratissimum and Hoslundia oopposita. mg (milligrams), kg (kilograms).

Table 4. Characteristics of known herbs in remainder of plant families.

Family (n taking)	Scientific Name	Local Names (n taking)	English Name	Taken in Rakai for:	Known Pharmacology	Known Liver Toxicity and/or ART Interaction
Anacardiaceae (2)	*Rhus vulgaris or Rhus natalenis*	Olukansokanso, akakwansokwanso (1)		Antenatal health, aphrodisiac, gastrointestinal ulcers, back pain	No published information about contents	
	Mangifera indica	Mango Tree Bark (1)	Mango tree bark		Leaves contains flavonoids [41], Peel contains phenolic compounds and carotenoids [42]	
Primulaceae (2)	*Maesa lanceolata*	Oluwongwa, Oluwongo (2)		Neonatal jaundice	Contains Saponins [43], benzoquinone [44]	
Euphorbiaceae (2)	*Sapium ellipticum*	Musasa, Omusiisa, Musanvuma (2)	Jumping tree seed	Hypertension, antenatal health, sexually transmitted infections, epigastric pain	Contains phenols [45]	
Amaryllidaceae (1)	*Allium sativum*	Garlic (1)	Garlic	—	Contians diallyl disulfide [46]	Induces CYP3A4 and Pgp and should not be taken with the following antiretrovirals: APV, ATV, AZT, EFV, IDV, LPV, NFV, NVP, SQV [27]
Bignoniaceae (1)	*Spathodea campanulata*	Ekifabakazi (1)	African tulip tree	Dysmennorrhea, antenatal health	Contains 3β-acetoxyoleanolic acid, siaresinolic acid, oleanolic acid, others [47]	
Solanaceae (1)	*Solanum incanum*	Akatengotengo (1)	Sodom apple	Cough, chest pain	Contains alkaloids, saponins, solanine; High concentrations cause hemolysis of erythrocytes [48]	Herbs containing pyrrolizidine alkaloids are associated with veno-occlusive liver disease [17].
Vitaceae (1)	*Cyphostemma adenocaule*	Kamombo (1)		Peptic ulcers	Contain carotenoids (carotenes), xanthophylls, Vitamin C, Tocopherols, and Tocotrienols [49]	
Myrtaceae (1)	*Callistemon citrinus*	Bottlebrush (1)	Bottlebrush tree	Rhino-sinusitis	Contains 1,8-cineole, apha-pinene [50]	
		Kagulukandayi, Katangulucumu (1)		Epilepsy		
		Kakubamusolo (1)				

APV (amprenavir), ATV (atazanavir), AZT (zidovudine), EFV (efavirenz), IDV indinavir), LPV (lopinavir), NFV (nelfinavir), NVP (nevirapine), SQV (saquinavir).

herb use were reclassified as not taking herbs because they only reported use of inert, non-plant substances including clay. Herb users did not differ by age ($p = 0.61$) or gender ($p = 0.15$) from those who did not report herb use (see table 2). Herb users were not more likely to work in the fishing industry ($p = 0.13$) or have chronic hepatitis B infection ($p = 0.73$). 7% of participants reporting herb use drank liquor heavily (≥1.25 L/week), compared to 2% of participants who did not report herb use ($p = 0.015$). 19 unique herbs from 13 families were used, and are characterized in tables 3 and 4. The most common families were Asteraceae, Fabaceae, and Lamiaceae, which were used by eight, six and five participants, respectively.

Herb Use and Liver Fibrosis

Among the 137/962 (14%) subjects with significant liver fibrosis, 12/137 (9%) reported herb use. Of the 825/962 (86%) subjects without significant liver fibrosis, 29/825 (4%) reported current herb use ($p = 0.005$). 56/494 (11%) of HIV-uninfected participants had significant fibrosis, compared to 81/468 (17%) of HIV-infected participants ($p = 0.008$).

In multivariable analysis that adjusted for age, fishing occupation, HIV infection, positive HBsAg, gender, and heavy liquor use, herb use was associated with two to five fold increases in significant liver fibrosis (see table 5). Among all participants, use of any herb (adjPRR = 2.2, 95% CI 1.3–3.5, $p = 0.002$), herbs from the Asteraceae family (adjPRR = 5.0, 95% CI 2.9–8.7, $p < 0.001$), and herbs from the Lamiaceae family (adjPRR = 3.4, 95% CI 1.2–

Table 5. Association of herbs with significant liver fibrosis in all participants.

	Univariate			Multivariate		
Herb (n taking)	**PRR**	**95% CI**	**P value**	**adjPRR**	**95% CI**	**P value**
Any current herb use (41)	2.2	1.3–3.6	0.003	2.2	1.3–3.5	0.002
Asteraceae (8)	5.5	3.6–8.4	<0.001	5.0	2.9–8.7	<0.001
Fabaceae (6)	1.2	0.19–7.1	0.86	1.6	0.26–10.3	0.60
Lamiaceae (5)	2.8	0.96.0–8.4	0.060	3.4	1.2–9.2	0.017
Unknown herb (21)	1.0	0.35–2.9	0.995	1.2	0.40–3.3	0.79

Multivariate model for all participants adjusts for: age, occupational fishing, HIV infection, positive Hepatitis B surface antigen, gender, heavy liquor use (≥1.25 L/week). Only participants with a valid TE scan (962/1000) were included in the model. CI (Confidence Interval).

9.2, p = 0.017) were associated with increased significant fibrosis. Use of herbs from the Fabaceae family was not associated with significant liver fibrosis (adjPRR = 1.6, 95% CI 0.26–10.3, p = 0.60).

Of 81 HIV-infected subjects with significant liver fibrosis, 4 (5%) reported herb use (see table 6). Among 387 HIV-infected subjects without significant liver fibrosis, 4 (1%) reported herb use (p = 0.014). In the multivariable analysis of HIV-infected participants adjusted for age, occupational fishing, positive HBsAg, gender, heavy liquor use, ART, and CD4 nadir, the associations between herb use and significant liver fibrosis were similar to findings among all participants. Among HIV-infected participants the use of any herb (adjPRR = 2.3, 95% CI 1.0–5.0, p = 0.044) and the use of herbs from the Asteraceae family (adjPRR = 5.0, 95% CI 1.7–14.7, p = 0.004) were associated with increased liver fibrosis.

Among all participants as well as HIV-infected participants, herb use was not associated with increased hepatotoxicity. 8/41 (20%) of participants reporting herb use had ACTG grade 1–4 ALT elevations, compared to 216/961 (23%) who did not report herb use (p = 0.56). Among HIV-infected participants reporting herb use, 6/33 (18%) had grade 1–4 ALT elevations, compared to 79/461 (17%) who did not report herb use (p = 0.88).

Table 7 shows the proportion of participants who took individual herbs in the Asteraceae, Lamiaceae, and Fabaceae families who had significant liver fibrosis. 6/8 participants taking herbs in the Asteraceae family had significant liver fibrosis. 4/6

Table 6. Association of herbs with significant liver fibrosis in HIV-infected participants.

	Univariate			Multivariate		
Herb (n taking)	**PRR**	**95% CI**	**P value**	**adjPRR**	**95% CI**	**P value**
Any current herb use (8)	3.0	1.4–6.2	0.003	2.3	1.0–5.0	0.044
Asteraceae (2)	6.0	4.9–7.3	<0.001	5.0	1.7–14.7	0.004
Unknown herb (5)	1.2	0.20–6.8	0.87	1.0	0.15–6.7	0.998

Multivariate model for HIV-infected participants adjusts for: age, occupational fishing, positive Hepatitis B surface antigen, gender, heavy liquor use (≥1.25 L/week), ART, and CD4 nadir. Only participants with a valid TE scan (468/500) were included in the model. CI (Confidence Interval).

Table 7. Use of specific herbs and significant liver fibrosis.

Herb used	Proportion of participants taking with significant liver fibrosis
Asteraceae Family	**6/8**
Vernonia amygdalina	2/4
Vernonia, species unknown	2/2
Microglossa densiflora	1/1
Aspilia Africana	1/1
Fabaceae Family	**2/6**
Pseudarthria hookeri	1/4
Indigofera congesta	1/2
Lamaceae Family	**2/5 ***
Ocimum gratissimum	1/3
Hoslundia opposita	1/3

*One participant took both Ocmum gratissimum and Hoslundia opposite. Only participants with a valid TE scans are shown.

subjects who used herbs in the *Vernonia* genus of the Asteraceae family had significant liver fibrosis.

Discussion

This study indicates that traditional herbal medicine use may contribute to liver disease in Uganda. Use of traditional herbal medicines was independently associated with two to five fold increases in significant liver fibrosis. Herbs from the Asteraceae family were the most often used and showed the strongest association with significant liver fibrosis: a five-fold increase in all participants ($p<0.001$) and HIV-infected participants ($p = 0.004$).

Six of eight participants who took herbs in the Asteraceae family had significant liver fibrosis (see table 5). Many plants in the Asteraceae and Fabaceae families contain pyrrolizidine alkaloids, a known risk factor for veno-occlusive liver disease [7,17]. Although none of the alkaloid-containing herbs used by participants in this study have been confirmed to contain pyrrolizidine alkaloids, ingestion of plants containing pyrrolizidine alkaloids caused outbreaks of veno-occlusive liver disease in Jamaica, India, Egypt, and South Africa [17,18]. No outbreaks of veno-occlusive liver disease associated with pyrrolizidine alkaloids have been reported to our knowledge in East Africa. Pyrrolizidine alkaloids are inert until dehydrogenation by cytochrome P450 3A4 (CYP3A4) in the liver [19], where reactive toxic pyrrolic and N-oxide metabolites directly damage liver sinusoidal endothelial cells and hepatocytes (zone III of the liver acinus) [20]. Pyrroles cause chromosomal damage in a dose-dependent manner, resulting in an inflammatory response that culminates in fibrin deposition [17,20,21].

Although plants in both the Asteraceae and Fabaceae families ingested by study participants may contain pyrrolizidine alkaloids, our data shows a strong association between significant liver fibrosis and use of herbs in the Asteraceae family but not the Fabaceae family. The literature about African traditional herbal medicines is limited and does not explain why this difference might exist. Traditional herbal medicine remedies used in Rakai and throughout Uganda are often mixtures containing multiple herbs [8,22]. It is possible that herbs in the Asteraceae family are taken at high doses, or potentiate the toxicity of other herbs or hepatotoxins.

Two participants with fibrosis reported use of *Vernonia amygdalina* in the Asteraceae family. This particular herb is commonly used in Africa is thought to have hepatoprotective properties [23]. However, animal studies show that at higher doses, this member of the Asteracaae family may be hepatotoxic. In an *in-vivo* rat CCl_4 liver injury model, low doses (250–500 mg/kg) of *Vernonia amygdalina* were hepatoprotective, but a high dose (750 mg/kg) caused increased hepatoxicity [24].

Herbs from the Lamiaceae family were associated with a 3.4 fold increase in significant liver fibrosis among all participants in our study (p = 0.017). Herbs in the Lamiaceae family have been associated with hepatoxicity in an *in-vivo* rabbit model [25]. In addition, Aloe, taken by two participants in our study, has been linked in case reports to severe hepatitis [26]. However, data about the potential hepatotoxicity of many herbs used by participants in this study do not exist, or come from animal model studies only that should be interpreted cautiously.

The risk of significant fibrosis associated with herb use was similar in the overall and HIV- infected study populations. Data on herb use was limited in the HIV-infected population, and plant family specific analysis was only possible for the Asteraceae family. Only two HIV- infected participants reported using herbs in the Asteraceae family.

Despite the small number of HIV-infected participants in this study who reported herb use, it is important to note that ART may alter the toxicity profile of co-administered herbs. CYP3A4 is a major pathway for metabolism of a wide range of chemically distinct foreign compounds including phytochemicals and antiretroviral drugs [27]. Antiretroviral drugs of the non- nucleoside reverse transcriptase inhibitor (NNRTI) and protease inhibitor (PI) classes are also inducers or inhibitors of CYP3A4 activity [28,29]. Therefore, these drugs have potential to influence phytochemical toxification or detoxification pathways in the liver. For example, commonly used NNRTI in initial ART regimens in Uganda (efavirenz and nevirapine) are inducers of CYP3A4 and therefore have potential to increase generation of toxic metabolites of pyrrolizidine alkaloids [27,28]. Inhibitors of CYP3A4 may lead to accumulation of phytochemicals or their metabolites in the liver which may also result in toxicity.

Conversely, herbs may potentiate ART toxicities by influencing antiretroviral drug disposition in the liver, kidney, and gut. Herbs may affect NNRTI and PI metabolism by CPY3A4 and alter activity of cellular drug transporters and glucuronidation pathways [27]. Existing evidence from Africa about herb-ART interactions is limited to two herb families commonly used in South Africa: *Hypoxis* (African potato) and *Sutherlandia*, neither of which were taken by participants in this study. Hypoxis causes a dose-dependent inhibition of CYP3A4 up to 86% of the normal activity of CYP3A4 and 50% reduction of the expression of P-glycoprotein. Sutherlandia *frutescens* also causes a dose dependent inhibition of CYP3A4 up to 96% of CYP3A4 activity [30]. One participant in this study reported garlic use, which is known to significantly reduce concentrations of a PI (saquinavir), most likely by induction of CYP3A4 [31]. Since nevirapine and efavirenz are also eliminated by CYP3A4, garlic may reduce plasma levels of these drugs, but there are no clinical data on these interactions.

Limitations

This study had limitations. The study was cross-sectional and only information about current herb use was available for analysis. Only 4% of participants in this study reported using herbs, compared to other studies in Uganda in which 60% of HIV-infected persons reported concurrent use of ART and herbs [2]. Some misclassification of herb exposure could have occurred due to a social desirability or reporting bias, especially among HIV-infected persons on ART who are counseled to avoid herbs in the communities around Rakai. Only 2% of HIV- infected participants reported herb use. While this lower number of HIV-infected participants reporting herb use could represent effective counseling, the difference in herb use among those on ART and those not on ART was not significant (1% vs. 2%, p = 0.42). The small number of participants reporting herb use limited many comparisons (e.g., herb-ART interactions) and suggests that our findings should be interpreted cautiously.

An important limitation of this study is the potential for reverse causality. Although the most frequently used families of herbs in this study contain known hepatotoxins (see table 3), it is possible that the association of fibrosis with herb use could represent reverse causality, or persons with symptomatic liver disease being more likely to use herbal medicines. According to consultations with local traditional practitioners, some of the herbs in Asteraceae and other families are sometimes prescribed for "fever with jaundice". However, none of the study participants had been previously diagnosed with liver disease within the formal medical system or by traditional healers. Most herbs used in this study to treat fever are usually taken for general fever ("fever" or "malaria"), not fever with jaundice ("yellow fever").

Conclusions

More studies are needed to assess the impact of traditional herbal medicines in sub-Saharan Africa. Phytochemical, pharmacokinetic and prospective clinical studies are needed to investigate herb contents, benefits, side effects, direct toxicity, and herb-ART interactions. Plants in the Asteraceae family reported in this study should be prioritized for these investigations.

The risk of liver disease associated with herb use was similar in the overall study population and among HIV-infected participants. Given the potential of at least additive risk of hepatotoxicity with long term use of some antiretroviral drugs, as well as the potential for herbs to alter the pharmacology of antiretroviral drugs, it may be prudent to counsel HIV-infected persons against herb use in sub-Africa until there is data about the safety of specific herbs. Counseling about herb use should be part of routine health counseling and counseling of HIV- infected persons in sub-Africa.

Author Contributions

Conceived and designed the experiments: LS SJR TCQ PO GDK. Performed the experiments: LS SJR IB PO. Analyzed the data: BJA LS GDK AN. Contributed reagents/materials/analysis tools: CKB. Wrote the paper: BJA LS. Provided additional technical assistance and contributed to interpretation of the data: BJA CKB ML CM AS PO VK IB FN AN MJW RHG DLT.

References

1. Hamill FA, Apio S, Mubiru NK, Mosango M, Bukenya-Ziraba R, et al. (2000) Traditional herbal drugs of southern Uganda, I. J Ethnopharmacol 70: 281–300.
2. Langlois-Klassen D, Kipp W, Rubaale T (2008) Who's talking? Communication between health providers and HIV-infected adults related to herbal medicine for AIDS treatment in western Uganda. Soc Sci Med 67: 165–176.
3. Tabuti J, Lye K, Dhillion S (2003) Traditional herbal drugs of Bulamogi, Uganda: plants, use, and administration. J Ethnopharmacol 88: 19–44.
4. Dara L, Hewett J, Lim JK (2008) Hydroxycut hepatotoxicity: a case series and review of liver toxicity from herbal weight loss supplements. World J Gastroenterol 14: 6999–7004.
5. Teschke R, Fuchs J, Bahre R, Genthner A, Wolff A (2010). Kava hepatotoxicity: comparative study of two structured quantitative methods for causality assessment. J Clin Pharm Ther 35: 545–563.

6. Ashafa AO, Sunmonu TO, Afolayan AJ (2010) Toxicological evaluation of aqueous leaf and berry extracts of Phytolacca dioica L. in male Wistar rats. Food Chem Toxicol 48: 1886–1889.
7. Asres K, Sporer F, Wink M (2007) Identification and quantification of hepatotoxic pyrrolizidine alkaloids in the Ethiopian medicinal plant Solanecio gigas (Asteraceae). Pharmazie 62: 709–713.
8. Lamorde M, Tabuti JR, Obua C, Kukunda-Byobona C, Lanyero H, et al. (2010) Medicinal plants used by traditional medicine practitioners for the treatment of HIV/AIDS and related conditions in Uganda. J Ethnopharmacol 130: 43–53.
9. Stabinski L, Reynolds S, Ocama P, Laeyendecker O, Ndyanabo A, et al. (2011) High Prevalence of Liver Fibrosis Associated with HIV Infection: A Study in Rural Rakai, Uganda. Antiviral Therapy 16: 405–411.
10. Wawer MJ, Gray RH, Sewankambo NK, Serwadda D, Paxton L, et al. (1998) A randomized, community trial of intensive sexually transmitted disease control for AIDS prevention, Rakai, Uganda. AIDS 12: 1211–1225.
11. AIDS Clinical Trials Group (1994) Table for grading the severity of adult and pediatric adverse advents. Rockville (Maryland): National Institutes of Health, Division of AIDS.
12. Prati D, Taioli E, Zanella A, Della Torre E, Butelli S, et al. (2002) Updated definitions of healthy ranges for serum alanine aminotransferase levels. Ann Intern Med 137: 1–10.
13. Ruhl CE, Everhart JE. (2012) Upper limits of normal for alanine aminotransferase activity in the United States population. Hepatology 55: 447–454.
14. Andersen ES, Christensen PB, Weis N (2009) Transient elastography for liver fibrosis diagnosis. Eur J Intern Med 20: 339–342.
15. Kirk GD, Astemborski J, Mehta SH, Spoler C, Fisher C, et al. (2009) Assessment of liver fibrosis by transient elastography in persons with hepatitis C virus infection or HIV- hepatitis C virus coinfection. Clin Infect Dis 48: 963–972.
16. Barros AJ, Hirakata VN (2003) Alternatives for logistic regression in cross-sectional studies: an empirical comparison of models that directly estimate the prevalence ratio. BMC Med Res Methodol 3: 21.
17. Chen Z, Huo JR (2010) Hepatic veno-occlusive disease associated with toxicity of pyrrolizidine alkaloids in herbal preparations. Neth J Med 68: 252–260.
18. Ridker PM, McDermott WV (1989) Comfrey herb tea and hepatic veno-occlusive disease. Lancet 1: 657–658.
19. Prakash AS, Pereira TN, Reilly PE, Seawright AA (1999) Pyrrolizidine alkaloids in human diet. Mutat Res 443: 53–67.
20. Chen T, Mei N, Fu PP (2010) Genotoxicity of pyrrolizidine alkaloids. J Appl Toxicol 30: 183–196.
21. Yeong ML, Wakefield SJ, Ford HC (1993) Hepatocyte membrane injury and bleb formation following low dose comfrey toxicity in rats. Int J Exp Pathol 74: 211–217.
22. Tabuti J, Collins B, Kukunda C, Waako P (2010) Medicinal plants used by traditional medicine practitioners in the treatment of tuberculosis and related ailments in Uganda. J Ethnopharmacol 127: 130–136.
23. Iwalokun BA, Efedede BU, Alabi-Sofunde JA, Oduala T, Magbagbeola OA, et al. (2006) Hepatoprotective and antioxidant activities of Vernonia amygdalina on acetaminophen- induced hepatic damage in mice. J Med Food 9: 524–530.
24. Adesanoye O, Farombi E (2009) Hepatoprotective effects of Vernonia amygdalina (Asteraceae) in rats treated with carbon tertachloride. Exp Toxicol Pathol 62: 197–206.
25. Effraim K, Jacks T, Sodipo O (2002) Histopathological studies on the toxicity of Ocimum gratissimum leave extract on some organs of rabbit. African Journal of Biomedical Research 6: 21–25.
26. Yang HN, Kim DJ, Kim YM, Kim BH, Sohn KM, et al. (2010) Aloe-induced toxic hepatitis. J Korean Med Sci 25: 492–495.
27. van den Bout-van den Beukel CJ, Koopmans PP, van der Ven AJ, De Smet PA, Burger DM (2006) Possible drug-metabolism interactions of medicinal herbs with antiretroviral agents. Drug Metab Rev 38: 477–514.
28. Barry M, Mulcahy F, Merry C, Gibbons S, Back D (1999) Pharmacokinetics and potential interactions amongst antiretroviral agents used to treat patients with HIV infection. Clin Pharmacokinet 36: 289–304.
29. Dickinson L, Khoo S, Back D (2010) Pharmacokinetics and drug-drug interactions of antiretrovirals: an update. Antiviral Res 85: 176–189.
30. Mills E, Foster BC, van Heeswijk R, Phillips E, Wilson K, et al. (2005) Impact of African herbal medicines on antiretroviral metabolism. AIDS 19: 95–97.
31. Piscitelli SC, Burstein AH, Welden N, Gallicano KD, Falloon J (2002) The effect of garlic supplements on the pharmacokinetics of saquinavir. Clin Infect Dis 34: 234–238.
32. Akah P, Okafor C (1992) Blood sugar lowering effect of Vernonia amygdalina (del) in an experimental rabbit model. Phytotherapy Research 6: 171–173.
33. Mukazayire MJ, Allaeys V, Buc Calderon P, Stevigny C, Bigendako MJ, et al. (2010) Evaluation of the hepatotoxic and hepatoprotective effect of Rwandese herbal drugs on in vivo (guinea pigs barbiturate-induced sleeping time) and in vitro (rat precision-cut liver slices, PCLS) models. Exp Toxicol Pathol 62: 289–299.
34. Tamokou JD, Kuiate JR, Tene M, Tane P (2009) Antimicrobial clerodane diterpenoids from Microglossa angolensis Oliv. et Hiern. Indian J Pharmacol 41: 60–63.
35. Kuiate J, Zollo PA, Lamaty G, Mentu C, Besseiere J (1999) Composition of essential oils from the leaves of two varieties of Aspilia africana (Pers) C.D Adams from Cameroon. Flavor and Fragrance 14: 167–169.
36. Taziebou LC, Etoa FX, Nkegoum B, Pieme CA, Dzeufiet DP (2006) Acute and subacute toxicity of Aspilia africana leaves. Afr J Tradit Complement Altern Med 4: 127–134.
37. Njamen D, Magne Nde CB, Tanee Fomum Z, Vollmer G (2008) Effects of the extracts of some tropical medicinal plants on estrogen inducible yeast and Ishikawa screens, and on ovariectomized Wistar rats. Pharmazie 63: 164–168.
38. Bakasso S, Lamien-Meda A, Lamien CE, Kiendrebeogo M, Millogo J, et al. (2008) Polyphenol contents and antioxidant activities of five Indigofera species (Fabaceae) from Burkina Faso. Pak J Biol Sci 11: 1429–1435.
39. Matias EF, Santos KK, Almeida TS, Costa JG, Coutinho HD (2010) Phytochemical screening and modulation of antibiotic activity by Ocimum gratissimum L. Biomed Pharmacother 23: 23.
40. Gundidza GM, Deans SG, Svoboda KP, Mavi S (1992) Antimicrobial activity of essential oil from Hoslundia opposita. Cent Afr J Med 38: 290–293.
41. Kanwal Q, Hussain I, Latif Siddiqui H, Javaid A (2010) Antifungal activity of flavonoids
42. Ajila CM, Rao LJ, Rao UJ (2010) Characterization of bioactive compounds from raw and ripe Mangifera indica L. peel extracts. Food Chem Toxicol 48: 3406–3411.
43. Foubert K, Cuyckens F, Vleeschouwer K, Theunis M, Vlietinck A, et al. (2010) Rapid quantification of 14 saponins of Maesa lanceolata by UPLC-MS/MS. Talanta 81: 1258–1263.
44. Arot Manguro LO, Midiwo JO, Kraus W, Ugi I (2003) Benzoquinone derivatives of Myrsine africana and Maesa lanceolata. Phytochemistry 64: 855–862.
45. Adesegun SA, Elechi NA, Coker HA (2008) Antioxidant activities of methanolic extract of Sapium ellipticum. Pak J Biol Sci 11: 453–457.
46. Nahdi A, Hammami I, Brasse-Lagnel C, Pilard N, Hamdaoui MH, et al. (2010) Influence of garlic or its main active component diallyl disulfide on iron bioavailability and toxicity. Nutr Res 30: 85–95.
47. Ngouela S, Tsamo E, Sondengam BL (1988) Extractives from bignoniaceae: constituents of the stem bark of Spathodea campanulata. Planta Med 54: 476.
48. Beaman-Mbaya V, Muhammed SI (1976) Antibiotic action of Solanum incanum Linnaeus.
49. Al-Duais M, Hohbein J, Werner S, Bohm V, Jetschke G (2009) Contents of vitamin C, carotenoids, tocopherols, and tocotrienols in the subtropical plant species Cyphostemma digitatum as affected by processing. J Agric Food Chem 57: 5420–5427.
50. Oyedeji OO, Lawal OA, Shode FO, Oyedeji AO (2009) Chemical composition and antibacterial activity of the essential oils of Callistemon citrinus and Callistemon viminalis from South Africa. Molecules 14: 1990–1998.

11

An Epidemiological Study of Concomitant Use of Chinese Medicine and Antipsychotics in Schizophrenic Patients: Implication for Herb-Drug Interaction

Zhang-Jin Zhang[1,2]*, Qing-Rong Tan[2]*, Yao Tong[1], Xue-Yi Wang[3], Huai-Hai Wang[2], Lai-Ming Ho[4], Hei Kiu Wong[1], Yi-Bin Feng[1], Di Wang[1], Roger Ng[5], Grainne M. McAlonan[6], Chuan-Yue Wang[7], Vivian Taam Wong[8]

1 School of Chinese Medicine, Faculty of Medicine, the University of Hong Kong, Hong Kong, China, **2** Department of Psychiatry, Fourth Military Medical University, Xijing Hospital, Xi'an, Shaanxi, China, **3** Mental Health Center, Hebei Medical University, Shijiazhuang, Hebei, China, **4** School of Public Health, the University of Hong Kong, Hong Kong, China, **5** Department of Psychiatry, Kowloon Hospital, Hong Kong, China, **6** Department of Psychiatry, the University of Hong Kong, Hong Kong, China, **7** Capital Medical University, Beijing Anding Hospital, Beijing, China, **8** Chinese Medicine Section, Hospital Authority, Hong Kong, China

Abstract

Background: Herb-drug interactions are an important issue in drug safety and clinical practice. The aim of this epidemiological study was to characterize associations of clinical outcomes with concomitant herbal and antipsychotic use in patients with schizophrenia.

Methods and Findings: In this retrospective, cross-sectional study, 1795 patients with schizophrenia who were randomly selected from 17 psychiatric hospitals in China were interviewed face-to-face using a structured questionnaire. Association analyses were conducted to examine correlates between Chinese medicine (CM) use and demographic, clinical variables, antipsychotic medication mode, and clinical outcomes. The prevalence of concomitant CM and antipsychotic treatment was 36.4% [95% confidence interval (95% CI) 34.2%–38.6%]. Patients using concomitant CM had a significantly greater chance of improved outcomes than non-CM use (61.1% vs. 34.3%, OR = 3.44, 95% CI 2.80–4.24). However, a small but significant number of patients treated concomitantly with CM had a greater risk of developing worse outcomes (7.2% vs. 4.4%, OR = 2.06, 95% CI 2.06–4.83). Significant predictors for concomitant CM treatment-associated outcomes were residence in urban areas, paranoid psychosis, and exceeding 3 months of CM use. Herbal medicine regimens containing Radix Bupleuri, Fructus Gardenia, Fructus Schisandrae, Radix Rehmanniae, Akebia Caulis, and Semen Plantaginis in concomitant use with quetiapine, clozapine, and olanzepine were associated with nearly 60% of the risk of adverse outcomes.

Conclusions: Concomitant herbal and antipsychotic treatment could produce either beneficial or adverse clinical effects in schizophrenic population. Potential herb-drug pharmacokinetic interactions need to be further evaluated.

Editor: Ehsan Syed, Pennsylvania State University, United States of America

Funding: This study was supported by the intramural research fund of the University of Hong Kong and Hospital Authority of Hong Kong. The funders had no role in study design, data collection and analysis, decision to publish, or preparation of the manuscript.

Competing Interests: The authors have declared that no competing interests exist.

* E-mail: zhangzj@hku.hk (ZJZ); tanqingr@fmmu.edu.cn (QRT)

Introduction

With the widespread use of various herbal products which are often concomitantly used with pharmaceutical drugs, herb-drug interactions have become an important issue in drug safety and clinical practice [1,2]. This was initially because of several case studies reporting nephrotoxic and hepatotoxic effects associated with herbal medicine use [3–5]. It is well documented that concomitant use of herbal medicine with conventional drug treatment can alter pharmacokinetic profiles of many classes of pharmaceutical drugs, including psychotropic agents, anticoagulants, oral contraceptives, immunosuppressants, cardiovascular drugs, anti-HIV, anticancer agents and antiepileptics [1,2,6]. However, whether such concomitant treatment with herbal and conventional medicine is associated with clinical outcomes in a defined population of patients remains to be determined.

Most patients with schizophrenia may develop a chronic course and are required for long-term maintenance treatment [7]. Although antipsychotic therapy is a mainstay in the maintenance treatment of schizophrenia, patients still often experience relapse and various adverse events caused by antipsychotic treatment [7]. In order to improve the therapeutic efficacy and reduce adverse side effects related to antipsychotic therapy, herbal medicine and other alternative therapies have been increasingly introduced into the treatment of schizophrenia [8]. This is particularly apparent in Chinese patients who have distinctive perceptions of Chinese medicine (CM), of which herbal materials account for about 85% preparations and products.

Numerous studies have shown therapeutic benefits of herbal medicine for persistent negative symptoms, cognitive impairment, and adverse side effects in schizophrenic patients [8]. Our recent study revealed that herbal medicine could alleviate hyperprolactinemia in schizophrenic patients [9]. Nevertheless, there are also case studies reporting acute and persistent psychosis caused by herbal supplementary use [10,11]. These data suggest that herbal medicine in combination with antipsychotic drugs may produce either positive or negative clinical effects, making it important to examine potential relationships between clinical outcomes and concomitant treatment with herbal and antipsychotic agents in schizophrenia.

The primary objective of this epidemiological survey was to determine the prevalence of CM concomitant use and its associations with demographic, clinical characteristics and treatment outcomes in a random sample of patients with schizophrenia through face-to-face interview using a structured questionnaire.

Methods

Study design and setting

This retrospective, cross-sectional epidemiological study was conducted in 17 psychiatric hospitals and mental health centers in China. The selection of the study sites was based on geographic and sociodemographic variations as previously described [12], with particular consideration of regions, local economic development levels, and overall educational levels, as these variables are heavily related to perceptions and beliefs for CM. The study was approved by Institutional Review Board (IRB) of the University of Hong Kong/Hospital Authority Hong Kong West Cluster and registered at www.HKClinicalTrials.com (HKCTR-874). All participants or their guardians were required to give written informed consent for participating in the survey. The survey was conducted between April 2009 and September 2009.

Population and sample

The study population was confined to patients with schizophrenia who visited psychiatric clinics or were hospitalized during the survey period. Patients who met the following criteria were eligible for the study: (1) aged 15 years or above; (2) had a primary diagnosis of schizophrenia or schizoaffective disorder based on *International Classification of Diseases (ICD), 10th Edition* [13]; (3) had been taking conventional antipsychotic treatment for at least 6 weeks; and (4) patients, their caregivers and/or doctors could provide necessary information about CM use if CM was used.

One key question that the present study attempted to answer was whether concomitant use of CM could affect the clinical outcomes of patients with schizophrenia, particularly adverse outcomes related to concomitant CM and antipsychotic use. Estimation of sample size was therefore based on the prevalence of CM use and the proportion of CM users with worse outcomes (see below). These two indices had been obtained from a pilot survey of 297 patients with schizophrenia [8], showing that nearly 36% of patients concomitantly used CM and 5.7% of CM users experienced worse outcomes, while only 2.8% of non-CM users had worse outcomes. In order to detect a 2.9% difference in the rate of worse outcomes between CM users and non-CM users, with a power (1-β) of 80% and a two-tailed level of $\alpha = 0.05$, 1750 participants were required to detect statistical difference in terms of worse outcomes associated with concomitant CM use. The number of surveyed subjects allocated to each study site was determined based on the volume of visits and annual admission numbers. The selection of eligible patients at each survey site was determined using random number tables.

Study instruments

A specifically designed structured questionnaire was administered in the survey. The questionnaire covered: (1) sociodemographic and clinical characteristics; (2) purpose, advice source, attitude, and awareness of CM use; (3) the concomitant use pattern including individual CMs, conventional medication modes, and duration of the concomitant use; and (4) clinical outcomes. Chinese medicine (CM) is defined as preparations and products in powder, tablet, capsule, soft-gel, or liquid form prepared from single or mixed herbal, mineral, and animal materials or extracts [8]. CM users were defined as those who had been using CM consecutively for at least one month or cumulatively for at least 3 months with no more than 45 days of absence in total and no more than 7 consecutive days of absence when the survey was conducted. Those who never or only occasionally used CM were defined as non-CM users. This definition of the length of CM use was based on CM clinical practice, demonstrating that CM therapy of most chronic mental-emotional conditions requires a considerable period before observable improvements are achieved [14].

Clinical outcomes were classified as improved, worse, and unchanged condition. Improved outcomes were defined as clinically meaningful improvements occurring in the preceding one month on one or more conditions as follows: (1) psychosis; (2) comorbid psychiatric symptoms, mainly anxiety, depression, cognitive impairment, and sleep disorders; (3) adverse side effects associated with antipsychotic therapy, frequently body weight gain, constipation, enuresis, hyperprolactinemia, hypersalivation, leukopenia, and tardive dyskinesia; and (4) comorbid non-psychiatric conditions, such as hypertension and diabetes. Worse outcomes were defined as hospitalization, emergency room visits, or changes in medication modes due to the worsening of psychosis, comorbid symptoms, intolerable side effects, or the occurrence of new comorbid symptoms in the preceding one month. Patients who did not experience either clinically meaningful improvement or worsening in the preceding one month were defined as subjects with unchanged conditions. The assessment of clinical outcomes was conducted by psychiatrists based on changes in the severity and frequency of episodes of related symptoms, physical examination, and laboratory tests as well as reports from patients and their guardians.

Survey procedures

The survey was performed by trained psychiatrists on site with face-to-face interview. To ensure consistency of the survey across sites and over time, two sessions of training workshop were conducted for interviewers who were practicing psychiatry. Upon completion of the training workshops, inter-rater reliability was assessed by calculating interrater agreement coefficients (κ value) for the designed questionnaire. All interviewers had achieved a κ value of at least 0.8 after training sessions. In addition, post-survey interviews were further conducted to verify missing and illogical data.

Data analysis

The prevalence of CM use was calculated using maximum likelihood estimation of logistic regression. Chi-square (χ^2) test was used to determine bivariate associations between CM use and demographic and clinical variables. Binary logistic regression model was further used for multivariate analyses to identify independent factors associated with CM use from the same variable tested in the bivariate analysis. The association between clinical outcomes and CM use was also examined using Chi-square (χ^2) test and binary logistic regression analysis, with adjustment for demographic and clinical variables that were found to be significantly associated with CM use.

Subgroup analyses were conducted in CM-using subjects to further determine associations between clinical outcomes and CM and antipsychotic concomitant use modes. Chi-square test and multinomial logistic regression model were respectively utilized to examine bivariate and multivariate associations of clinical outcomes with demographic and clinical variables. Multinomial logistic regression model was also applied to evaluate associations of clinical outcomes with individual CMs and antipsychotic regimens that were used in at least 5% of CM-using respondents with either improved or worsened conditions, with adjustment for demographic and clinical variables that were shown to be significantly associated with clinical outcomes.

Odds ratio (OR) and 95% confidence interval (95% CI) were obtained from binary and multinomial logistic regression analysis. In association analyses of clinical outcomes, the unchanged outcome served as reference for improved and worse outcome in the calculation of OR values. All analyses were performed with SPSS version 16 software (Chicago, IL, USA). Statistical significance was defined as $p<0.05$ and all tests were two-sided.

Results

The characteristics of the sample

In a total of 1795 eligible subjects surveyed, seven were excluded from the analyses due to missing basic demographic and clinical data (gender, age, and the illness duration). In the remaining 1788 subjects who were included in the final analyses, 51% were males and the mean ($\pm$SD) age was 32 ± 12 years. Fifty-three percent were diagnosed with paranoid schizophrenia. These demographic and clinical characteristics were similar to those reported in previous epidemiological surveys of schizophrenic population in China [15].

The characteristics of antipsychotic medication modes

Thirty-five psychotropic drugs were identified. Medication regimens of 99.3% subjects included antipsychotics and 43% had two or more antipsychotics. The remaining 0.7% subjects were medicated with mood stabilizers occasionally combined with antipsychotics. The most commonly used antipsychotics in all subjects were risperidone (50.8%), quetiapine (21.0%), clozapine (17.2%), olanzapine (8.2%), and phenothiazines (7.0%). This medication mode was similar to that previously reported in China [16]. No significant differences were observed in frequency distribution of these antipsychotic regimens between CM- and non-CM-using subjects (see below), except for risperidone monotherapy. For the latter the proportion of CM-using respondents treated was significantly higher than non-CM-using respondents (30.8% vs. 23.4%, $p<0.001$, Chi-square test).

The prevalence and characteristics of CM use

Direct observation showed a prevalence of 37.5% (671/1788) of the concomitant use. Re-calculation using maximum likelihood estimation yielded a similar prevalence of 36.4% (95% CI: 34.2%–38.6%). One hundred and twenty different CM materials used were identified: 92 herbal materials, 12 mineral materials, and 16 animal materials. But 33.7% of CM-using subjects were unable to provide full information about their CM formulae or prescriptions for identifying individual CMs. Only a small portion (6.4%, 43/671) of CM-using patients used single-herbal preparations.

There were 86% of CM-users who used CM therapy initially in order to enhance antipsychotic efficacy, reduce antipsychotic-induced adverse side effects and comorbid psychiatric symptoms (mainly anxiety, depression, cognitive and sleep problems). Sixty-six percent of CM users reported that CM use was recommended by their psychiatrists. Most CMs were prescribed by CM practitioners. Nearly 47% of CM-users were entirely unaware of potential risks of concomitant use of herbal and antipsychotic agents; only 16.4% realized such potential risks. In non-CM-using patients, 35.1% did not know much about CM and 58.1% did not think CM was helpful for their conditions, while only 5.1% were aware of the potential risks of the concomitant treatment.

Demographic and clinical correlates of CM use

Bivariate analysis displayed significant associations of CM use with gender ($p=0.002$), household income ($p=0.001$), the illness duration ($p<0.001$), number of episode ($p<0.001$), and number of hospitalization ($p<0.001$) (Table 1). Multivariate analysis further revealed that CM use was significantly associated with male (OR = 1.32, 95% CI 1.09-1.62, $p=0.006$), residence in rural areas (OR = 1.48, 95% CI 1.18–1.85, $p=0.001$), average (OR = 1.56, 95% CI 1.19–2.06, $p=0.001$) and high (OR = 2.36, 95% CI 1.58–3.53, $p<0.001$) household income, and greater than one year of illness duration (OR = 1.95, 95% CI 1.45–2.63, $p<0.001$).

CM use correlates of clinical outcomes

While 61.1% (410/671) of CM-using patients and 34.3% (383/1117) of non-CM-using patients displayed improved outcomes, 7.2% (48/671) CM users and 4.4% (49/1117) of non-CM users experienced worse outcomes in the preceding one month (Table 2). Chi-square tests showed that clinical outcomes were significantly associated with whether CM was concomitantly used with antipsychotic drugs ($p<0.001$). In a binary logistic regression model, CM users had significantly greater odds of improved (OR = 3.44, 95% CI 2.80–4.24, $p<0.001$) and worse outcomes (OR = 3.15, 95% CI 2.06–4.83, $p<0.001$) compared to non-CM users.

Demographic and clinical correlates of clinical outcomes in CM users

Chi-square tests showed that clinical outcomes were significantly associated with resident areas ($p<0.001$), diagnostic types ($p<0.001$), and duration of CM use ($p=0.007$). Multinomial logistic regression analysis further revealed significant associations of improved outcomes with residence in urban areas (OR = 4.81, 95% CI 3.14–7.36, $p<0.001$), paranoid schizophrenia (OR = 2.65, 95% CI 1.83–3.84, $p<0.001$) and more than 3 months of CM use (OR = 1.35, 95% CI 0.91–1.98, $p=0.036$). In CM users who experienced worse conditions, similar significant multivariate associations were also observed with residence in urban areas (OR = 6.91, 95% CI 3.09–15.43, $p<0.001$), paranoid schizophrenia (OR = 1.89, 95% CI 0.96–3.71, $p=0.012$), and more than 3 months of CM use (OR = 3.28, 95% CI 1.44–7.46, $p=0.005$) (Table 3).

Antipsychotic medication correlates of clinical outcomes in CM users

Five different antipsychotic agents and five antipsychotic treatment regimens that were used in at least 5% of CM-using patients with either improved or worse outcomes were identified (Table 4). Multinomial logistical regression analyses, with adjustment for resident areas, diagnostic types, and duration of CM use, variables that were significantly associated with clinical outcomes, revealed no significant associations with any antipsychotic treatment regimens favoring improve outcomes, but significantly lower odds of improved outcomes were observed in patients whose antipsychotic regimens included olanzapine (OR = 0.48, 95% CI 0.27–0.85, $p=0.035$). There were significantly higher odds of worse outcomes in subjects whose

Table 1. Bivariate and multivariate associations of CM use with demographic and clinical variables in patients with schizophrenia under antipsychotic medication.[a]

Variable	bivariate			Multivariate	
	n	CM use (%)	p	OR (95% CI)	p
Gender			0.002		
Female	879	33.9		1	
Male	909	41.0		1.32 (1.09–1.62)	0.006
Age, yrs			0.108		
<18	92	31.5		1	
18–45	1478	37.1		1.04 (0.58–1.37)	0.899
>45	218	43.1		1.17 (0.71–1.94)	0.540
Marital status			0.109		
Single/divorce/widow	1004	35.9		1	
Married	784	39.7		1.06 (0.86–1.32)	0.589
Education, yrs			0.391		
≤10	1064	36.8		1	
11–13	458	40.2		1.27 (0.99–1.63)	0.062
≥14	266	36.1		1.01 (0.72–1.42)	0.941
Occupation			0.645		
Unemployed	368	38.9		1	
Non-professional	927	37.9		0.92 (0.68–1.24)	0.568
Professional and students	493	35.9		0.81 (0.62–1.08)	0.153
Resident areas			0.135		
Urban	1120	36.2		1	
Rural	668	39.8		1.48 (1.18–1.85)	0.001
Household income [b]			0.001		
Low	330	30.6		1	
Average	1242	37.9		1.56 (1.19–2.06)	0.001
High	216	45.8		2.36 (1.58–3.53)	
<0.001					
Diagnostic subtype			0.143		
Paranoid	942	39.2		1	
Non-paranoid [c]	846	35.7		0.89 (0.73–1.09)	0.245
Duration of the illness, yrs			<0.001		
≤1	396	25.0		1	
>1	1392	41.1		1.95 (1.45–2.63)	
<0.001					
Number of episodes			<0.001		
≤2	895	32.2		1	
>2	893	42.9		1.14 (0.84–1.53)	0.402
Number of hospitalization			<0.001		
≤2	1142	33.9		1	
>2	646	44.0		1.18 (0.88–1.58)	0.270

a. CM, Chinese medicine. Data analyses were based on CM users (n = 671) with non-CM users (n = 1117) as reference. Chi-square test was used for bivariate analysis and binary logistic regression mode for multivariate analysis.
b. Household income was compared to local average levels.
c. Non-paranoid psychosis includes disorganized, undifferentiated, residual, and tonic types of schizophrenia and schizoaffective disorder.

Table 2. Bivariate and multivariate associations between clinical outcomes and CM use in patients with schizophrenia.[a]

Outcomes	Bivariate			Multivariate	
	n	CM users (%)	p	OR (95% CI) [b]	p
			<0.001		
Unchanged	898	23.7		1	
Improved	793	51.7		3.44 (2.80–4.24)	<0.001
Worse	97	49.5		3.15 (2.06–4.83)	<0.001

a. CM, Chinese medicine. Data analyses were based on CM users (n = 671) with non-CM users (n = 1117) as reference. Chi-square test was used for bivariate analysis and binary logistic regression for multivariate analysis.
b. Binary logistic regression analysis was adjusted for sex, resident areas, household income, duration of illness, number of episode, and number of hospitalization, variables significantly associated with CM use as shown in Table 1.

antipsychotic regimens included quetiapine (OR = 1.90, 95% CI 0.88–4.08, p = 0.013), quetiapine alone (OR = 2.16, 95% CI 0.95–4.95, p = 0.031) or clozapine alone (OR = 3.02, 95% CI 0.94–9.70, p = 0.025) (Table 4).

Individual CM correlates of clinical outcomes

Of 120 different CM materials identified, 21 (20 herbal materials and one animal material) were used in at least 5% of CM-using subjects with either improved or worse outcomes (Table 5). Multinomial logistic regression model analysis showed no significant associations of improved outcomes with any individual CMs identified, but the inclusion of Acorus gramineus in CM treatment regimens significantly reduced odds of worse outcomes compared to improved outcomes (OR = 0.11, 95% CI 0.01–0.88, p = 0.037). Significantly higher odds of worse outcomes were observed in subjects whose CM treatment regimens included Radix Bupleuri (OR = 2.49, 95% CI 1.10–5.62, p = 0.028), Fructus Gardenia (OR = 9.16, 95% CI 4.19–20.02, p<0.001), Fructus Schisandrae (OR = 3.90, 95% CI 1.42–10.73, P = 0.008), Radix Rehmanniae (OR = 3.48, 95% CI 1.03–11.70, p = 0.044), Akebia Caulis (OR = 14.6, 95% CI 2.50–31.87, p<0.001), and Semen Plantaginis (OR = 21.10, 95% CI 4.32–103.05, p<0.001). Frequency distributions revealed that concomitant treatment regimens containing these six herbal materials and worse outcome-associated antipsychotics accounted for 59.8% (49/82) of total identified concomitant treatment regimens in patients with worse outcomes (Table 6).

Discussion

In our survey of a representative sample of patients with schizophrenia, nearly 36% of them had concomitant CM and antipsychotic treatment. This prevalence rate of CM use is somewhat lower than that observed in other commonly occurring chronic conditions in Chinese communities [17–19]. In non-CM-using patients, nearly 58% did not believe CM could help their condition, suggesting that the lower prevalence of CM use in schizophrenic population is mainly related to their negative attitude towards this traditional remedy. Unlike patients in Western society where a minority of them informed their doctors of their use of alternative medicine [20,21], CM use in most patients in this study was recommended by their psychiatrists. However, only about one-third of patients were aware of the

Table 3. Bivariate and multivariate associations of clinical outcomes with demographic and clinical variables in schizophrenic patients in Chinese medicine and antipsychotic concomitant treatment.[a]

	Bivariate				Multivariate-IM		Multivariate-WS	
	n	IM (%)	WS (%)	p	OR (95% CI)	p	OR (95% CI)	p
Gender				0.344				
Male	373	62.2	8.0		1		1	
Female	298	59.7	6.0		0.77 (0.53–1.12)	0.173	0.55 (0.28–1.10)	0.091
Age, yrs				0.625				
<18	29	72.4	6.9		1		1	
18–45	548	61.1	7.3		0.76 (0.24–2.43)	0.304	0.73 (0.09–5.81)	0.325
>45	74	57.5	6.4		0.40 (0.14–1.16)	0.231	0.66 (0.10–4.19)	0.438
Marital status				0.349				
Single/divorce/widow	360	58.9	6.9		1		1	
Married	311	63.7	7.4		1.23 (0.83–1.82)	0.816	1.30 (0.63–2.65)	0.478
Education, yrs				0.270				
≤10	391	62.7	8.4		1		1	
11–13	184	58.7	4.9		0.72 (0.46–1.12)	0.183	0.52 (0.21–1.24)	0.299
≥14	96	59.4	6.3		0.92 (0.50–1.69)	0.476	0.90 (0.30–2.73)	0.335
Occupation				0.345				
Unemployed	143	55.2	8.4		1		1	
Non-professional	351	63.3	7.7		1.69 (1.03–2.78)	0.183	1.39 (0.58–3.32)	0.186
Professional/students	177	61.6	5.1		1.17 (0.68–2.02)	0.835	0.70 (0.25–1.93)	0.460
Resident areas				<0.001				
Rural	266	48.9	8.2		1		1	
Urban	405	69.1	5.6		4.81 (3.14–7.36)	<0.001	6.91 (3.09–15.43)	<0.001
Household income [b]				0.302				
Low	101	56.4	11.9		1		1	
Average	471	62.6	6.4		1.57 (0.74–3.29)	0.213	0.66 (0.18–2.41)	0.191
High	99	58.6	6.1		1.41 (0.82–2.42)	0.136	0.44 (0.18–1.06)	0.291
Diagnostic subtype				<0.001				
Non-paranoid [b]	302	50.7	7.2		1		1	
Paranoid	369	69.7	7.0		2.65 (1.83–3.84)	<0.001	1.89 (0.96–3.71)	0.012
Duration of illness, yrs				0.991				
≤1	99	60.6	7.1		1		1	
>1	572	61.2	7.2		1.02 (0.56–1.84)	0.958	1.17 (0.40–3.42)	0.769
Number of episodes				0.747				
≤2	288	60.1	8.0		1		1	
>2	383	61.9	6.5		1.13 (0.65–1.97)	0.663	0.75 (0.27–2.13)	0.594
Number of hospitalization				0.780				
≤2	387	61.8	7.5		1		1	
>2	284	60.2	6.7		0.88 (0.51–1.52)	0.655	0.86 (0.31–2.40)	0.775
Duration of CM use, months				0.007				
1–3	233	58.4	3.9		1		1	
>3	438	62.6	8.9		1.35 (0.91–1.98)	0.036	3.28 (1.44–7.46)	0.005

a. CM, Chinese medicine; IM, improved; WS, worse. Data analyses were based on CM users (N = 671) who had clinical outcomes with improved (n = 410), worse (n = 48), and unchanged (n = 213) conditions. The unchanged condition served as reference. Chi-square test was used for bivariate analysis and multinomial logistic regression for multivariate analysis.
b. The definitions of household income and non-paranoid schizophrenia are the same as Table 1.

potential risks of concomitant treatment with CM. These findings may reflect an underestimation of both potential benefits and risks of CM use among patients and their psychiatrists.

We found that concomitant CM use was significantly associated with male, residence in rural areas, relatively higher household income, longer duration of illness, and more episodes and

Table 4. Multivariate associations between clinical outcomes and antipsychotic medication modes in patients with schizophrenia who were treated concomitantly with CM.[a]

	Improved (n = 410)			Worse (n = 48)		
	%	OR (95% CI)	p	%	OR (95% CI)	p
The most frequently used antipsychotics						
Risperidone	56.1	1.22 (0.86–1.75)	0.900	41.7	0.81 (0.42–1.56)	0.696
Quetiapine	19.5	0.75 (0.49–1.16)	0.463	27.1 [b]	1.90 (0.88–4.08)	0.013
Clozapine	20.7	1.40 (0.90–2.19)	0.542	22.9	1.29 (0.63–2.66)	0.068
Olanzapine	7.1	0.48 (0.27–0.85)	0.035	12.5	0.97 (0.37–2.54)	0.463
Phenothiazines	6.5	0.92 (0.47–1.81)	0.819	2.1	0.25 (0.03–1.95)	0.837
The most frequently used antipsychotic regimens						
Risperidone alone	33.9	1.34 (0.90–1.99)	0.276	33.3	1.14 (0.56–2.31)	0.424
Quetiapine alone [b]	11.7	0.69 (0.41–1.17)	0.063	27.1 [b]	2.16 (0.95–4.95)	0.031
Clozapine + risperidone	6.3	1.43 (0.65–3.17)	0.527	8.3	2.63 (0.74–9.38)	0.064
Clozapine alone	4.6	1.37 (0.60–3.12)	0.438	12.5	3.02 (0.94–9.70)	0.025
Olanzapine alone	4.1	0.57 (0.27–1.22)	0.213	12.5	1.88 (0.66–5.34)	0.399

a. CM, Chinese medicine. Unchanged outcomes (n = 213) served as reference. Multinomial logistical regression analysis was adjusted for resident areas, diagnostic subtype, and duration of CM use, variables significantly associated with clinical outcomes as shown in Table 3.
b. It is noted that all quetiapine-including treatment regimens are quetiapine monotherapy.

hospitalizations. These associations suggest that the men living in rural areas may have greater positive beliefs about CM for their illnesses. Previous studies also showed that people who had persistent and recurrent mental-emotional problems more often sought alternative therapies than populations with other chronic diseases [21,22].

While it was similar in most antipsychotic treatment regimens in CM- and non-CM-using patients, there exist significant bivariate and multivariate associations between CM use and clinical outcomes. Patients in CM concomitant treatment had a significantly greater chance of improved clinical outcomes compared to non-CM use (61.1% vs. 34.3%, OR = 3.44, 95% CI 2.80–4.24). However, a small but significant number of patients treated concomitantly with CM had a greater risk of developing worse outcomes (7.2% vs. 4.4%, OR = 2.06, 95% CI 2.06–4.83). These data clearly indicate that CM concomitant treatment could produce either beneficial or adverse effects on clinical outcome, probably depending on different combinations of CM and antipsychotics.

Furthermore, bivariate and multivariate analyses of CM-using subgroup revealed that both improved and worse outcomes were significantly associated with residence in urban areas, suggesting that patients living in urban areas may have greater impacts with CM therapy than those in rural areas. This is likely due in part to the fact that urban patients generally have more unconventional and conventional treatment options compared to rural patients [16]. This perhaps results in an increase in unpredictable positive and negative clinical effects, as the therapeutic properties of most CM preparations are not yet well identified. Meanwhile, the addition of CM significantly increased the chances of improved outcomes in paranoid patients compared to non-paranoid subtype. Several studies have demonstrated differences in neuropsychological character and clinical response to antipsychotic treatment between paranoid and non-paranoid subtypes [23,24] as well as subtype specificity of genetic profile [25,26]. Thus, the greater chance of alteration in treatment outcomes observed in paranoid patients may reflect a similar subtype difference in clinical effects of CM treatment.

Our results demonstrated that exceeding 3 months of CM use is a significant predictor for both improved and worse clinical outcomes. This finding confirms empirical evidence, suggesting that CM therapy of most chronic conditions requires a considerable duration in order to achieve observable improvement [14]. However, the finding is also consistent with those of case studies, revealing that most nephrotoxic and hepatotoxic effects associated with herbal medicine use are observed after 1–5 months of intake [4,5,27]. Considering difficulties in monitoring herbal toxicity and potential herb-drug interactions due to complex mixtures of unknown and unidentified ingredients in CM, the determination of an optimal length of the treatment might be a feasible strategy in minimizing adverse and toxic effects while maximizing beneficial effects. For this purpose, correlations between different length of CM use and changes in pharmacokinetic profile of conventional drugs may deserve to be further determined.

We found that CM-using patients whose antipsychotic regimens included olanzapine had significantly lower chance of improved outcomes. Meanwhile, quetiapine and clozapine monotherapy significantly heightened the risk of developing worse outcomes, suggesting associations of these three atypical antipsychotics with adverse clinical outcomes when used concomitantly with CM. On the other hand, among seven individual CM materials identified to be significantly associated with clinical outcomes, six were found to be significantly associated with adverse outcomes. They were Radix Bupleuri, Fructus Gardenia, Fructus Schisandrae, Radix Rehmanniae, Akebia Caulis, and Semen Plantaginis. Moreover, the concomitant treatment regimens including these herbal materials and antipsychotics associated with adverse outcomes accounted for nearly 60% of total identified treatment regimens in patients with worse outcomes. These data suggest that the heightened risk of adverse outcomes observed is closely associated with these herbal agents in combination with antipsychotic regimens.

As the identified herbal medicines have been well demonstrated to have high safety profiles [28], the adverse outcomes observed seem to be attributable to herb-drug pharmacokinetic interactions in which the pattern of drug metabolism is altered. Despite lack of information about the interactions between herbal and antipsychotic agents, early case studies reported that ginseng combined with phenelzine and betel nut with fluphenazine caused broad adverse effects in schizophrenic patients [29–31]. Our recent study of bipolar patients also found that combination treatment with the mood stabilizer carbamazepine and an herbal preparation for 26 weeks resulted in a significantly lower level of serum carbamazepine compared to carbamazepine alone, suggesting that the

Table 5. Multivariate associations of clinical outcomes with individual CMs in concomitant use with antipsychotics in schizophrenic patients.[a]

Individual Chinese medicine	Improved (n = 410)			Worse (n = 48)		
	%	OR (95% CI)	p	%	OR (95% CI)	p
Radix Glycyrrhizae (Gan-Cao)	26.8	1.59 (1.06–2.38)	0.232	12.5	0.53 (0.21–1.35)	0.181
Acorus gramineus (Shi-Chang-Pu)	17.3	1.11 (0.66–1.87)	0.699	2.1	0.11 (0.01–0.88)	0.037
Ziziphus jujuba (Suan-Zao-Ren)	14.1	0.63 (0.39–1.01)	0.056	18.8	0.83 (0.36–1.90)	0.660
Curcuma root (Yu-Jin)	13.9	1.76 (0.98–3.17)	0.058	14.6	1.84 (0.70–4.79)	0.214
Radix Angelica Sinensis (Dang-Gui)	13.9	1.03 (0.63–1.70)	0.901	8.3	0.63 (0.21–1.92)	0.422
Poria cocos (Fu-Ling)	13.2	1.30 (0.76–2.24)	0.335	12.5	1.28 (0.48–3.40)	0.620
Radix Bupleuri (Chai-Hu)	12.2	1.14 (0.68–1.93)	0.616	22.9	2.49 (1.10–5.62)	0.028
Radix Polygalae (Yuan-Zhi)	10.0	0.86 (0.50–1.49)	0.599	20.8	1.82 (0.77–4.31)	0.173
Salvia Miltrorrhiza (Dan-Shen)	9.8	0.87 (0.49–1.53)	0.625	10.4	0.92 (0.33–2.61)	0.881
Lumbricus (Di-Long)	9.8	0.95 (0.54–1.68)	0.863	4.2	0.17 (0.02–1.30)	0.088
Rhizoma Atractylodes (Bai-Zhu)	9.8	1.31 (0.69–2.47)	0.408	4.2	0.51 (0.11–2.34)	0.388
Dried tangerine peel (Chen-Pi)	9.5	1.16 (0.63–2.12)	0.635	8.3	0.94 (0.30–2.97)	0.921
Fructus Gardenia (Zhi-Zi)	8.3	1.02 (0.55–1.90)	0.947	45.8	9.16 (4.19–20.02)	<0.001
Flos Carthami (Hong-Hua)	8.3	0.99 (0.57–1.75)	0.984	4.2	0.47 (0.11–2.08)	0.318
Rhizoma Chuan Xiong (Chuan-Xiong)	7.6	0.73 (0.40–1.33)	0.306	4.2	0.38 (0.09–1.69)	0.204
Semen Persicae (Tao-Ren)	7.3	0.92 (0.49–1.75)	0.808	4.2	0.53 (0.12–2.41)	0.413
Magnolia officinalis (Hou-Po)	4.3	0.59 (0.26–1.30)	0.190	8.3	1.05 (0.31–3.52)	0.938
Fructus Schisandrae (Wu-Wei-Zi)	4.1	0.89 (0.38–2.07)	0.782	22.9	3.90 (1.42–10.73)	0.008
Radix Rehmanniae (Di-Huang)	3.4	1.22 (0.49–3.06)	0.669	12.5	3.48 (1.03–11.70)	0.044
Akebia Caulis (Mu-Tong) [b]	1.0	0.49 (0.12–2.04)	0.326	25.0	8.92 (2.50–31.87)	<0.001
Semen Plantaginis (Che-Qian-Zi)	0.7	1.64 (0.17–16.20)	0.671	33.3	21.10 (4.32–103.05)	<0.001

a. CM, Chinese medicine. The unchanged outcomes (n = 213) served as reference. Models were adjusted for resident areas, diagnostic subtype, and duration of CM use, variables significantly associated with clinical outcomes as shown in Table 3.
b. Akebia Caulis includes the two species: Akebia quinata (Thunb.) Decne. and Akebia trifoliate (Thunb.) Koidz.

addition of herbal medicine accelerates carbamazepine metabolism and lowers its blood concentration [32]. Like carbamazepine, most antipsychotic drugs, including clozapine, olanzapine, and quetiapine, are metabolized as substrates for cytochrome P450s (CYPs) [33,34]. Therefore, pharmacokinetic interactions may play an important role in influencing clinical outcomes in patients with

Table 6. Frequency distribution of herbal and antipsychotic concomitant treatment regimens associated with adverse outcome in schizophrenic patients.

	Risperidone alone	Quetiapine alone [a,b]	Clozapine alone [a]	Olanzepine-including [a]	Risperidone +clozapine	Others
Radix Bupleuri	4	1	3	2	1	0
Fructus Gardenia	7	7	2	3	3	0
Fructus Schisandrae	4	4	2	1	0	0
Radix Rehmanniae	2	2	2	0	0	0
Akebia Caulis	4	5	1	1	1	0
Semen Plantaginis	3	7	3	3	0	0
Others [c]	2	0	0	1 [c]	0	1
Subtotal	**26**	**26**	**13**	**11**	**5**	**1**
		49				
Total	82					

a. These antipsychotic regimens are significantly associated with adverse outcome as shown in Table 4.
b. It is noted that all quetiapine-including treatment regimens are quetiapine monotherapy.
c. Other herbal material-including regimens were not counted in subtotal regimens associated with adverse outcomes.

schizophrenia under concomitant treatment of herbal and antipsychotic agents observed in the present study.

There are several limitations in the present study. First, as patients who sought CM treatment may have distinctive perceptions about herbal medicine, psychological or "placebo" factors could not be excluded. The use of structured assessment instruments, including symptom scales and laboratory tests, should be helpful in further clarifying treatment effects of CM therapy. Second, since a considerable portion of CM-users were unable to provide full information about their CM formulae, it may lead to an underestimation of individual CMs associated with clinical outcomes. On the other hand, due to difficulties in collecting information about dosages of herbal and antipsychotic agents as well as the quality of herbal preparations, these factors were not considered in the present study. However, it should be noted that there have been extensive reports about severe adverse events caused by overdosing, heavy metal contaminations, and adulterants with conventional drugs of herbal supplements [5,35,36], all of which might account for the presumed adverse effects of herbal and antipsychotic combinations. Fourth, as the majority of CM treatments were recommended by psychiatrists to their patients, obtaining information about psychiatrists' attitudes and knowledge of CM would be helpful in devising safe and effective strategies of concomitant CM and antipsychotics in the treatment of schizophrenia. Finally, although there are many statistically significant results found in the study, "chance significances" may not be excluded. Additional cautions should be paid when the results are considered with reference in future studies.

In conclusion, a relatively small proportion of patients with schizophrenia have concomitant CM and antipsychotic treatment. Such concomitant treatment may heighten the risk of developing worse clinical outcomes in a small number, but increase the chance of improving treatment outcomes in a much greater number of patients. Better identification of the concomitant herbal and antipsychotic treatment regimens that are associated with clinical outcomes provides useful hints for further clarifying herb-drug pharmacokinetic interactions.

Acknowledgments

We thank the following research members for conducting on-site survey and data collection: Yun-Chun Chen, Rui-Guo Zhang, Hua-Ning Wang, Ya-Hong Zhang, and Li Guo at Department of Psychiatry of the Fourth Military Medical University, Zeng-Rong Gong at Xinfeng Psychiatric Hospital of Lintong City, La-Ke Li at Baoji Psychiatric Hospital, Xiang Wang at Yulin Psychiatric Hospital, Zhen Peng at Xianyan Psychiatric Hospital, Ling Dong at Xi'an Dongfang Psychiatric Hospital, Hui Wang at Mianxian Psychiatric Hospital, Bo Zhang at Ankang Psychiatric Hospital, Cui-Xia An, Gui-Xing Jin and Shao-Min Yao at Mental Health Center of Hebei Medical University, Xiao-Dong Zhou at PLA 256 Hospital, Guo-Zheng Li at Xingtai Qiaodong Psychiatric Hospital, Bing-Li Wang at Nangong Minghua Township Hospital, Jun-Jie Feng at Handan Integrative Hospital, Jian-Jie Qiao at Jize Licaozhuang Mental Health Clinic, Xiao-Ying Wang at Langfang Psychiatric Hospital, Shuang-Qian Xie at Hengshui Psychiatric Hospital, Yong-Jun Cui at Cangzhou Anding Hospital, and Zheng Li at Huanghua Anding Psychiatric Hospital. Ms. Lilly Lee helped with data input.

Author Contributions

Conceived and designed the experiments: ZJZ QRT YT XYW. Performed the experiments: QRT XYW HHW CYW. Analyzed the data: LMH HKW DW. Wrote the manuscript: ZJZ QRT YT YBF RN GMM CYW VTW.

References

1. Fugh-Berman A (2002) Herb-drug interactions. Lancet 355: 134–138.
2. Izzo AA, Ernst E (2009) Interactions between herbal medicines and prescribed drugs: an updated systematic review. Drugs 69: 1777–1798.
3. Isnard Bagnis C, Deray G, Baumelou A, Le Quintrec M, Vanherweghem JL (2004) Herbs and the kidney. Am J Kidney Dis 44: 1–11.
4. Vanherweghem JL, Depierreux M, Tielemans C, Abramowicz D, Dratwa M, et al. (1993) Rapidly progressive interstitial renal fibrosis in young women: association with slimming regimen including Chinese herbs. Lancet 341: 387–391.
5. Yuen MF, Tam S, Fung J, Wong DK, Wong BC, et al. (2006) Traditional Chinese medicine causing hepatotoxicity in patients with chronic hepatitis B infection: a 1-year prospective study. Aliment Pharmacol Ther 24: 1179–1186.
6. Yang XX, Hu ZP, Duan W, Zhu YZ, Zhou SF (2006) Drug-herb interactions: eliminating toxicity with hard drug design. Curr Pharm Des 12: 4649–4664.
7. Csernansky JG, Schuchart EK (2002) Relapse and rehospitalisation rates in patients with schizophrenia: effects of second generation antipsychotics. CNS Drugs 16: 473–484.
8. Zhang ZJ, Tan QR, Zhen XC, Tong Y (2010) The potential benefits of herbal medicines for schizophrenia: from empirical observations to clinical trials (chapter 16) In: Hertzman M, Adler L, eds. Clinical Trials in Psychopharmacology. UK: Wiley-Blackwell. pp 311–335.
9. Yuan HN, Wang CY, Sze CW, Tong Y, Tan QR, et al. (2008) A randomized crossover comparison of herbal medicine and bromocriptine against risperidone-induced hyperprolactinemia in patients with schizophrenia. J Clin Psychopharmacol 28: 264–370.
10. Peterson E, Stoebner A, Weatherill J, Kutscher E (2008) Case of acute psychosis from herbal supplements. S D Med 61: 173–177.
11. Przekop P, Lee T (2009) Persistent psychosis associated with salvia divinorum use. Am J Psychiatry 166: 832.
12. Zhang ZX, Zahner GE, Román GC, Liu XH, Wu CB, et al. (2006) Socio-demographic variation of dementia subtypes in China: Methodology and results of a prevalence study in Beijing, Chengdu, Shanghai, and Xian. Neuroepidemiology 27: 177–187.
13. World Health Organization (1992) The ICD-10 classification of mental and behavioural disorders: clinical descriptions and diagnostic guidelines .
14. Maciocia G (1994) The practice of Chinese medicine: the treatment of diseases with acupuncture and Chinese herbs. Edinburgh, UK: Churchill Livingstone. pp 342–385.
15. Xiang YT, Ma X, Cai ZJ, Li SR, Xiang YQ, et al. (2008) Prevalence and socio-demographic correlates of schizophrenia in Beijing, China. Schizophr Res 102: 270–277.
16. Xiang YT, Weng YZ, Leung CM, Tang WK, Ungvari GS (2007) Clinical and social determinants of antipsychotic polypharmacy for Chinese patients with schizophrenia. Pharmacopsychiatry 40: 47–52.
17. Chen Z, Gu K, Zheng Y, Zheng W, Lu W, et al. (2008) The use of complementary and alternative medicine among Chinese women with breast cancer. J Altern Complement Med 14: 1049–1055.
18. Wu B, Liu M, Liu H, Li W, Tan S, et al. (2007) Meta-analysis of traditional Chinese patent medicine for ischemic stroke. Stroke 38: 1973–1979.
19. Ma K, Lee SS, Chu EK, Tam DK, Kwong VS, et al. (2008) Popular use of traditional Chinese medicine in HIV patients in the HAART era. AIDS Behav 12: 637–642.
20. Druss BG, Rosenheck RA (1999) Association between use of unconventional therapies and conventional medical services. JAMA 282: 651–656.
21. Eisenberg DM, Davis RB, Ettner SL, Appel S, Wilkey S, et al. (1998) Trends in alternative medicine use in the United States, 1990-1997: results of a follow-up national survey. JAMA 280: 1569–1575.
22. Eisenberg DM, Kessler RC, Foster C, Norlock FE, Calkins DR, et al. (1993) Unconventional medicine in the United States. Prevalence, costs, and patterns of use. N Engl J Med 328: 246–252.
23. Bersani G, Valeri M, Bersani I, Piazza A, Adorno D, et al. (1989) HLA antigens and neuroleptic response in clinical subtypes of schizophrenia. J Psychiatr Res 23: 213–220.
24. Zalewski C, Johnson-Selfridge MT, Ohriner S, Zarrella K, Seltzer JC (1998) A review of neuropsychological differences between paranoid and nonparanoid schizophrenia patients. Schizophr Bull 24: 127–145.
25. Fanous AH, Kendler KS (2008) Genetics of clinical features and subtypes of schizophrenia: a review of the recent literature. Curr Psychiatry Rep 10: 164–170.
26. Jablensky A (2006) Subtyping schizophrenia: implications for genetic research. Mol Psychiatry 11: 815–836.
27. Tanaka A, Nishida R, Yoshida T, Koshikawa M, Goto M, et al. (2001) Outbreak of Chinese herb nephropathy in Japan: are there any differences from Belgium? Intern Med 40: 296–300.
28. Feng YB, (ed.) (2009) Basic and clinical toxicology of Chinese medicine (Chinese version). Hong Kong: Public House of Commercial Affairs.
29. Deahl M (1989) Betel nut-induced extrapyramidal syndrome: an unusual drug interaction. Mov Disord 4: 330–332.
30. Jones BD, Runikis AM (1987) Interaction of ginseng with phenelzine. J Clin Psychopharmacol 7: 201–202.

31. Shader RI, Greenblatt DJ (1985) Phenelzine and the dream machine—ramblings and reflections. J Clin Psychopharmacol 5: 65.
32. Zhang ZJ, Kang WH, Li Q, Tan QR (2007) The beneficial effects of the herbal medicine Free and Easy Wanderer Plus (FEWP) for mood disorders: double-blind, placebo-controlled studies. J Psychiatr Res 41: 828–836.
33. Sheehan JJ, Sliwa JK, Amatniek JC, Grinspan A, Canuso CM (2010) Atypical Antipsychotic Metabolism and Excretion. Curr Drug Metab 11: 516–25.
34. Wang B, Zhou SF (2009) Synthetic and natural compounds that interact with human cytochrome P450 1A2 and implications in drug development. Curr Med Chem 16: 4066–4218.
35. Ernst E (2002) Toxic heavy metals and undeclared drugs in Asian herbal medicines. Trends Pharmacol Sci 23: 136–139.
36. Ernst E (2004) Risks of herbal medicinal products. Pharmacoepidemiol Drug Saf 13: 767–771.

How Current Clinical Practice Guidelines for Low Back Pain Reflect Traditional Medicine in East Asian Countries: A Systematic Review of Clinical Practice Guidelines and Systematic Reviews

Hyun-Woo Cho[1], Eui-Hyoung Hwang[1,2], Byungmook Lim[3], Kwang-Ho Heo[1], Jian-Ping Liu[4], Kiichiro Tsutani[5], Myeong Soo Lee[6], Byung-Cheul Shin[1,2]*

1 Department of Rehabilitation Medicine of Korean Medicine, Spine and Joint Center, Pusan National University Korean Medicine Hospital, Yangsan, Republic of Korea, 2 Division of Clinical Medicine, School of Korean Medicine, Pusan National University, Yangsan, Republic of Korea, 3 Division of Humanities and Social Medicine, School of Korean Medicine, Pusan National University, Yangsan, Republic of Korea, 4 Center for Evidence-Based Chinese Medicine, Beijing University of Chinese Medicine, Beijing, China, 5 Department of Drug Policy and Management, Graduate School of Pharmaceutical Sciences, The University of Tokyo, Tokyo, Japan, 6 Brain Disease Research Center, Korea Institute of Oriental Medicine, Daejeon, Republic of Korea

Abstract

Objectives: The aims of this study were to investigate whether there is a gap between evidence of traditional medicine (TM) interventions in East-Asian countries from the current Clinical Practice Guidelines (CPGs) and evidence from current systematic reviews and meta-analyses (SR-MAs) and to analyze the impact of this gap on present CPGs.

Methods: We examined 5 representative TM interventions in the health care systems of East-Asian countries. We searched seven relevant databases for CPGs to identify whether core CPGs included evidence of TM interventions, and we searched 11 databases for SR-MAs to re-evaluate current evidence on TM interventions. We then compared the gap between the evidence from CPGs and SR-MAs.

Results: Thirteen CPGs and 22 SR-MAs met our inclusion criteria. Of the 13 CPGs, 7 CPGs (54%) mentioned TM interventions, and all were for acupuncture (only one was for both acupuncture and acupressure). However, the CPGs did not recommend acupuncture (or acupressure). Of 22 SR-MAs, 16 were for acupuncture, 5 for manual therapy, 1 for cupping, and none for moxibustion and herbal medicine. Comparing the evidence from CPGs and SR-MAs, an underestimation or omission of evidence for acupuncture, cupping, and manual therapy in current CPGs was detected. Thus, applying the results from the SR-MAs, we moderately recommend acupuncture for chronic LBP, but we inconclusively recommend acupuncture for (sub)acute LBP due to the limited current evidence. Furthermore, we weakly recommend cupping and manual therapy for both (sub)acute and chronic LBP. We cannot provide recommendations for moxibustion and herbal medicine due to a lack of evidence.

Conclusions: The current CPGs did not fully reflect the evidence for TM interventions. As relevant studies such as SR-MAs are conducted and evidence increases, the current evidence on acupuncture, cupping, and manual therapy should be rigorously considered in the process of developing or updating the CPG system.

Editor: Sonia Brucki, University Of São Paulo, Brazil

Funding: The authors have no support or funding to report.

Competing Interests: The authors have declared that no competing interests exist.

* E-mail: drshinbc@gmail.com

Introduction

Low back pain (LBP) is a common condition that affects a significant proportion of the population, with an estimated prevalence of 70%–85% [1]. Current Clinical Practice Guidelines (CPGs) recommend various LBP treatments, such as pharmacotherapy, physical therapy, manual therapy, educational therapy, psychological therapy, and invasive therapy [2,3].

Traditional medicine (TM) is defined as indigenous medicine used to maintain health and to prevent, diagnose, and treat physical and mental illnesses and is distinct from allopathic medicine based on theories, beliefs, and experiences [4]. In East-Asian countries, especially China, Korea, and Japan, the main therapeutic methods of TM consist of acupuncture, moxibustion, cupping therapy, herbal medicines, and manual therapies (called Tuina in China, Chuna in Korea, and Shiatsu in Japan) [5]. In East-Asian countries, 80% of the population depends on TM for primary health care, and 70% to 80% of the population in many developed countries has used some form of alternative or complementary medicine (e.g., acupuncture) [4]. Although studies on the use of TM are increasing [6,7], differences in medical circumstances, culture, or poor evidence in support of TM seem to complicate the inclusion of TM in CPGs.

CPGs are systematically developed to assist practitioners and patients in making decisions about appropriate healthcare in specific clinical circumstances [8]. In contrast with previous approaches that were often based on tradition or authority, modern CPGs are based on an examination of current evidence within the paradigm of evidence-based medicine [9]. SR-MAs are literature reviews focused on a research question that attempts to identify, appraise, select, and synthesize all high-quality research evidence relevant to that question. SR-MAs of high-quality randomized controlled trials (RCTs) are crucial for evidence-based medicine [10]. Although it seems easy to write an SR-MA, good SR-MAs take time, and they frequently encounter delays but do not update the literature review. The additional typical delays for peer review and publishing add extra time, and SR-MAs may be printed two to four years after the end of the information retrieval. Finally, most SR-MAs are published worldwide without an accompanying CPG [11].

The purpose of this review was to investigate whether there is a gap between evidence of traditional medicine (TM) interventions in East-Asian countries from the current Clinical Practice guideline (CPGs) and evidence from current systematic reviews and meta-analyses (SR-MAs) and to analyze the impact of this gap on present CPGs.

Methods

Data Sources and Searches

Two types of databases were searched according to their database content. The first database was a CPG-related database for LBP that was used to understand the current status of LBP management. The other database included systematic reviews or meta- analyses (SR-MAs) and was used to compare the current evidence to current CPGs. Following the core, standard, ideal search (CoSI) model [12], we searched the following electronic databases from database inception to December 2012.

Our CPG database searches were the core searches because representative databases were more highly recommended than ideal searches. The CPG databases included the National Guideline Clearinghouse (NGC), Guidelines International Network (G-I-N), National Institute for Health and Clinical Excellence (NICE), and Scottish Intercollegiate Guidelines Network (SIGN). Additionally, we searched 3 representative East-Asian countries' databases: the Chinese National Knowledge Infrastructure (CNKI) for China, the Korean Medical Guideline Information (KoMGI) for Korea, and the Medical Information Network Distribution Service (MINDS) for Japan.

For SR-MAs, we conducted an ideal search because all relevant SR-MAs of LBP were needed for the TM area. We found TM in the following databases: The Cochrane Database of Systematic Review (CDSR), PubMed, MEDLINE, EMBASE, DH-DATA, AMED, Chinese databases (China Knowledge Resource Integrated Database, Wanfang database, and Chinese VIP information), a Korean database (Oriental Medicine Advanced Searching Integrated System), and a Japanese database (Japan Medical Abstracts Society).

Each East-Asian country's CPG and SR-MA databases were searched by authors from their own county.

The search keywords for CPG were (back pain OR low back pain OR lumbago) in each CPG database mentioned above. The search keywords for SR-MAs were (acupuncture OR acup*) for acupuncture, (moxa OR moxibustion) for moxibustion, (cupping) for cupping therapy, (herbal medicine OR traditional Chinese medicine OR Chinese herbal medicine) for herbal medicine, (manual therapy OR manipulation OR massage OR Chinese massage OR Tuina OR Chuna OR Shiatsu) for manual therapy, (low back pain OR back pain OR lumbago) for LBP, and (systematic review OR meta analysis OR meta analyze) for SR-MAs in each language. These search terms were combined in the form of [(LBP) AND (TM interventions) AND (SR-MA)]. This search strategy was adjusted for each database.

In addition, the bibliographies of relevant CPGs and SR-MAs were manually searched. Gray literature, consisting of theses, dissertations, letters, government documents, research reports, conference proceedings, and abstracts, was searched to avoid publication bias. The reference section for each study was searched. Personal contacts were made with the original authors of the searched studies to identify any data that were potentially missing from the publications.

The title and abstract of searched articles were read by a single primary researcher (H-WC), who conducted the screening process. Articles that were not written in English were translated into Korean or English prior to screening. The articles for potential inclusion in our review were checked by 2 independent reviewers (H-WC, E-HH). After screening the titles and abstracts retrieved in our search, we excluded all articles that did not meet our pre-defined inclusion/exclusion criteria. Then, the full text of the articles for inclusion was carefully read. The final inclusion was determined by two independent reviewers (H-WC, E-HH), who used the matching method.

Study Selection

Types of CPG and SR-MA. Current CPGs regarding the treatment of non-specific LBP, which were used universally and considered the standard, were evaluated. When we conducted the preliminary search, there were few CPGs not written in English, and they were from the Netherlands, Spain, Germany, France, Finland, and Brazil. The CPGs' development dates were relatively older than the English versions, and the relevance of their content was low. Thus, we concluded that they would have no effect on the analysis. Because we wanted to show the current state of TM through the representative CPGs, the authors reached a consensus to limit the language of the CPGs to English.

Non-specific LBP was searched and evaluated to understand the current evidence from SR-MAs research studies on the effectiveness of 5 major TM interventions (acupuncture, moxibustion, cupping therapy, manual therapy, and herbal medicine). Language was not restricted during the selection of SR and MA.

Types of participants in CPG and SR-MA. LBP was defined as pain localized to the area between the costal margin or the 12th rib to the inferior gluteal fold. Non-specific LBP indicated the lack of a detectable specific cause, such as infection, neoplasm, metastasis, osteoporosis, rheumatoid arthritis, fracture, or inflammatory process [13].

The CPGs and SR-MAs in our review included all stages of non-specific LBP with or without radiating pain, such as acute (lasting up to six weeks), sub-acute (lasting six to 12 weeks), or chronic (lasting longer than 12 weeks) non-specific LBP [14].

Types of interventions in SR and MA. We analyze the TM of the primary therapeutic interventions, including acupuncture, moxibustion, cupping therapy, herbal medicines, and manual therapies, found in East-Asian countries. We selected these 5 types of interventions because they were medical insurance reimbursement items in East-Asian countries [15].

Table 1. Comparison of Clinical Practice Guidelines for Low Back Pain.

Database	Guideline & Year	Target population	Interventions and practices considered	Presence of Traditional Medicine Interventions	Recommendation	AGREE II Overall Assessment
NGC (USA)	NGC-8959/2012 [21]	(Sub)acute/Non-specific LBP with or without radiculopathy/ including pregnant women	1, 2, 3, 5	None	NA	6/Y
	NGC-8744/2011 [24]	(Sub)acute/Non-specific LBP with or without back-related leg symptoms	1, 2, 3	None	NA	5/YWM
	NGC-8517/2011 [28]	(Sub)acute & chronic/ Non- specific LBP	1, 2, 3, 5, 6	Yes (acupuncture/ Acupressure)	Acupuncture/Acupressure considered, but are not recommended	6/Y
	NGC-8193/2010 [22]	(Sub)acute & chronic/ Non- specific LBP with or without radiculopathy	1,2,3,4	None	NA	3/YWM
	NGC-8009/2010 [26]	(Sub)acute/Non-specific LBP	1,2,3,6	None	NA	3/YWM
	NGC-7704/2009 [25]	(Sub)acute & chronic/ Non-specific LBP	(sub)acute LBP : 1, 2, 3, 5, 6/ Chronic LBP : 1, 2, 5, 6	Yes (acupuncture)	1. (Sub)acute: acupuncture - Do Not Know/2. Chronic: acupuncture - Do	3/YWM
	NGC-7510/2009 [27]	Work-related injuries or illnesses related to the low back, elbow, shoulder, forearm, wrist, or hand	2, 3, 4	None	NA	3/YWM
	NGC-7428/2009 [2]	Chronic/Non-specific LBP	6	None	NA	4/YWM
	NGC-6456/2007 [23]	Work-related low back disorders with radiculopath	1, 2, 3, 5, 6	Yes (acupuncture)	1.(Sub)acute LBP:acupuncture - Not recommended (Insufficient)/ 2.Chronic LBP: acupuncture for select use during a limited course with a clear objective and functional goals –Recommended (C-weak)/acupuncture - Notrecommended (Insufficient)	4/YWM
	NGC-5968/2007 [20]	(Sub)acute & chronic/ Non- specific LBP	1, 2, 3, 4, 5, 6	Yes (acupuncture)	Moderate quality evidence, Weak recommendation	3/YWM
NICE (UK)	CG-88/2009* [29]	(Sub)acute & chronic/ Non-specific LBP	1, 2, 3, 4, 5, 6	Yes (acupuncture)	Consider offering a course of acupuncture needling comprising up to a maximum of 10 sessions over a period of up to 12 weeks.	5/YWM
G-I-N (International)	Prodigy(UK) Back pain - low (without radiculopathy) /2009 [3]	(Sub)acute & chronic/ Non-specific LBP without radiculopathy(sciatica) (including sprains and strains)	1, 2, 3, 4, 5, 6	Yes (acupuncture)	The course should have up to 10 sessions given over a period of up to 12 weeks	3/YWM
MINDS (Japan)	Clinical Practice guideline for the management of LBP/2012 [30]	(Sub)acute & chronic/ Non-specific LBP	1, 2, 3, 4, 5, 6	Yes (acupuncture)	(Sub)acute – Do not know/ Chronic- It is hard to say acupuncture is better than other conservative therapies.	4/YWM

Abbreviations: LBP, low back pain; AT, acupuncture; NA, Not applicable YMA, yes with modification; Y, yes.
Items of Interventions and practices: 1 = pharmacological therapy, 2 = physical therapy, 3 = education, 4 = psychological therapy, 5 = manual therapy, 6 = invasive therapy; Items of outcomes considered: 1 = pain, 2 = Global measure, 3 = functional status, 4 = Quality of Life, 5 = Safety, 6 = Cost effectiveness, 7 = Other outcomes.; All AGREE II items are rated with the following 7-point scale: Score of 1 (Strongly Disagree) = There is no information relevant to the AGREE II item or very poor reporting of the concept.; Score of 7 (Strongly Agree) = quality of reporting is exceptional and the full criteria and considerations articulated in the User's Manual have been met.; Scores between 2 and 6 = The reporting of the AGREE II item does not meet the full criteria or considerations. A score is assigned depending on the completeness and quality of reporting. Scores increase as more criteria are met and considerations are addressed. We classified scores of 1 or 2 as low quality, scores of 3, 4 or 5 were moderate quality and 6 or 7 were high quality.; Domain scores are calculated by summing all the scores of the individual items in a domain and by scaling the total as a percentage of the maximum possible score for that domain. The scaled domain score will be: (Obtained score – Minimum possible) score/(Maximum possible score – Minimum possible score)*100.
*: NGC-7269 was originated from CG88 and it was summary of CG-88; thus, it was excluded.

Table 2. Systematic Reviews of Low Back Pain.

Type of Traditional Medicine	Stage of LBP	First Author & Year	Intervention	Outcome measurement	Direction of Outcome (Number of RCTs)	Level of Evidence/ Recommendation (SIGN)	Total AMSTA R score
Acupuncture							
	(Sub)acute						
		McIntosh 2008 [45]	Acupuncture	1, 2, 3, 7	P+(3)	1−/A	5
	Chronic						
		Hutchinson 2012 [44]	Acupuncture	1, 3, 4, 6, 7	P+ (7)	1+/A	4
		Trigkilidas 2010 [40]	Acupuncture	1, 3, 4, 6	I (4)	Not applicable	2
		Rubinstein 2010 [42]	Acupuncture	1, 3	P+ (18)	1+/A	10
		Yuan 2009 [39]	Acupuncture	1, 3, 4	Chronic LBP: P+ (23)	1+/A	7
		Ammendolia 2008 [37]	Acupuncture	1, 3, 4, 5, 7	I (19)	1+/A	4
		McIntosh 2008 [38]	Acupuncture	1, 2, 3, 7	P+ (32)	1−/A	4
		Henderson 2002 [34]	Acupuncture	Not reported	I (5)	2+/C	2
	Mixed						
		Furlan 2012 [41]	Acupuncture	1, 3, 5, 6	(Sub)acute LBP : I/chronic LBP : P+ (33)	1−/B	9
		Lu 2011 [43]	Acupuncture	1, 3, 4, 6, 7	P+ (5)	1+/A	8
		Furlan 2005 [35]	Acupuncture	1, 2, 3, 4, 5, 7	(Sub)acute LBP : I (3)/chronic LBP : P+ (32)	1+/A	3
		Maurits 2005 [46]	Acupuncture	1, 3, 7	acute LBP : I (2)/chronic LBP : P+ (13)	1+/A	9
		Manheimer 2005 [36]	Acupuncture	1, 2, 3, 7	P+ (33)	1+/B	8
		Ernst 2002 [33]	Acupuncture	1, 3	I (12)	1−/A	10
		Smith 2000 [32]	Acupuncture	1, 2, 7	(sub)acute LBP : N+ (2)/chronic LBP : N+ (8)	1+/A	7
		Tulder 1999 [31]	Acupuncture	1, 3, 7	I (11)	1−/A	8
Cupping Therapy							
	Mixed						
		Kim 2011 [52]	Dry/Wet cupping	1, 5	(sub)acute & chronic LBP : P+ (2)	1−/B	8
Manual Therapy							
	Chronic						
		Kim 2012 [50]	Acupressure	1, 3, 7	P++ (3)	1−/B	10
		Imamura 2008 [47]	Acupuncture massage, Acupressure	1, 2, 3, 4, 5, 6, 7	P+ (4)	1+/A	5
	Mixed						
		Moon 2012 [51]	Chuna	1	P+ (2)	1−/B	6
		Robinson 2011 [49]	Shiatsu, Acupressure	1, 3	Shiatsu: I (1)/Acupressure : P+ (3)	1−/B	6
		Furlan 2009 [48]	Acupuncture massage, Acupressure	1, 2, 3, 4, 5, 6, 7	P++ (5)	1+/A	10

Abbreviations: LBP, low back pain; I, insufficient; P, positive; N, negative;
+ = weak; ++ = moderate; +++ = strong.
Items of outcomes measurement: 1 = pain; 2 = Global measure; 3 = functional status; 4 = Quality of Life; 5 = Safety; 6 = Cost effectiveness; 7 = Other outcomes.
The total AMSTAR score was calculated by adding the average scores for all 11 items. We averaged item scores across guidelines. Item scores were classified such that 0–3 indicated low quality, 4–7 indicated moderate quality and 8–11 indicated high quality.

1. Acupuncture: only included needle acupuncture with or without electrical stimulation. Acupuncture without needling, such as laser or TENS on acupoints, was excluded.
2. Moxibustion: included when acupoints were heated with moxibustion.
3. Cupping therapy: included both dry and wet cupping.
4. Manual therapy: included Tuina in China or Chuna in Korea. Massage techniques were included, such as Chinese massage, acupressure, acupuncture massage, or Shiatsu when applied to acupoints or meridians.
5. Herbal medicine: included herbal medicine according to the TM diagnosis.

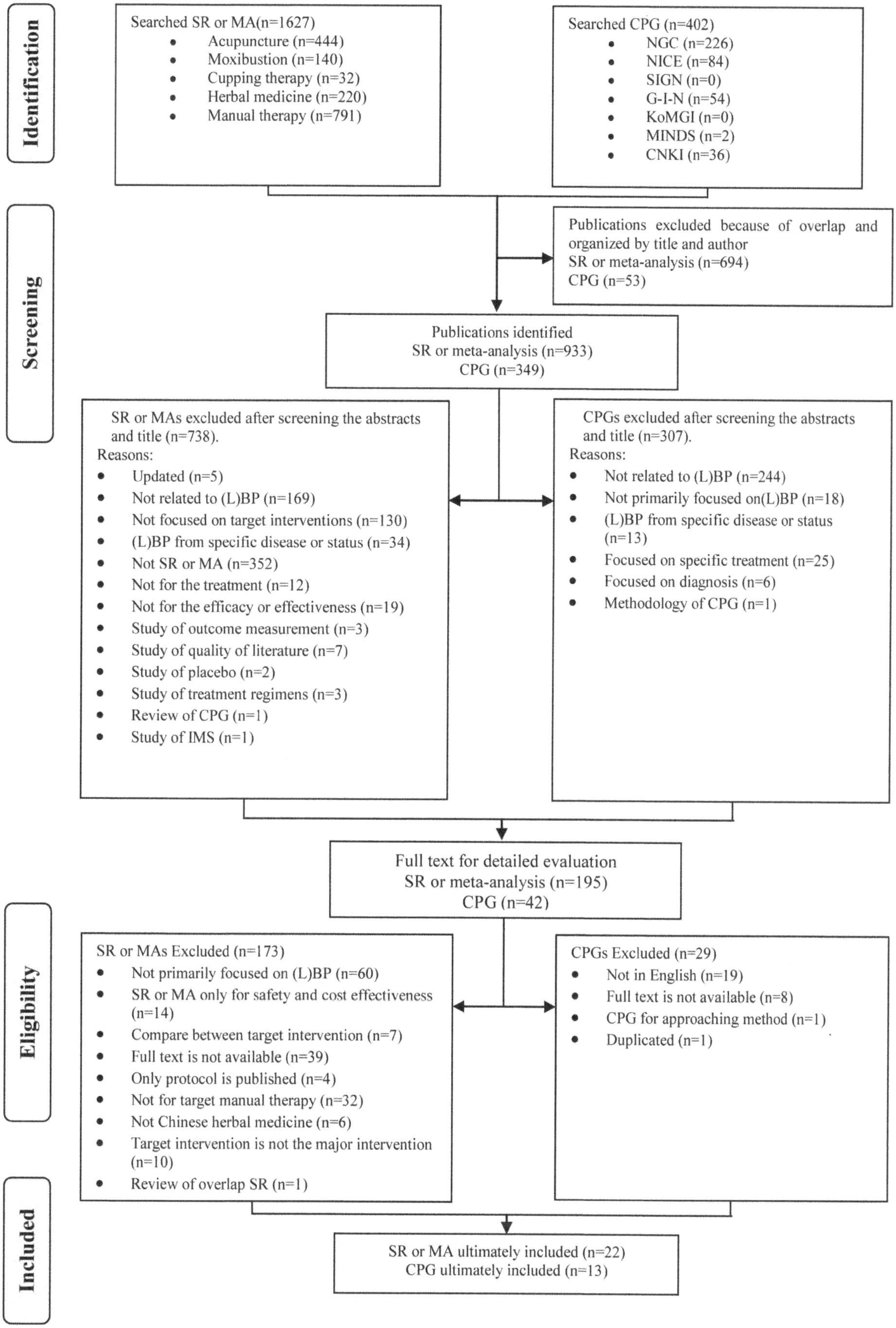
Identification
Searched SR or MA(n=1627)
Acupuncture (n=444)
Moxibustion (n=140)
Cupping therapy (n=32)
Herbal medicine (n=220)
Manual therapy (n=791)
Searched CPG (n=402)
NGC (n=226)
NICE (n=84)
SIGN (n=0)
G-I-N (n=54)
KoMGI (n=0)
MINDS (n=2)
CNKI (n=36)
Screening
Publications excluded because of overlap and organized by title and author
SR or meta-analysis (n=694)
CPG (n=53)
Publications identified
SR or meta-analysis (n=933)
CPG (n=349)
SR or MAs excluded after screening the abstracts and title (n=738).
Reasons:
Updated (n=5)
Not related to (L)BP (n=169)
Not focused on target interventions (n=130)
(L)BP from specific disease or status (n=34)
Not SR or MA (n=352)
Not for the treatment (n=12)
Not for the efficacy or effectiveness (n=19)
Study of outcome measurement (n=3)
Study of quality of literature (n=7)
Study of placebo (n=2)
Study of treatment regimens (n=3)
Review of CPG (n=1)
Study of IMS (n=1)
CPGs excluded after screening the abstracts and title (n=307).
Reasons:
Not related to (L)BP (n=244)
Not primarily focused on(L)BP (n=18)
(L)BP from specific disease or status (n=13)
Focused on specific treatment (n=25)
Focused on diagnosis (n=6)
Methodology of CPG (n=1)
Full text for detailed evaluation
SR or meta-analysis (n=195)
CPG (n=42)
Eligibility
SR or MAs Excluded (n=173)
Not primarily focused on (L)BP (n=60)
SR or MA only for safety and cost effectiveness (n=14)
Compare between target intervention (n=7)
Full text is not available (n=39)
Only protocol is published (n=4)
Not for target manual therapy (n=32)
Not Chinese herbal medicine (n=6)
Target intervention is not the major intervention (n=10)
Review of overlap SR (n=1)
CPGs Excluded (n=29)
Not in English (n=19)
Full text is not available (n=8)
CPG for approaching method (n=1)
Duplicated (n=1)
Included
SR or MA ultimately included (n=22)
CPG ultimately included (n=13)

Figure 1. Flow chart of the study selection process. SR = systematic review; MA = meta-analysis; CPG = clinical practice guideline; (L)BP = (low) back pain; IMS = Intra Muscular Stimulation.

When studies addressed various symptoms or interventions in one acupuncture SR, we limited the inclusion criteria if the majority (>50%) of the participants and the intervention were acceptable for predefined criteria because there were numerous acupuncture SR-MAs. However, there were few available SR-MAs of moxibustion, cupping, manual therapy, and herbal medicine. Therefore, we included the SR-MAs when the RCTs of those interventions were greater than 10% of all RCTs when the data could be separately extracted.

When it was difficult to evaluate the independent effectiveness of TM intervention, such as comparing the same interventions or mixed treatments, the SR-MAs were excluded.

Data Extraction and Quality Assessment

Two reviewers (H-WC, E-HH) independently extracted the data based on predefined characteristics to describe each study (refer to Tables 1, 2). In CPG, we extracted the type of interventions, the presence of TM, and the recommendation. In SR-MAs, we extracted outcome measures and their directions of outcome for each intervention and condition of LBP.

Outcome measures. The outcome measures that we considered are described below. SR-MAs that used at least one outcome measure related to pain were included. The other outcome measures were considered, and their inclusion may be important for the study of LBP.

1. Primary outcome: Pain intensity
2. Secondary outcome: Global measure of improvement or recovery/Back-specific functional status/Quality of life/Safety/Cost-effectiveness/Other outcomes

Level of Evidence and Recommendation

We reassessed the evidence level and recommendations of the SR-MAs using the SIGN grading system [16]. All disagreements were resolved through discussion and consensus or by the first author (H-WC).

Quality Assessment of CPGs and SR-MAs

The SR-MAs of 24 different appraisal tools and some studies have shown that the Appraisal of Guidelines for Research & Evaluation (AGREE) instrument is an acceptable standard for guideline evaluation. Therefore, the AGREE Instrument for reporting the quality of CPGs was used [17,18], and the Assessment of Multiple Systematic Reviews (AMSTAR) checklist for reporting the quality of SR-MAs was used to evaluate the methodological quality of the included publications. The AMSTAR instrument has recently been used in another study [19].

Four reviewers (H-WC, E-HH, K-HH, and B-CS) were fully trained in the quality assessment and data extraction methodology.

Data Synthesis and Analysis

We identified the directions for future CPG of LBP through deep discussion and expert consensus among authors. All authors were CPG-related experts from East-Asian countries (China, Korea, and Japan). The authors discussed and reached consensus through e-mail contact. In cases of disagreement, the final recommendation was made by consensus. Per the authors' recommendations, we recommend studies based on the results in Table 1 and Table 2.

Results

Study Description

A total of 402 CPGs and 1627 SR-MAs were identified. After manually removing the duplicates and screening the titles and abstracts, 42 CPGs and 195 SR-MAs were identified as potentially relevant. After a detailed evaluation of the full text, 29 CPGs and 173 SR-MAs were excluded. Finally, 13 CPGs and 22 SR-MAs met our inclusion criteria. The literature search process is summarized in Figure 1, following the Preferred Reporting Items for Systematic Reviews and Meta-Analysis (PRISMA) flow diagram. The key data are summarized in Table 1.

Current Clinical Practice Guidelines

Of the 13 CPGs, 10 originated in the USA [2,20–28], 2 were from the UK [3,29], and 1 was from Japan [30]. There were no CPGs from any East-Asian country. There were 7 CPGs for both (sub)acute and chronic LBP [3,20,22,25,28–30], 1 for chronic LBP [2], 3 for (sub)acute LBP [21,24,26], and 2 for work-related LBP [23,27]. The CPGs addressed various interventions, such as pharmacological therapy, physical therapy, education, psychological therapy, manual therapy, and invasive therapy. However, TM interventions were only included in 7 CPGs [3,20,23,25,28–30]. All TM interventions were for acupuncture, and only 1 CPG [28] mentioned both acupuncture and acupressure.

Of 7 CPGs, 6 recommended acupuncture, but all of these CPGs had weak recommendation strength or made the recommendation with session limitations [3,20,23,25,29,30]. However, 3 CPGs did not recommend acupuncture for (sub)acute LBP [23,25,28]. Only 1 CPG [28], which analyzed acupressure, did not recommend the treatment (Table 1).

Quality Assessment of Clinical Practice Guidelines

The overall assessment mean of the included CPGs was 4±1 (range: 3–6), indicating that CPGs have moderate quality. There were 2 high-quality CPGs [21,28], 11 moderate-quality CPGs [2,3,20,22–27,29,30], and no low-quality CPGs. We assessed 2 CPGs [21,28] as "recommend without modification" due to high quality and 11 other CPGs as "recommend with modifications" (Table 1). In each domain, the CPGs showed comparatively more than moderate quality (Table S1).

Evidence of Systematic Review and Meta-analysis

Of 22 SR-MAs, 16 were for acupuncture [31–46], 5 were for manual therapy (Chuna, acupressure, acupuncture massage, shiatsu) [47–51], and 1 was for cupping therapy [52]. For chronic LBP, 1 SR reported a moderately negative conclusion [32], 5 SR-MAs reported an insufficient conclusion [31,33,34,37,40], and 9 SR-MAs reported weakly positive effects of acupuncture [35,36,38,39,41–44,46]. For (sub)acute LBP, 1 SR reported a moderate negative conclusion [32], 5 SR-MAs reported insufficient conclusions [31,33,35,41,46], and 3 SR-MAs reported weakly positive effects of acupuncture [36,38,43]. The evidence level and recommendation strength were reassessed using the SIGN grading system. For the level of evidence, 5 SR-MAs were assessed 1− [31,33,38,41,45], 9 SR-MAs were 1+ [32,35–37,39,42–44,46], 1 SR was 2+ [34], and 1 SR was not applicable [40]. For recommendation strength, 12 SR-MAs were assessed as grade A [31–33,35,37–39,42–46], 2 SR-MAs were grade B [36,41], 1 was grade C [34],and 1 was not applicable [40].

Table 3. Directions for future Clinical Practice Guideline of Low Back Pain.

Database	Guideline & Year	Acupuncture		Moxibustion		Cupping Therapy		Manual Therapy		Herbal Medicine	
Current											
NGC (USA)	NGC-8959 2012	–		–		–		–		–	
	NGC-8744 2011	–		–		–		–		–	
	NGC-8517 2011	U		–		–		U		–	
	NGC-8193 2010	–		–		–		–		–	
	NGC-8009 2010	–		–		–		–		–	
	NGC-7704.2009	E		–		–		–		–	
	NGC-7510 2009	–		–		–		–		–	
	NGC-7428 2009	–		–		–		–		–	
	NGC-6456 2007	U		–		–		–		–	
	NGC-5968 2007	U		–		–		–		–	
NICE (UK)	CG-88 2009	U		–		–		–		–	
G-I-N (International)	Prodigy (UK) 2009	U		–		–		–		–	
MINDS (Japan)	CPG for the management of LBP 2012	E		–		–		–		–	
Future											
Authors Recommendation	Condition of LBP	Level of Evidence	Grade of Recommendation	Level of Evidence	Grade of Recommendation	Level of Evidence	Grade of Recommendation	Level of Evidence	Grade of Recommendation	Level of Evidence	Grade of
Recommendation											
	(Sub)acute	1−	B	–	–	1−	B	1−	B	–	–
	Chronic	1+	A	–	–	1−	B	1−	B	–	–
		Moderate recommendation for chronic LBP/Inconclusive for (Sub)acute LBP		Do not know		Weak recommendation for both (Sub)acute and chronic LBP		Weak recommendation for both (Sub)acute and chronic LBP		Do not know	

Abbreviations: U, underestimated; E, enough.
–:There were no available data, and assessments were not applicable.

Only 1 SR-MA on cupping for pain, including 2 RCTs for both (sub)acute and chronic LBP, reported weakly positive conclusions. The study partially considered pain and safety (adverse effect). The evidence level was assessed to be 1−, and the recommendation strength received a grade of B [52].

Of 5 SR-MAs of manual therapy, 1 considered Chuna [51], and 4 considered acupressure (including acupuncture massage and Shiatsu) [47–50]. All of these SR-MAs were compared with other interventions and reported positive conclusions, except for an inconclusive conclusion reported in 1 study of Shiatsu [49]. The study evidence level was assessed to be 1−, and the recommendation strength received a grade of B [51]. In 4 studies of acupressure, 2 were on chronic LBP alone [47,50], and the other 2 included both (sub)acute LBP and chronic LBP [48,49]. The evidence level was assessed to be 1− in 2 studies [49,50] and 1+ in the other 2 studies [47,48]. The recommendation strength received a grade of A in 2 studies [47,48] and B in the other 2 studies [49,50] (Table 2).

Quality Assessment of Systematic Reviews

The mean (± standard deviation) score of total quality assessment of the SR-MAs was 6.59±2.65 (range: 2–10) (Table S2). A total of 10 SR-MAs (47.6%) were assessed to be high quality [31,33,36,41–43,46,48,50,52], 9 SR-MAs (38.1%) were moderate quality [32,37–39,44,45,47,49,51], and 3 SR-MAs (14.3%) were low quality [34,35,40](Table 2).

Directions for Future CPG of LBP

Of the 7 CPGs that included acupuncture, 2 showed a similar recommendation compared with current research on SR-MAs [25,30], but 5 CPGs were underestimated [3,20,23,28,29]. Only 1 CPG included manual therapy and showed effectiveness underestimation [28]. Similar to moxibustion, cupping therapy and herbal medicine were not discussed in current CPGs and thus could not be compared.

We moderately recommended acupuncture for chronic LBP with a 1+/A evidence level and recommendation grade. However, we inconclusively recommended acupuncture for (sub)acute LBP due to the current SR-MA evidence. We weakly recommended cupping therapy for both (sub)acute and chronic LBP with a 1−/B evidence level and recommendation grade. We weakly recommend manual therapy for both (sub)acute and chronic LBP with a 1−/B evidence level and recommendation grade. Moxibustion and herbal medicine were not applicable due to the lack of data available at this time (Table 3).

Discussion

The main aim of our review was to analyze TMs in East-Asian countries (China, Korea, and Japan) in the current CPGs for LBP. The results showed that TMs in East-Asian countries were not sufficiently included in current CPGs.

Notably, moxibustion, cupping therapy, and herbal medicine are not mentioned in current CPGs. The lack of eligible RCTs and the aggregation of SR of moxibustion for LBP might be the primary causes of this lack of inclusion. This omission leads to a lack of evidence for the CPG. The use of moxibustion has become more common; 67% of Korean Oriental medical doctors have used moxibustion [53]. Additionally, 40% of health care in China is currently based on traditional Chinese medicinal approaches that include moxibustion [54]. The adverse effects and difficulties of placebo moxibustion that are reported in the literature [55] may have emerged due to the limited moxibustion studies.

The relevant studies on cupping therapy were of poor quality [56], which might lead to a lack of inclusion in current CPGs. However, the only SR showed a positive effect for both sub(acute) and chronic LBP.

The heterogeneity of herbal medicine products may be a considerable problem. The various types of preparation and the amount of chemical constituents per dose influence the pharmacokinetics and relative efficacy of the herbal medicine [57]. These differences may make it difficult to conduct a high-quality study.

Some acupuncture recommendations had both favorable and unfavorable conclusions. Of all of the studies, 7 CPGs (54%) mentioned acupuncture, but only 1 study recommended acupuncture for chronic LBP without use limitations. The other studies recommended acupuncture for limited treatment sessions or did not recommend acupuncture. These results demonstrate a gap with the results of current SR-MAs. Negative or insufficient effects in SR-MAs were dominant for (sub)acute LBP [31–33,35,41]. However, the positive effects were dominant for chronic LBP [35,36,38,39,41–44]. Similar results were reported for the evidence-based medicine approach to LBP [58]. Therefore, we conclude that the recommendations for (sub)acute LBP seem appropriate, and the recommendations for chronic LBP are underestimated.

Regarding manual therapy, 1 CPG mentioned acupressure but did not recommend acupressure for both (sub)acute and chronic LBP. However, we found some gaps in SR-MAs. There were 5 SR-MAs with a positive result [47–51] (1 on Chuna [51] and 4 on acupressure or acupuncture massage [47–50]) and 1 insufficient SR on Shiatsu [49]. Additionally, 1 related SR-MA that was not included in this study supported the possibility of Tuina-integrated treatment t for LBP [59]. Thus, we find that the current CPGs underestimate the effectiveness of TM manual therapy for LBP.

The overall evidence available was usually published in the US and European countries, Thus, a lack of familiarity with East-Asian TM may influence the lack of interventions. These problems may explain the underpowered evidence for TM.

One important thing to consider is the need for more objective methods in TM practice. In contradistinction to classical approaches in Eastern medicine, where the methodology is much more concrete, TM is mainly considered an "art". This understanding complicates an objective study of the results.

We also conducted a quality assessment that included CPGs and SR-MAs. The AGREE assessment showed that the quality of included CPGs was acceptable. The average scores of 5 domains (with the exception of 1 domain) were greater than 60%, and the mean score in the overall assessment was 4±1 [range: 3–6], indicating a moderate quality of CPG (Table 1). The domains of applicability obtained the lowest score, suggesting that more attention should be paid to quality enhancement during CPG development (Table S1).

The SR-MAs were assessed using the AMSTAR instrument [19]. Although the item "Was a priori design provided?" received the lowest score, the overall scores were quite high. The total mean score showed moderate quality of 6.59 [range: 2–10] for included SR-MAs (Table S2). Therefore, future authors should conduct an a priori design to ensure better study quality.

The strength of our study is its successful completion of the first review of TM in current CPGs for LBP. Previous CPGs of Traditional Chinese Medicine [60] did not focus on specific diseases or make further suggestions to address the lack of evidence. To prevent this bias, we attempted to determine whether current TM interventions were adequately included in current, rigorous CPGs of LBP. Thus, we searched current available CPGs and SR-MAs with systematic search methods and assessed CPG and SR-MA quality. In this study, we reanalyzed the evidence level and grade of recommendation of SR-MAs and aimed to identify directions for future research via a CPG-related expert consensus.

Several study limitations should be considered. Despite our best efforts to retrieve all CPGs and SR-MAs on this subject, we are not convinced that our search was inclusive. Notably, the definition of manual therapy categories in Oriental medicine is a considerable problem. Because we selected the subjects for TM in East-Asian countries, there is a potential question regarding whether the 5 types of intervention represent all TM interventions. To address this problem, we selected the interventions that consider the use of traditional Chinese medicine [61]. Although we suggested recommendation reassessments, we did not follow the entire procedure involved in crafting CPGs [62]. Instead, we made decisions via the expert consensus method. Therefore, biased conclusions are possible.

To address these weaknesses, we suggest important recommendations for future research in this area. First, high-quality RCTs were not conducted despite the use of TM, and there is a remarkable lack of studies on moxibustion, cupping therapy, Tuina (or Chuna), and herbal medicine, which deserve increased interest and further study. Second, a broader scope of TM interventions should be searched in further studies, and accurate recommendations for TM interventions should be drawn via proper procedures by larger organizations or teams. The increasing TM evidence should be included in the process of updating CPGs, and TM interventions based on LBP CPGs should be developed in collaboration with TM experts.

Conclusion

Although interest in and use of TM is increasing, the CPGs identified did not fully reflect the TM interventions in East-Asian countries. In particular, acupuncture, cupping therapy, and manual therapy were underestimated or not mentioned despite their current evidence. The current evidence on acupuncture for chronic LBP and evidence on cupping and manual therapy for both (sub)acute and chronic LBP should be rigorously considered in the process of developing or updating the CPG system. However, a lack of evidence on moxibustion and herbal medicine prevented us from providing recommendations in these areas.

Supporting Information

Table S1 Assessment of Clinical Practice Guidelines (CPG) by AGREEII.
(DOCX)

Table S2 Assessment of Systematic Reviews by AMSTAR.
(DOCX)

Checklist S1 PRISMA checklist.
(DOCX)

Author Contributions

Conceived and designed the experiments: H-WC E-HH K-HH B-CS. Performed the experiments: H-WC E-HH. Analyzed the data: H-WC BML B-CS. Wrote the paper: H-WC. Contributed to assess the level of evidence, grade of recommendation and methodological quality of the CPGs and SR-MAs: H-WC J-PL KT. Contributed to search the CPGs and SRs from each countries: H-WC E-HH K-HH B-CS. Contributed to the consensus of recommendation of future CPGs: H-WC E-HH B-CS BML K-HH J-PL KT MS-L.

References

1. Andersson GB (1999) Epidemiological features of chronic low-back pain. Lancet 354: 581–585.
2. Manchikanti L, Boswell MV, Singh V, Benyamin RM, Fellows B, et al. (2009) Comprehensive evidence-based guidelines for interventional techniques in the management of chronic spinal pain. Pain Physician 12: 699–802.
3. SCHIN - Sowerby Centre for Health Informatics at Newcastle (2009) Back pain - low (without radiculopathy) (Prodigy).
4. World Health Organization Media Centre (2012) "Traditional medicine,". World Health Organization Media Centre.
5. Cheung F (2011) TCM: Made in China. Nature 480: S82–S83.
6. Frass M, Strassl RP, Friehs H, Mullner M, Kundi M, et al. (2012) Use and acceptance of complementary and alternative medicine among the general population and medical personnel: a systematic review. Ochsner J 12: 45–56.
7. Ernst E, Schmidt K, Wider B (2005) CAM research in Britain: the last 10 years. Complement Ther Clin Pract 11: 17–20.
8. Field MJ, Lohr KN (1990) Committee to Advise the Public Health Service on Clinical Practice Guidelines IoM. Clinical practice guidelines: directions for a new program. Washington: National Academy Press.
9. Graham R, Mancher M, Wolman DM, Greenfield S, Steinberg E (2011) Committee on Standards for Developing Trustworthy Clinical Practice Guidelines Institute of Medicine. Clinical Practice Guidelines We Can Trust: The National Academies Press.
10. Sackett DL, Rosenberg WM, Gray JA, Haynes RB, Richardson WS (1996) Evidence based medicine: what it is and what it isn't. BMJ 312: 71–72.
11. Dijkers M (2013) Want your systematic review to be used by practitioners? Try this! KT Update 1: Available from http://www.ktdrr.org/products/update/v1n4.
12. Bidwell S, Jensen MF (2004) Chapter 3: Using a search protocol to identify sources of information: the COSI model. In: Topfer L-A, Auston I, editors. Etext on Health Technology Assessment (HTA) Information Resources. Bethesda, MD: National Information Center on Health Services Research and Health Care Technology (NICHSR).
13. Waddell G (1996) Low back pain: a twentieth century health care enigma. Spine (Phila Pa 1976) 21: 2820–2825.
14. Koes BW, van Tulder M, Lin CW, Macedo LG, McAuley J, et al. (2010) An updated overview of clinical guidelines for the management of non-specific low back pain in primary care. Eur Spine J 19: 2075–2094.
15. Park HL, Lee HS, Shin BC, Liu JP, Shang Q, et al. (2012) Traditional medicine in china, Korea, and Japan: a brief introduction and comparison. Evid Based Complement Alternat Med 2012: 429103.
16. Harbour R, Miller J (2001) A new system for grading recommendations in evidence based guidelines. BMJ 323: 334–336.
17. AGREE Collaboration (2003) Development and validation of an international appraisal instrument for assessing the quality of clinical practice guidelines: the AGREE project. Qual Saf Health Care 12: 18–23.
18. MacDermid JC, Brooks D, Solway S, Switzer-McIntyre S, Brosseau L, et al. (2005) Reliability and validity of the AGREE instrument used by physical therapists in assessment of clinical practice guidelines. BMC Health Serv Res 5: 18.
19. Shea BJ, Grimshaw JM, Wells GA, Boers M, Andersson N, et al. (2007) Development of AMSTAR: a measurement tool to assess the methodological quality of systematic reviews. BMC Med Res Methodol 7: 10.
20. Chou R, Qaseem A, Snow V, Casey D, Cross JT, Jr., et al. (2007) Diagnosis and treatment of low back pain: a joint clinical practice guideline from the American College of Physicians and the American Pain Society. Ann Intern Med 147: 478–491.
21. Goertz M, Thorson D, Bonsell J, Bonte B, Campbell R, et al. (2012 Jan) Institute for Clinical Systems Improvement (ICSI). Adult acute and subacute low back pain. Bloomington (MN): Institute for Clinical Systems Improvement (ICSI).
22. Goertz M, Thorson D, Bonsell J, Bonte B, Campbell R, et al. (2010 Nov) Institute for Clinical Systems Improvement (ICSI). Adult low back pain. Bloomington (MN): Institute for Clinical Systems Improvement (ICSI).
23. Hegmann K (2007) Low back disorders. Occupational medicine practice guidelines: evaluation and management of common health problems and functional recovery in workers. 2nd ed. Elk Grove Village (IL): American College of Occupational and Environmental Medicine (ACOEM).
24. Michigan Quality Improvement Consortium (2011 Sep) Management of acute low back pain. Southfield (MI): Michigan Quality Improvement Consortium.

25. Toward Optimized Practice (2009 Mar 2) Guideline for the evidence-informed primary care management of low back pain. Edmonton(AB): Toward Optimized Practice. 21 p.
26. University of Michigan Health System (2010 Jan) Acute low back pain. Ann Arbor (MI): University of Michigan Health System.
27. National Guideline Clearinghouse (2009) Occupational therapy practice guidelines for individuals with work-related injuries and illnesses. Rockville MD: Agency for Healthcare Research and Quality (AHRQ).
28. National Guideline Clearinghouse (2011) Low back - lumbar & thoracic (acute & chronic). Rockville MD: Agency for Healthcare Research and Quality (AHRQ).
29. National Collaborating Centre for Primary Care (2009 May) Low back pain. Early management of persistent non-specific low back pain. London (UK): National Institute for Health and Clinical Excellence (NICE). pp. 25.
30. Japanese Orthopaedic Association (2012) Clinical Practice Guideline for the Management of Low Back Pain. Tokyo: Nankodo Co., Ltd.
31. van Tulder MW, Cherkin DC, Berman B, Lao L, Koes BW (1999) The effectiveness of acupuncture in the management of acute and chronic low back pain. A systematic review within the framework of the Cochrane Collaboration Back Review Group. Spine (Phila Pa 1976) 24: 1113–1123.
32. Smith LA, Oldman AD, McQuay HJ, Moore RA (2000) Teasing apart quality and validity in systematic reviews: an example from acupuncture trials in chronic neck and back pain. Pain 86: 119–132.
33. Ernst E, White AR, Wider B (2002) Acupuncture for back pain: Meta-analysis of randomised controlled trials and an update with data from the most recent studies. Schmerz 16: 129–139.
34. Henderson H (2002) Acupuncture: evidence for its use in chronic low back pain. Br J Nurs 11: 1395–1403.
35. Furlan AD, van Tulder M, Cherkin D, Tsukayama H, Lao L, et al. (2005) Acupuncture and Dry-Needling for Low Back Pain: An Updated Systematic Review Within the Framework of the Cochrane Collaboration. Spine (Phila Pa 1976) 30: 944–963.
36. Manheimer E, White A, Berman B, Forys K, Ernst E (2005) Meta-analysis: acupuncture for low back pain. Ann Intern Med 142: 651–663.
37. Ammendolia C, Furlan AD, Imamura M, Irvin E, van Tulder M (2008) Evidence-informed management of chronic low back pain with needle acupuncture. Spine J 8: 160–172.
38. Hall H, McIntosh G (2008) Low back pain (chronic). Clin Evid (Online) 2008.
39. Yuan J, Purepong N, Kerr DP (2009) Effectiveness of acupuncture for low back pain: A systematic review (Spine (2008) 33, (E887–E900)). Spine (Phila Pa 1976) 34: 1630.
40. Trigkilidas D (2010) Acupuncture therapy for chronic lower back pain: a systematic review. Ann R Coll Surg Engl 92: 595–598.
41. Furlan AD, Yazdi F, Tsertsvadze A, Gross A, Van Tulder M, et al. (2012) A systematic review and meta-analysis of efficacy, cost-effectiveness, and safety of selected complementary and alternative medicine for neck and low-back pain. Evid Based Complement Alternat Med 2012: 953139.
42. Rubinstein SM, van Middelkoop M, Kuijpers T, Ostelo R, Verhagen AP, et al. (2010) A systematic review on the effectiveness of complementary and alternative medicine for chronic non-specific low-back pain. Eur Spine J 19: 1213–1228.
43. Lu SC, Zheng Z, Xue CC (2011) Does acupuncture improve quality of life for patients with pain associated with the spine? A systematic review. Evid Based Complement Alternat Med 2011: 301767.
44. Hutchinson AJ, Ball S, Andrews JC, Jones GG (2012) The effectiveness of acupuncture in treating chronic non-specific low back pain: a systematic review of the literature. J Orthop Surg Res 7: 36.
45. Hall H, McIntosh G (2008) Low back pain (acute). Clin Evid (Online) 2008.
46. van Tulder MW, Furlan AD, Gagnier JJ (2005) Complementary and alternative therapies for low back pain. Best Pract Res Clin Rheumatol 19: 639–654.
47. Imamura M, Furlan AD, Dryden T, Irvin E (2008) Evidence-informed management of chronic low back pain with massage. Spine J 8: 121–133.
48. Furlan AD, Imamura M, Dryden T, Irvin E (2009) Massage for low back pain: an updated systematic review within the framework of the Cochrane Back Review Group. Spine (Phila Pa 1976) 34: 1669–1684.
49. Robinson N, Lorenc A, Liao X (2011) The evidence for Shiatsu: a systematic review of Shiatsu and acupressure. BMC Complement Altern Med 11: 88.
50. Kim YC, Lee MS, Park E-S, Lew J-H, Lee B-J (2012) Acupressure for the Treatment of Musculoskeletal Pain Conditions: A Systematic Review. J Musculoskelet Pain 20: 116–121.
51. Moon TW, Choi TY, Park TY, Lee MS (2012) Chuna therapy for musculoskeletal pain: A systematic review of randomized clinical trials in Korean literature. Chin J Integr Med 19: 228–232.
52. Kim JI, Lee MS, Lee DH, Boddy K, Ernst E (2011) Cupping for treating pain: a systematic review. Evid Based Complement Alternat Med 2011: 467014.
53. Han CH, Shin MS, Shin SH, Kang KW, Park SH, et al. (2007) Telephone survey for grasping clinical actual state of moxibustion therapeutics in Korea. J Meridian Acupoint 24: 17–31.
54. Hesketh T, Zhu WX (1997) Health in China. Traditional Chinese medicine: one country, two systems. BMJ 315: 115–117.
55. Park JE, Lee SS, Lee MS, Choi SM, Ernst E (2010) Adverse events of moxibustion: a systematic review. Complement Ther Med 18: 215–223.
56. Cao H, Li X, Liu J (2012) An updated review of the efficacy of cupping therapy. PLoS ONE 7: e31793.
57. Gagnier JJ, van Tulder M, Berman B, Bombardier C (2006) Herbal medicine for low back pain. Cochrane Database Syst Rev: CD004504.
58. Dagenais S, Haldeman S (2011) Evidence-Based management of low back pain: Elsevier Health Sciences.
59. Kong LJ, Fang M, Zhan HS, Yuan WA, Pu JH, et al. (2012) Tuina-focused integrative chinese medical therapies for inpatients with low back pain: a systematic review and meta-analysis. Evidence-based complementary and alternative medicine : eCAM 2012: 578305–578305.
60. Yu WY, Xu JL, Shi NN, Wang LY, Han XJ, et al. (2011) Assessing the quality of the first batch of evidence-based clinical practice guidelines in traditional Chinese medicine. J Tradit Chin Med 31: 376–381.
61. Xu J, Yang Y (2009) Traditional Chinese medicine in the Chinese health care system. Health Policy 90: 133–139.
62. Moret L, Lefort C, Terrien N (2012) [How to write, how to implement and how to evaluate a practice guideline in order to improve quality of care?]. Transfus Clin Biol 19: 174–177.

13

Anticonvulsive Effect of Paeoniflorin on Experimental Febrile Seizures in Immature Rats: Possible Application for Febrile Seizures in Children

Hitomi Hino[1], Hisaaki Takahashi[2,3], Yuka Suzuki[1], Junya Tanaka[2,3], Eiichi Ishii[1], Mitsumasa Fukuda[1,3]*

1 Department of Pediatrics, Ehime University Graduate School of Medicine, Shitsukawa, Toon, Ehime, Japan, **2** Department of Molecular and Cellular Physiology, Ehime University Graduate School of Medicine, Shitsukawa, Toon, Ehime, Japan, **3** Ehime Proteo-Medicine Research Center, Department of Basic and Clinical Neuroscience, Ehime University, Toon, Ehime, Japan

Abstract

Febrile seizures (FS) is the most common convulsive disorder in children, but there have been no clinical and experimental studies of the possible treatment of FS with herbal medicines, which are widely used in Asian countries. Paeoniflorin (PF) is a major bioactive component of Radix Paeoniae alba, and PF-containing herbal medicines have been used for neuromuscular, neuropsychiatric, and neurodegenerative disorders. In this study, we analyzed the anticonvulsive effect of PF and Keishikashakuyaku-to (KS; a PF-containing herbal medicine) for hyperthermia-induced seizures in immature rats as a model of human FS. When immature (P5) male rats were administered PF or KS for 10 days, hyperthermia-induced seizures were significantly suppressed compared to control rats. In cultured hippocampal neurons, PF suppressed glutamate-induced elevation of intracellular Ca^{2+} ($[Ca^{2+}]_i$), glutamate receptor-mediated membrane depolarization, and glutamate-induced neuronal death. In addition, PF partially suppressed the elevation in $[Ca^{2+}]_i$ induced by activation of the metabotropic glutamate receptor 5 (mGluR5), but not that mediated by α-amino-3-hydroxy-5-methyl-4-isoxazolpropionic acid (AMPA) or N-methyl-D-aspartate (NMDA) receptors. However, PF did not affect production or release of γ-aminobutyric acid (GABA) in hippocampal neurons. These results suggest that PF or PF-containing herbal medicines exert anticonvulsive effects at least in part by preventing mGluR5-dependent $[Ca^{2+}]_i$ elevations. Thus, it could be a possible candidate for the treatment of FS in children.

Editor: Anthony E. Kline, University of Pittsburgh, United States of America

Funding: This study was supported by a Grant-in-Aid for Scientific Research (C) of the Ministry of Education, Culture, Sports, Science and Technology of Japan, a Research Grant of the Japan Epilepsy Research Foundation, and a Research Promotion Award of Ehime University. The funders had no role in study design, data collection and analysis, decision to publish, or preparation of the manuscript.

Competing Interests: The authors have declared that no competing interests exist.

* E-mail: fukumits@m.ehime-u.ac.jp

Introduction

FS is the most common convulsive disorder in children; more than 5% of the normal population experience at least one attack of FS, and the incidence is estimated as high as 7–14% in Japan and the Pacific islands [1]. FS can be divided into subtypes according to severity, with 30–40% of patients having a complex type with seizures that are partial, prolonged, or repeated in the same illness. Although FS does not generally induce long-term brain damage or cognitive deficits, a relationship between a history of complex FS, especially prolonged FS, during early childhood and temporal lobe epilepsy with hippocampal sclerosis has been reported [2,3]. Therefore, it is important to prevent the recurrence of FS during childhood. Prophylactic use of antiepileptic drugs, especially phenobarbital and valproic acid, has previously been shown to reduce the recurrence of FS [4]. Unfortunately, long-term use of these drugs increases the incidence of adverse effects, such as drowsiness, hyperactivity, or learning difficulties by phenobarbital [5], and fatal liver damage by valproic acid [6]. Thus, less toxic therapeutic agents are urgently required for patients with complex FS.

Herbal medicines have been used in the treatment of several neurological disorders including epilepsy for many years [7,8]. PF, a major component of Radix Paeoniae alba, has been used for neuromuscular blocking, cognition enhancement, and immune-regulatory function [9–11]. A double-blind comparative study confirmed the usefulness of PF-containing herbal medicine for adult epileptic patients [7]. However, there have been no clinical or experimental studies of herbal medicines in children with FS.

The aim of this study was to assess the efficacy of PF and a PF-containing herbal medicine against hyperthermia-induced seizures in immature rats as a model of human FS [12,13]. Further, we investigated possible mechanisms underlying the effects of PF using cultured hippocampal neurons. We showed that PF suppressed hyperthermia-induced seizures, and that this action was associated with prevention of Ca^{2+} mobilization induced by stimulation of the metabotropic glutamate receptor (mGluR) 5. These findings suggest that PF has potential in the treatment of FS, and that the mGluR5 may be a new target for the development of new therapies for complex FS.

Results

Suppression of hyperthermia-induced seizures by KS and PF in immature rats

We evaluated the effects of PF and the PF-containing herbal medicine Keishikasyakuyaku-to (KS) on hyperthermia-induced seizures in immature rats. Oral PF, KS, or distilled water was administered for 10 days from P5, and the threshold temperature of hyperthermia-induced seizure onset was measured on P15 (Fig. 1A). Our preliminary data showed that hyperthermia induced a seizure in all rats, and that recovery was complete following the seizure. The hyperthermia-induced seizures were stereotyped, consisting of a sudden arrest of hyperthermia-induced hyperkinesias, together with facial automatism, and occasionally followed by body flexion. When the sudden immobility and facial automatism appeared at the onset of seizures, cortical EEG recordings showed moderately sustained semi-rhythmic activities or only sporadic spikes. However, deep electrodes implanted in the dorsal hippocampus revealed rhythmic ictal discharges concurrent with the onset of behavioral events (Fig. 1B). The brain temperature at the onset of the hippocampal ictal discharge was defined as the temperature at seizure onset.

As shown in Fig. 1C, the brain temperature at the onset of seizure was significantly higher in the KS group (median: 42.6°C, range: 41.9–43.0) than that in the control group (median: 40.7°C, range: 39.7–42.7°C) ($P = 0.008$), indicating that KS can suppress hyperthermia. The upper limit of brain temperature during hyperthermia was set at 43.0°C to avoid unphysiological hyperthermia, and one of the 6 rats in the KS group exhibited no seizure during the heating period.

We then investigated the effect of PF on seizures. The brain temperature at the onset of seizures was significantly higher in the PF group (median: 43.0°C, range: 41.9–43.0°C) than in the control group (median: 41.1°C, range: 40.5–41.8) ($P = 0.001$). Four of the 7 rats in the PF group did not have a seizure during the heating period (Fig. 1D). In rats of the KS and PF groups, the severity of some seizures was mild compared to the control group, with sudden immobility and facial automatism but without body flexion.

Effect of PF on GABA concentration in cultured hippocampal neurons

We previously demonstrated that reduced activity of the GABAergic system plays the role in the pathogenesis of hyperthermia-induced seizures in immature rats [14]. We here analyzed the protein levels of the GABA synthesizing enzymes GAD65/67, to confirm whether PF suppressed hyperthermia-induced seizures via the GABAergic system. Western blotting revealed that the protein level of GAD65/67 in the cultured hippocampal neurons did not change with PF treatment (Fig. 2A). We next assessed whether PF could affect GABA release from cultured hippocampal neurons. The GABA concentration in the medium was not affected by PF treatment, whereas it was elevated 2.45 fold upon addition of glutamate, which is known to induce seizures during hyperthermia (Fig. 2B).

Effect of PF on glutamate-induced intracellular Ca^{2+} elevation and neurotoxicity in cultured hippocampal neurons

The balance between glutamatergic and GABAergic neurotransmission is important in the pathophysiology of convulsive disorders and the pharmacological mechanism of anticonvulsants. As shown in Fig. 2, PF treatment did not influence the GABAergic system. Therefore, to assess the effect of PF on the excitatory system, we investigated whether PF could change the $[Ca^{2+}]_i$ elevation induced in hippocampal neurons by exposure to glutamate. As shown in Fig. 3, glutamate exposure induced an elevation of $[Ca^{2+}]_i$ in hippocampal neurons. When the neurons were pretreated with PF (200 μM) for 48 h before the glutamate exposure, the $[Ca^{2+}]_i$ was significantly decreased.

It is well known that aberrant elevations of $[Ca^{2+}]_i$ has neurotoxic effects [15]. In the current study, we observed cell damage, such as reduction of processes and shrinkage of somata, after glutamate stimulation. PF decreased this cell damage in a dose-dependent manner (Fig. 4A). We further performed a lactate dehydrogenase (LDH) cytotoxicity assay to analyze the effect of PF on cell damage. LDH release was measured to evaluate total glutamate-induced cell death. LDH release occurred during excessive glutamate stimulation, and PF decreased this LDH release in a dose-dependent manner (Fig. 4B). These results suggest that PF has an ability to suppress glutamate-induced neuronal hyperexcitability caused by aberrant elevations of $[Ca^{2+}]_i$.

We further assessed changes in membrane potential using the voltage-sensitive dye $DiBAC_4(3)$. Glutamate caused a significant depolarization of hippocampal neurons. When neurons were treated with PF prior to glutamate stimulation, the change in membrane potential was significantly suppressed compared to control (Fig. 5A). In contrast to glutamate, KCl increases $[Ca^{2+}]_i$ through the opening of voltage-dependent calcium channels (VDCC). Fig. 5B shows that the same degree of depolarization was seen in PF-treated and control neurons during KCl stimulation, indicating that the effect of PF is dependent on glutamate receptors, but not on VDCCs.

Effect of PF on elevations in intracellular Ca^{2+} concentration caused by exposure to mGluR5 agonist

We next used agonists of the NMDA receptor, AMPA receptor and mGluR5, which are the main glutamate receptors in the hippocampus, to reveal the point of action of PF [16]. PF inhibited the Ca^{2+} response induced by mGluR5 agonist, (R, S)-2-chloro-5-hydroxyphenylglycine (CHPG), but did not affect the response to NMDA or AMPA (Fig. 6).

Discussion

Prophylactic use of antiepileptic drugs has been considered to reduce the recurrence of complex FS [4], but it can also induce several side effects, such as drowsiness, hyperactivity, or learning difficulties by phenobarbital [5] and weight gain, nausea, hair loss, or liver injury by valproic acid [6,17–19]. The development of less toxic prophylactic treatments for complex FS is thus necessary to help children with FS, and we therefore analyzed the effect of a herbal medicine that has been widely used in Asian countries.

Previous studies have shown that PF-containing herbal medicines or PF metabolites inhibit experimental seizures in EL mice, a natural model of multifactorial idiopathic generalized epilepsy [20–22]. In addition, metabolites of PF showed not only an inhibitory effect on pentylenetetrazole (PTZ)-induced EEG power spectrum changes, but also had a protective effect on hippocampal neuronal damage in the cobalt-induced epilepsy model in adult rats [23,24]. However, the effect of PF in infant or immature rats is still unknown.

We used rats of an immature age (P14–15) as a model of human FS [25]. Neville et al. [26] reported that the majority of FS show a focal origin and arise from the hippocampus, although FS are usually recognized as a generalized seizure type. In our immature

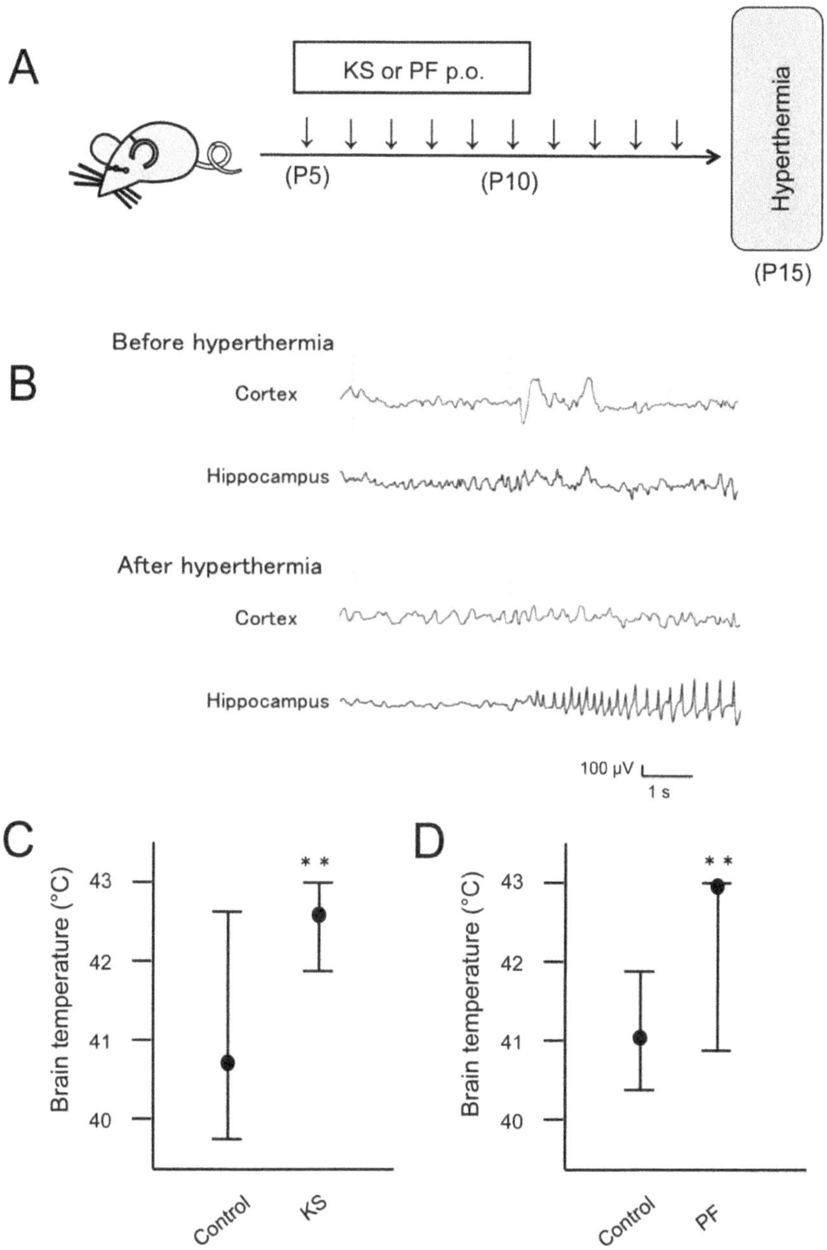

Figure 1. Effects of KS and PF on hyperthermia-induced seizures in immature rats. (A) Experimental schedule of drug administration. P5, P10 and P15 indicate the age of rats. (B) EEGs from cortex and hippocampus before and after hyperthermia. Before hyperthermia, EEG in both areas showed slight sustained irregular activities and a movement artifact. During hyperthermia, rhythmic ictal discharges concurrent with behavioral events were observed on hippocampal recording, and the start of this ictal discharges was defined as the onset of seizure. (C) and (D) Brain temperature at the seizure onset. The data are represented as median and range. KS, Keishikasyakuyaku-to; PF, Paeoniflorin. ** indicate $P<0.01$.

rat model, ictal discharges during behavioral seizures originated from the hippocampus when the brain temperature was within a physiological range, consistent with previous studies [27]. Therefore, our model is thought to be suitable for the analysis of the mechanism of human FS and its prevention by less toxic drugs.

The anticonvulsive mechanisms of PF remain to be fully elucidated. Among several factors, the balance between glutamatergic and GABAergic neurotransmission may contribute to the pathogenesis of convulsive disorders. It was reported that the GABA concentration in the cerebrospinal fluid (CSF) was lower in children with complex FS than in control groups [28]. Some patients with FS-related disorders were found to have a mutation in the $GABA_A$ receptor $\gamma 2$ subunit [29]. The fact that the $GABA_A$ receptor agonists benzodiazepine and phenobarbital are clinically effective against FS supports this possibility. We previously showed that a GABA agonist suppressed hyperthermia-induced seizures in developing rats, whereas blockade of $GABA_A$ receptors or GABA synthesis enhanced them [14]. In addition, whole-cell patch clamp recordings showed that hyperthermia could suppress $GABA_A$-receptor-mediated inhibition in the immature rat hippocampus [30]. These findings indicate that inadequate GABAergic function is involved in the pathogenesis of FS. On the other hand, Knight et

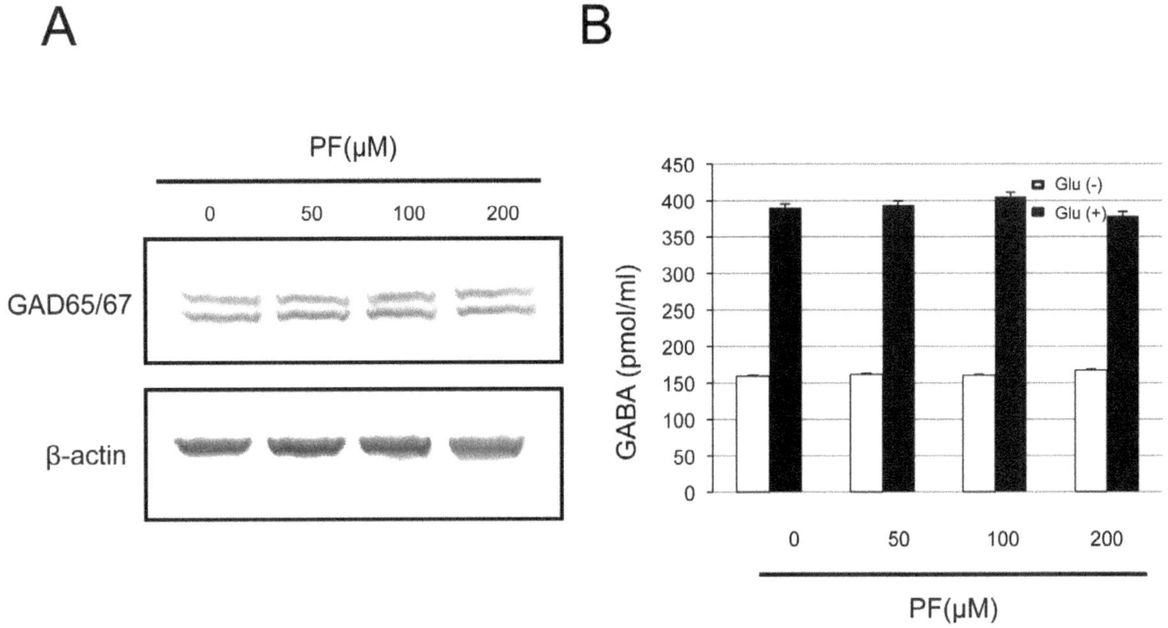

Figure 2. Effect of PF on the GABA production of cultured hippocampal neurons. (A) Western blot analysis of GAD65/67 protein level in cell lysates of cultured hippocampal neurons cultured in the presence of PF at the indicated concentration for 2 days. β-actin was used as a loading control. (B) Hippocampal neurons at 9 DIV were cultured in the presence of PF at the indicated concentration for 2 days. The GABA concentration was measured in the culture medium as described in Materials and Methods. The induction by L-glutamate (125 μM) was performed for 30 min in cultured hippocampal neurons. Each column represents the mean ± SE (n = 4).

al. [31] suggested that the CSF levels of GABA did not change in patients with first-time febrile seizures. Although further studies are needed to elucidate the GABA-dependent mechanisms of PF anticonvulsant action, we found no effects of PF treatment on GABA production or release in hippocampal neurons.

Excessive neuronal stimulation by glutamate may also be related to convulsive disorders, and is known to play an important role in the induction of experimental FS [32]. It was reported that glutamate levels in the immature rat cortex increased with the elevation in body temperature during hyperthermia-induced seizures, and the NMDA receptor blocker MK-801 inhibited the seizures [33]. Excess glutamate is toxic by increasing $[Ca^{2+}]_i$, free radicals and protease activity, then inducing cell death [34]. Evidence for a role of Ca^{2+} in epileptogenesis has been shown in hippocampal slices and cultured hippocampal neurons [35,36]. Furthermore, pharmacological studies on anticonvulsant properties of Ca^{2+} antagonists in mouse have provided a direct link between Ca^{2+} channel function and susceptibility to PTZ-induced seizures [37]. Concerning the pharmacological actions of PF, it was reported that PF treatment suppressed the $[Ca^{2+}]_i$ elevation induced by glutamate stimulation in rat pheochromocytoma (PC12) cells [38]. However, there have been no previous reports of an involvement of Ca^{2+} signaling in the anticonvulsant actions of PF. In the current study, we showed that PF suppressed the glutamate-induced $[Ca^{2+}]_i$ increase and membrane depolarization in cultured hippocampal neurons, suggesting that the anticonvulsant effect of PF is Ca^{2+}-dependent. This inhibiting effect of PF on $[Ca^{2+}]_i$ elevations may reduce the neuronal hyperexcitability induced by glutamate.

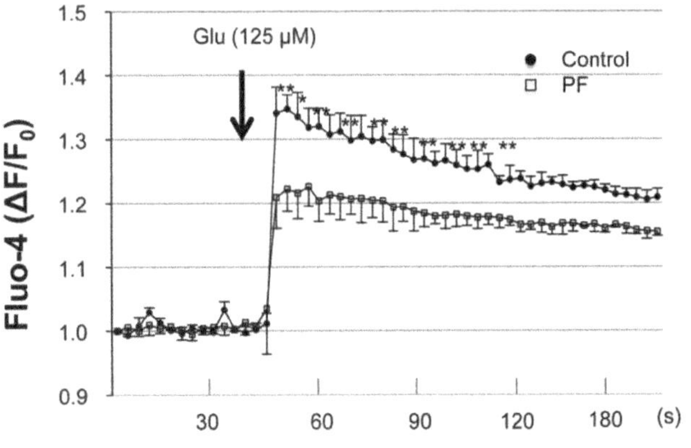

Figure 3. Reduction of glutamate-induced intracellular Ca^{2+} response in cultured hippocampal neurons by PF. Intracellular Ca^{2+} levels in Fluo-4-loaded cultured hippocampal neurons were monitored as the change of fluorescence intensity at 2 s intervals. Arrow indicates the time point of glutamate (125 μM) addition. Values represent mean ± SE of three independent experiments. *$P<0.05$ compared to control group.

Although excessive glutamate stimulation during seizures may lead to neuronal death, hyperthermia-induced seizures themselves do not cause neuronal death in rat hippocampus [39]. However, retrospective studies have demonstrated a significant relationship between a history of prolonged FS during early childhood and TLE-HS as sequel to hippocampal neuronal death [40]. In the current study, PF suppressed cell death induced by glutamate in cultured hippocampal neurons. Continuous PF treatment in patients with complex FS might contribute to the prevention of TLE-HS.

We demonstrated that PF significantly suppressed the $[Ca^{2+}]_i$ elevation induced by glutamate, but not that induced by AMPA or NMDA. These results suggest that PF influences Ca^{2+} levels via mGluRs. The mGluR family comprises eight G protein-coupled

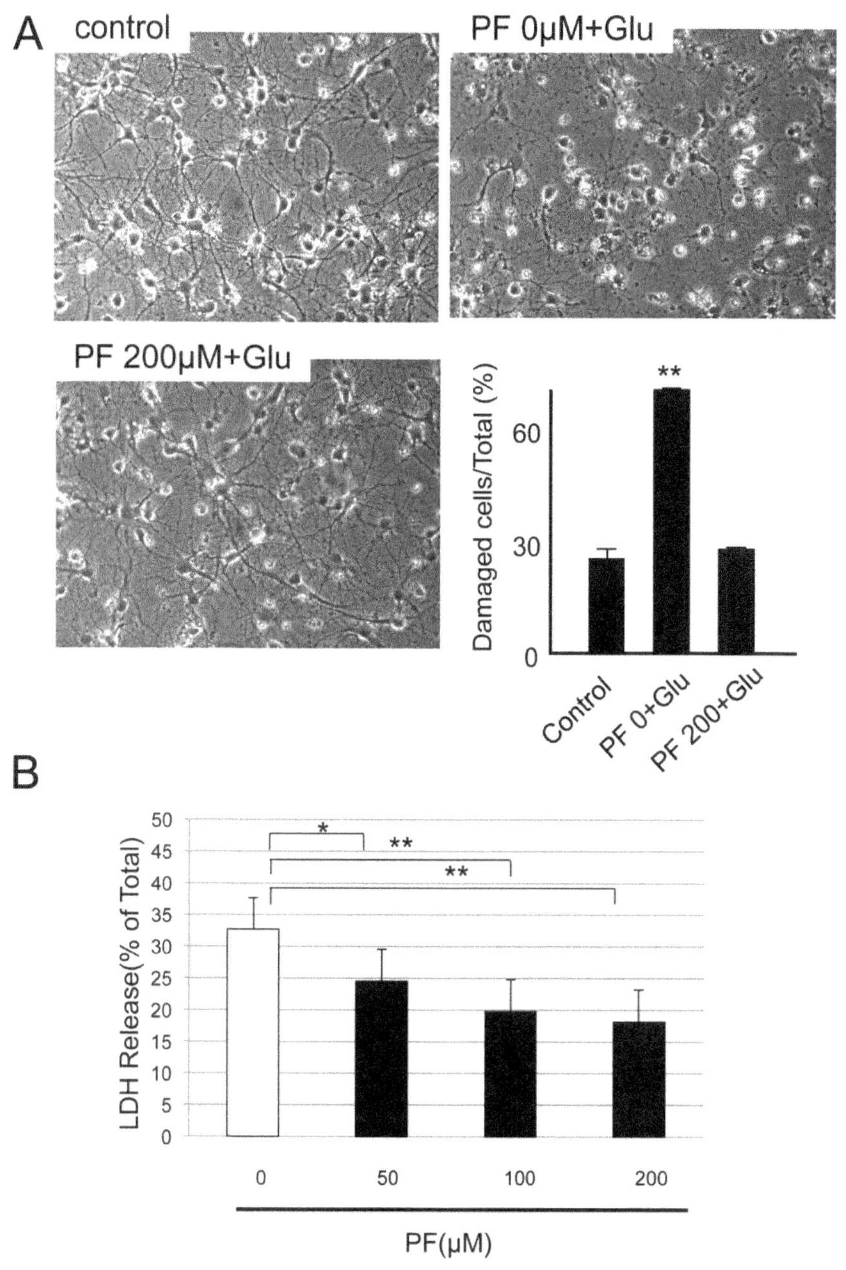

Figure 4. Protective effect of PF against glutamatergic neurotoxicity on cultured hippocampal neurons. Hippocampal neurons at 9 DIV were cultured in the presence of PF at indicated concentration for 2 days, treated with glutamate (500 μM) for 30 min, then the medium was replaced with culture medium followed by further culture for one day. (A) Cells were photographed under a phase contrast microscope, and quantitation of damaged hippocampal neurons with somata shrinkage after glutamatergic neurotoxicity was counted. The column indicates percentage (%) of damaged cells in total cells. Each column represents mean ± SE (n = 3). (B) Cell viability was measured by LDH assay. Each column indicates a percentage (%) of released LDH into the medium compared to total LDH. Values represent by mean ± SE (n = 4). $^{*}P<0.02$, $^{**}P<0.001$ compared to control group.

receptors, which are classified into three groups (Groups I–III) according to sequence homology, effector coupling, and agonist selectivity. Group I mGluRs (mGluR1 and mGluR5) are coupled to phosphatidylinositol hydrolysis/Ca^{2+} signal transduction, and activation leads to a variety of cellular responses, including inhibition of Ca^{2+} and K^{+} currents, presynaptic modulation of synaptic transmission, and postsynaptic interaction with ionotropic glutamate receptors [41]. Group I mGluRs are especially important for the regulation of neuronal excitability. In general, activation of group I receptors enhances or facilitates the excitatory effects of glutamate by modulation of ion channel activity. Antagonists of group I mGluRs have been proposed to exhibit potential positive therapeutic effects in CNS disorders related to excessive excitatory neurotransmission, such as epilepsy, ischemia, and pain [42]. A previous study using mGluR5 knock-out mice indicated an involvement of the receptor in hippocampus-dependent learning and memory [43]. In the current study, PF treatment suppressed the $[Ca^{2+}]_i$ elevation caused by a selective

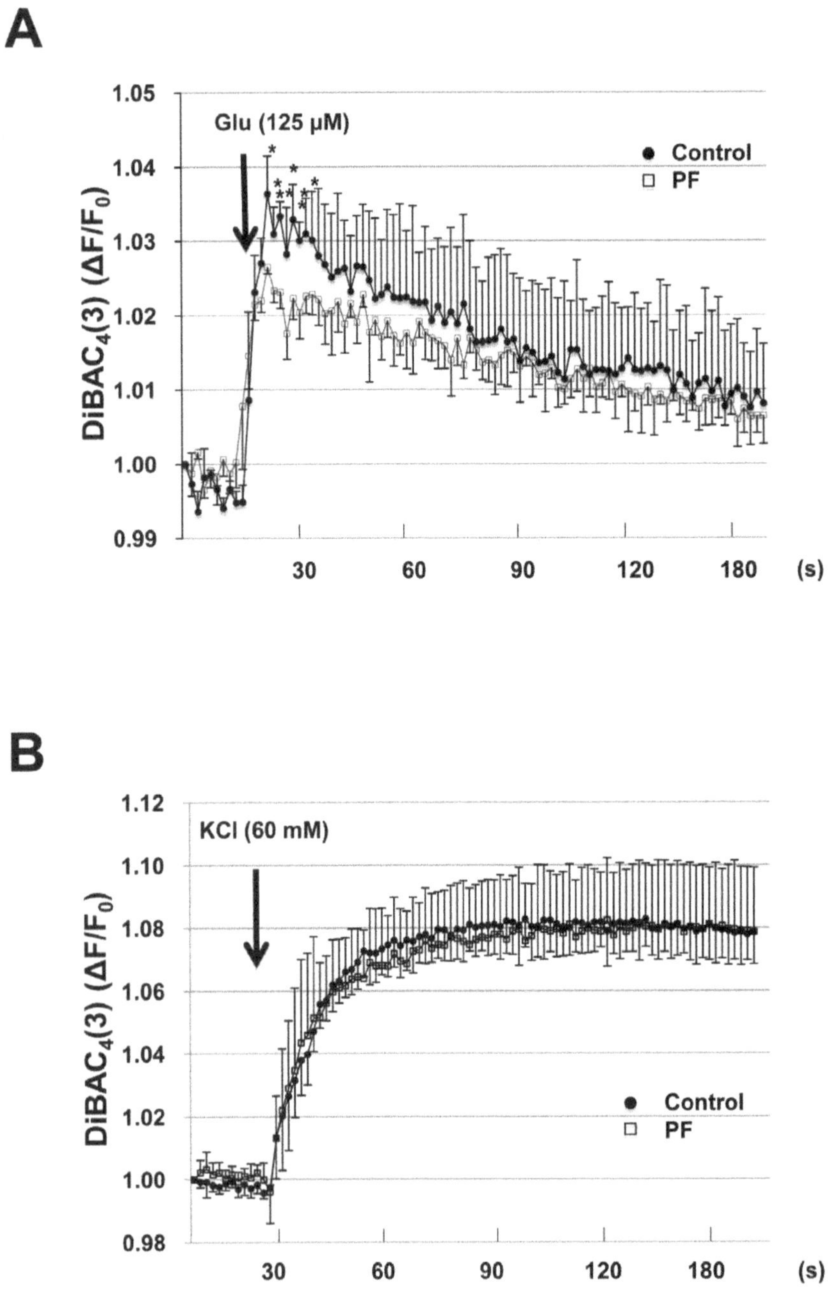

Figure 5. Effect of PF on the membrane depolarization of cultured hippocampal neurons. The membrane depolarization of cultured hippocampal neurons by 125 μM glutamate (A) and 60 mM KCl (B) detected as the change of fluorescence intensity of $DiBAC_4(3)$ at 2 s intervals. Values represent mean ± SE (n = 4). *$P<0.05$ compared to control group.

mGluR5 agonist to about 10% of the peak in the control group. This suggests that PF might be a negative modulator of the mGluR5 and PF treatment might not cause severe side effect.

In summary, PF suppressed hyperthermia-induced seizures in immature rats, and inhibited glutamate-mediated $[Ca^{2+}]_i$ elevation, depolarization, and cell death via a mechanism involving the mGluR5. Our results indicate that PF may be a negative modulator of mGluR5, shedding new light on its potential in the development of new prophylactic treatments for complex FS.

Materials and Methods

Animals

Male Lewis rats (Charles River Laboratories Japan, Yokohama, Japan) were kept with their mothers on a 12-h light/12-h dark cycle, with free access to food and water. All experimental procedures conformed to guidelines from the Ministry of Education of Japan, and were approved by the animal experimental committee of Ehime University.

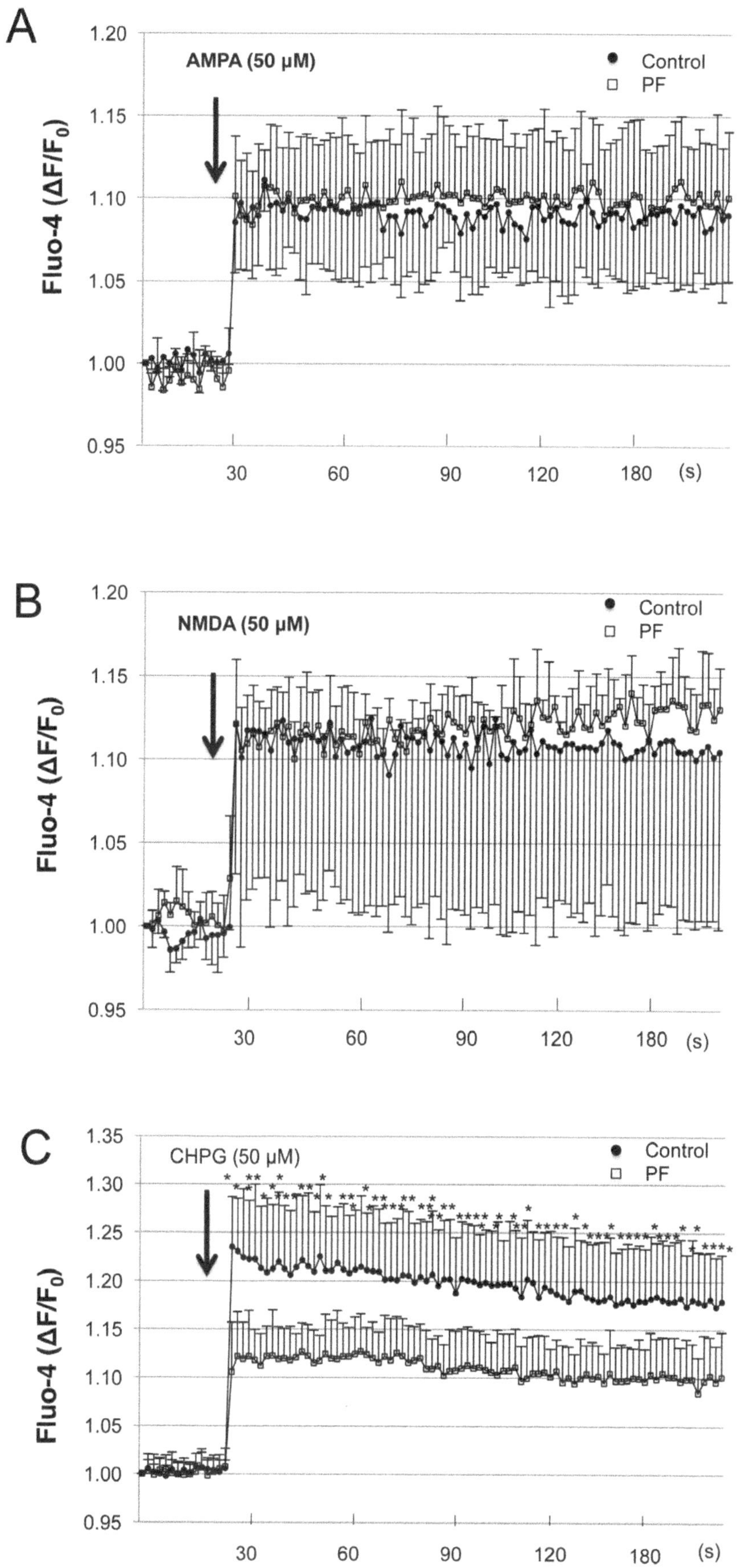
A
AMPA (50 μM)
Control
PF
Fluo-4 (ΔF/F0)
1.20
1.15
1.10
1.05
1.00
0.95
30
60
90
120
180
(s)
B
NMDA (50 μM)
Control
PF
Fluo-4 (ΔF/F0)
1.20
1.15
1.10
1.05
1.00
0.95
30
60
90
120
180
(s)
C
CHPG (50 μM)
Control
PF
Fluo-4 (ΔF/F0)
1.35
1.30
1.25
1.20
1.15
1.10
1.05
1.00
0.95
30
60
90
120
180
(s)

Figure 6. Effect of PF on intracellular Ca^{2+} response in cultured hippocampal neurons stimulated by AMPA, NMDA and CHPG. Intracellular Ca^{2+} levels in Fluo-4-loaded cultured hippocampal neurons were monitored as the change of fluorescence intensity at 2 s intervals. Arrow indicates the time point of AMPA (50 μM), NMDA (50 μM), and CHPG (50 μM) addition. Values represent mean ± SE of three independent experiments. *P<0.05 compared to control group.

Monitoring of electroencephalography and brain temperature

On P12, male rats were implanted with silver electroencephalography (EEG) electrodes under anesthesia with an intraperitoneal (i.p.) injection of pentobarbital sodium (25 mg/kg). Cefotaxime sodium was injected to prevent bacterial infections (500 mg/kg, i.p.). The head was fixed in a stereotaxic frame (Narishige, Tokyo, Japan), and two holes were made in the skull over the right frontal and left central regions for placement of silver cortical EEG electrodes. A stereotaxic depth EEG electrode (0.3 mm diameter; Unique Medical, Tokyo, Japan) was inserted through a central hole into the dorsal hippocampus (AP = −4.0, L = 3.0, V = −4.0 mm relative to bregma). Another hole was made over the right central cortex for placement of the needle brain temperature thermometer (Unique Medical).

Drug administration and induction of hyperthermia-induced seizures

On P5, male Lewis rats were divided into two groups: KS (n = 7) and control (n = 8). KS (600 mg/kg; Tsumura, Tokyo, Japan) was dissolved in distilled water to a total volume of 25 μl and administered orally once a day, for 10 days starting at P5. Rats in the control group received only distilled water. On P15, rats were placed in a plastic cage and seizures were induced by moist warm air (42–43°C) while monitoring EEG activity (Fig. 1A). The brain temperature was measured at seizure onset, which was defined based on EEG and behavior. After seizure induction, rats were removed and placed on a cool surface. The upper limit of brain temperature during hyperthermia was set at 43.0°C. We carried out a similar experiment using PF. For this, rats were divided into two groups: PF (n = 8) and control (n = 8). PF (100 mg/kg; Wako, Osaka, Japan) was dissolved in distilled water to a total volume of 25 μl and orally administered daily for 10 days starting from P5. Rats in the control group received distilled water only.

After the hyperthermia-induced seizure, we applied a 10-s direct current (100 μA) to the electrodes using a current rectifier (SEN-7103; Nihon Kohden, Tokyo, Japan) to mark up the location of the electrode. Rats were anesthetized with diethyl ether (Kanto Chemical, Tokyo, Japan), and the brains were quickly removed and fixed with 4% paraformaldehyde overnight at 4°C. After dehydration in 30% sucrose for at least 24 h, the brains were sectioned coronally and stained to confirm the electrode orientation. Three rats were excluded from analysis due to inappropriate location of electrodes (one in the KS group, one in the PF group, and one in the control group).

Hippocampal neuron culture

Rat embryos were removed from the uterus of pregnant Lewis rat at E20 and decapitated. Hippocampal tissues were carefully dissected out under the dissection microscope. Manipulations were performed under inhalation anesthesia with diethyl ether (Wako). Mechanically minced hippocampi were incubated with 0.05% trypsin/EDTA to dissociate cells for 10 min at 37°C. After the incubation, 100 μg/ml DNase I was added, and the cell suspension was triturated with pipettes. The trypsinization was quenched by fetal bovine serum. The cell suspension was filtered with a 75 μm mesh and centrifuged at 1,000 rpm. The cells were re-suspended in Neurobasal medium (Life technologies Japan, Tokyo, Japan) supplemented with B27 supplement (Life technologies Japan), 500 μM glutamine, and a penicillin/streptomycin/amphotericin B mixture (Sigma-Aldrich, St. Louis, MO, USA), and were grown for 9–11 days *in vitro* (DIV) on poly-L-lysine-coated cell culture plates.

GABA production

Hippocampal neurons were treated with PF (0, 50, 100, 200 μM) for 48 h. To assess the effect of PF on GABA neurons, we measured GABA release in the culture supernatant of cultured hippocampal neurons before and after stimulation by glutamate (500 μM) for 30 min. GABA was detected with high performance liquid chromatography (SRL, Tokyo, Japan).

We also assessed the levels of the GABA synthesis enzyme glutamic acid decarboxylase (GAD) by western blotting. Hippocampal neurons were re-suspended in Laemmli's sample solution after treatment with PF. The lysates were electrophoresed, transferred to nitrocellulose membranes, and incubated with antibodies against β-actin (mouse monoclonal, 1:1,000, Sigma-Aldrich) and GAD65/67 (rabbit polyclonal, 1:1,000, Sigma-Aldrich). The blots were visualized with alkaline phosphatase-labeled secondary antibodies (Promega, Tokyo, Japan) with nitroblue tetrazolium (Sigma-Aldrich) and 5-bromo-4-chloro-3-indolyl phosphate (Sigma-Aldrich) serving as the substrates.

LDH assay

Hippocampal neurons were exposed to a medium containing 500 μM glutamate (Wako) for 30 min. After treatment, cells were washed with culture medium or medium supplemented with PF. After 48 h, phase images of neurons were taken. To measure glutamate-induced cell death, LDH release was measured using a cytotoxicity detection kit (Roche Diagnostics, Tokyo, Japan), as previously described [44]. Briefly, hippocampal neurons at 8 DIV in 96-well plates were stimulated by glutamate (500 μM) for 30 min at 37°C. Neurons were washed in extracellular solution and incubated in cell culture medium for 16 h. Five microliters of cell lysis solution was added to cells, and the LDH activity in this sample was taken as the maximum LDH activity. After 15 min, 100 μl of the supernatant of each cell culture well was transferred to the corresponding well of a fresh 96-well plate and mixed with 100 μl of the LDH substrate. After incubation with protection from light at room temperature for 10 min, the reaction was stopped by adding 50 μl of stop buffer, and the absorbance was measured at 490 nm with a plate reader (Bio-Rad, Tokyo, Japan). The LDH release percentage was calculated by the formula: 100×(experimental culture medium background)/(maximum LDH release culture medium background). All experiments were repeated four times and the average LDH release percentage is shown in the figures.

Ca^{2+} assay

Hippocampal neurons were seeded at a density of 50,000 cells/ml into 96-well plates. After 10 DIV, the cells were loaded with a medium supplemented with 5 μM of the Ca^{2+}-sensitive fluorescent dye Fluo-4 AM (DOJINDO, Kumamoto, Japan) and 0.04% pluronic acid for 30 min at 37°C. The loading solution was then aspirated and 100 μl/well of assay buffer—Hank's balanced salt solution supplemented with 20 mM HEPES—was added. Cells were stimulated with glutamate (125 μM), NMDA (Merck, Tokyo, Japan), or AMPA (Wako), diluted in distilled H_2O, and CHPG (Tocris Bioscience, Bristol, UK) diluted in 0.1 M NaOH. After placing both plates (cell culture and compound plate) into the FlexStation3 (Molecular Devices Japan, Tokyo, Japan), fluorescence changes were measured at 37°C. Online additions were carried out in a volume of 20 μl/well. Agonists were incubated for 5 min before addition of the agonist. The traces represent the light emission alterations of Fluo-4 (recorded between 495 nm and 518 nm), with an increase in the fluorescence ratio reflecting an elevation in cytosolic free Ca^{2+}. The relative fluorescence change over time was calculated relative to the fluorescence measured at the beginning of the glutamate stimulation ($\Delta F/F_0$), and was expressed as relative $[Ca^{2+}]_i$.

Membrane potential changes

Changes in membrane potential were measured using $DiBAC_4(3)$ (DOJINDO), which is a bis-barbituric acid oxonol dye with an excitation maximum at approximately 488 nm. The cells were incubated in 5 μM $DiBAC_4(3)$ in a HEPES-buffered solution at 37°C for 30 min prior to the fluorescence measurement. The stained cells were used for experiments without washing. Fluorescence was monitored with Flexstation3 using the excitation and emission wavelengths of 488 and 517 nm, respectively. For the experiments, background fluorescence was measured every 2 s for 2 min before addition of KCl (60 mM) or glutamate (125 μM). After adding KCl or glutamate, fluorescence was measured every 2 s for 18 min in the $DiBAC_4(3)$ solution.

Statistics

To assess changes in brain temperature, GABA, and LDH, one-way ANOVA with Scheffe's multiple comparisons test were used. When data were not normally distributed, the Mann-Whitney U-test, Kruskal-Wallis test, and Dunn's post hoc test were used. For the Ca^{2+} assay and membrane potential measurements, unpaired two-tailed student's t-tests were used. SPSS version 15.0J was used for all analysis. Data were expressed as mean ± standard error (SE) or as median (range), and $P<0.05$ was considered to be significant.

Acknowledgments

We thank the Department of Bioscience and Biological Resources, INCS, Ehime University for technical assistance.

Author Contributions

Conceived and designed the experiments: HH HT JT EI MF. Performed the experiments: HH HT YS MF. Analyzed the data: HH HT MF. Contributed reagents/materials/analysis tools: HH HT MF. Wrote the paper: HH HT EI MF.

References

1. Hauser WA (1994) The prevalence and incidence of convulsive disorders in children. Epilepsia 35: S1–S6.
2. Camfield C, Camfield P (2005) Febrile seizures. In: Roger J, Bureau M, Dravet C, Genton P, Tassinari CA, Wolf P, editors. Epileptic syndrome in infancy, childhood and adolescence 4th edition: Montrouge: John Libbey Eurotext. pp. 159–169.
3. Cendes F, Kahane P, Brodie M, Andermann F (2005) The mesio-temporal lobe epilepsy syndrome. In: Rojer J, Bureau M, Dravet C, Genton P, Tassinari CA, Wolf P, editors. Epileptic syndromes in infancy, childhood and adolescence 4th edition. Montrouge: John Libbey Eurotext. pp. 555–575.
4. Lux AL (2010) Treatment of febrile seizures: historical perspective, current opinions, and potential future directions. Brain Dev 32: 42–50.
5. Zhang LL, Zeng LN, Li YP (2011) Side effects of phenobarbital in epilepsy: a systematic review. Epileptic Disord 13: 349–365.
6. Anderson GD (2002) Children versus adults: pharmacokinetic and adverse-effect differences. Epilepsia 43: 53–9.
7. Nagakubo S, Niwa S, Kumagai N, Fukuda M, Anzai N, et al. (1993) Effects of TJ-960 on Sternberg's paradigm results in epileptic patients. Jpn J Psychiatry Neurol 47: 609–620.
8. Hiratsuka T, Matsuzaki S, Miyata S, Kinoshita M, Kakehi K, et al. (2010) Yokukansan inhibits neuronal death during ER stress by regulating the unfolded protein response. PLoS One. 5: e13280.
9. Dezaki K, Kimura I, Miyahara K, Kimura M (1995) Complementary effects of paeoniflorin and glycyrrhizin on intracellular Ca^{2+} mobilization in the nerve-stimulated skeletal muscle of mice. Jpn J Pharmacol 69: 281–284.
10. Watanabe H (1997) Candidates for cognitive enhancer extracted from medicinal plants: paeoniflorin and tetramethylpyrazine. Behav Brain Res 83: 135–141.
11. Tang NY, Liu CH, Hsieh CT, Hsieh CL (2010) The anti-inflammatory effect of paeoniflorin on cerebral infarction induced by ischemia-reperfusion injury in Sprague-Dawley rats. Am J Chin Med 38: 51–64.
12. Hjeresen DL, Diaz J (1988) Ontogeny of susceptibility to experimental febrile seizures in rats. Dev Psychobiol 21: 261–275.
13. Baram TZ, Schultz L (1991) Corticotropin-releasing hormone is a rapid and potent convulsant in the infant rat. Dev Brain Res 61: 97–101.
14. Fukuda M, Morimoto T, Nagao H, Kida K (1997) The effect of GABAergic system activity on hyperthermia-induced seizures in rat. Dev Brain Res 104: 197–199.
15. Siesjö BK, Bengtsson F, Grampp W, Theander S. (1989) Calcium, excitotoxins, and neuronal death in the brain. Ann N Y Acad Sci 568: 234–251.
16. Shigemoto R, Kinoshita A, Wada E, Nomura S, Ohishi H, et al. (1997) Differential presynaptic localization of metabotropic glutamate receptor subtypes in the rat hippocampus. J Neurosci 17: 7503–7522.
17. Verrotti A, D'Egidio C, Mohn A, Coppola G, Chiarelli F (2011) Weight gain following treatment with valproic acid: pathogenetic mechanisms and clinical implications. Obes Rev 12: 32–43
18. Zarate CA, Jr Tohen M, Narendran R, Tomassini EC, McDonald J, et al. (1999) The adverse effect profile and efficacy of divalproex sodium compared with valproic acid: a pharmacoepidemiology study. J Clin Psychiatry 60: 232–236.
19. Castro-Gago M, Pérez-Gay L, Gómez-Lado C, Castiñeiras-Ramos DE, Otero-Martínez S, et al. (2011) The influence of valproic acid and carbamazepine treatment on serum biotin and zinc levels and on biotinidase activity. J Child Neurol 26: 1522–1524.
20. Sugaya E, Ishige A, Sekiguchi K, Iizuka S, Sugimoto A, et al. (1988) Inhibitory effect of a mixture of herbal drugs (TJ-960, SK) on pentylenetetrazol-induced convulsions in E1 mice. Epilepsy Res 2: 337–339.
21. Sugaya E, Ishige A, Sekiguchi K, Iizuka S, Ito K, et al. (1988) Inhibitory effect of TJ-960 (SK) on pentylenetetrazol-induced EEG power spectrum changes. Epilepsy Res 2: 27–31.
22. Abdel-Hafez AA, Meselhy MR, Nakamura N, Hattori M, Watanabe H, et al. (1999) Anticonvulsant activity of Paeonimetabolin-I Adducts obtained by incubation of paeoniflorin and thiol compounds with Lactobacillus brevis. Chem Pharm Bull (Tokyo) 22: 491–497.
23. Sugaya A, Suzuki T, Sugaya E, Yuyama N, Yasuda K, et al. (1991) Inhibitory effect of peony root extract on pentylenetetrazol-induced EEG power spectrum changes and extracellular calcium concentration changes in rat cerebral cortex. J Ethnopharmacol 33: 159–167.
24. Tsuda T, Sugaya A, Ohguchi H, Kishida N, Sugaya E (1997) Protective effects of peony root extract and its components on neuron damage in the hippocampus induced by the cobalt focus epilepsy model. Exp Neurol 146: 518–525.
25. Dobbing J (1973) Nutrition and the developing brain. Lancet 1:48
26. Neville B, Gindner D (2010) Febrile seizures are a syndrome of secondarily generalized hippocampal epilepsy. Dev Med Child Neurol 52: 1151–1153.
27. Dube C, Vezzani A, Behrens M, Bartfai T, Baram TZ (2005) Interleukin-1beta contributes to the generation of experimental febrile seizures. Ann Neurol 57: 152–155.
28. Rating D, Siemes H, Löscher W (1983) Low CSF GABA concentration in children with febrile convulsions, untreated epilepsy, and meningitis. J Neurol 230: 217–225.
29. Audenaert D, Schwartz E, Claeys KG, Claes L, Deprez L, et al. (2006) A novel GABRG2 mutation associated with febrile seizures. Neurology 67: 687–690.
30. Qu L, Leung LS (2008) Mechanisms of hyperthermia-induced depression of GABAergic synaptic transmission in the immature rat hippocampus. J Neurochem 106: 2158–2169.
31. Knight M, Ebert J, Parish RA, Berry H, Fogelson MH (1985) Gamma-Aminobutyric acid in CSF of children with febrile seizures. Arch Neurol 42: 474–475.
32. Freeman AR (1976) Polyfunctional role of glutamic acid in excitatory synaptic transmission. Prog Neurobiol 13:137–153.
33. Morimoto T, Kida K, Nagao H, Yoshida K, Fukuda M, et al. (1995) The pathogenic role of the NMDA receptor in hyperthermia-induced seizures in developing rats. Dev Brain Res 84: 204–207.

34. Frandsen A, Schousboe A (1993) Excitatory amino acid-mediated cytotoxicity and calcium homeostasis in cultured neurons, J Neurochem 60:1202–1211.
35. Raza M, Pal S, Rafiq A, DeLorenzo RJ (2001) Long-term alteration of calcium homeostatic mechanisms in the pilocarpine model of temporal lobe epilepsy. Brain Res 903: 1–12.
36. Pal S, Sun D, Limbrick D, Rafiq A, DeLorenzo RJ (2001) Epileptogenesis induces long-term alterations in intracellular calcium release and sequestration mechanisms in the hippocampal neuronal culture model of epilepsy. Cell Calcium 30: 285–296.
37. Shitak R, Sahai AK, Hota D, Chakrabarti A (2007) Evaluation of the modulatory role of nimodipine in seizures induced by kainic acid and pentylenetetrazole in mice. Methods Find Exp Clin Pharmacol 29: 11–17.
38. Mao QQ, Zhong XM, Feng CR, Pan AJ, Li ZY, et al. (2010) Protective effects of paeoniflorin against glutamate-induced neurotoxicity in PC12 cells via antioxidant mechanisms and Ca^{2+} antagonism. Cell Mol Neurobiol 30: 1059–1066.
39. Bender RA, Dubé C, Gonzalez-Vega R, Mina EW, Baram TZ (2003) Mossy fiber plasticity and enhanced hippocampal excitability, without hippocampal cell loss or altered neurogenesis, in an animal model of prolonged febrile seizures. Hippocampus 13: 399–412.
40. Tanabe T, Hara K, Shimakawa S, Fukui M, Tamai H (2011) Hippocampal damage after prolonged febrile seizure: one case in a consecutive prospective series. Epilepsia 52: 837–840.
41. Nakanishi S, Nakajima Y, Masu M, Ueda Y, Nakahara K, et al. (1998) Glutamate receptors: brain function and signal transduction. Brain Res Rev 26: 230–235.
42. Nicoletti F, Bruno V, Copani A, Casabona G, Knopfel T (1996) Metabotropic glutamate receptors: a new target for the therapy of neurodegenerative disorders? Trends Neurosci 19: 267–271.
43. Lu YM, Jia Z, Janus C, Henderson JT, Gerlai R, et al. (1997) Mice lacking metabotropic glutamate receptor 5 show impaired learning and reduced CA1 long-term potentiation (LTP) but normal CA3 LTP. J Neurosci 17: 5196–5205.
44. Suzuki Y, Takahashi H, Fukuda M, Hino H, Kobayashi K, et al. (2009) Beta-hydroxybutyrate alters GABA-transaminase activity in cultured astrocytes. Brain Res 1:17–23.

14

Chinese Herbal Medicines for the Treatment of Type A H1N1 Influenza: A Systematic Review of Randomized Controlled Trials

Wei Chen[1], Chi Eung Danforn Lim[2], Hong-Jun Kang[3], Jianping Liu[1,4]*

1 Centre For Evidence-Based Chinese Medicine, Beijing University of Chinese Medicine, Beijing, China, **2** Faculty of Medicine, South Western Sydney Clinical School, University of New South Wales, Sydney, Australia, **3** Intensive Care Unit, Chinese PLA General Hospital, Beijing, China, **4** NAFKAM, University of Tromso, Tromso, Norway

Abstract

Background: Chinese herbs are thought to be effective for type A H1N1 influenza. Series of Chinese herbs have been authorized recommended by the Chinese government, and until now a number of clinical trials of Chinese herbs for H1N1 influenza have been conducted. However, there is no critically appraised evidence such as systematic reviews or meta-analyses on potential benefits and harms of medicinal herbs for H1N1 influenza to justify their clinical use and their recommendation.

Methods and Findings: CENTRAL, MEDLINE, EMBASE, CBM, CNKI, VIP, China Important Conference Papers Database, China Dissertation Database, and online clinical trial registry websites were searched for published and unpublished randomized controlled trials (RCTs) of Chinese herbs for H1N1 influenza till 31 August, 2011. A total of 26 RCTs were identified and reviewed. Most of the RCTs were of high risk of bias with flawed study design and poor methodological quality. The combination of several Chinese herbal medicines with or without oseltamivir demonstrated positive effect on fever resolution, relief of symptoms, and global effectiveness rate compared to oseltamivir alone. However, only one herbal medicine showed positive effect on viral shedding. Most of the trials did not report adverse events, and the safety of herbal medicines is still uncertain.

Conclusions: Some Chinese herbal medicines demonstrated potential positive effect for 2009 type A H1N1 influenza; however, due to the lack of placebo controlled trial and lack of repeated test of the intervention, we could not draw confirmative conclusions on the beneficial effect of Chinese herbs for H1N1 influenza. More rigorous trials are warranted to support their clinical use.

Editor: Benjamin J. Cowling, University of Hong Kong, Hong Kong

Funding: This work was supported by a 2009 Specific Professional Research Grant in Traditional Chinese Medicine (TCM) funded by the State Administration of TCM of China: Clinical Study on Traditional Chinese Medicine for Severe Cases of (H1N1) Influenza A (No. 200907001-2A), and partly supported by an international collaboration project funded by the Ministry of Science and Technology of China (No. 2009DFA31460). The funders had no role in study design, data collection and analysis, decision to publish, or preparation of the manuscript.

Competing Interests: The authors have declared that no competing interests exist.

* E-mail: jianping_l@hotmail.com

Introduction

The influenza virus, known to be a circulating pathogen in the human population since the 16th century, is notable for its unique ability to cause recurrent epidemics and global pandemics. The ability of this virus to undergo genetic reassortments causes unpredictable changes in its antigens and the consequent immune response leads to recurrent epidemics of febrile respiratory disease every 1–3 years. In the 20th, three influenza pandemics occurred and killed tens of millions of people, with each of these pandemics being caused by the appearance of a new strain of the virus in humans [1]. In April 2009 a novel flu strain evolved that combined genes from human, pig, and bird flu, initially dubbed 'swine flu' and also known as influenza A/H1N1, emerged in Mexico, the United States, and several other nations. The World Health Organization officially declared the outbreak to be a pandemic on June 11, 2009 [2].

Presently, two classes of antiviral drugs have been approved by the US Food and Drug Administration (FDA) in treating or preventing influenza virus infections: M2 ion channel blockers and neuraminidase inhibitors (NAIs). The M2 blockers, amantidine and rimantidine, are effective against influenza A viruses, but not influenza B viruses, which lack the M2 protein. However, use of the M2 blockers has been associated with the rapid emergence of drug-resistance mutations of the M2 protein among human influenza A viruses of H3N2 subtype and H1N1 subtypes circulating in certain geographic areas [3]. Two NAIs, oseltamivir (Tamiflu) and zanamivir (Relenza) are approved by US FDA for use against type A and type B influenza infections. The NAIs target the active site of the NA protein, inhibiting its sialidase activity that is essential for virus release. Most of the influenza virus strains are sensitive to oseltamivir. However, it has been thought that the development of drug resistance may limit the clinical utility of the drug in the future [4].

Chinese herbs, which are the most important component of Traditional Chinese medicine (TCM), are widely used in China. Due to the limitation of healthcare resources and high cost of antiviral drugs, Chinese herbs have been recommended for preventing and treating influenza in China, especially for poor regions. In October 2009, the Ministry of Health of China issued 'Guidelines for Management of Pandemic (H1N1) 2009 Influenza', and recommended series of Chinese herbs for the treatment of type A H1N1 influenza, including herbal products extracted from natural herbs, Chinese patent medicine (including herbal injection), and principles for individually prescribed herbal decoction [5].

Until now, a number of clinical trials of Chinese herbs for H1N1 influenza have been conducted and reported with positive findings. However, there is no critically appraised evidence such as systematic reviews or meta-analyses on potential benefits and harms of medicinal herbs for H1N1 influenza to justify their clinical use and their recommendation.

Methods

The supporting PRISMA checklist is available as supporting information; see Checklist S1.

Search strategy and study selection

Literature searches were conducted in the Cochrane Central Register of Controlled Trials (CENTRAL) in the Cochrane Library (January, 2011), MEDLINE, EMBASE, Chinese Bio-Medical Literature Database (CBM), Chinese National Knowledge Infrastructure (CNKI), Chinese Scientific Journal Database (VIP), China's Important Conference Papers Database, and China's Dissertation Database from their inception to 31 August, 2011. Ongoing registered clinical trials were searched in the website of Chinese clinical trial registry (http://www.chictr.org/) and international clinical trial registry by U.S. national institutes of health (http://clinicaltrials.gov/). The following search terms were used individually or combined: 'influenza', 'H1N1 influenza', 'Chinese Traditional', 'Chinese Herbal', 'Oriental Traditional', 'herb', 'herbal medicine', 'clinical trial', and 'randomized controlled trial'.

Two authors conducted the literature searching (WC, CEDL), study selection (WC, CEDL), and data extraction (WC, HJK) independently. The extracted data included authors and title of study, year of publication, study size, age and sex of the participants, details of methodological information, name and component of Chinese herbs, treatment process, details of the control interventions, outcomes (for example, total effective rate), and adverse effects for each study. Disagreement was resolved by discussion and reached consensus through a third party (JPL).

Inclusion criteria

Parallel randomized controlled trials (RCTs) of Chinese herbs compared with no treatment, symptomatic treatment, placebo, or antivirus for H1N1 patients were included. Combined therapy of Chinese herbs and other interventions compared with other interventions in RCTs was also included. Chinese herbs included herbal products extracted from natural herbs, Chinese patent medicine, or individually prescribed herbal formula. The primary outcome measures were duration of fever (the average time for fever to clear), duration of flu-like symptoms (the average time for flu-like symptoms to disappear), and global effectiveness rate (defined as a three-class measurement including 'cure', 'effective', and 'ineffective' according to the degree of overall symptom improvement). The secondary outcome measures were hospital stay (number of days in hospital), viral shedding, and adverse events. Multiple publications reporting the same groups of participants were excluded. There was no limitation on language and publication type.

Trial quality assessment

Two authors (WC, CEDL) evaluated the quality of included trials. The quality of included trials were assessed by using the 'risk of bias' assessment tool according to the 'Cochrane Handbook of Systematic Reviews of Interventions' (Chapter 8.5) to address the following five criteria [6]: sequence generation, allocation concealment, blinding, incomplete outcome data, and selective outcome reporting. The quality of all the included trials was categorized to low/unclear/high risk of bias. Trials which met all criteria were categorized to low risk of bias, trials which met none of the criteria were categorized to high risk of bias, and other trials were categorized to unclear risk of bias if insufficient information acquired to make judgment.

Data analysis

Data were summarized using relative risk (RR) with 95% confidence intervals (CI) for binary outcomes or mean difference (MD) with 95% CI for continuous outcomes. Revman 5.0.17 software was used for data analyses. Meta-analysis was used if the trials had a good homogeneity on study design, participants, interventions, control, and outcome measures, which assessed by examining I^2 (a quantity that describes approximately the proportion of variation in point estimates due to heterogeneity rather than sampling error). Publication bias would explored by funnel plot analysis if sufficient studies were found. If we had identified a sufficient number of randomized trials, we had planned to perform sensitivity analyses to explore the influence of trial quality on effect estimates. The quality components of methodology included adequacy of generation of allocation sequence, concealment of allocation, double blinding, and the use of intention -to -treat (yes or no).

Results

Description of studies

A flow chart depicted the search process and study selection (Fig. 1). After primary searches from the seven databases, 270 citations were screened. After reading the titles and abstracts, a majority of them was excluded. Full text of 46 papers were retrieved, and finally 26 RCTs were included [7–32] including two three-armed RCTs [16,31] and four four-armed RCTs [17,21,24,27]. All the RCTs were conducted in China and published in Chinese, except one published in English [24]. Twenty papers were excluded [33–52], and the reasons for excluded studies were listed in Table S3.

The search for ongoing registered trials identified four trials: three RCTs from the website of Chinese clinical trial registry: No. ChiCTR-TRC-10000828 investigating herbal anti-virus liquid for H1N1 influenza A; No. ChiCTR-TRC-10000814 investigating Reduning herbal injection for H1N1 influenza A; and ChiCTR-TRC-10000779 investigating TCM treatment for H1N1 influenza. All the three RCTs were either under participant recruitment or not initiated and thus the data were not available. One RCT was identified from www.clinicaltrials.gov: NCT01053533 investigating Chinese herbal medicines (details not provided) plus western medicine for H1N1 influenza A. This trial was under recruitment and data were not available.

The characteristics of included trials were listed in Table S1. A total of 2946 participants with H1N1 influenza were involved with

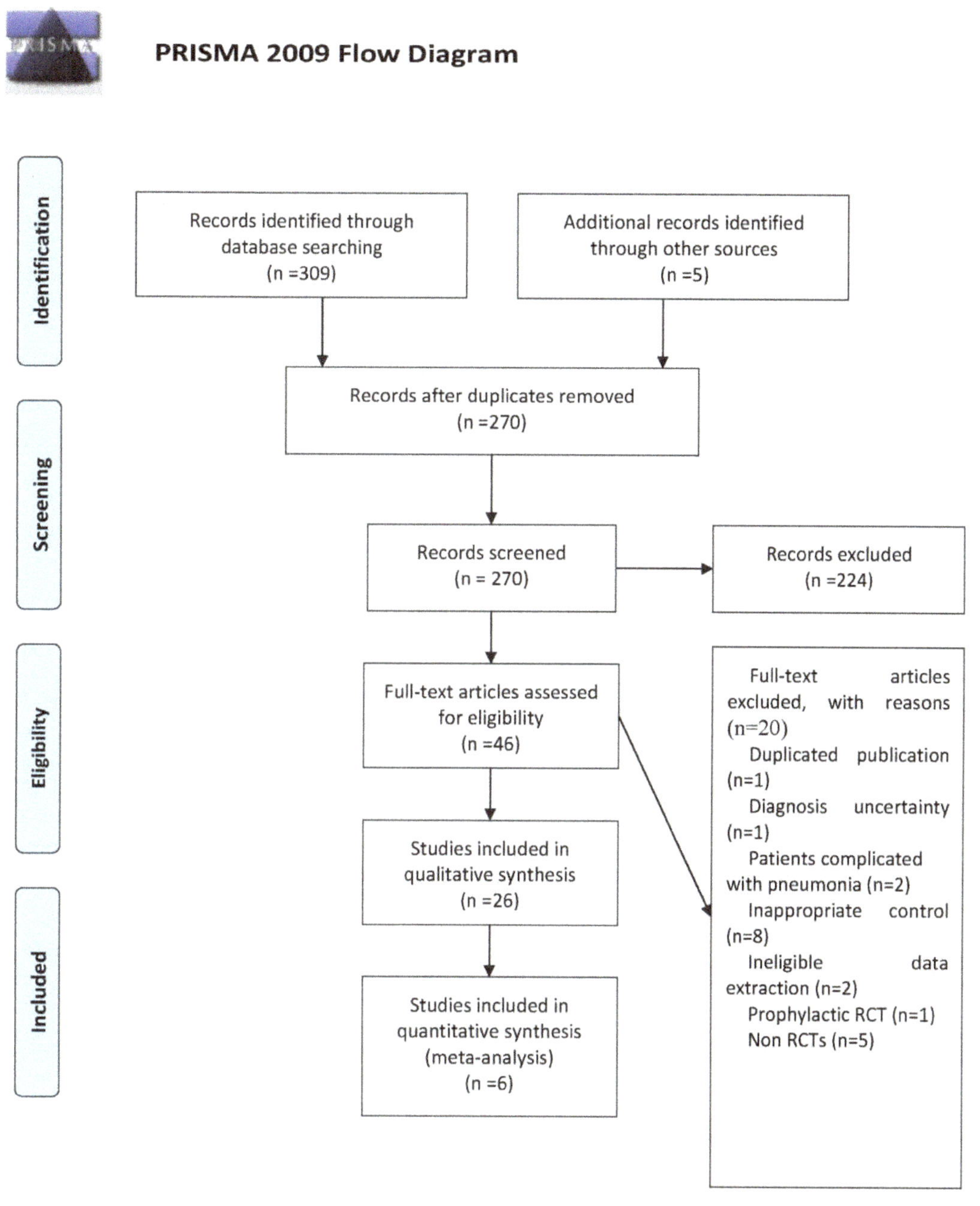

Figure 1. PRISMA 2009 Flow Diagram.

the average number of 113 per trial, ranging from 43 to 410. All participants got influenza during the H1N1 influenza epidemic year of 2009 and were virologically confirmed as having 2009-H1N1 influenza according to Chinese Center For Disease Control And Prevention (CDC). Seven trials [7,8,10,14,18,28,32] provide information on patients' syndrome differentiation (Bianzheng, TCM diagnosis) as the basis for individualized herbal preparations. A total of 27 different Chinese herbs were investigated. The Chinese herbs investigated included Chinese patent medicine including single herb extract [9,10,11,16,23,25,29], and individually prescribed herbal formula [8,12–15,18–20,22,24,26–28,30,32], in some trials [7,17,21,31], mixed herbal medicines including multiple Chinese herbal prescription or Chinese patent medicines were tested. The specific compositions of these Chinese herbs varied as shown in Table S4. Only one trial reported the quality standard of the herbal preparations [24]. The total treatment duration ranged from 3 to 14 days. The controls included symptomatic treatment [8,21], placebo [16,27], and oseltamivir [7,9–15,17–20,22,23,25–32]. The reported outcome measures included duration of fever, duration of flu-like symptoms, global effectiveness rate, hospital stay, viral response, and adverse events.

Methodological quality

The majority of the included trials were assessed to be of general poor methodological quality according to the predefined quality assessment criteria. The randomized allocation of participants was mentioned in all trials; however, only 6 trials stated the methods for sequence generation including random number table

[8,16,21,24], drawing [31], and computer software [7]. However, insufficient information was provided to judge whether or not it was conducted properly. Allocation concealment was only mentioned in one RCT [24]. Double-blind was not mentioned in all trials. Single blind was mentioned in one trial [7] without providing further information as to who was blinded. However, as the testing Chinese herbs and controlled drug were in different forms (liquid versus tablet), neither the participants nor the investigators were likely to be blinded. Only two trials reported drop-out or withdraw [7,24], however the trial did not intend to analyze the cause, and no trials used intention-to-treat analysis. Only one trial [24] had a pre-trial estimation of sample size, which indicated the lack of statistical power to ensure appropriate estimation of the therapeutic effect. Selective reporting was generally unclear in the RCTs due to the inaccessibility to the trial protocol.

Effect estimates

All the trials claimed positive effect favoring Chinese herbs though some of the trials turned out to be negative when analyzed by standard statistical techniques using risk ratios or mean differences. The effect estimates of Chinese herbs were shown in the Table S2.

1. Duration of fever. A total of seventeen trials [7–9,12,13,15–17,19–21,23,24,27,28,29,31,32] reported the effect of Chinese herbs individually or in combination with oseltamivir on defervescence. Among them, eight trials demonstrated better effect favoring Chinese herbs: Fanggan Granule [8] mildly shortened fever duration than symptomatic treatment; Bingyanqing formula Ten [20] and Chinese herbal formula [17] had shorter fever duration than oseltamivir; the combination of Maxingshigan-yinqiaosan and oseltamivir had more proportion of patients who became afebrile than no intervention [24], Maxingshigan decoction combined with oseltamivir had shorter fever duration than placebo of oseltamivir [27]; Maxingshigan decoction combined with placebo of oseltamivir had shorter fever duration than placebo of oseltamivir [27]; self-prescribed herbal medicines had shorter fever duration than oseltamivir [28]; the combination of Gegen Granule [32] and oseltamivir, Tanreqing Injection [13,19] and oseltamivir, Chinese herbal formula [17] and oseltamivir had mildly shorter fever duration than oseltamivir alone.

The forest plot of comparison of CHM versus oseltamivir for the outcome of duration of fever was shown in the Figure S1.

2. Duration of flu-like symptoms. Nine trials [7–9,14,16,23,27,29,31] reported the effect of Chinese herbs individually or in combination with oseltamivir on the duration of flu-like symptoms. Among them, two trials demonstrated better effect favoring Chinese herbs: Qingwen Tuire Decoction combined with oseltamivir shortened the duration of flu-like symptoms compared to oseltamivir alone [29], and Fanggan Granule had shorter duration of flu-like symptoms compared to symptomatic treatment [8].

3. Global effectiveness rate. Eleven trials [8,10,11,13,17,18,22,25–28] reported the effect of Chinese herbs individually or in combination with oseltamivir on the global effectiveness rate. Among them, six trials demonstrated better effect favoring Chinese herbs: Qingfei Jiedu Decoction [10] showed better effect compared to oseltamivir, the combinations of oseltamivir and Tanreqing Injection [11,13], oseltamivir and Xiyanping Injection [22] had better effect compared to oseltamivir alone, Qingjie Huashi decoction showed better effect compared to oseltamivir [25], and the combination of Reduning Injection [26] and ribavirin plus oseltamivir had better effect compared to ribavirin plus oseltamivir.

4. Hospital stay. Six trials [7,14,16,17,19,27] reported the effect of Chinese herbs individually or in combination with oseltamivir on hospital stay. Among them, two trials demonstrated better effect favoring Chinese herbs: one herbal formula showed shorter hospital stay compared to oseltamivir [17], and Tanreqing Injection combined with oseltamivir had shorter hospital stay compared to oseltamivir alone [19].

5. Viral shedding. Ten trials [9,12,14,15,17,19,21,28,30,31] reported the effect of herbal medicines individually or in combination with oseltamivir on viral shedding. Among them, one self-prescribed herbal medicines showed better effect compared with oseltamivir [28].

6. Adverse events. As shown in Table S2, the outcome of adverse events were reported in fifteen trials [7,8,10,12,14–18,22,24,25,27,30,31]. Among them, no adverse events were found in three trial [12,14,15,31]. Six trials reported adverse events in Chinese herbs group, which included diarrhea [7,8,16], arrhythmia [8], mild nausea [17,24], vomit [24], mild upper abdominal discomfort [17], and lung infection [18]. In the trial of Tang 2010 [22], two cases of wheal were identified, but did not report in which group it occurred.

We conducted funnel plots to investigate the publication bias (see Figure S2). It demonstrated asymmetrical funnel plots, suggesting potential publication bias.

Discussion

In this review, several Chinese herbal medicines demonstrated potential positive effect for 2009 type A H1N1 influenza on fever resolution, relief of flu-like symptoms, and global effectiveness rate. However, due to the lack of placebo controlled trial and lack of repeated test, we could not make confirmative conclusions on the therapeutic effect of Chinese herbs for H1N1 influenza. In addition, we found out that few Chinese herbs recommended in the 'Guidelines for Management of Pandemic (H1N1) 2009 Influenza' issued by the Ministry of Health of China were supported in this review, which revealed the lack of evidence for clinical use and policy making in China.

The following reasons might contribute to the inconclusive results of Chinese herbs. Firstly, all the included trials were of poor methodology quality, which were in accordance with previous studies [53,54]. Only six RCTs stated randomization procedure, however, most of them provided insufficient information to judge whether randomization was conducted properly. For the rest fourteen trials, they just mentioned that 'the patients were randomized into two groups' with no further information. Allocation concealment was only mentioned in one RCT. Therefore, we could not exclude the possibility that some of these claimed RCTs are not real RCTs. This possibility came to forefront in the trial of Han 2011 and Li 2010 [11,13]; these trials only has one author, which is impossible for a RCT to be done properly in terms of randomization procedure and the allocation concealment. In addition, no trials claimed double-blind. We understood that it was difficult to perform double-blinding because of certain features associated with Chinese herbs, for example, aroma and appearance, but blinding to the outcome assessors and data analyzer could be feasible. Unfortunately, none of the RCTs mentioned blinding to the outcome assessors or data analyzer. All the trials did not report pre-sample size estimation except one [24], and for majority trials, the sample size was small. Therefore we are not sure if they could provide enough power to detect the difference between groups. It is well known that methodologically poorly designed trials show larger differences between experimental and control groups than those conducted rigorously [55–57] and as such the small improvements in outcomes should be regarded with caution.

Secondly, there was lack of knowledge for placebo control in the included trials. Two trials [16,27] claimed that they used placebo control. However, in these trials the placebo is for oseltamivir, not for Chinese herbs. It is not an appropriate control for the estimation of the effect of Chinese herbs. Because of the lack of placebo controls, the interpretation of the positive findings of treatment with Chinese herbs should be made with caution. In addition, the potential positive placebo effect of an injection should also be highlighted. In the review a total of three Chinese herbal injections were used, that is, Tanreqing Injection [11,13], Xiyanping Injection [22], and Reduning Injection [26]; and all demonstrated positive results in terms of defervescence and global symptoms improvement. However, no adequate placebo control was used to offset the effect of injection alone. It is known that an injection alone has a strong potential placebo effect, therefore the overall effect of Chinese herbal injection could not rule out the effect that the injection itself produced. These positive effects should also be interpreted conservatively.

Thirdly, in most of the trials, the patients were not treated according to syndrome differentiation. In the practice of TCM, herbal preparations should match the type of syndrome differentiation, that is, 'bianzheng', a specific diagnosis in TCM. This approach is also known as treatment based on individualized (tailored) syndrome pattern, and is thought to be the advantages of TCM. However, in this review, only seven trials provide information on patients' syndrome differentiation. Chinese medicine practitioners believed that treating patients without syndrome differentiation will impair the advantages of Chinese herbs, and this might be another reason for the unsatisfactory therapeutic effect of Chinese herbs for H1N1 influenza in the review. Emphasis should be paid to encourage authors to explain each 'Bianzheng' by using common medical terms in the future trials, therefore making it understandable by physicians and consumers.

Finally, there existed great heterogeneity in the Chinese herbs investigated in the review. A total of 27 different Chinese herbs were investigated in the 26 trials. As a result, it is impossible to conduct meaningful meta-analysis for a specific Chinese herb, or difficult to undertake subgroup analyses to explore specific factors that may have an impact on the effects of the treatment regimen. What is more interesting is that although diversified Chinese herbs were investigated, most of them were not the authoritatively recommended Chinese herbs for the H1N1 influenza. In October 2009, the Ministry of Health of China issued 'Guidelines for Management of Pandemic (H1N1) 2009 Influenza A' and recommended series of Chinese herbs for the treatment of H1N1 influenza A [5]. These Chinese herbs included herbal products extracted from natural herbs, Chinese patent medicines (including herbal injection), and principles for prescribing individually herbal decoction. However, only three Chinese patent medicines (Lianhuaqingwen Capsule [12,15,17,18], Xiyanping Injection [22], Tanreqing Injection [11,13,19]) and two prescript Chinese herbal decoction (unnamed Self-prescribed Chinese herbal decoction [9], and Qingfei Jiedu Decoction [10]) in the guideline had been investigated by RCTs, and only two of them (Tanreqing Injection [11,13,19] and Qingfei Jiedu Decoction [10]) demonstrated positive results. World Health Organization (WHO) calls for evidence-based practice of TCM, that is, any medical decision-making of TCM should be based on clinical research evidence. In the era of evidence-based medicine (EBM), TCM is facing a big challenge because of the lack of a rigorous research evidence base. Our review revealed the lack of evidence for clinical use and policy making of Chinese herbs for H1N1 influenza in China. There is still a long way to go for evidence-based practice of TCM.

In addition, our review found inadequate reporting on adverse events in the included trials. Eleven trials did not mention whether they had monitored adverse effects at all. Conclusions about the safety of herbal medicines cannot be drawn from this review due to the limited, inadequate recording and reporting of adverse events. Even for the trials that reported adverse events, their report was very brief, providing limited information. In China, there is a general perception that it is safe to use herbal medicines for various conditions. However, with the increasing reports of liver toxicity and other adverse events associated with Chinese herbal medicines [58–60], more emphasis should be placed on the monitoring and reporting of adverse events to justify the safety of Chinese herbs in clinical trials in the future.

The funnel plot analysis showed asymmetry which suggests the possibility of publication bias of Chinese herbs for H1N1 influenza. Almost all the trials claimed positive effect of Chinese herbs though some of them turned out to be negative when analyzed by standard statistical techniques using risk ratios or mean differences. We undertook extensive searches for unpublished material, but found no unpublished 'negative' studies as in previous study [61]. We thought this might be attributed to the lack of awareness to register clinical trials in China, the rejection of journal editors to negative trials, and the inaccessibility to unpublished data. We hope that with increasing awareness of prospective registration of clinical trials, publication of clinical trial protocol and reporting of negative clinical trials, the picture may change in the future.

The mechanism of Chinese herbs in the treatment of influenza is complex. In traditional Chinese medicine (TCM), H1N1 influenza belongs to the scope of 'cold'. In TCM, cold is differentiated into two types: Wind-cold Syndrome and Wind-heat Syndrome. The principles behind treating these two types were different. Generally speaking, the principles behind treating wind-cold syndrome are to: relieve external symptoms with drugs which are pungent in flavour and warm in property; ventilate the lungs and expel the pathogenic cold. The principles behind treating wind-heat syndrome are to: relieve external symptoms with drugs which are pungent in flavour and cool in property and promote the dispersing function of the lungs and clear up pathogenic wind heat [62,63]. In addition, previous studies showed that administration of some Chinese herbs may have beneficial immunomodulatory effects for rapid recovery of viral infections [64,65]. However, in this review, it seems that compared with oseltamivir, Chinese herbs might have better potential effects on fever solution than viral shedding, which suggested that most of Chinese herbs might not act as an antiviral.

Last but not least, there is a lack of information about quality control for the development of the herbal preparations or for the manufacture of the herbal products, which is a quite common problem in Chinese clinical trials. Future trials should provide information about standardization including compositions, quality control, detailed regimen, and duration of treatment.

In summary, the reported beneficial effect from Chinese herbs for H1N1 influenza can not be taken as confirmative conclusion. To ensure evidence-based clinical practice, further rigorous placebo-controlled, randomized trials are warranted. The following methodological issues should be addressed: (i) methods used to generate allocation sequence and allocation concealment; (ii) double blinding with the use of adequate placebo; (iii) clear descriptions of withdrawal/dropout during the trial and use of intention-to-treat analysis; and (iv) reporting trials according to the

CONSORT Statement (www.consort_statement.org) [57]. In the literature searching, we identified several registered trials of Chinese herbs for H1N1 influenza. We hope with the publication of these ongoing trials in the future, new high-qualified evidence will arise to provide clinical evidence for the use of Chinese herbs for the H1N1 influenza.

Supporting Information

Figure S1 Forest plot of comparison of CHM versus oseltamivir for the outcome of duration of fever.
(TIF)

Figure S2 Funnel plot of comparison of CHM versus oseltamivir for the outcome of duration of fever.
(TIF)

Table S1 Characteristics of included RCTs.
(DOC)

Table S2 Effect estimates of Chinese herbs for treatment of H1N1 influenza in included trials.
(DOC)

Table S3 Excluded studies with reasons.
(DOC)

Table S4 Compositions of Chinese herbs in the included trials.
(DOC)

Checklist S1 PRISMA 2009 checklist.
(DOC)

Author Contributions

Conceived and designed the experiments: WC JL. Performed the experiments: WC CEDL. Analyzed the data: WC H-JK. Contributed reagents/materials/analysis tools: WC CEDL H-JK. Wrote the paper: WC.

References

1. Narain JP, Bhatia R (2009) Influenza A (H1N1): responding to a pandemic threat. Indian J Med Res 129: 465–7.
2. World Health Organization (2009) Pandemic (H1N1) 2009 - update 84. Available: http://www.who.int/csr/don/2010_01_22/en/index.html. Accessed 2010 Jan 24.
3. Center for Desease Control and Prevention (2010) Seasonal Influenza (Flu). 2009–2010 Influenza Season Week 19 ending May 15, 2010 Antiviral Resistance. Available: http://www.cdc.gov/flu/weekly/. Accessed 2010 May 20.
4. Moscona A (2005) Oseltamivir resistance-disabling our influenza defenses. N Engl J Med 353: 2633–2636.
5. Ministry of Health of the People's Republic of China (2009) Guidelines for Management of Pandemic (H1N1) 2009 Influenza. Available: http://www.moh.gov.cn/publicfiles/business/htmlfiles/H1N1/s10628/index.htm. Accessed 2009 Oct 13.
6. Higgins JPT, Green S, eds. (2008) Cochrane Handbook for Systematic Reviews of Interventions Version 5.0.2 [updated September 2009]. The Cochrane Collaboration. Available: www.cochrane-handbook.org. Accessed 2009 Sep.
7. Chen H, Zeng YL, Liu DF, Liu YL, Ye Q, et al. (2010) The randomized controlled trial of Chinese herbs in treating influenza A/H1N1 compared with oseltamivir [in Chinese]. Sichuan Medical Journal 31: 1050–1052.
8. Chen F, Song K, Zhu XH, Chen H (2010) The clinic study of the H1N1 influenza virus with Fanggan granule [in Chinese]. Journal of Zhejiang University of Traditional Chinese Medicine 34: 658–660.
9. Dou AH, Li DZ, Liu YZH, Yu F, OuYang Y, et al. (2010) Curative effect of oseltamivir combined with traditional Chinese medicine on type A H1N1 influenza [in Chinese]. Modern Journal of Integrated Traditional Chinese and Western Medicine 19: 3289–3290.
10. Jin F, Zhang JH, Jin PL (2010) Clinical study of Qingfei Jiedu decoction for the treatment of influenza A (H1N1) patients with syndrom of toxic heat attack on lung [in Chinese]. Journal of Sichuan Traditional Chinese Medicine 28: 81–82.
11. Han JT (2011) Clinical study of Tanreqing Injection combined with oseltamivir in treating type A H1N1 influenza [in Chinese]. Jilin Medicine 32: 1491–1492.
12. Li BF, Zhang CQ, Fu M, Bai W, Liu BH, et al. (2009) Clinical study of Lianhuaqingwen capsule in treating A/H1N1 influenza patients [in Chinese]. Journal of Medical Forum 30: 91–92.
13. Li G (2010) Clinical study of Tanreqing injection combined with oseltamivir in influenza A (H1N1) [in Chinese]. Journal of Emergency in Traditional Chinese Medicine 19: 1681–1682.
14. Lin CZ, Wang J, Zhou ZS, Jiang HD (2011) Curative effect of modified Xiaochaihu decoction on influenza A/H1N1 [in Chinese]. Acta Academiae Medicinae Qingdao universities 47: 132–134.
15. Liu GX, Zhang YX, Yang JQ, Gao ZQ, Meng YC (2010) The randomized controlled study of Lianhuaqingwen capsule in treating A/H1N1 Influenza [in Chinese]. Chinese Journal of Difficult and Complicated Cases 9: 14–16.
16. Liu DF, Liu YL, Chen H, Zeng YL, Wen XM, et al. (2011) Evaluation on the curative effect and safety of Chinese traditional medicine in treatment of mild A/H1N1 influenza in Sichuan area [in Chinese]. Modern Preventive Medicine 38: 338–343.
17. Ma YP, Guo YL, Kang L, Zhao L, Peng J, et al. (2010) Clinical study of Chinese herbs for the treatment of A/H1N1 influenza [in Chinese]. Shanxi Journal of Traditional Chinese Medicine 31: 1351–1353.
18. OuYang HX, Tang QY, Chen YZ, Wei Y, Li GS (2010) Clinical study of Lianhuaqingwen capsules in treatment of the influenza A/H1N1 [in Chinese]. China Medical Herald 7: 6–8.
19. Qian J, Xu JR, Shi LQ (2011) Clinical study of Tanreqing injection combined with oseltamivir in influenza A (H1N1) [in Chinese]. Jilin Medicine 32: 266–267.
20. Qu JL, Gao X, Su YH (2010) Clinical study of Bingyanqing Formula Ten for treatment of Seasonal H1N1 [in Chinese]. Chinese Medicine Modern Distance education of China 8: 196–197.
21. Tan XH, Liu YX, Xia Z, Li HJ (2010) Clinical research of combined Chinese medicine and Western medicine for A/H1N1 influenza [in Chinese]. Journal of Guangzhou University of Traditional Chinese Medicine 27: 441–444.
22. Tang CB, Bo YN (2010) Xiyanping injection combined with Western medicine in treating 30 cases of high fever in A/H1N1 influenza patients [in Chinese]. Chinese Community Doctors 12: 141.
23. Tian G, Wang J, Kang LH, Yang HQ (2011) Clinical study of Qingkailing Oral Liquid for A/H1N1 influenza [in Chinese]. Chinese Journal of Information on TCM 18: 81,112.
24. Wang C, Cao B, Liu QQ, Zou ZQ, Liang ZA (2011) Oseltamivir compared with the Chinese traditional therapy Maxingshigan-Yinqiaosan in the treatment of H1N1 influenza: A randomized trial. Ann Intern Med 155: 217–225.
25. Weng BX, Cai Y, Lu J (2010) Clinical study of Qingjie Huashi Decoction for A/H1N1 influenza on 150 patients [in Chinese]. International Medicine & Health Guidance News 16: 979–980.
26. Ye YM, Tu JJ, Zhu XY (2010) Clinical study of Reduning injection combined with oseltamivir on 190 children with H1N1 influenza [in Chinese]. Sichuan Medical Journal 31: 1533–1534.
27. Zeng YF, Liu DF, Liu YL, Chen H, Bai Y, et al. (2011) The Randomized Controlled Trial on the Efficacy and Safety of Modified Maxingshigan Decoction in Treatment of the Light Influenza A Pandemic (H1N1) in Sichuan [in Chinese]. Modern Preventive Medicine 38: 2227–2230,2239.
28. Zhang WS, He CS, Wang YL (2011) Clinical Study on prescription of Chinese medicine administration in Sichuan province in treating H1N1 Influenza A [in Chinese]. Gansu Journal of TCM 24: 20–22.
29. Zhao ZL, Liu HY, Wang YZ, Lei ZY (2010) Clinical study of Qingwen Tuire Decoction on the treatment of 30 cases of H1N1 influenza [in Chinese]. Ningxia Med J 32: 376–377.
30. Zhao JR, Wang S, Fan YS, Lou JC, Li HQ, et al. (2011) Traditional Chinese medicine therapy for mild patients with influenza A (H1N1) [in Chinese]. Infect Dis Info 24: 46–48.
31. Zheng HP, Yang Z, Zhang FC, Zhang AM, Wang J, et al. (2010) Effectiveness analysis of Chinese herbs for the treatment of influenza A (H1N1) [in Chinese]. China Journal of Traditional Chinese Medicine and Pharmacy 25: 780–782.
32. Zhu YH, Tian L, Xu N (2010) Gegen granule and oseltamivir for treatment of 38 cases of H1N1 influenza [in Chinese]. Shandong Journal of Traditional Chinese Medicine 29: 535–536.
33. Chai LX, Sun J, Ma QM, Gou HH, Zhang J (2010) Clinical observation of curative effect of Chinese herbs in the treatment of A/H1N1 influenza [in Chinese]. Critical Journal of Chinese Medicine 2: 36–37.
34. Hu J, Yu Y, Ye N, Li LQ, Qiu WJ, et al. (2011) Observation of Reduning Injection for children patients with H1N1 influenza A complicated with pneumonia [in Chinese]. Chinese Journal of Practical Pediatrics 26: 388.
35. Huang M, Jiang SY (2010) Clinical analysis of Chan Su injection in the treatment of suspected H1N1 influenza patients with high fever [in Chinese]. Chinese Journal of Misdiagnostics 10: 2079–2080.
36. Kou GX, Han AH, Chen MM, Xiong FM, Luo DY (2011) Observation of Tanreqing Injection for H1N1 influenza A complicated with pneumonia [in Chinese]. JETCM 20: 872,876.
37. Li XQ, Liu JY, Hu Q (2010) The combination of ribavirin and Shuanghuanglian oral liquid in the treatment of mild influenza A (H1N1) patients [in Chinese]. National Chinese and Western integrative medicine conference on critical illness and emergency medicine.

38. Li TX, Zhou ZS, Ji HL, Zou SM, Li HY (2010) Clinical observation of 84 cases of A/H1N1 influenza [in Chinese]. China Journal of Modern Medicine 20: 3479–3482.
39. Liu YL, Zeng YL, Chen H, Liu DF, Wen XM, et al. (2010) The combination of Chinese herbs and oseltamivir in the treatment of 56 H1N1 influenza patients [in Chinese]. Clinical Focus 25: 439–440.
40. Liu J (2010) Evaluation of curative effect of combined Chinese and Western medicine in the treatment of clinical diagnosed A/H1N1 influenza [in Chinese]. Contemporary Medicine 16: 158–159.
41. Qin XY, Lu QF, Qin HJ, Huang GX (2010) Clinical trial of Reduning injection in the treatment of influenza A (H1N1) [in Chinese]. Medicine information 23: 155.
42. Qiu YJ, Xia WH, Wang ZX (2010) Clinical observation of Baoyun Kangdu Decoction in the prevention of A/H1N1 influenza in pregnant women [in Chinese]. Guiding Journal of Traditional Chinese Medicine and Pharmacy 16: 36–37.
43. Ru GX, Song MD, Su YN (2010) Clinical observation of curative effect of Self-prescribed Chinese herbs in the treatment of A/H1N1 influenza [in Chinese]. International Medicine & Health Guidance News 16: 1897–1898.
44. Song K, Chen F, Zhu XH, Chen H (2010) The clinical study of the H1N1 influenza virus with Fanggan Granules [in Chinese]. Medical forum on role of Chinese medicine in public health system.
45. Wei Q, Luo H (2010) Clinical study of Lianhuaqingwen capsule combined with oseltamivir in the treatment of mild influenza A (H1N1) [in Chinese]. Guangming Journal of Chinese Medicine 25: 2318–2319.
46. Wen XM, Liu DF, Zeng YL, Ye Q, Chen SH, et al. (2010) Comparison of Self-prescribed Chinese herbs with Chinese herbs recommended by the Ministry of Health of China in treatment of mild A/H1N1 influenza in Sichuan area [in Chinese]. Journal of Sichuan of Traditional Chinese Medicine 28: 56–59.
47. Xia BS, Shi J, Jia N, Wang HX, Zhang X (2010) The Combination of Kangbingdu oral liquid and Gannao Qingre granule for the prevention of A/H1N1 influenza [in Chinese]. People's Military Surgeon 53: 645–646.
48. Xie YZ, Wang DB (2010) Clinical observation of 136 cases of H1N1 influenza [in Chinese]. China Foreign Medical Treatment 33: 38.
49. Xie Y (2010) The combination of Tanreqing injection and oseltamivir in the treatment of influenza A (H1N1) [in Chinese]. China Modern Doctor 48: 47–49.
50. Yang C, Li BZ, Yang SW (2010) Clinical study of Shashen Maidong Decoction combined with oseltamivir in 31 cases of influenza A (H1N1) [in Chinese]. Journal of Community Medicine 8: 69–70.
51. Zhang ZQ, Zheng HJ, Liu DH, Li JS, Yin FR, et al. (2010) Clinical study of Julan Qingdu Decoction combined with Western medicine in the treatment of mild influenza A (H1N1) on 28 patients [in Chinese]. Hebei Journal of Traditional Chinese Medicine 32: 1192–1193.
52. Zheng HJ, Dai EH, Zhang ZQ, Li JS, Wu L, et al. (2010) Clinical study of Julan Qingdu Decoction in the treatment of mild influenza A (H1N1) on 52 patients [in Chinese]. Hebei Journal of Traditional Chinese Medicine 32: 1621–1622.
53. Tang JL, Zhan SY, Ernst E (1999) Review of randomised controlled trials of traditional Chinese medicine. BMJ 319: 160–61.
54. Liu JP (2009) What should we do with the growing amount of TCM research published in the Chinese literature? Focus on Alternative and Complementary Therapies 14: 92–93.
55. Kjaergard LL, Villumsen J, Gluud C (2001) Reported methodological quality and discrepancies between large and small randomized trials in meta-analyses. Annals of Internal Medicine 135: 982–9.
56. Schulz KF, Chalmers I, Hayes R, Altman D (1995) Empirical evidence of bias. JAMA 273: 408–12.
57. Moher D, Hopewell S, Schulz KF, Montori V, Gøtzsche PC, et al. (2010) CONSORT 2010 Explanation and Elaboration: updated guidelines for reporting parallel group randomised trial. BMJ 340: c869.
58. Gottieb S (2000) Chinese herb may cause cancer (news). BMJ 320: 1623.
59. Ishizaki T, Sasaki F, Ameshima S, Shiozaki K, Takahashi H, et al. (1996) Pneumonitis during interferon and/or herbal drug therapy in patients with chronic active hepatitis. European Respiratory Journal 9: 2691–2696.
60. Melchart D, Linde K, Weidenhammer W, Hager S, Shaw D, et al. (1999) Liver enzyme elevations in patients treated with traditional Chinese medicine. JAMA 282: 28–29.
61. Vickers A, Goyal N, Harland R, Rees R (1998) Do certain countries produce only positive results? A systematic review of controlled trials. Control Clin Trials 19: 159–66.
62. Deng WL (1998) Pharmacology of Traditional Chinese Medicine. 1st Edition. Beijing: People Health Publishing House.
63. Liu GW (2001) Chinese Herbal Medicine. 1st Edition. Beijing: Hua Xia Publishing House.
64. Zhao WN, Lu FG, Zhang W, Zhu YW, He YC (2007) Effect of maxing shigan decoction and its alteration on mice T-cell subpopulation exposed to influenza virus A. Practical Preventive Medicine 14: 178–280.
65. Poon PM, Wong CK, Fung KP, Fong CY, Wong EL, et al. (2006) Immunomodulatory effects of a traditional Chinese medicine with potential antiviral activity: a self-control study. Am J Chin Med 2006;34: 13–21.

15

Traditional Chinese Medicine in Cancer Care: A Review of Controlled Clinical Studies Published in Chinese

Xun Li[1,2], Guoyan Yang[1], Xinxue Li[1], Yan Zhang[3], Jingli Yang[4]❡, Jiu Chang[3]❡, Xiaoxuan Sun[3]❡, Xiaoyun Zhou[5], Yu Guo[5], Yue Xu[6], Jianping Liu[1]*, Alan Bensoussan[2]*

1 Centre for Evidence-based Chinese Medicine, Beijing University of Chinese Medicine, Beijing, China, **2** Centre for Complementary Medicine Research (CompleMED), University of Western Sydney, Sydney, New South Wales, Australia, **3** School of Preclinical Medicine, Beijing University of Chinese Medicine, Beijing, China, **4** School of Management, Beijing University of Chinese Medicine, Beijing, China, **5** School of Acupuncture and Moxibustion, Beijing University of Chinese Medicine, Beijing, China, **6** School of Humanities, Beijing University of Chinese Medicine, Beijing, China

Abstract

Background: Traditional Chinese medicine (TCM) has been widely applied for cancer care in China. There have been a large number of controlled clinical studies published in Chinese literature, yet no systematic searching and analysis has been done. This study summarizes the current evidence of controlled clinical studies of TCM for cancer.

Methods: We searched all the controlled clinical studies of TCM therapies for all kinds of cancers published in Chinese in four main Chinese electronic databases from their inception to November 2011. We bibliometrically analyzed the included studies and assessed the reporting quality.

Results: A total of 2964 reports (involving 253,434 cancer patients) including 2385 randomized controlled trials and 579 non-randomized controlled studies were included. The top seven cancer types treated were lung cancer, liver cancer, stomach cancer, breast cancer, esophagus cancer, colorectal cancer and nasopharyngeal cancer by both study numbers and case numbers. The majority of studies (72%) applied TCM therapy combined with conventional treatment, whilst fewer (28%) applied only TCM therapy in the experimental groups. Herbal medicine was the most frequently applied TCM therapy (2677 studies, 90.32%). The most frequently reported outcome was clinical symptom improvement (1667 studies, 56.24%) followed by biomarker indices (1270 studies, 42.85%), quality of life (1129 studies, 38.09%), chemo/radiotherapy induced side effects (1094 studies, 36.91%), tumor size (869 studies, 29.32%) and safety (547 studies, 18.45%). Completeness and adequacy of reporting appeared to improve with time.

Conclusions: Data from controlled clinical studies of TCM therapies in cancer treatment is substantial, and different therapies are applied either as monotherapy or in combination with conventional medicine. Reporting of controlled clinical studies should be improved based on the CONSORT and TREND Statements in future. Further studies should address the most frequently used TCM therapy for common cancers and outcome measures should address survival, relapse/metastasis and quality of life.

Editor: Wael El-Rifai, Vanderbilt University Medical Center, United States of America

Funding: This work was supported by Program for Innovative Research Team of Beijing University of Chinese Medicine (No.2011-CXTD-09), and grant number 2011ZX09302-006 from the Ministry of Science and Technology of China and 101207007 from the State Administration of Traditional Chinese Medicine. The funders had no role in study design, data collection and analysis, decision to publish, or preparation of the manuscript.

Competing Interests: The authors have declared that no competing interests exist.

* E-mail: jianping_l@hotmail.com (JL); a.bensoussan@uws.edu.au (AB)

❡ These authors contributed equally to this work.

Introduction

With an ageing worldwide population coupled with unhealthy lifestyles and increased medical intervention, the burden of disease and overall mortality has shifted gradually to primarily non-communicable diseases such as cardiovascular disease and cancer [1]. It is estimated that about 12.7 million cancer cases and 7.6 million cancer deaths occurred in 2008 [2], and the World Health Organization (WHO) estimates that 84 million people would die of cancer between 2005 and 2015 [3].

The earliest records of tumors can be traced back to inscriptions on bones and tortoiseshells in the 16th–11th century B.C., and the "malignant sores" with "swelling but without ulceration" recorded by traditional Chinese medicine (TCM) doctors in Qin Dynasty (221-207 B.C.) already presented various theories and approaches to treat cancer. [4].

TCM has increasingly become popular in the West including in cancer patients [5]. Chinese medicine plays an important role in minimizing disability, protecting cancer patients against suffering from complications, and helping patients to live well [6]. Chinese medicine may also assist in supportive and palliative care by reducing side-effects of conventional treatment or improving quality of life [7]. It is estimated the United States National Cancer

Institute (NCI) spends around $120 million each year on CAM related research projects [8].

A recent review of surveys of complementary and alternative medicine use for cancer [9] identified 74 studies over the last 15 years, with 70% of publications occurring after 2005.

Previous reviews of TCM for cancer care in Chinese publications have identified 716 case reports involving 1,198 patients [10], and 1,217 case series reports involving 92,945 patients [11], which showed a large prevalence of a diversity of TCM clinical application for cancer patients. However, controlled clinical studies were not included in these two reviews. In order to catch a more comprehensive picture on TCM clinical usage for cancer care in China, we systematically reviewed Chinese literature to summarize the clinical evidence of controlled clinical studies in this area.

Materials and Methods

Literature Search

We searched four major Chinese electronic databases including China National Knowledge Infrastructure (CNKI) (1911-November 2011), Chinese Scientific Journal Database (VIP) (1989-November 2011), Chinese BioMedical Literature Database (CBM) (1978-November 2011), and Wanfang Database (1994-November 2011).

The Chinese searching terms were zhong yi (Chinese medicine), zhong yao (Chinese medicine/Chinese herbal medicine), zhong yi yao (Chinese medicine), zhong cheng yao (Chinese proprietary medicine), zhen (needling/acupuncture), jiu (moxibustion), tui na (tui na/massage), gua sha (scraping), ba guan (cupping), xue wei (acupoint), qi gong, min zu yao (ethnomedicine), min jian (folk); terms related to cancer disease including ai (cancer), liu (tumor), e (malignant), bai xue (leukemia), gu sui (bone marrow) and lin ba (lymph). Based on pilot searches, we noted improved outcomes by searching for any match with study citation, abstract, keyword or subject word.

Study Selection

Randomized controlled trials (RCT) or non-randomized (clinical) clinical studies (CCS) with at least one group involving TCM treatment for all types of cancer-related patients including malignant tumor, malignant hematologic disease and patients with precancerous condition were included. Controlled studies reporting "random allocation" were regarded as RCT, while controlled studies without mentioning randomization were regarded as CCS, including non-randomized controlled clinical trial (CCT) and prospective/retrospective observational study.

Two authors (XL and GYY) screened the titles and abstracts of the hits from literature searching, and full papers were retrieved by downloading electronic versions (JC, JLY, XYZ, and YG) and hand searching when electronic versions were unavailable (GYY).

Data Extraction

A structured data extraction form was designed (XL and XXL), and 10 authors (YZ, GYY, JLY, YG, XXS, XYZ, JC, XXL, YX and XL) participated in data extraction. The data extraction involved study information as followed:

We extracted bibliometric information, including citation information, publication types and funding information if available.

Clinical related indices consisted: 1) Disease and diagnosis: we recorded the cancer types according to International Statistical Classification of Diseases and Related Health Problems 10th Revision [12]. We extracted clinical-related conditions which the study addressed as the primary diagnosis of the included patients in the studies. Studies about prevention were specially categorized. Studies reported primary diagnosis related to TCM syndrome differentiation were specially recorded. We recorded the reporting completeness of diagnostic criteria, syndrome differentiation (bianzheng) and application of diagnostic gold standard (pathological diagnosis or cytological diagnosis). 2) Treatment and control: We distinguished conventional treatments and TCM, administration routes of TCM information both in treatment group and control group, further classification of herbal medicine and acupoint stimulation, and the reporting of treatment method, dosage and treatment duration for both TCM and conventional medicine. 3) Outcome measures: We extracted and classified clinical-related outcomes. If quality of life was reported, the tool for measuring was extracted if available. If the authors defined the graded effectiveness by combining a number of outcomes, for example, obvious improvement of quality of life and obvious reduction of tumor size meant "very effective" while obvious improvement of quality of life or obvious reduction of tumor size meant "effective", rather than reporting each original outcome, we recorded this as "combined outcome". Whether the author recommended the clinical application as the study report conclusion was also extracted.

We assessed the completeness of reporting according to CONSORT Statement [13] for RCTs and TREND Statement [14] for CCSs. We assessed the reporting of diagnosis criteria, inclusion/exclusion criteria, allocation methods, blinding, details of interventions and level of controls, and use of outcomes measures for quality of life. We identified whether the study was randomized and whether the method of randomization as reported by authors. We identified blinding as either to patients, physicians, evaluators and/or statisticians. If placebo was reported and "double blind" was mentioned, we classified the blinding as "blinding to physicians and patients", while if placebo was reported without mentioning the details of blinding, we classified the blinding as "blinding to the patients".

We summarised well designed (reporting both randomization methods and blinding details) studies reporting positive survival outcomes to identify any significant evidence for the TCM treatments.

All the extraction was verified by one author (XL), and any discrepancies were discussed with the other authors for consensus.

Data Analysis

Data were presented by counts, percentage and frequency. Epidata (Version 13.02) was applied for data extraction, and Microsoft Excel and SPSS for Windows (version 17.0, Chicago, Illinois, USA) were applied for data analysis (XL, XXL, GYY).

Results

Bibliometric Information

A total of 137,510 citations were identified and screened based on searching in the four electronic databases, and 3737 full papers were retrieved. A final 2,964 articles involving 253,434 (10-1700, 85.50±70.59) participants were included after exclusion due to duplication, non-controlled clinical studies, non-cancer related studies or insufficient information (Figure 1).

A total of 2385 RCTs and 579 CCSs were identified. The earliest controlled clinical study was a retrospective clinical report about integrative medicine treating esophageal cancer published in 1984 [15]. The earliest RCTs we identified were one study of herbal injection for cancer pain in 513 advanced-staged cancer patients [16] and another study of herbal decoction for bone

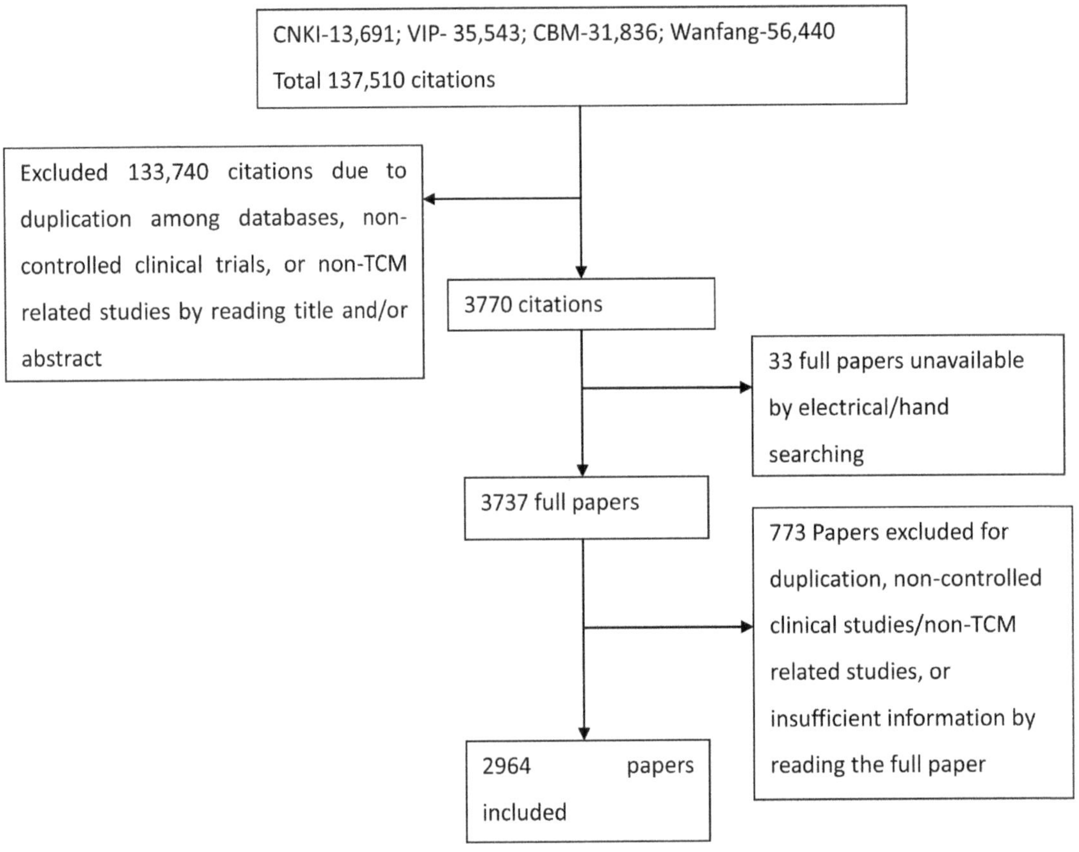

Figure 1. Flow chart of Literature searching and study selection. Presentation of the procedure of literature searching and study selection with numbers of articles at each stage.

marrow and immune function-related side effects induced by chemotherapy involving 40 patients [17], both of which were published in 1985. The quantity of publications increased especially after the year 2000. The publication types were further divided into journal articles, dissertations and conference proceedings. Studies reporting the funding information were specifically summarised in order to present the quantity change tendency, too. (Figure 2).

Participants and Diseases

Among the 2964 controlled clinical studies, 1490 studies focused on the treatment of cancer, and the other studies focused on precancerous condition, cancer-related clinical conditions, post-surgery conditions and radio/chemotherapy induced side effects (Table S2). Leucopenia was the most frequently reported primary diagnosis in radio/chemotherapy-induced side effects (119 studies out of 991), and cancer pain showed the highest frequency in cancer-related conditions (123 studies out of 283).

Out of the total 2964 studies, 292 (9.85%) involving 26,585 (10.49%) patients focused on cancer or cancer-related conditions prevention. Prevention of relapse and/or metastasis took up 16 studies out of 17 for relapse and/or metastasis, occupying the largest percentage (94.12%) of prevention. There were also more studies related to the prevention of radiation injury (61.19%), and prevention of other drug induced side effects (60.00%) than the studies about treatment of the same clinical conditions. (Table S1).

Cancer types were summarised into 17 categories according to ICD-10 (Table S2, Figure 3). Calculating by case numbers and study numbers, the highest prevalence cancer types treated, included in descending order of priority, were respectively lung cancer, liver cancer, stomach cancer, breast cancer, esophagus cancer, colorectal cancer, and nasopharyngeal cancer (Figure 4).

Interventions in Different Groups

Among the total 2964 studies, the majority of 2770 (93.45%) studies reported studies with 2 arms, 175 (5.90%) studies reported 3 arm studies, while 19 (0.64%) reported 4 or more arms in one study.

Interventions in treatment groups involved purely TCM intervention in 836 (28.21%) studies, while TCM combined with conventional treatment in 2128 (71.79%) studies. The interventions in control groups involved purely conventional treatment in 2570 (86.71%) studies, TCM combined with conventional treatment in 204 (6.88%) studies, and purely TCM intervention in 182 (6.14%) studies.

TCM intervention. TCM interventions reported in the total 2964 studies were classified into herbal medicine, acupoint stimulation, dietary therapy, massage, TCM psychological intervention, TCM five element music therapy and qigong. Herbal medicine, including oral decoction, injection, external usage, perfusion, aerosol inhalation, mouth rinsing and nasal feeding, was the most frequently applied intervention in both treatment group (2667 studies, 89.98%) and control group (327 studies, 11.03%). Among all the types of herbal medicine, herbal medicine decoction was the majority. More than half (1145 out of 1720, 66.57%) decoctions were individualized, and most of the studies

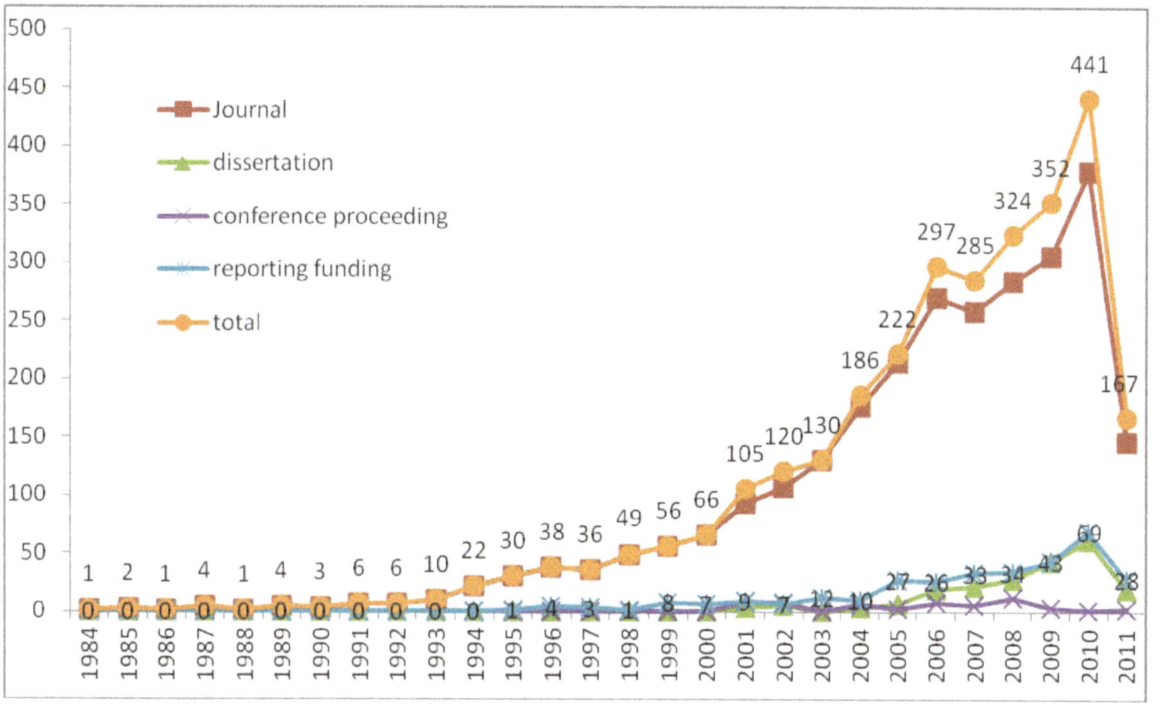

Figure 2. Publication number of controlled clinical studies of TCM for cancer published in Chinese. Presentation of the number of Chinese publication of controlled clinical studies of TCM for cancer in each year. The publication numbers of all the studies, journal articles, conference proceedings, dissertations, and the publications reporting funding information are shown respectively.

reported the detailed ingredients of the decoctions (Table 1). No study reported quality assessment of herbs or final herbal products.

Out of 379 (12.79%) and 56 (1.89%) studies reporting acupoint stimulation as the TCM treatment in treatment groups and control groups respectively, needling acupuncture and acupoint injection were dominating. Most of the studies related to acupoint stimulation reported acupoint composition (treatment group 372 studies, 86.28%, control group 50 studies, 89.29%) (Table 1).

Conventional treatment. Conventional treatment reported in the 2964 studies included chemotherapy, Western medicine as routine treatment, radiotherapy, interventional therapy and surgery. Chemotherapy was the dominating conventional treatment in both treatment group (1170 studies, 54.98% in the 2128 studies reporting TCM+conventional medicine) and control group (1328 studies, 47.87% in the 2774 studies reporting TCM+con-

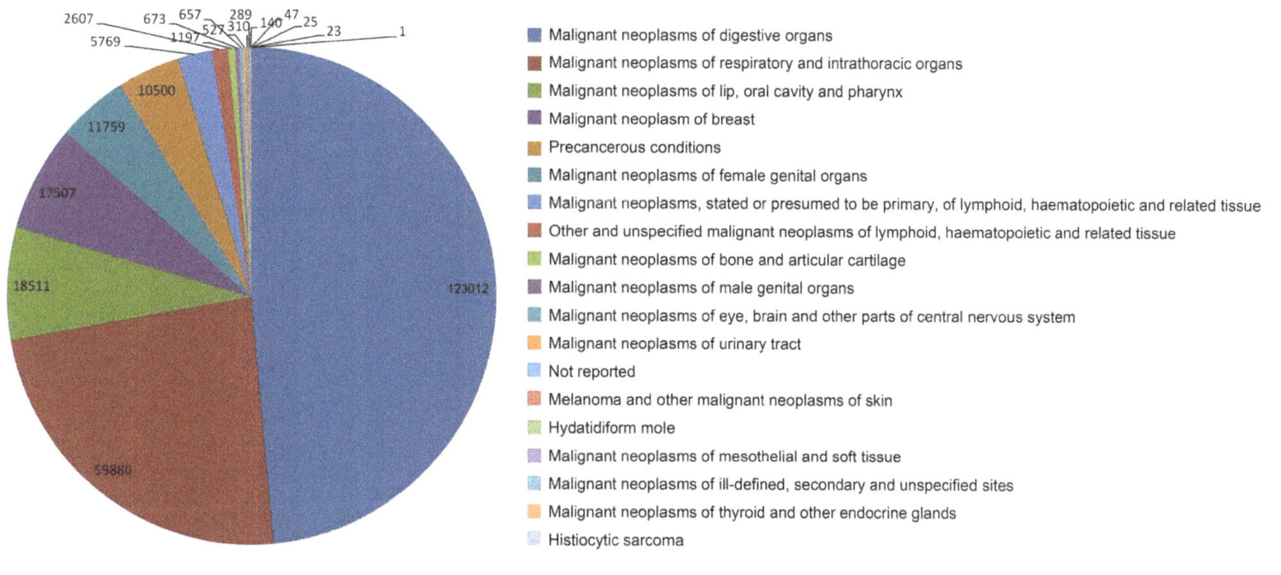

Figure 3. Cancer categories in controlled clinical studies of TCM for cancer published in China. Presentation of the categories of cancers reported in the include studies according to ICD-10.

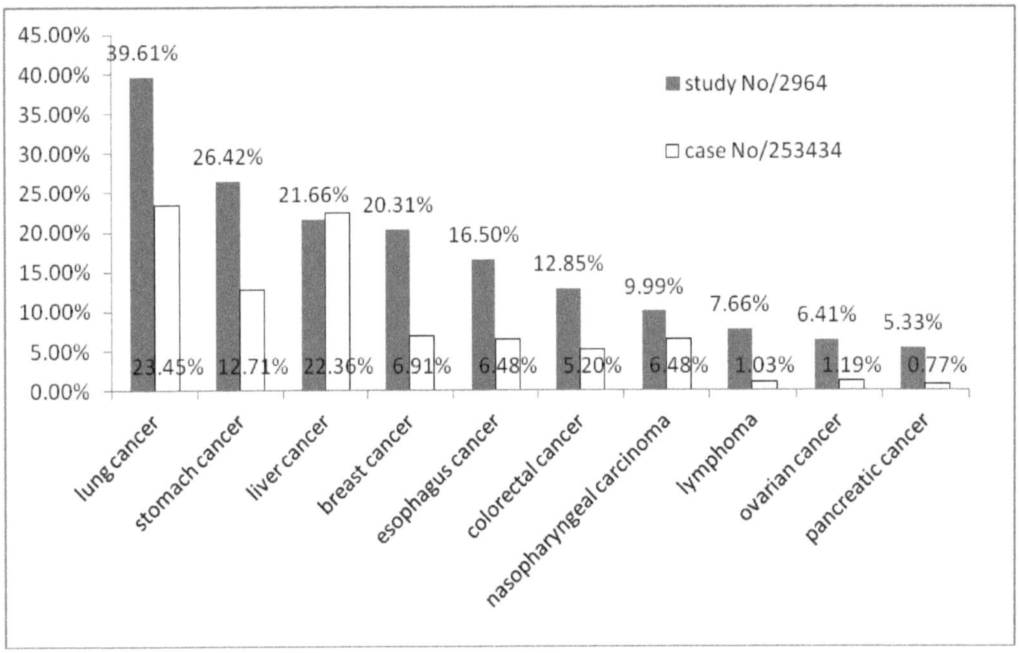

Figure 4. Top 10 cancer types with study numbers. Presentation of the top 10 most frequently reported cancer types calculate by study numbers. The numbers of participants ware also presented.

ventional medicine or conventional medicine only), followed by western medicine or other routine treatments (Table 1).

Control types. There were 25 studies applied placebo and 2 applied sham acupuncture as the control, and another 6 studies did not give any treatment to the patients in the control groups.

Detailed information of the intervention. Most studies reported the details of treatment such as method description, dosage and treatment duration. There were 410 (13.83%) studies failed to present any treatment information for treatment group and 376 (12.69%) for control group (Table 1).

Outcome Measurement

The most-frequently reported outcome measurement was clinical symptom (1667 studies, 56.24%), followed by laboratory indices (1270 studies, 42.85%), quality of life (1129 studies, 38.09%), chemo/radiotherapy induced side effects (1094, 36.91%), tumor size (869 studies, 29.32%) and safety (547 studies, 18.45%). Survival was reported in 433 (14.61%) studies while metastasis and relapse were reported in 109 (3.68%) and 101 (3.41%). Among the total 1129 studies reporting quality of life as the outcome measurement, Karnofsky Score was applied in most of the studies (942 studies, 83.44%). There were 41 studies reported quality of life measured by "QOL Score" without giving any other detailed information, and we could not identify the exact tool by any of the information provided by the publication and references. (Table 2).

There were totally 516 studies (17.41%) reported clinical effectiveness levels graded by several outcomes together without giving adequate information for each of the original outcome. (Table 2).

Overall Recommendation of Treatments

Among the total 2964 studies, 756 (25.51%) studies recommended generalizing the treatment to the broader community based on treatment effectiveness. Commonly seen recommendations included: "this treatment method is very effective with good safety, and is very suitable for generalization in the clinical applications".

Completeness of Reporting

Out of 2964 studies, 2136 (72.06%) reported diagnosis criteria of the included patients, 2315 (78.10%) reported golden standard for cancer diagnosis, such as pathological diagnosis or cytologic diagnosis, 1020 (34.41%) reported inclusion and/or exclusion criteria for the participants, while 1339 (45.18%) reported the stages of cancer.

The reporting rates across different publication types were different in diagnosis criteria, golden standard of cancer, inclusion/exclusion criteria, cancer staging and randomization method. Dissertations more frequently reported all of the detailed information mentioned above. (Table 3, Table 4).

Studies with funding information more frequently reported inclusion/exclusion criteria, cancer staging and blinding details than those without funding information. (Table 3, Table 4).

Reporting of inclusion/exclusion criteria, randomization method and details of blinding increased over time. (Figure 5).

There were 679 (22.91%) studies reported TCM diagnosis based on syndrome differentiation as diagnosis standards as selection criteria, reference for treatment or for outcome measuring.

Randomization. Among the 2385 RCTs, 394 (16.52%) reported adequate randomization methods, such as random table, computer software randomization, drawing lots and throwing coin. There were 33 studies reported "envelope method" or "random envelop "as the randomization method, and we counted them as adequate randomization method, too. Conference proceedings and dissertations had higher rate of reporting randomization methods out of studies mentioning "randomization" (Table 4).

Table 1. Intervention and control for cancer patients in controlled clinical studies of TCM for cancer published in Chinese.

Therapy	Treatment group	% (/2964)	Control group	% (/2964)
Herbal medicine	**2667**	**89.98%**	**327**	**11.03%**
oral medication	2098	70.78%	273	9.21%
decoction (reporting ingredients)	1720 (1631)	58.03%	149 (131)	5.03%
individualized prescription (reporting ingredients)	1145 (1089)	38.63%	103 (90)	3.48%
proprietary herbal products (reporting ingredients)	758 (564)	25.57%	185 (111)	6.24%
hospital prepared herbal medicine (reporting ingredients)	303 (278)	10.22%	22 (19)	0.74%
injection	450	15.18%	51	1.72%
external	200	6.75%	15	0.51%
perfusion	15	0.51%	1	0.03%
aerosol inhalation	5	0.17%	0	0.00%
mouth rinsing	5	0.17%	1	0.03%
nasal feeding	1	0.03%	0	0.00%
Acupoint stimulation (acupoint composition)	**379 (372)**	**12.79%**	**56 (50)**	**1.89%**
needling	131	4.42%	22	0.74%
acupoint injection	122	4.12%	20	0.67%
moxibustion	71	2.40%	5	0.17%
electronic acupuncture	44	1.48%	3	0.10%
acupoint application	28	0.94%	3	0.10%
ear acupuncture	18	0.61%	1	0.03%
acupressure	16	0.54%	0	0.00%
laser or microwave stimulation	4	0.13%	2	0.07%
cupping	2	0.07%	0	0.00%
acupoint nerve stimulation	2	0.07%	0	0.00%
bee-sting therapy	2	0.07%	0	0.00%
point embedding therapy	1	0.03%	0	0.00%
sham acupuncture (control group)			2	0.07%
Other types of TCM intervention	**31**	**1.05%**	**6**	**0.20%**
dietary therapy	15	0.51%	2	0.07%
massage	10	0.34%	3	0.10%
TCM psychological intervention	3	0.10%	0	0.00%
TCM five element music therapy	2	0.07%	0	0.00%
qigong	1	0.03%	1	0.03%
Conventional medicine				
chemotherapy	1170	39.47%	1328	44.80%
radiotherapy	354	11.94%	367	12.38%
western medicine or other routine treatment	622	20.99%	1228	41.43%
interventional therapy	162	5.47%	155	5.23%
surgery	73	2.46%	68	2.29%
Reporting completeness of interventions				
no information about medication duration	410	13.83%	376	12.69%
no information about dosage	133	4.49%	190	6.41%
no information about medication	38	1.28%	114	3.85%

Blinding. A total of 63 studies reported blinding to the participants, and 40 studies out of them (63.49%) reported the people who were blinded, such as participants, physicians, outcome measurers and statisticians. The other 23 studies just mentioned "blinding", "single blinding" or "double blinding" without providing any further information. Again, conference proceeding and dissertations reported the people who were blinded more frequently if "blinding" was mentioned (Table 4).

Significant Evidence of TCM Treatments

There were five studies [18–22] reporting relatively well designed RCTs with positive survival findings using Chinese herbal medicine. One study used herbal extract granules, another

Table 2. Outcome measurements reported in controlled clinical studies of TCM for cancer published in Chinese.

Outcome measurement	No.	Frequency (/2964)
clinical symptom	1667	56.24%
biomarker indices	1270	42.85%
quality of life	1129	38.09%
Karnofsky Score	942	31.78%
EORTC-QLQ	58	1.96%
QOL score without specific information	41	1.38%
FACT	27	0.91%
ECOG Score	5	0.17%
WHOQOL	5	0.17%
SF-36	4	0.13%
self-description	3	0.10%
FLIC Scale	2	0.07%
GQLI (Gastrointestinal Quality of Life Index)	2	0.07%
TCM quality of life scale	2	0.07%
other	15	0.51%
not reported	27	0.91%
chemo/radiotherapy induced side effects	1094	36.91%
tumor size	869	29.32%
safety	547	18.45%
survival	433	14.61%
post-surgery side effects	156	5.26%
body weight	126	4.25%
metastasis	109	3.68%
relapse	101	3.41%
pain	71	2.40%
imaging indexes	47	1.59%
fever	29	0.98%
depression indexes	10	0.34%
appetite	8	0.27%
economic indexes	6	0.20%

used a herbal capsule, and 3 used conventional Chinese herbal decoctions. Two of the studies reported TCM alone as the treatment intervention and the other 3 involved integrative TCM and conventional medicine. (Table S3).

Discussion

This study systematically identified and analyzed controlled clinical studies of TCM for cancer, and included 2964 studies from 1984 to 2011. This is the continuous part of previous reviews on case reports and case series [10,11] with the same topic. Unlike case reports and case series, Chinese publications of controlled clinical studies of TCM for cancer did not commence until 1984. This was consistent with the starting time of clinical trials in China, as a previous searching found that the earliest clinical trial in China started in the end of 1970s, and the first clinical trial in TCM area was a study of Chinese herbal injection for angina published in 1983 [23]. The number of publications increased with time, especially after 2000, which paralleled significant

Table 3. Completeness of Reporting across different types of publications.

	Total No. of the studies	Reporting funding	*Impact of reporting with or without funding reporting (p value)* Δ	Journal articles	Dissertation	*Compared with journal article (chi-square, p value)*	C onference proceeding	*Compared with journal article (chi-square, p value)*
Total	2964	322		2698	209		57	
Diagnosis criteria	2136	242	*0.191*	1895	201	*64.863, <0.001**	40	*<0.001, 0.992*
Golden standard	2315	251	*0.944*	2082	186	*15.821, <0.001**	47	*0.889, 0.425*
Inclusion/exclusion Criteria	1020	158	*<0.001* (OR = 1.99)*	789	204	*403.083, <0.001**	27	*8.796, 0.003**
Staging	1339	169	*0.005* (OR = 1.31)*	1152	154	*75.271, <0.001**	33	*5.295, 0.021*

*: statistically significant difference.
Δ: based on logistic regression.

Table 4. Overall picture of methodology quality of RCT and CCS of TCM for cancer.

	Total No. of the studies	Reporting funding	Impact of reporting with or without funding reporting (p value) Δ	Journal articles	Dissertation	Compared with journal article (chi-square, p value)	Conference proceeding	Compared with journal article (chi-square value, p value)
Total	2964	322		2698	209		57	
RCT	2385	289		2191	157		37	
Randomization method	394	95	<0.001* (OR = 2.94)	326	58	52.134, <0.001*	10	4.193, 0.041
Blinding	63	17		53	9		1	
Who is blinded	40	14	0.069	34	5	0.894,0.819**	1	0.894,0.819**

*statistically significant difference.
**p value of chi-square across journal articles, dissertation and conference proceeding.
Δ: based on logistic regression.

development of controlled clinical studies in China, and also possibly of the establishment of Chinese medical databases. Publication numbers fall in 2011 which may be partially due to the time lag in recording of trials by the databases.

The most frequently reported cancer types were consistent with the most common types of cancer (lung, stomach, liver, colon and breast cancer) causing deaths each year according to WHO [24] and basically consistent with the estimation of the new cancer diagnosis for developing countries (lung & bronchus cancer, stomach cancer, liver cancer, breast cancer and colon & rectum cancer) [2] Leukemia was ranked 10th as calculated by patient cases numbers, and was not ranked within the top 10 cancer types if calculated by study numbers, which was quite different from case series (5th rank) and case reports (2nd rank). One possibility is that the treatment of leukemia is quite individualized, and there tends to be more publications of case series and case reports where more flexible and variable treatments are allowed than strict standardized interventions expected in RCTs. Both clinical observations and controlled clinical trials should be implemented to confirm the effectiveness and safety in the future.

The clinical application of TCM is of high clinical interest not only in the treatment of cancer and cancer related conditions, but also in its prevention. We identified 292 studies involving 26,585 patients using TCM treatment for prevention of relapse/metastasis of cancer or other cancer related conditions. Compared to treatment interventions, TCM seems to have higher impact in the prevention of relapse and/or metastasis, hemorrhage, radiotherapy induced inflammation, radiation injury, chemo/radiotherapy induced nausea and/or vomiting or other gastrointestinal disorder, other chemotherapy included side effects, and other drug-induced side effects. This is consistent with previously identified role of TCM as complementary medicine adjuvant or postal to conventional treatment [6–7,9].

In our literature search, whilst we did not apply any terms directly related to precancerous lesions; we nevertheless identified 98 studies involving 11,759 patients with precancerous conditions. A more comprehensive search with more precise search terms including specific names of each precancerous condition should be implemented for a complete view of studies of TCM in cancer prevention.

Reporting completeness, including recording of inclusion/exclusion criteria, randomization method for RCTs, and recording of blinding improved with time. However, around half of the studies still did not provide adequate information around patient diagnosis and recruitment. This could be directly due to the poor reporting of studies, or indeed that some of these studies were actually retrospective clinical records summary instead of prospective clinical trials although the published article claimed itself as "clinical trial" or "clinical study". It is necessary and essential for a prospective clinical study to recruit participants based on pre-defined standardized diagnosis criteria and clear selection criteria.

As far as the methodology is concerned, according to CONSORT Statement [13], a randomized controlled trial must report the details of randomization methods and blinding if blinding was implemented, and for non-randomized clinical study, TREND (Improving the Reporting Quality of Nonrandomized Evaluations of Behavioral and Public Health Interventions) Statement [14] requires that the authors report whether or not participants, those administering the interventions, and those assessing the outcomes were blinded to study condition assignment. We recommend that future publications give detailed information of randomization methods including sequence generation and randomization concealment and blinding information

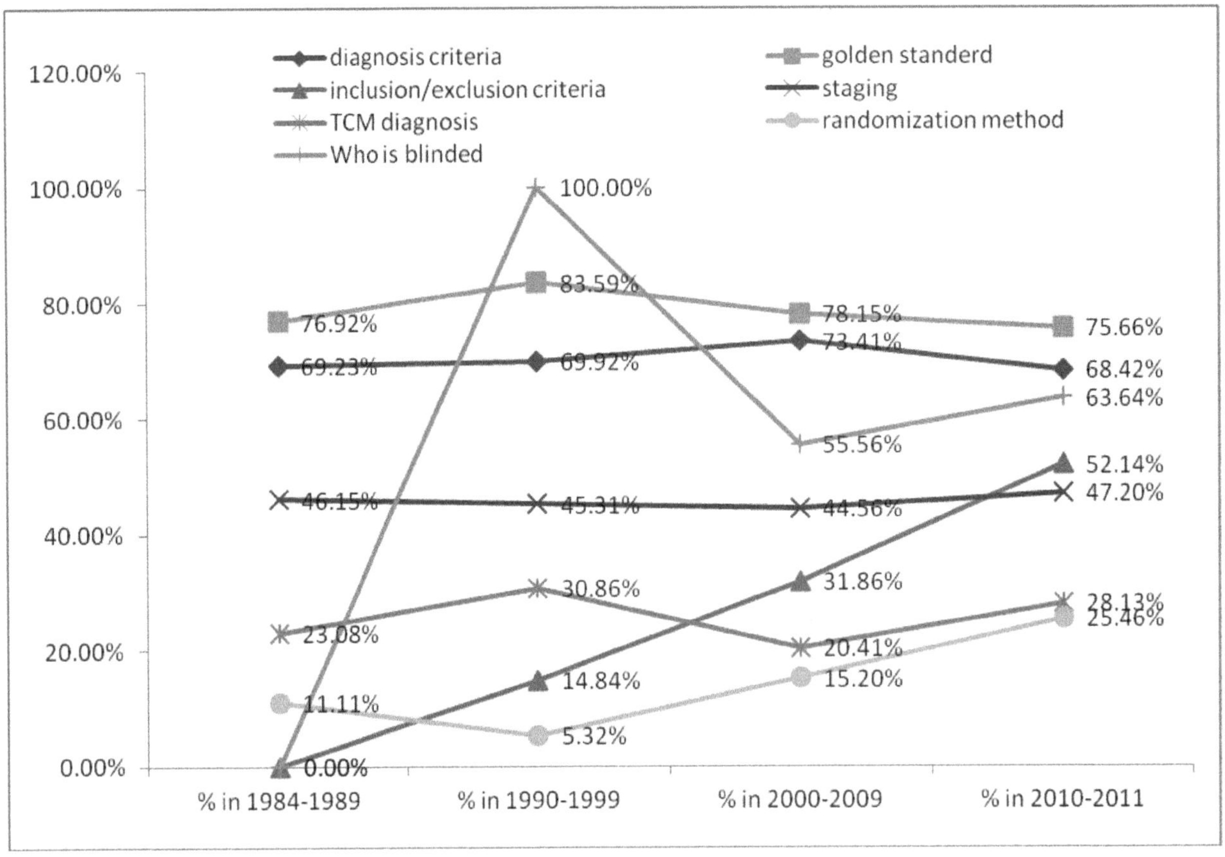

Figure 5. Reporting completeness, randomization methods and blinding across years. Percentage of reporting diagnosis criteria, inclusion/exclusion criteria, TCM diagnosis, golden standard of cancer, cancer staging, randomization method and blinding in the time order. Years are presented by the clusters of 1984–1989, 1990–1999, 2000–2009 and 2010–2011.

including whether blinding is used and who are blinded if available. If the report is based on existing previous data, the article should clearly articulate that it is a retrospective report so as todistinguish itself from prospective clinical studies.

If TCM syndrome differentiation is applied, the standard for judgment should be clearly stated.

Quality of life as one of the most important clinical outcomes and closely related to the patient wellbeing and increasingly included in studies. However the tools for measuring quality of life should have been more thoroughly reported with standard references in order to ensure clearer contribution to clinical decision making and design of further studies.

Funded studies, conference proceedings and dissertations seemed to generate higher report quality, which indicates that peer reviews is important for reporting of clinical studies, and the researchers in China are aware and able to do better research, however many of the Chinese journals haven't paid enough attention to the standard and strict requirement when accepting submissions. It is urgently suggested that journals in China endorse international standards such as CONSORT for randomized controlled trials and TREND for non-randomized controlled trials in their author guidelines to improve the quality of clinical studies and reporting.

More than 20% of the studies failed to provide adequate gold standard diagnosis for cancers, which could creates risks in interpretation of data. As an essential element of cancer studies, we suggest every clinical studyreport clear methods of cancer diagnosis in the future. We searched the Chinese publications based on general searching terms for example zhong yi (Chinese medicine) and zhong yao (Chinese herbal medicine), publications only labeled by the exact treatment such like the name of the herbal formula would have been missed out. More standard labelling is responsible for a more complete searching. We recommend that the future publication have at least one label related to Chinese medicine or herbal medicine for keyword or subject word if the study is TCM-related.

It was difficult to judge whether papers were reports of a prospective clinical studies without adequate information such as randomization methods and inclusion/exclusion criteria. Thus we combined together all clinical studies which involved comparison between different groups of patients receiving different interventions. Whilst most of studies mentioned "randomization", we could not assess more than 2,000 studies for study type (retrospective or prospective), and could not apply strict methodological evaluation as described in Cochrane Handbook [25]. Future studies should focus on specific types of TCM treatment for certain cancer with more detailed evaluation and analysis to ensure conclusions around effectiveness and safety and contribute to evidence-based clinical recommendations.

With regards to reviews of case series and case reports of TCM for cancer, individualized Chinese herbal medicine was the most frequently reported intervention. We suggest that the future studies focus on tailoring of treatment in cancer care.

Among the studies published in Chinese, herbal medicine is the main TCM intervention for cancer, comprising almost 90% in the total 2964 studies, which is also 7 times the number of acupuncture studies. This difference is much larger compared to a review based on English publications (acupuncture in 71 studies while Chinese herbal medicine in 11 studies) [9], which might reflect policy and levels of use of herbal medicine in different countries as well as publication bias. Although most of the included studies involved herbal medicine, there is no study reporting quality assessment of herbs or herbal products. Since the quality of herbal medicine is closely related to the clinical effectiveness and safety, and also essential for the quality of clinical study [26], this issue should be addressed in the future.

There have been a large number of controlled clinical studies of TCM for cancer, especially certain types with higher frequency such as lung cancer, liver cancer, stomach cancer, colorectal cancer, breast cancer, esophagus cancer, nasopharyngeal cancer, cervical cancer, ovarian cancer and pancreatic cancer. Systematic reviews could be implemented in order to access the effectiveness and safety of the TCM treatments for thesis types of cancers so that higher quality of evidence could be brought about based on the existing clinical information, the money and time have been spent, for the contribution to the clinical practice. One literature review of systematic reviews of TCM published in PubMed and Cochrane Library during the year 1999 to 2009 [26] identified 4 systematic reviews of TCM for cancer care including nasopharyngeal cancer, esophageal cancer, unrespectable hepatocellular cancer, and cancer pain respectively. We also identified Cochrane systematic reviews or protocols about Chinese herbal medicine for certain types of cancer including gastric precancerous lesions [27], Chinese herbal medicine for advanced pancreatic cancer [28], Chinese herbal medicine for chemotherapy side effects in colorectal cancer [29], Chinese herbal medicine for side effects of breast cancer [30], and herbal medicine for advanced colorectal cancer [31].

Conclusions

In future standard and adequate reporting of TCM cancer studies is essential. More attention should be paid to reporting clinical outcomes of importance to patient care and clinical decision making including survival times, extent of relapse/metastasis and quality of life.

Supporting Information

Table S1 Cancer-related clinical condition of the cancer patients treated by TCM in the controlled clinical studies. The study numbers and case numbers of cancer-related clinical conditions of the cancer patients treated by TCM. The clinical diagnosis is further classified as treated by TCM and prevented by TCM.
(DOC)

Table S2 Types of cancer treated by TCM in controlled clinical studies published in Chinese journals. Types of cancer treated by TCM in controlled clinical studies according to the category of. ICD-10 codes of all the cancers are presented in the table.
(DOC)

Table S3 Characteristics of studies with significant evidence of TCM treatments for cancer published in Chinese. The characteristics of 5 RCTs of TCM for cancer reporting randomization methods and blinding information with outcomes of survival, relapse and/or metastasis and quality of life.
(DOC)

Acknowledgments

We thank Associate Prof. Zhaolan Liu and PhD student Qing Li from Centre for Evidence-based Chinese Medicine, Beijing University of Chinese Medicine for their suggestions in statistic analysis, and Prof. Kelvin Chan from Herbal Medicine Group, Faculty of Pharmacy, University of Sydney, and Centre for Complementary Medicine Research, University of Western Sydney for his suggestions in drafting the manuscript.

Author Contributions

Substantial contribution to the study design and manuscript revision: JL AB. Conceived and designed the experiments: JL Xun Li. Performed the experiments: Xun Li GY Xinxue Li YZ JY JC XS XZ YG YX. Analyzed the data: Xun Li GY Xinxue Li. Wrote the paper: Xun Li.

References

1. World Health Organization (2009) Global health risks: mortality and burden of disease attributable to selected major risk.
2. Jemal A, Bray F, Center MM, Ferlay J, Ward E, et al. (2011) Glabal cancer statistics. CA Cancer j Clin 61: 69–90.
3. Danhier F, Feron O, Préat V (2010) To exploit the tumor microenvironment: Passive and active tumor targeting of nanocarriers for anti-cancer drug delivery. J Control Release 148: 135–146.
4. Li PW (2003) Management of cancer with Chinese medicine. Donica Publishing.
5. Boon HS, Olatunde F, Zick SM (2007) Trends in complementary/alternative medicine use by breast cancer survivors: comparing survey data from 1998 and 2005. BMC Womens Health 30: 4.
6. Yoder LH (2005) Let's talk 'cancer prevention'. MedSurg Nursing 14: 195–198.
7. Ernst E (2009) Complementary and alternative medicine (CAM) and cancer: the kind face of complementary medicine. Int J Surg 7: 499–500.
8. Jia L (2012) Cancer complementary and alternative medicine research at the US National Cancer Institute. Chin J Integr Med 18: 325–332.
9. Carmady B, Smith CA (2011) Use of Chinese medicine by cancer patients: a review of surveys. Chin Med 9: 22.
10. Liu J, Li X, Liu J, Ma L, Li X, et al. (2011) Traditional Chinese medicine in cancer care: a review of case reports published in Chinese literature. Forsch Komplementmed 18: 257–263.
11. Yang GY, Li X, Li XL, Wang L, Li J, et al. (2012) Traditional Chinese medicine in cancer care: a review of case series published in the Chinese literature. Evid Based Complement Alternat Med 2012: 751046. Epub 2012 May 31.
12. ICD-10 Version 2010. Available: http://apps.who.int/classifications/icd10/browse/2010/en. Accessed 2012 Nov 3.
13. Schulz KF, Altman DG, Moher D, for the CONSORT Group (2010) CONSORT 2010 Statement: updated guidelines for reporting parallel group randomised trials. Ann Int Med 2010 152: 726–732.
14. Des Jarlais DC, Lyles C, Crepaz N, TREND Group (2004) Improving the reporting quality of nonrandomized evaluations of behavioral and public health interventions: the TREND statement. Am J Public Health 94: 361–366.
15. Bao YH, Fang SY, Li G (1984) [Clinical analysis of integrative medicine for treating pancreatic cancer]. Zhong Xi Yi Jie He Za Zhi (Journal of Integrative Chinese and Western Medicine) 4: 16–18.
16. Xie BH, Huang KJ, Wang FM (1985) [Clinical observation of Chinese herbal medicine plus chemotherapy for pain in advanced stage cancer patients]. Zhong Xi Yi Jie He Za Zhi (Chinese Journal of Integrated Traditional and Western Medicine) 10: 586.
17. Wang TX, Du XG (1985) [The use of Chinese traditional medicine and herbs in prevention of immune-myelo-suggpressive effects in chemotherapy of malignant lymphoma]. Zhong Liu Lin Chuang (Chinese Journal of Clinical Oncology) 2: 144–146.
18. Huang S, Li DY (2011) [Clinical observation of Fufang Zhebei Keli in improving the survival of acute leukemia patients]. Master thesis. Beijing University of Chinese Medicine.
19. Xu ZY, Jin CJ, Shen DE, Li M, Zhou WD, et al. (2007) [Clincal study on treatment of advanced non-small-celllung cancer with Chinese herbal medicine in different stages combined with chemotherapy]. Zhong Guo Zhong Xi Yi Jie He Za Zhi (Chinese Journal of Integrative Traditional and Western Medicine) 27: 874–878.
20. Wang LF, Xu ZY, Jin CJ, Wang ZQ, Deng HB, et al. (2010) [Clinical study on treatment of advanced lung adenocarcinoma with staged Chinese herbal

medicine and chemotherapy]. Zhanghai Zhong Yi Yao Za Zhi (Shanghai Journal of Traditional Chinese Medicine) 6: 41–43.
21. Liu HT, Li JH (2009) [Evidence-based medicine analysis of Chinese herbal medicine in improving survival of post-surgery breast cancer patients]. Zhong Wai Yi Xue Wen Zhai (World Health Digest Medical Periodical) 8: 26–29.
22. Li LN, Liu WS, Xu K, Wu WY, Liu YL, et al. (2003) [Prognostic factor study of traditional Chinese medicine treatment based on syndrome differentiation for treating III,IV stage non-small cell lung cancer]. Shaanxi Zhong Liu Yi Xue (Shaanxi Journal of Oncology Medicine) 11: 44–47.
23. Wu T, Zhan SY, Li LM (2004) [History of the development of epidemiology experimental study]. Chin J Epidemiol (Zhong Hua Liu Xing Bing Xue Za Zhi) 25: 633–636.
24. World Health Organization (2012) Cancer Fact Sheets. Available: http://www.who.int/mediacentre/factsheets/fs297/en/. Accessed 2012 Nov 3.
25. Higgins JPT, Green S (editors) (2011) Cochrane Handbook for Systematic Reviews of Interventions Version 5.1.0 [updated March 2011]. The Cochrane Collaboration.
26. Jiang M, Yang J, Zhang C, Liu B, Chan K, et al. (2012) Clinical studies with traditional Chinese medicine in the past decade and future research and development. Planta Med 76: 2048–2064.
27. Tang X, Liu G, Wang P, Wu T (2008) Chinese herbal medicine alone or combined with vitamins for gastric precancerous lesions (Protocol). Cochrane Database of Systematic Reviews.
28. Ni YH, Li X, Xu Y, Liu JP (2012) Chinese herbal medicine for advanced pancreatic cancer (Protocol). Cochrane Database of Systematic Reviews.
29. Wu T, Munro AJ, Guanjian L, Liu GJ (2005) Chinese medical herbs for chemotherapy side effects in colorectal cancer patients. Cochrane Database of Systematic Reviews.
30. Zhang M, Liu X, Li J, He L, Tripathy D (2007) Chinese medicinal herbs to treat the side-effects of chemotherapy in breast cancer patients. Cochrane Database of Systematic Reviews.
31. Guo Z, Jia X, Liu JP, Liao J, Yang Y (2012) Herbal medicines for advanced colorectal cancer. Cochrane Database of Systematic Reviews.

16

Cochrane Systematic Reviews of Chinese Herbal Medicines

Jing Hu[1,2], Junhua Zhang[1], Wei Zhao[1], Yongling Zhang[1], Li Zhang[1], Hongcai Shang[1]*

1 Research Institute of Traditional Chinese Medicine, Tianjin University of Traditional Chinese Medicine, Tianjin, China, **2** Department of Epidemiology and Biostatistics, School of Public Health, Peking University, Beijing, China

Abstract

Objectives: Our study had two objectives: a) to systematically identify all existing systematic reviews of Chinese herbal medicines (CHM) published in Cochrane Library; b) to assess the methodological quality of included reviews.

Methodology/Principal Findings: We performed a systematic search of *the Cochrane Database of Systematic Reviews* (CDSR, Issue 5, 2010) to identify all reviews of CHM. A total of fifty-eight reviews were eligible for our study. Twenty-one of the included reviews had at least one Traditional Chinese Medicine (TCM) practitioner as its co-author. 7 reviews didn't include any primary study, the remaining reviews (n = 51) included a median of 9 studies and 936 participants. 50% of reviews were last assessed as up-to-date prior to 2008. The questions addressed by 39 reviews were broad in scope, in which 9 reviews combined studies with different herbal medicines. For OQAQ, the mean of overall quality score (item 10) was 5.05 (95% CI; 4.58-5.52). All reviews assessed the methodological quality of primary studies, 16% of included primary studies used adequate sequence generation and 7% used adequate allocation concealment. Of the 51 nonempty reviews, 23 reviews were reported as being inconclusive, while 27 concluded that there might be benefit of CHM, which was limited by the poor quality or inadequate quantity of included studies. 58 reviews reported searching a median of seven electronic databases, while 10 reviews did not search any Chinese database.

Conclusions: Now CDSR has included large numbers of CHM reviews, our study identified some areas which could be improved, such as almost half of included reviews did not have the participation of TCM practitioners and were not up-to-date according to Cochrane criteria, some reviews pooled the results of different herbal medicines and ignored the searching of Chinese databases.

Editor: Jos H. Verbeek, Finnish Institute of Occupational Health, Finland

Funding: This study was supported in part by the National Significant Projects of New Drugs Creation (No. 2008ZX09312-001) and the program of New Century Excellent Talents in University (NCET-09-0900). The funders had no role in study design, data collection and analysis, decision to publish, or preparation of the manuscript.

Competing Interests: The authors have declared that no competing interests exist.

* E-mail: shanghongcai@foxmail.com

Introduction

Traditional Chinese Medicine (TCM) is an essential part of the healthcare system in several Asian countries, and is considered a complementary or alternative medical system in most Western countries [1]. Chinese herbal medicines (CHM) are an essential part of TCM [2]. The 2002 National Health Interview Survey showed that 18.6% of adults used CHM in the United States, while it was 12.1% in 1997 [3]. With the increased use of CHM, questions arise from clinicians, patients, and policymakers as to the effectiveness of these interventions [4]. In an era of evidence-based healthcare, systematic reviews of randomized controlled trials (RCTs) are becoming increasingly important as a source of evidence for decision-making. As the number of systematic reviews of CHM increase, the quality of which has been highlighted and called into question. Some studies have assessed the quality of CHM reviews published in Chinese journals, in general, they have been criticized for lacking a comprehensive search for clinical trials, ignoring the characteristics of TCM, using inappropriate criteria to assess the methodological quality of included studies, and addressing too broadly defined questions [5–7]. All [8] these aspects could have contributed to a poor quality review.

The Cochrane Collaboration is an international organization that aims to prepare and maintain rigorous systematic reviews in order to help people make well-informed decisions about health care [8]. Compared with reviews published in paper-based journals, Cochrane reviews are noted to have greater methodological quality [9]. Ever since 1999 when the first Cochrane review of CHM was published, a sharp increase has been observed in the number of similar reviews. However, no previous studies have systematically assessed the methodological quality of Cochrane reviews of CHM. Therefore, we did this overview of systematic reviews. Our study had two objectives: a) to systematically identify all existing Cochrane reviews of CHM; b) to assess the methodological quality of included reviews.

Methods

Ethics

Data for this study was acquired through previously published work, no patient or hospital data was accessed. Therefore, written consent and institutional ethical review was not required for this research. The PRISMA checklist and flow diagram are available as supporting information; see PRISMA Checklist S1 and PRISMA Flow Diagram S1.

Literature search

In order to identify reviews focusing on CHM, we searched the titles and abstracts of all reviews contained within *the Cochrane Database of Systematic Reviews* (CDSR) (Issue 5, 2010) using the following terms: *Chinese* or *herb** or *traditional* or *plant* or *medic**.

Inclusion and exclusion criteria

We included all Cochrane reviews of CHM. Protocols and reviews which have been withdrawn from publication were excluded. We defined CHM as preparations derived from plants or parts of plants (e.g. leaves, stems, buds, flowers, roots or tubers) that grow in China and have been widely used for medical purpose. CHM include single herbs (or extracts from single herbs) and compound formulas of several herbs in all forms of preparation formulation (e.g. oral liquid, tablet, capsule, pill, powder, plaster or injection liquid). It should be noted that our definition of CHM does not include plant-derived chemicals or synthetic chemicals which contain constituents of plants. For example, although Huperzia serrata has its origin in China, according to our definition, Huperzine A does not belong to CHM because it is a kind of alkaloid extracted from Huperzia serrata. In addition, we only included reviews discussing herbs which originated from China, reviews on herbs such as Passiflora and Echinacea, both of American origin, were invariably excluded.

Oxman-Guyatt Overview Quality Assessment Questionnaire (OQAQ) [10]

The OQAQ instrument was selected as the quality appraisal tool, which was designed to evaluate whether the authors of a systematic review conducted a comprehensive search, minimized bias in the selection of primary studies, evaluated the primary literature, and pooled the results appropriately. It consists of 10 questions, the first 9 questions are designed to assess different aspects of methodological quality and have set answers of "yes", "partially/can't tell", or "no", question 10 is an assessment of the overall scientific quality of the systematic review on a scale of 1 to 7, it is answered based on how well the review scored on the first 9 questions.

Data extraction

We established a database (using Microsoft Excel 2007) to extract data. The database had two components: 1) general characteristics, including country of first author and number of authors, whether the review had the participation of TCM practitioners, number of trials and participants included, disease, the year of review last assessed as up-to-date, conclusions drawn by the reviewers (by assessing the reviewers' abstract conclusions statements), interventions in experimental groups, number of herbs included, and whether the results of different herbal medicines were pooled; 2) methodological quality of included reviews, including OQAQ scale, the approach to assessment of methodological quality of primary studies, the number of trials with adequate sequence generation and allocation concealment, and type and number of English and Chinese databases searched. Two reviewers (Jing Hu and Wei Zhao) independently extracted the information of each review, disagreements between the two reviewers were resolved by discussion.

The questions addressed by a review may be broad or narrow in scope, each review was assigned into one of the following two categories: 1) narrowly focused reviews, intervention in each review was single herb or herbal preparation, as an example of "Chinese herbal medicine suxiao jiuxin wan for angina pectoris"; 2) broadly focused reviews, including reviews concerned multiple Chinese herbs or a family of herbal medicines sharing similar efficacy, such as "Chinese herbal medicine for premenstrual syndrome" and "Chinese herbal medicine Huangqi type formulations for nephrotic syndrome". For broadly focused reviews, we listed the number of herbs included and assessed whether the results of different herbal medicines were pooled.

A review was believed to have the participation of TCM practitioners if at least one author works in TCM department, university or hospital, or it stated that it had got suggestion from TCM practitioners.

When we assessed the type and number of English and Chinese databases searched, we only listed the databases which at least 4 reviews searched. In addition, the Cochrane Specialized Register and databases/websites for ongoing trials were also searched in some reviews, we did not list them in our study.

Results

278 potentially relevant reviews were obtained, after selection (according to inclusion and exclusion criteria), a total of 58 Cochrane reviews [11–68] were eligible for our study, a full list of reviews is included in Table S1. Of the 58 reviews, one review [49] included herbs originated in China, India and Japan; interventions in another review [55] concerned both herbal and chemical medicines. In these two cases, we extracted and analyzed the information relating to CHM.

General characteristics of included reviews

The number of authors in the 58 reviews ranged from 1 to 10, the first authors were most often from China (46 [79%]), followed by UK (n = 8), and Netherlands, Canada, USA and Australia each have one first-authored review. Twenty-one (36%) of the included reviews had at least one TCM practitioner as its co-author. 7 (12%) reviews didn't include any primary study, of the remaining reviews (n = 51), a total of 671 studies and 75,609 participants were included, the median number of studies and participants included were 9 (Quartile: 3, 15) and 936 (Quartile: 492, 1567) respectively. 50% of the reviews were last assessed as up-to-date prior to 2008, of reviews considered out-of-date, one was last updated in 2000. In total, 44 diseases were investigated in the included reviews, 18 (31%) reviews addressed cerebral vascular and cardiovascular diseases (9 reviews focused on stroke), followed by reviews focused on respiratory diseases (n = 6) and gynecological/pregnancy diseases (n = 6).

Of the 51 nonempty reviews, only one review concluded positively, 27 (53%) concluded that there might be benefit of CHM for treating specific health conditions, which was limited by the poor quality or inadequate quantity of studies, 23 (45%) reviews concluded that the currently available data do not allow any conclusion to be drawn, generally because of low methodological quality of studies, small number of studies and participants included or publication bias.

Nineteen reviews focused on 13 single herbs or herbal preparations, while the remainder (39 [67%]) addressed broad questions, in which 34 reviews concerned multiple Chinese herbs or multiple formulations of Chinese herbs, 5 reviews involved a family of herbal medicines sharing similar efficacy, including Huangqi type formulations (including Huangqi injection and

Table 1. Summary of OQAQ questions in included reviews.

OQAQ question	Yes(%)	Partially/Can't tell(%)	No(%)
1. Were the search methods used to find evidence reported?	58(100)	0(0)	0(0)
2. Was the search strategy for evidence reasonably comprehensive?	51(88)	1(2)	6(10)
3. Were the criteria used for deciding which studies to include reported?	58(100)	0(0)	0(0)
4. Was bias in the selection for studies avoided?	41(71)	13(22)	4(7)
5. Were the criteria used for assessing validity of included studies reported?	57(98)	1(2)	0(0)
6. Was the validity of included studies assessed using appropriate criteria?	56(97)	2(3)	0(0)
7. Were the methods used to combine the findings of studies reported?	49(84)	9(16)	0(0)
8. Were the Findings of studies combined appropriately?	48(83)	9(15)	1(2)
9. Were the conclusions made by authors supported by the reported data?	58(100)	0(0)	0(0)
10. How would you rate the scientific quality of this overview?	5.05(1.78)*, (95% CI: 4.58, 5.52)		

OQAQ, Oxman-Guyatt Overview Quality Assessment Questionnaire.
*Mean (SD).

Huangqi-Danggui mixture), Chuanxiong preparations (including Nao-an capsule, Xifeng wan and Apoplexy Preventing Dry Ointment Powder), Dan Shen agents (including Compound Danshen Dripping Pill, Compound Danshen injection, Danshen injection, Yiqi huoxue injection, and Quyu huatan xiezhuo fang) and Sanchi (including Xinnaotai, Sanchitongshu capsule, Naoming injection, Xuesaitong soft capsule, Sanqitongshu capsule, Xuesaitong and Xueshuantong injection). Of the 39 reviews, 4 didn't include any primary study, of the remaining reviews (n = 35), the median number of herbal medicines involved was 6 within a range of 1 to 71, results of different herbal medicines were pooled in 9 reviews, in which 7 reviews pooled the results of all Chinese herbal medicines, one review pooled all Danshen agents, and one pooled Sanchi.

Methodological quality of included reviews

Table 1 presents a summary of OQAQ items of the included reviews, the mean score (item 10) was 5.05, 95% CI (4.58, 5.52). 41 of 58 reviews attempted to minimize bias during the selection of studies by at least two reviewers independently select eligible studies.

All reviews reported assessing the methodological quality of included primary studies, 21 (36%) reviews used the Cochrane Collaboration's 'Risk of Bias' tool, the Jadad scale was used in 6 reviews, 12 (21%) reviews used unnamed checklist. Among 671 included studies, 108 (16%) used adequate sequence generation, allocation concealment was adequate in 50 (7%) studies.

The median number of databases searched in 58 reviews was 7 within a range of 4 to 15. Regarding to the English language databases, the most searched was MEDLINE (98%), followed by EMBASE (97%) and CENTRAL (97%). CBM was the most searched Chinese database (78%), the second most used was CNKI (45%) and the third was VIP (24%) (Table 2). All reviews searched at least 2 English databases, while 10 reviews did not search any Chinese database. 41 (71%) reviews searched at least 3 English databases, while only 6 (10%) reviews searched at least 3 Chinese databases (Table 3).

Discussion

Evidence-based health care involves the systematic collection, synthesis and application of scientific evidence to guide clinical practice and policy-making. Systematic reviews are a key

Table 2. Databases searched in included reviews.

English databases searched	Number of reviews (%) n = 58	Chinese databases searched	Number of reviews (%) n = 58
MEDLINE*	57(98%)	CBM(Chinese Biomedical Database)	45(78%)
CENTRAL(The Cochrane Central Register of Controlled Trials)	56(97%)	CNKI(China National Knowledge Infrastructure)	26(45%)
EMBASE	56(97%)	VIP (a full text database of China)	14(24%)
AMED(Allied and Complementary Medicine Database)	28(48%)	The Chinese Cochrane Centre Controlled Trials Register	11(19%)
Cochrane Complementary Medicine Field Trials Register	20(34%)	TCMLARS(Traditional Chinese Medical Literature Analysis and Retrieval System)	6(10%)
CINAHL(Cumulative Index to Nursing and Allied Health Literature)	15(26%)		
LILACS(Latin American and Caribbean Health Science Literature)	11(19%)		
SIGLE(System for Information on Grey Literature in Europe)	7(12%)		
PsycINFO	4(7%)		

*including two reviews which used PubMed.

Table 3. Number of English and Chinese databases searched.

Number of English databases	Number of reviews (%) n = 58	Number of Chinese databases	Number of reviews (%) n = 58
0	0(0%)	0	10(17%)
1	0(0%)	1	15(26%)
2	2(3%)	2	19(33%)
3	15(26%)	3	8(14%)
>3	41(71%)	>3	6(10%)

component of evidence-based health care. Currently, CDSR has included 58 systematic reviews of CHM.

Almost seventy percent of included reviews' topics were too broad, the percentage was much higher than that of similar reviews published in Chinese journals, which was 38 percent (41 among 107 reviews) [69]. It is difficult to develop a comprehensive search strategy for broadly focused reviews, for instance, one hundred and sixty herbal medicines are now available for coronary heart diseases treatment, a systematic review of CHM for coronary heart disease will have to include clinical trials of all these herbal medicines, it is easily to cause the incomplete identification of relevant studies. Choosing broad topics for reviews will require more resources in data collection and analysis, the results may also be too complicated to interpret. So topic selection of CHM reviews should focus on specific clinical problems, the extensive titles are not recommended.

As broad questions of reviews may be addressed by large sets of heterogeneous studies, the data synthesis may be particularly challenging. In our study, 9 reviews (among the 39 broadly focused reviews) pooled the results of different herbs, which did not identify potentially important differences in effects across different interventions. Systematic reviews can, but do not have to use meta-analysis when combining data from primary studies, prior to conducting a meta-analysis, reviewers should examine the consistency of the interventions. It is recommended that the data of each intervention should be analyzed and presented separately if several different interventions for the same condition were tested in one review.

The goal of a systematic review is to identify relevant studies completely and unbiasedly [70]. It has been demonstrated [71,72] that significant amounts of evidence would potentially be missed if the search is limited to English-only sources. Because a considerable number of clinical trials on CHM were published only in the Chinese language journals, so a comprehensive search of Chinese databases is essential for a systematic review of CHM. However, we were disappointed to find that almost twenty percent of reviews did not search any Chinese database in our study. One study [73] compared four Chinese databases and concluded that CBM is the preferred database for systematic reviewers to retrieve relevant Chinese studies, while CNKI is recommended for non-Chinese-speaking researchers due to its free searched English version website (www.global.cnki.net) and "Cross-Language Search" functions. CBM has no English website and a fee is charged for searching, now many Chinese medical universities have got the permission to search CBM, so maybe the most cost- and time-efficient way to search it is to enhance collaboration with Chinese researchers.

In doing a review of CHM, professional advice from TCM practitioners is of great value. It is generally assumed that the characteristics of TCM would be well taken into account in a review if one or some of its reviewers majored in TCM. In our study, we found that more than sixty percent of reviews did not have one TCM practitioner in the authors list, which might lead to insufficient consideration of the characteristics of TCM (e.g. determination of treatment based on pathogenesis obtained through differentiation of symptoms and signs) and incorrect results. We suggest that future reviews should be authored by a group of individuals with both clinical expertise and methodological expertise.

Of the 671 primary studies included, less than twenty percent of studies used adequate sequence generation, and only seven percent used adequate allocation concealment. Because of the poor methodological quality of primary studies, nearly half of reviews were reported as being inconclusive, while 27 reviews provided preliminary evidence of CHM's benefits to certain conditions, which should be considered tentative and need to be confirmed with rigorous RCTs. The Chinese government has been aware of the importance of conducting scientifically sound RCTs and has made substantial investments into funding clinical researches of CHM, now many well-designed RCTs of CHM with rigorous methodology are in progress or have been completed in China [74], we believe future updates of currently inconclusive Cochrane reviews of CHM may reach more definitive conclusions.

Limitations of the study

Although we believed a review has a greater chance of considering the characteristics of TCM if at least one author works in TCM department, university or hospital, or it stated that it had got suggestion from TCM practitioners, it is quite possible that some reviewers had consulted TCM experts while designing and doing the review, but did not report it in articles. As cases of this kind could not be ruled out, we therefore might have underestimated the proportion of reviews getting support from TCM practitioners. In addition, we restricted our search to Cochrane reviews because they are generally less prone to bias than systematic reviews published in paper-based journals [9,75,76]. However, this might cause the results of this study to be only applicable to review articles in the Cochrane database. Further evaluation is needed in order to know whether the systematic reviews of CHM published in English paper-based journals even in the leading journals have the same problem.

Supporting Information

Table S1 List of all included Cochrane reviews of CHM.
(DOC)

PRISMA Checklist S1
(DOC)

PRISMA Flow Diagram S1
(DOC)

Acknowledgments

The authors thank Mu Wei, Ph.D., Tianjin University of TCM, China, and Xiao Lu, M.S., Tianjin University of TCM, China, for their help with reviewing and revising the entire manuscript for English Language editing.

Author Contributions

Conceived and designed the experiments: JH JZ HS. Performed the experiments: JH HS. Analyzed the data: JH LZ YZ. Contributed reagents/materials/analysis tools: LZ YZ. Wrote the paper: JH JZ. Searched and selected studies: JH WZ. Extracted the data: JH WZ.

References

1. Chan E, Tan M, Xin JN, Sudarsanam S, Johnson DE (2010) Interactions between traditional Chinese medicines and Western therapeutics. Curr Opin Drug Discov Devel 13: 50–65.
2. Vickers A, Zollman C (1999) ABC of complementary medicine: herbal medicine. BMJ 319: 1050–1053.
3. Tindle HA, Davis RB, Phillips RS, Eisenberg DM (2005) Trends in use of complementary and alternative medicine by US adults: 1997-2002. Altern Ther Health Med 11: 42–49.
4. Firenzuoli F, Gori L (2007) Herbal Medicine Today: Clinical and Research Issues. Evid Based Complement Alternat Med 4: 37–40.
5. Liu JP, Xia Y (2007) Quality appraisal of systematic reviews or meta-analysis on traditional Chinese medicine published in Chinese journals. Zhongguo Zhong Xi Yi Jie He Za Zhi 27: 306–311.
6. Li TQ, Liu XM, Zhang MM, Ma JX, Du L, et al. (2007) Assessment of Systematic Reviews and Meta-analyses on Traditional Chinese Medicine Published in Chinese Journals. Chin J Evid-based Med 7: 180–188.
7. Hu D, Kang DY, Hong Q (2010) Heterogeneity Analysis of Systematic Reviews on Traditional Chinese Medicine. Chin J Evid-based Med 10: 488–491.
8. Green S, Higgins JPT, Alderson P, Clarke M, Mulrow CD, et al. (2008) Cochrane Handbook. The Cochrane Library. Version 5.0.2.
9. Jadad AR, Cook DJ, Jones A, Klassen TP, Tugwell P, et al. (1998) Methodology and Reports of Systematic Reviews and Meta-analyses: A Comparison of Cochrane Reviews with Articles Published in Paper-Based Journals. JAMA 280: 278–280.
10. Oxman AD, Guyatt G (1991) Validation of an index of the quality of review articles. J Clin Epidemiol 44: 1271–8.
11. Liu JP, McIntosh H, Lin H (2009) Chinese medicinal herbs for chronic hepatitis B. Cochrane Database of Systematic Reviews 1: CD001940.
12. Li WZ, Liu M, Feng SJ, Wu B, Zhang SH, et al. (2009) Acanthopanax for acute ischaemic stroke. Cochrane Database of Systematic Reviews 3: CD007032.
13. Zhang WY, Leonard T, Bath-Hextall FJ, Chambers C, Lee CF, et al. (2009) Chinese herbal medicine for atopic eczema. Cochrane Database of Systematic Reviews 4: CD002291.
14. Cui XJ, Trinh K, Wang YJ (2010) Chinese herbal medicine for chronic neck pain due to cervical degenerative disc disease. Cochrane Database of Systematic Reviews 1: CD006556.
15. Flower A, Liu JP, Chen SS, Lewith G, Little P (2009) Chinese herbal medicine for endometriosis. Cochrane Database of Systematic Reviews 3: CD006568.
16. Jing Z, Yang XZ, Khaled MK, Chen XY, Wu TX (2009) Chinese herbal medicine for premenstrual syndrome. Cochrane Database of Systematic Reviews 3: CD006414.
17. Zhu ZS, Proctor M, Bensoussan A, Wu E, Smith CA (2009) Chinese herbal medicine for primary dysmenorrhoea. Cochrane Database of Systematic Reviews 1: CD005288.
18. Rathbone J, Zhang L, Zhang MM, Xia J, Liu XH, et al. (2008) Chinese herbal medicine for schizophrenia. Cochrane Database of Systematic Reviews 3: CD003444.
19. uan W, Wang J, Wu TX (2009) Chinese herbal medicine Huangqi type formulations for nephrotic syndrome. Cochrane Database of Systematic Reviews 3: CD006335.
20. Duan X, Zhou LK, Wu TX, Liu GJ, Qiao JQ, et al. (2009) Chinese herbal medicine suxiao jiuxin wan for angina pectoris. Cochrane Database of Systematic Reviews 4: CD004473.
21. Wang Q, Guo Z, Zhao PC, Wang YP, Gan T, et al. (2009) Chinese herbal medicines for acute pancreatitis. Cochrane Database of Systematic Reviews 3: CD003631.
22. Zeng XX, Yuan Y, Wu TX, Yan L, Su H (2009) Chinese herbal medicines for hyperthyroidism. Cochrane Database of Systematic Reviews 1: CD005450.
23. Gan T, Wu ZY, Tian L, Wang YP (2010) Chinese herbal medicines for induction of remission in advanced or late gastric cancer. Cochrane Database of Systematic Reviews 1: CD005096.
24. Grant SJ, Bensoussan A, Chang D, Kiat H, Klupp NL, et al. (2009) Chinese herbal medicines for people with impaired glucose tolerance or impaired fasting blood glucose. Cochrane Database of Systematic Reviews 4: CD006690.
25. Li WJ, Tang LL, Wu TX, Zhang J, Liu GJ, et al. (2010) Chinese herbal medicines for treating pre-eclampsia. Cochrane Database of Systematic Reviews 1: CD005126.
26. Liu JP, Zhang M, Wang WY, Grimsgaard S (2009) Chinese herbal medicines for type 2 diabetes mellitus. Cochrane Database of Systematic Reviews 1: CD003642.
27. Wang DF, Hu LN, Marjoribanks J, Jia HJ, Sun Y, et al. (2009) Chinese herbal medicines in the treatment of ectopic pregnancy. Cochrane Database of Systematic Reviews 1: CD006224.
28. Liu XM, Zhang MM, He L, Li YP, Kang YK (2008) Chinese herbs combined with Western medicine for severe acute respiratory syndrome (SARS). Cochrane Database of Systematic Reviews 4: CD004882.
29. Wu TX, AJ, Liu GJ (2008) Chinese medical herbs for chemotherapy side effects in colorectal cancer patients. Cochrane Database of Systematic Reviews 4: CD004540.
30. Wei JF, Ni J, Wu TX, Chen XY, Duan X, et al. (2010) Chinese medicinal herbs for acute bronchitis. Cochrane Database of Systematic Reviews 2: CD004560.
31. Liu JP, McIntosh H, Lin H (2009) Chinese medicinal herbs for asymptomatic carriers of hepatitis B virus infection. Cochrane Database of Systematic Reviews 1: CD002231.
32. Chen XY, Wu TX, Liu GJ, Wang Q, Zheng J, et al. (2010) Chinese medicinal herbs for influenza. Cochrane Database of Systematic Reviews 2: CD004559.
33. Zheng YL, Gu R, Wu TX (2010) Chinese medicinal herbs for measles. Cochrane Database of Systematic Reviews 2: CD005531.
34. Shi YY, Gu R, Liu C, Ni J, Wu TX, et al. (2010) Chinese medicinal herbs for sore throat. Cochrane Database of Systematic Reviews 2: CD004877.
35. Zhang XG, Wu TX, Zhang J, Yan Q, Xie LX, et al. (2010) Chinese medicinal herbs for the common cold. Cochrane Database of Systematic Reviews 2: CD004782.
36. Zhang MM, Liu XM, Li J, He L, Tripathy D (2009) Chinese medicinal herbs to treat the side-effects of chemotherapy in breast cancer patients. Cochrane Database of Systematic Reviews 1: CD004921.
37. Yang XZ, Zeng XX, Wu TX (2010) Chuanxiong preparations for preventing stroke. Cochrane Database of Systematic Reviews 1: CD006765.
38. Yuan Y, Zeng XX, Luo YK, Li ZG, Wu TX (2008) Chuanxiong-type preparations for acute ischemic stroke. Cochrane Database of Systematic Reviews 4: CD005569.
39. Wu B, Liu M, Zhang SH (2008) Dan Shen agents for acute ischaemic stroke. Cochrane Database of Systematic Reviews 4: CD004295.
40. Wu TX, Ni J, Wei JF (2009) Danshen (Chinese medicinal herb) preparations for acute myocardial infarction. Cochrane Database of Systematic Reviews 1: CD004465.
41. Cao WZ, Liu WM, Wu TX, Zhong DC, Liu GJ (2008) Dengzhanhua preparations for acute cerebral infarction. Cochrane Database of Systematic Reviews 4: CD005568.
42. Dong R, Chen XY, Wu TX, Liu GJ (2009) Elemene for the treatment of lung cancer. Cochrane Database of Systematic Reviews 1: CD006054.
43. Evans JR (2009) Ginkgo biloba extract for age-related macular degeneration. Cochrane Database of Systematic Reviews 2: CD001775.
44. Zeng XR, Liu M, Yang YS, Li Y, Asplund K (2009) Ginkgo biloba for acute ischaemic stroke. Cochrane Database of Systematic Reviews 1: CD003691.
45. Birks J, Grimley EJ (2009) Ginkgo biloba for cognitive impairment and dementia. Cochrane Database of Systematic Reviews 2: CD003120.
46. Nicolaï SPA, Kruidenier LM, Bendermacher BLW, Prins MH, Teijink JAW (2009) Ginkgo biloba for intermittent claudication. Cochrane Database of Systematic Reviews 2: CD006888.
47. Hilton MP, Stuart EL (2010) Ginkgo biloba for tinnitus. Cochrane Database of Systematic Reviews 3: CD003852.
48. Guo RL, Pittler MH, Ernst E (2009) Hawthorn extract for treating chronic heart failure. Cochrane Database of Systematic Reviews 1: CD005312.
49. Arnold E, Clark CE, Lasserson TJ, Wu TX (2008) Herbal interventions for chronic asthma in adults and children. Cochrane Database of Systematic Reviews 4: CD005989.
50. Gagnier JJ, Tulder MW, Berman BM, Bombardier C (2010) Herbal medicine for low back pain. Cochrane Database of Systematic Reviews 2: CD004504.
51. Liu JP, Manheimer E, Yang M (2009) Herbal medicines for treating HIV infection and AIDS. Cochrane Database of Systematic Reviews 1: CD003937.
52. Liu JP, Yang M, Liu YX, Wei ML, Grimsgaard S (2008) Herbal medicines for treatment of irritable bowel syndrome. Cochrane Database of Systematic Reviews 4: CD004116.
53. Liu JP, Yang M, Du XM (2009) Herbal medicines for viral myocarditis. Cochrane Database of Systematic Reviews 1: CD003711.
54. Liu JP, Yang H, Xia Y, Cardini F (2009) Herbal preparations for uterine fibroids. Cochrane Database of Systematic Reviews 2: CD005292.
55. Wu HM, Tang JL, Sha ZH, Li YP (2009) Interventions for preventing infection in nephrotic syndrome. Cochrane Database of Systematic Reviews 2: CD003964.
56. Yang WM, Hao ZL, Zhang SH, Dong W, Wu TX, et al. (2009) Mailuoning for acute ischaemic stroke. Cochrane Database of Systematic Reviews 2: CD007028.
57. Liu JP, Manheimer E, Tsutani K, Gluud C (2009) Medicinal herbs for hepatitis C virus infection. Cochrane Database of Systematic Reviews 1: CD003183.

58. Tan Y, Liu M, Wu B (2009) Puerarin for acute ischaemic stroke. Cochrane Database of Systematic Reviews 1: CD004955.
59. Wang Q, Wu TX, Chen XY, Duan X, Zheng J, et al. (2009) Puerarin injection for unstable angina pectoris. Cochrane Database of Systematic Reviews 1: CD004196.
60. Chen XY, Zhou MK, Li QF, Yang J, Zhang Y, et al. (2008) Sanchi for acute ischaemic stroke. Cochrane Database of Systematic Reviews 4: CD006305.
61. Chen J, Wu G, Li SQ, Yu T, Xie Y, et al. (2009) Shengmai (a traditional Chinese herbal medicine) for heart failure. Cochrane Database of Systematic Reviews 1: CD005052.
62. Wu TX, Harrison RA, Chen XY, Ni J, Zhou LK, et al. (2009) Tongxinluo (Tong xin luo or Tong-xin-luo) capsule for unstable angina pectoris. Cochrane Database of Systematic Reviews 1: CD004474.
63. Zhuo Q, Yang XZ, Wu TX, Liu GJ, Zhou LK (2008) Tongxinluo capsule for acute stroke. Cochrane Database of Systematic Reviews 4: CD004584.
64. Adams D, Wu TX, Yang XZ, Tai SS, Vohra S (2009) Traditional Chinese medicinal herbs for the treatment of idiopathic chronic fatigue and chronic fatigue syndrome. Cochrane Database of Systematic Reviews 4: CD006348.
65. Li QF, Chen XY, He L, Zhou D (2009) Traditional Chinese medicine for epilepsy. Cochrane Database of Systematic Reviews 3: CD006454.
66. Wu TX, Li QP, Yuan ZY (2009) Yizhi capsule for vascular dementia. Cochrane Database of Systematic Reviews 2: CD005382.
67. Yue JR, Yang XY, Wu TX, Shu DF, Dong BR (2008) Zhiling decoction for vascular dementia. Cochrane Database of Systematic Reviews 3: CD004670.
68. Zhuo Q, Yuan ZY, Chen HX, Wu TX (2010) Traditional Chinese herbal products for stable angina. Cochrane Database of Systematic Reviews 5: CD004468.
69. Zhang JH, Shang HC, Gao XM, Zhang BL, Xiang YZ, et al. (2007) Methodology and Reporting Quality of Systematic Review/Meta-Analysis of Traditional Chinese Medicine. J Altern Complement Med 13: 797–805.
70. Lui S, Smith EJ, Terplan M (2010) Heterogeneity in search strategies among Cochrane acupuncture reviews: is there room for improvement? Acupunct Med 28: 149–53.
71. Moher D, Fortin P, Jadad AR, Juni P, Klassen T, et al. (1996) Completeness of reporting of trials published in languages other than English: implications for conduct and reporting of systematic reviews. Lancet 347: 363–6.
72. Ezzo J, Berman B, Vickers A, Linde K (1998) Complementary medicine and the Cochrane Collaboration. JAMA 280: 1628–1630.
73. Ai CL, Duan YR, Wiffen P, Zhang MM, Li J (2010) Chinese Biomedical Databases: Selection and Search for Trials to Conduct Systematic Reviews. Chin J Evid-based Med 10(6): 749–53.
74. Shang HC, Zhang BL (2010) To improve the overall level of traditional chinese medicine research by government leading and multiple participation. Chin J Evid-based Med 10(6): 640–41.
75. Delaney A, Bagshaw SM, Ferland A, Laupland K, Manns B, et al. (2007) The quality of reports of critical care meta-analyses in the Cochrane Database of Systematic Reviews: an independent appraisal. Crit Care Med 35(2): 589–94.
76. Moseley AM, Elkins MR, Herbert RD, Maher CG, Sherrington C (2009) Cochrane reviews used more rigorous methods than non-Cochrane reviews: survey of systematic reviews in physiotherapy. Journal of Clinical Epidemiology 62: 1021–1030.

17

Oral Chinese Herbal Medicine Combined with Pharmacotherapy for Stable COPD: A Systematic Review of Effect on BODE Index and Six Minute Walk Test

Xiankun Chen[1,2], Brian May[3], Yuan Ming Di[3], Anthony Lin Zhang[3], Chuanjian Lu[2,4], Charlie Changli Xue[2,3,4], Lin Lin[5]*

1 Evidence-Based Medicine & Clinical Research Service Group, Guangdong Provincial Academy of Chinese Medical Sciences, Guangzhou, China, **2** Guangdong Provincial Hospital of Chinese Medicine, Guangzhou, China, **3** Traditional & Complementary Medicine Research Program, Health Innovations Research Institute, School of Health Sciences, RMIT University, Melbourne, Australia, **4** Guangdong Provincial Academy of Chinese Medical Sciences, Guangzhou, China, **5** Department of Respiratory Medicine, Guangdong Provincial Hospital of Chinese Medicine, Guangzhou, Guangdong Province, China

Abstract

This systematic review evaluated the effects of Chinese herbal medicine (CHM) plus routine pharmacotherapy (RP) on the objective outcome measures BODE index, 6-minute walk test (6MWT), and 6-minute walk distance (6MWD) in individuals with stable chronic obstructive pulmonary disease (COPD). Searches were conducted of six English and Chinese databases (PubMed, EMBASE, CENTRAL, CINAHL, CNKI and CQVIP) from their inceptions until 18th November 2013 for randomized controlled trials involving oral administration of CHM plus RP compared to the same RP, with BODE Index and/or 6MWT/D as outcomes. Twenty-five studies were identified. BODE Index was used in nine studies and 6MWT/D was used in 22 studies. Methodological quality was assessed using the Cochrane Risk of Bias tool. Weaknesses were identified in most studies. Six studies were judged as 'low' risk of bias for randomisation sequence generation. Twenty-two studies involving 1,834 participants were included in the meta-analyses. The main meta-analysis results showed relative benefits for BODE Index in nine studies (mean difference [MD] −0.71, 95% confidence interval [CI] −0.94, −0.47) and 6MWT/D in 17 studies (MD 54.61 meters, 95%CI 33.30, 75.92) in favour of the CHM plus RP groups. The principal plants used were *Astragalus membranaceus*, *Panax ginseng* and *Cordyceps sinensis*. *A. membranaceus* was used in combination with other herbs in 18 formulae in 16 studies. Detailed sub-group and sensitivity analyses were conducted. Clinically meaningful benefits for BODE Index and 6MWT were found in multiple studies. These therapeutic effects were promising but need to be interpreted with caution due to variations in the CHMs and RPs used and methodological weakness in the studies. These issues should be addressed in future trials.

Editor: Cordula M. Stover, University of Leicester, United Kingdom

Funding: This study is funded by a project grant from the International Science & Technology Cooperation Project of the Ministry of Science and Technology of China (Project Grant Number: 2012DFA31760, Project Title: Evaluation of Traditional and Scientific Evidence of Chinese Medicine). The project is partially supported by the China-Australia International Research Centre for Chinese Medicine, funded by Guangdong Provincial Academy of Chinese Medical Sciences & Guangdong Provincial Hospital of Chinese Medicine (GPACMS & GPHCM), Guangdong China, and RMIT University, Australia. The authors also acknowledge the support provided by the GPHCM and the School of Health Sciences, RMIT University to the first author (XKC). The funders had no role in study design, data collection and analysis, decision to publish, or preparation of the manuscript.

Competing Interests: The authors have declared that no competing interests exist.

* E-mail: drlinlin620@163.com

Introduction

Chronic obstructive pulmonary disease (COPD) is a disorder characterized by progressive development of airflow limitation and an enhanced chronic inflammatory response in the airways [1]. It is predicted to become the third most frequent cause of death in the world by 2020 [2]. The aim of current routine pharmacotherapy (RP) for stable COPD is to control disease progression by using bronchodilators and anti-inflammatory drugs [1]. However the treatment outcomes remain less than satisfactory and some RPs have been associated with adverse events such as cardiovascular events, oropharyngeal candidiasis and risk of pneumonia [1].

The use of the complementary and alternative medicine (CAM) is relatively common among stable COPD sufferers. One survey in Australia found that 41% of respondents had used some form of CAM to improve their health, counteract side effects of medications and/or compensate for dietary deficiencies [3]. Chinese herbal medicine (CHM) is currently considered a complementary or alternative medicine in most Western countries and has become increasingly accepted worldwide [4]. CHMs are prescribed as single herbs or made into formulae according to the therapeutic actions of each herb and also their effects in combination [5]. Studies have indicated that some plants have anti-inflammatory effects [6–9], can improve immune functions [10–14] and can assist in expelling phlegm [15,16]. CHMs can be administered as oral decoctions or prepared into pills, powders or capsules. They are commonly combined with routine pharmacotherapy in an attempt to improve outcomes [17].

A recent review of clinical trials of CHM reported that CHM plus RP had a better effect on quality of life (QoL) for patients with stable COPD compared to RP alone [18]. However, QoL measures largely depend on patients' perception, so the additional benefit of CHM that was reported may have been due to the effect of an additional therapy rather than to the specific effects of the CHMs. Therefore, this review focuses on trials that used more objective outcome measures in order to determine whether adding CHMs to pharmacotherapy produced clinical benefits for patients with stable COPD.

Six-Minute Walk Test

Objectively measured exercise impairment is reported to be a powerful indicator of health status impairment and a predictor of prognosis [19]. The Six-Minute Walk Test (6MWT) is a well-validated standardised test of exercise capacity that has been used as an outcome measure in clinical trials of COPD, is well tolerated, and reflects everyday life like activities [20].

Change in 6MWT is a predictor of survival in COPD [21] and low values on 6MWT have been shown to be predictive of mortality [22]. It was found that 6MWT was a significant predictor of survival with longer times to death observed in patents with longer walking distances [21]. The minimal clinically important difference for the 6MWT in COPD has been estimated using various methods as 54 meters [23] and more recently as 25 meters [24]. In a 3-year prospective multicentre observational study, the mean six minute walk distance (6MWD) declined by 1.6 meters per year in moderate COPD patients, defined as stage II according to the Global Initiative for Chronic Obstructive Lung Disease (GOLD) classification, 9.8 meters per year in GOLD III, and 8.5 meters per year in GOLD IV [25]. A longer observational study showed that COPD mortality was much higher for patients walking less than 350 meters [26].

BODE Index

The BODE Index is a multidimensional scoring system that has gained broad acceptance and has been developed as a prognostic marker for COPD patients in an attempt to integrate not only the respiratory but also the systemic expressions of COPD. It is composed of: body mass (B), degree of airflow obstruction (O), level of functional dyspnea (D) and exercise capacity (E) [27]. Body mass is calculated as body mass index (BMI), airflow obstruction is measured as forced expiratory volume in one second (FEV1%) predicted, dyspnoea is measured using the modified Medical Research Council (MMRC) dyspnoea scale, and exercise capacity is measured as 6MWT [27]. Of the BODE Index components, 6MWT was found to have a better predictive ability for mortality than the other three components [28].

In this 10 point scale, higher scores indicate a higher risk of death. For a one-point increase in the BODE Index, the hazard ratio for all-cause mortality was found to be 1.34 [27]. The minimal clinically important difference for the BODE Index has been set at 1 point [29]. Cohort studies have found that the BODE Index had superior predictive power for mortality and hospitalization than the GOLD stage over a median period of 16.2 months [28], and had similar clinical utility to the GOLD stage in predicting the risk for exacerbations during one year [30]. In a long-term study (mean 52 months), BODE Index was found to correlate well with COPD mortality and with scores on the St. George's Respiratory Questionnaire (SGRQ), although BODE Index was the better predictor of mortality [31].

BODE Index has been used in clinical trials as an outcome measure. In a study of the effects of lung volume reduction surgery, post-operative reduction in BODE Index was found to correlate with survival and a decrease to a lower BODE Index quartile was associated with a reduction in mortality (hazard ratio 0.497) [32].

The aim of this review was to evaluate the evidence for efficacy of therapies using CHM plus RP versus the same RP in stable COPD based on RCTs that used the objective outcome measures 6MWT/D and/or BODE Index. In addition, the review aimed to assess the safety of the combined treatments.

Methods

Search strategy

The electronic databases PubMed, Cochrane Central Register of Controlled Trials (CENTRAL), EMBASE, CINAHL, China National Knowledge Infrastructure (CNKI) and Chinese Scientific Journals Full text Database (CQVIP) were searched from their inceptions until 18th November, 2013, without language restriction. Search terms were in three groups: condition (COPD, chronic bronchitis and related terms); intervention (CHM, Traditional Medicine and related terms) and study type (Table S1). The three groups of terms were combined and the search results downloaded into Endnote libraries for each data-base. The results for all searches were combined, and duplicates were removed. Relevant review articles were examined to identify any additional studies.

Inclusion criteria

CHMs were defined as preparations originating from plants or parts of plants (such as seeds, roots, stems, leaves, flowers, fruits, or tubers) that have been used therapeutically in China. Plant-derived purified compounds were not included within this definition of CHM. For example, Tanshinone IIA which is a compound isolated from *Salvia miltiorrhiza* was not considered a CHM [33]. Also, herbs such as Echinacea which is of American origin were considered as beyond the scope of CHM.

Studies included in this review are randomized controlled trials (RCTs) published in English or Chinese that meet all the following criteria: (1) Participants: patients diagnosed with COPD in the stable stage and had no current infection, exacerbation or hospitalization; (2) Types of intervention and control: interventions were orally administered CHM in any form combined with RP (i.e. beta2-agonist, anticholinergic, theophylline, inhaled corticosteroid, mucolytic, or other routine therapy) with the same RP being used in the control arm. Non-pharmacologic respiratory therapy (i.e. smoking cessation, pulmonary rehabilitation, oxygen therapy or pulmonary exercise) was allowed as a co-intervention; (3) Types of outcome measurement: only studies using BODE Index and/or 6MWD/T as outcome measures were considered.

Exclusion criteria

Clinical trials were excluded if they did not meet the above criteria. In addition, the following types of studies were excluded: (1) Oral CHM used in combination with other non-oral interventions such as acupuncture or injections of a CHM preparation; (2) Studies that included participants with respiratory failure, pulmonary hypertension or *cor pulmonale*; (3) Studies using antibiotics as RP were excluded since antibiotics are recommended for exacerbations and not for stable COPD [34].

Study selection, data extraction and quality assessment

Study selection. One researcher (XC) conducted the searches. The resultant titles and abstracts were screened independently by XC and YD. Irrelevant citations were excluded. The full texts of potentially relevant articles were obtained. Two researchers (XC and YD) independently assessed the eligibility of these articles against the inclusion and exclusion criteria. Issues were resolved by agreement after discussion with a third reviewer (BM).

Data extraction and management. Two researchers (XC and YD) extracted data from each study using a standard data extraction form which included details of author, year, country, source of patients, trial design, treatment duration, follow-up period, number of participants, age of patients, severity of COPD, differentiation of syndrome, dropouts, adverse events, and methodological aspects. Attempts were made to contact the original investigators regarding any missing data or to obtain data clarification but no responses were obtained. The extracted data were checked against the full text articles by BM. Any discrepancies were resolved by agreement after rechecking the source papers and further discussion with BM.

Assessment of risk of bias in included studies. In accordance with recommendations in the Cochrane Handbook [35], the methodological quality of trials was independently evaluated by two researchers (XC and YD) using the Cochrane risk of bias assessment tool. For each study the following domains were assessed: random sequence generation; allocation concealment; blinding of participants and personnel; blinding of outcome assessors; incomplete outcome data; and selective outcome reporting.

Data analysis

Data were analysed using Review Manager version 5.2, developed by the Cochrane Collaboration. Mean difference (MD) was used for continuous data and risk ratio (RR) was calculated for dichotomous data, both with 95% confidence intervals (CI). Heterogeneity was tested with I^2. I^2 values of 50% or more indicated a substantial level of heterogeneity, so data were pooled using a random effect model (REM). Otherwise, a fixed effect model (FEM) was applied. Sensitivity analysis was used to explore heterogeneity. Possible publication bias was checked using funnel plots when ten or more studies reported the same outcome measure [35]. Egger's test was conducted using STATA 12.0 software (StataCorp LP, USA) to determine whether the funnel plots were symmetrical. Correlation analysis was conducted in IBM SPSS 20.

Results

Description of studies

The study selection process is outlined in Figure 1. Of the 4,948 records screened, 328 full text articles were considered and 25 studies met all criteria and were included in this review [36–60]. One study was indexed in the English language databases [43], two were indexed in both English and Chinese databases [38,54] and the other 23 studies were indexed exclusively in Chinese databases [36,37,39–42,44–53,55–60]. The characteristics of the included studies are shown in Table S2. All the trials were conducted in China from 2004 to 2013. Two trials were reported in English [43,54]. Treatment duration ranged from 1 month to 12 months (median: 3 months) and 7 out of 25 studies had a treatment duration of six months or more [36,40,42,43,47,51,53]. Five studies mentioned a follow-up period [41,43,46,51,55]. Two studies had a 6-month follow-up [41,42] and four had a one-year follow-up [43,46,51,55]. Fifteen studies specified participants' COPD stage [39–41,43,45,47,48,50,52,54–58,60] and 17 studies gave information on the number of years that patients had suffered from COPD [36,41–49,51–53,55–58]. Thirteen studies described the Chinese medicine differentiation of syndrome [38,40,43–45,48–51,53,55,56,58]. Nine studies used BODE Index [37,40,42,47,49,50,54,58,60] and 22 studies used 6MWT/D [36–46,48,49,51–59] as outcome measures.

In total, there were 2,385 participants in the 25 studies. Study size ranged from 40 to 352 participants with nine studies having more than 100 participants [39,40,43,46,51–53,55,59]. Nine studies reported dropouts during the treatment with or without reasons totalling 54 participants [42,43,47,49,50,53,54,56,58]. One study used intention-to-treat analysis (last case carried forward) [43]. Three studies (involving 497 participants) did not provide numerical data suitable for meta-analysis [43,56,57], so 22 studies involving 1,834 participants (56% male, age range 36~83 years) were included in the meta-analyses. Meta-analysis of BODE Index was based on 9 studies [37,40,42,47,49,50,54,58,60] and 6MWT/D was based on 17 studies [36–39,41,44–46,48,49,51–55,58,59], four of which also reported data on BODE Index [37,49,54,58].

Interventions

The interventions used in the included studies are shown in Table S3.

Types of CHM. Six studies used two or three herbal formulae in combination [40,41,43,45,49,53], while the others used one formula [36–39,42,44,46–48,50–52,54–60]. In total, 29 different CHM formulae were used in the form of decoction, capsule or granule. Two studies selected the formulae according to patients' traditional Chinese medicine (TCM) syndrome differentiation [43,49]. Fourteen studies provided information on the quality control of the herbal ingredients [36,39–46,51,54,55,58,59].

The most commonly used formulae were: 'Bai-Ling Capsule' aka 'Jin-Shui-Bao Capsule' in five studies [40,41,45,46,51] followed by 'Yu-Ping-Feng' decoction or granule in three studies [41,43,44]. Both 'Bai-Ling Capsule' and 'Jin-Shui-Bao Capsule' contained cultured *Cordyceps sinensis* (*Dongchongxiacao*) mycelia [40,41,45,46,51]. 'Yu-Ping-Feng' decoction or granule contained *Astragalus membranaceus (Huangqi)*, *Atractylodes macrocephala (Baizhu)* and *Saposhnikovia divaricata (Fangfeng)*.

Eighty distinct herbs were used in total. The ten most frequently used were: *Astragalus membranaceus* (*Huangqi*) [36–38,40,41,43–45,48,49,53,55,57–60], *Panax ginseng* (*Renshen*) [38,39,41–43,52,60], *Atractylodes macrocephala* (*Baizhu*) [36,37,41,43,44,47,48,55–57,60], *Glycyrrhiza uralensis* (*Gancao*) [36,38,47,48,50,53,55,57,60], *Poria cocos* (*Fuling*) [37,38,45,47,48,53], *Codonopsis pilosula* (*Dangshen*) [36,37,43,45,47,49,55,57,59], *Cordyceps sinensis* (*Dongchongxiacao*) [40,41,45,46,51,59], *Citrus tangerina* (*Chenpi*) [2,26,31,55,57,60], *Ophiopogon japonicus* (*Maimendong*) [38,41,43,48,50,56], and *Epimedium grandiflorum* (*Yinyanghuo*) [43,48,54,55].

Astragalus membranaceus (*Huangqi*) was used in combination with other herbs in 18 formulae in 16 studies [36–38,40,41,43–45,48,49,53,55,57–60]. Ten of these formulae were decoctions [36–38,45,48,53,55,57,58,60], seven were granules [41,43,44,49,59], and one was made into capsules [40]. The most frequently used herbal combination was *A. membranaceus* plus *A. macrocephala* which was used in ten formulae [36,37,41,43,44,48,55,57,60].

Types of routine pharmacotherapy (RP) and other routine therapy. Three studies did not provide detailed information about the routine treatment [44,54,59]. Two of these mentioned pulmonary rehabilitation in addition to unspecified routine pharmacotherapy [54,59]. Comprehensive pulmonary rehabilitation programs generally have four major components: exercise training, education, psychosocial/behavioural intervention, and outcome assessment [61]. In 7 studies [41,43,45,48–50,55], patients were treated based on severity according to the

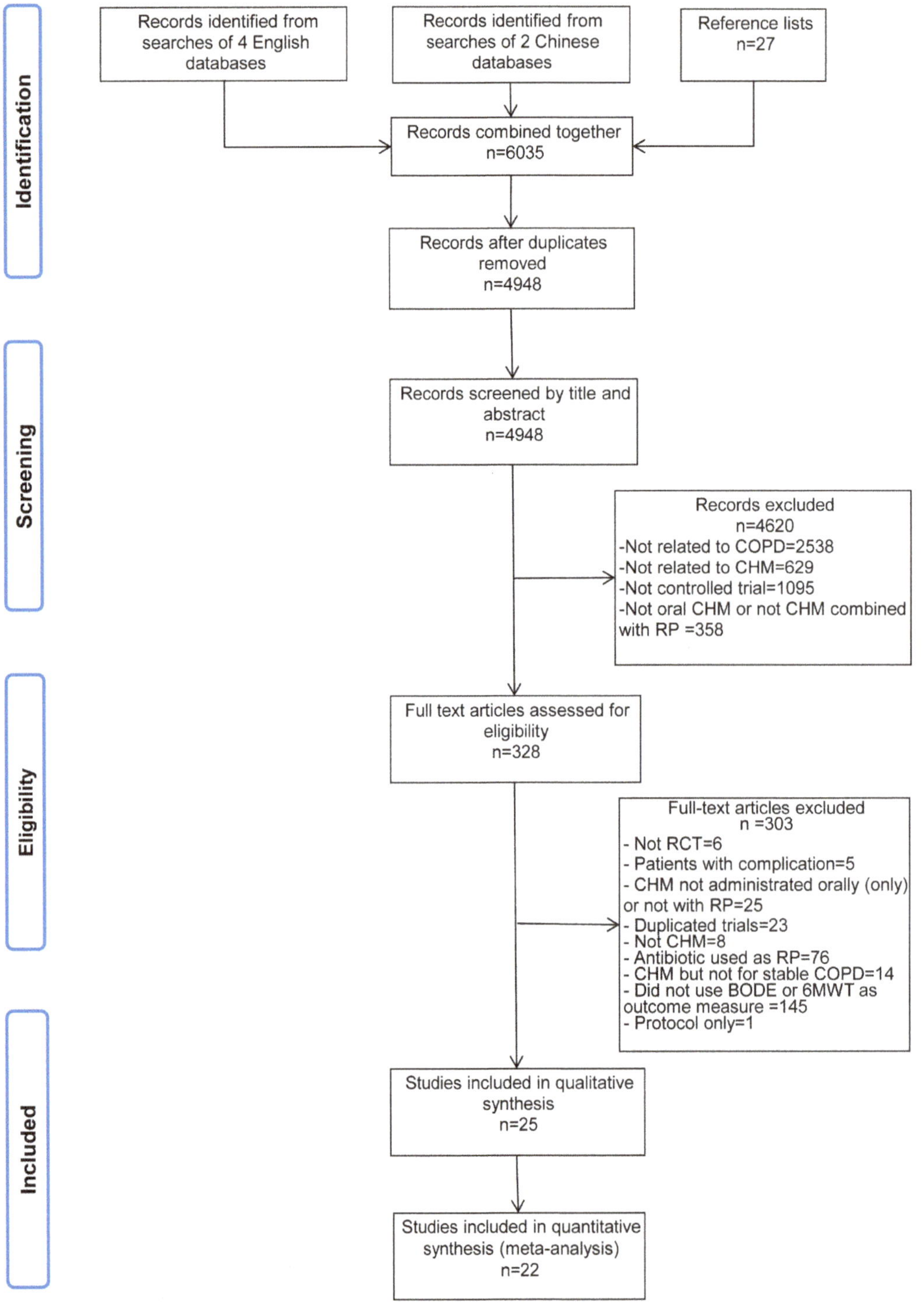

Figure 1. Flowchart of the search and study selection process.

recommendations of the GOLD guideline or the Guideline of the Chinese Society of Respiratory Disease (CSRD) [62]. Fifteen studies specified the medications used [36–40,46,47,51–53,56–60]. Inhalation of ipratropium bromide was used in three studies [38,42,51] one of which also used oxygen therapy [38]. Salbutamol was used alone in one study [40], and combined with ipratropium and pulmonary exercise in one study [36]. Four studies used inhalation of salmeterol plus fluticasone [37,53,56,60]. Theophylline was used orally alone in one study [47], in combination with pulmonary rehabilitation in one study [58], with inhaled salmeterol plus fluticasone in one study [57], and with oral Mucosolvan and inhaled long-acting β2 agonists in two studies [39,52]. One study used a compound oral medication which contained aminophylline, bromhexine and chlorphenamine [46].

Risk of bias

Risk of bias assessment details are provided in Table 1. All 25 studies were described by the original authors as 'randomised'. Three of these studies reported that the random sequence was generated by a random number table [36,42,44], one used a 'stratified and block randomization design' with detailed information on the sequence generation [43], one used 'drawing of lots' [46] and one used a 'computer random number generator' [58]. For allocation concealment, one study used 'sealed envelopes' [43] which was judged as low risk of bias, while the remainder did not describe this aspect [36–42,44–60]. One study specified that the randomisation process was conducted by an independent person [43].

Four studies mentioned that they were single blind [44,45,50,54], with one study using a CHM placebo [54]. However, blinding of participants and personnel were judged as unclear risk of bias for these four studies as they had no descriptions of the blinding procedures. There was one 'open-label' study [43], which was judged as high risk of bias for blinding of participants and personnel. The other twenty studies did not mention any blinding method for participants or personnel [36–42,46–49,51–53,55–60]. One study claimed independent assessors [43]. Another study specified that data were collected by an unblinded investigator [54]. The remaining studies did not provide information on the binding of outcome assessors [36–42,44–53,55–60].

There was no withdrawal in fourteen studies [36,38–41,44,45,48,51,52,55,57,59,60]. Seven studies reported withdrawals with reasons [42,43,47,53,54,56,58], and one of these applied intention-to-treat analysis [43]. Two studies reported withdrawals without reasons [49,50] and two did not provide information [37,46]. Three studies provided data which were not suitable for meta-analysis, so were judged as high risk of bias for selective outcome reporting [43,56,57].

Publication bias

The number of studies reporting BODE Index was less than ten, so a funnel plot was not applicable. For 6MWT/D studies, as seen in Figure S1, the funnel plot is not symmetric and there are outliers on both sides of the distribution. Egger's test was not significant ($t = 1.42$, 95% CI -2.15 to 10.75, $p = 0.176$) suggesting that the risk of publication bias is not high.

Correlation analysis

In COPD, there are different levels of severity and patients' conditions tend to deteriorate over time (Figure 2, Figure 3). These factors may affect meta-analyses. To investigate any correlations between severity at baseline and change at the end of treatment (EoT), data were grouped by duration and by treatment or control group and weighted by number of participants in SPSS. In order to focus on the effects of the CHMs and the pharmacotherapies, correlation analysis was conducted after excluding the studies that applied pulmonary rehabilitation as a co-intervention in addition to the RP [54,58,59].

For the test groups in the studies that used BODE Index, a negative correlation was found for the three 3-month studies ($n = 91$) ($r = -0.988$, $p < 0.001$, two tailed) and for the two 6-month studies ($n = 80$) ($r = -1.000$, $p < 0.001$, two tailed). Overall, for the seven studies ($n = 225$), the higher the BODE Index was at baseline for the CHM plus RP groups, the greater was the benefit gained at the end of treatment ($r = -0.707$, $p < 0.001$, two tailed). For the control groups, there was a significant negative correlation for the two 6-month studies ($n = 78$) ($r = -1.000$, $p < 0.001$, two tailed), for the 3-month studies ($n = 88$) ($r = -0.867$, $p < 0.001$, two tailed) and for all seven studies ($n = 206$) ($r = -0.345$, $p < 0.001$, two tailed). Therefore there was a greater relative improvement when the patients' COPD was more severe at baseline.

For the three 6-month studies that used 6MWT/D, there was a significant negative correlation for the test groups ($n = 143$) ($r = -0.979$, $p < 0.001$, two tailed) and for the control groups ($n = 145$) ($r = -0.985$, $p < 0.001$, two tailed). For the 9 studies of 3 to 4 months duration, there was a negative correlation for the test groups ($n = 332$) ($r = -0.31$, $p = 0.571$, two tailed) and for the control groups ($n = 324$) ($r = -0.145$, $p = 0.09$, two tailed). For the 3 studies of one month duration, there was a significant negative correlation for the test groups ($n = 130$) ($r = -0.741$, $p < 0.001$, two tailed) but a positive correlation for the control groups ($n = 130$) ($r = 0.963$, $p < 0.001$, two tailed). Overall, for the test groups, the longer the distance walked at baseline, the less the benefit conferred by the combined CHM plus RP intervention ($n = 605$, $r = -0.278$, $p < 0.001$, two tailed). The same effect was evident for the RP control groups ($n = 599$, $r = -0.115$, $p = 0.005$, two tailed).

Meta-analyses of outcomes and sensitivity analyses

For the two outcome measures, studies were grouped according to the type of RP used and the duration of the study in order to enable more valid comparisons. Data were pooled when possible. Comparisons between groups at baseline and EoT and within-group differences from baseline to EoT were all investigated.

BODE Index. The BODE Index was used in nine studies [37,40,42,47,49,50,54,58,60]. Seven studies provided the mean and standard deviation (SD). Two presented data as the number of patients for each BODE Index score [47,60], so the data were transformed into mean and SD to enable meta-analysis. One study did not provide the baseline data but complete data for the other eight were available [37,40,47,49,50,54,58,60]. Six studies used a clearly defined RP [37,40,42,47,58,60]. The BODE Index scores and SDs are presented in Figure 2 and numerical results for the meta-analyses are presented in Figure 4, Table 2 and Table S4.

The longest study employed ipratropium (inhaled) for 12 months but the lack of baseline data meant that it could not be determined whether the BODE Index declined or improved over this period. At EoT there was a significant benefit for the CHM plus ipratropium group of -0.68 points compared to ipratropium alone (Table S4) [42].

Two studies were conducted for 6 months [40,47]. One study, used salbutamol (inhaled) in patients with a mean BODE Index of 7.1. There was neither improvement nor decline in the salbutamol only group but there was a clinically significant improvement of -1.70 in the group that used *Cordyceps sinensis* mycelia plus salbutamol [40]. The other study used oral theophylline in participants with a much lower mean BODE Index at baseline (T: 3.38, C: 3.18). No significant change was found in the theophylline group at the end of 6 months but a significant benefit was found in the CHM plus theophylline group of -1.35. At EoT there was a clinically significant reduction in BODE Index in favour of the CHM plus theophylline group (MD -1.08) [47] (Figure 4, Table S4).

In the study that used salmeterol/fluticasone (inhaled) for 3 months, the mean BODE Index was 6.31 in the RP group at baseline and there was a significant decrease at EoT (MD -1.44). In the test group, the addition of the CHM produced an improvement of -2.64 over the baseline mean of 6.30 points. At EoT, there was a clinically significant difference between groups of -1.21 in favour of CHM plus salmeterol/fluticasone [37]. Another study also used salmeterol/fluticasone as the RP but the treatment duration was only 1 month. After 1 month there was a non-significant decrease (MD -0.27) in the RP group and a

Table 1. Assessment of risk of bias for 19 studies based on the Cochrane Handbook.

	Sequence Generation	Allocation Concealment	Blinding of Participants	Blinding of Personnel	Blinding of Outcome Assessment	Incomplete Outcome Data	Selective Outcome Reporting
Chen, 2009 [37]	U	U	U	U	U	U	L
Chen, 2012[36]	L	U	U	U	U	L	L
Cui, 2004 [38]	U	U	U	U	U	L	L
Guo, 2008 [39]	U	U	U	U	U	L	L
Hu, 2012 [40]	U	U	U	U	U	L	L
Huang, 2005 [41]	U	U	U	U	U	L	L
Jian, 2012 [42]	L	U	U	U	U	L	L
Li, 2012 [43]	L	L	H	H	L	L	H
Liao, 2011 [44]	L	U	U	U	U	L	L
Liu, 2009 [45]	U	U	U	U	U	L	L
Mao, 2009 [46]	L	U	U	U	U	U	L
Shan, 2011 [47]	U	U	U	U	U	L	L
Xu(2), 2012 [48]	U	U	U	U	U	L	L
Xu (1), 2012 [49]	U	U	U	U	U	U	L
Yu, 2011 [50]	U	U	U	U	U	U	L
Zhang (2), 2007 [51]	U	U	U	U	U	L	L
Zhang (1), 2007 [52]	U	U	U	U	U	L	L
Zhang, 2011 [53]	U	U	U	U	U	L	L
Zhao, 2012 [54]	U	U	U	U	H	L	L
Fan, 2012 [55]	U	U	U	U	U	L	L
Liang, 2013 [56]	U	U	U	U	U	L	H
Lin, 2013 [57]	U	U	U	U	U	L	H
Peng, 2013 [58]	L	U	U	U	U	L	L
Yang, 2013 [60]	U	U	U	U	U	L	L
Zeng, 2013 [59]	U	U	U	U	U	L	L

Risk of Bias Judgements: L: Low risk, U: Unclear risk, H: High risk.

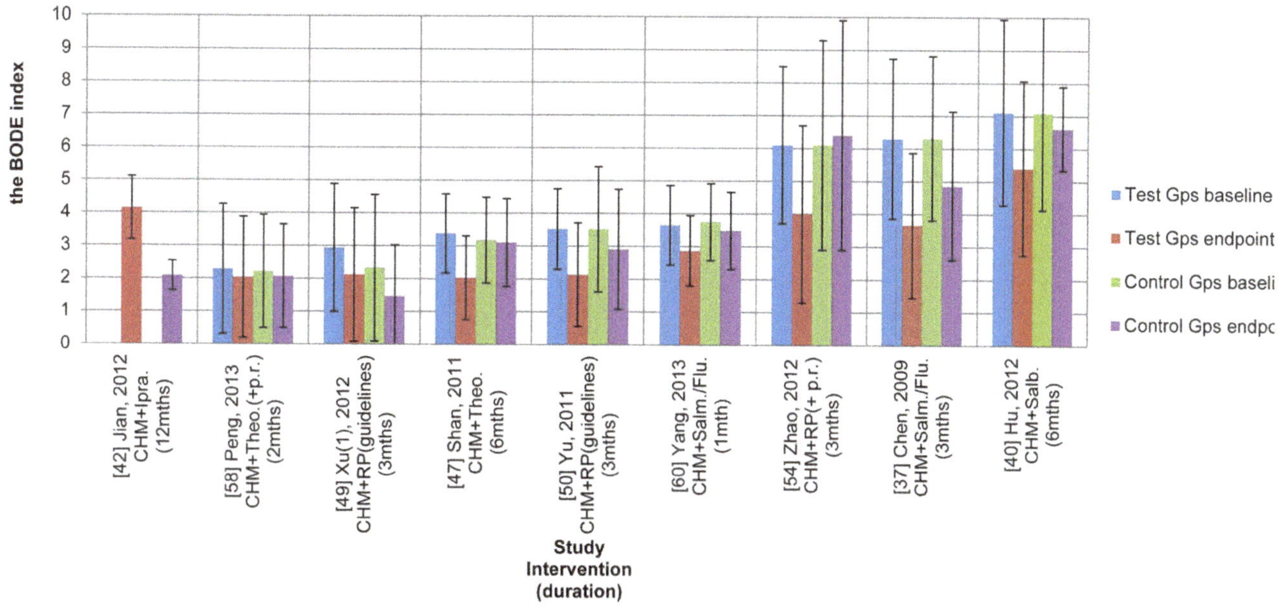

Figure 2. BODE Index mean and SD scores at baseline and end of treatment for 9 studies of CHM plus RP for stable COPD (showing type of intervention). Legend: SD: standard deviation, CHM: Chinese Herbal Medicine, RP: routine pharmacotherapy, mths: months, Gps: groups, Ipra.: ipratropium (inhaled), Theo.(+p.r.): oral theophylline (plus pulmonary rehabilitation), RP (guidelines): routine pharmacotherapy (adjusted for severity according to guidelines), Theo.: theophylline (oral), Salm./Flu.: salmeterol/fluticasone (inhaled), RP(+p.r.): routine pharmacotherapy (pharmacotherapy plus pulmonary rehabilitation), Salb.: salbutamol (inhaled).

significant decrease in the CHM plus RP group (MD −0.78). At EoT there was a significant difference between groups in favour of the CHM plus RP group (MD −0.61) [60]. There was a significant decrease in the pooled data (MD −0.70) for the two studies in this subgroup [37,60] (Figure 4, Table 2).

Two studies used RP adjusted according to the guidelines for 3 months [49,50]. In one study, both groups had a mean BODE Index of 3.52 at baseline and there was a non-significant decline in the RP group at EoT. In the CHM plus RP group, there was a significant decline (MD −1.39), so there was a significant difference between groups at 3 months (MD −0.78) [50]. In the other study, there was a difference in baseline BODE Index mean scores (T: 2.94, C: 2.33) but this was not significant (MD 0.61). After 3 months there were non-significant declines in BODE Index in the RP group and in the CHM plus RP group [49] (Table S4). There was no difference between groups in the pooled data but the heterogeneity was high (Figure 4).

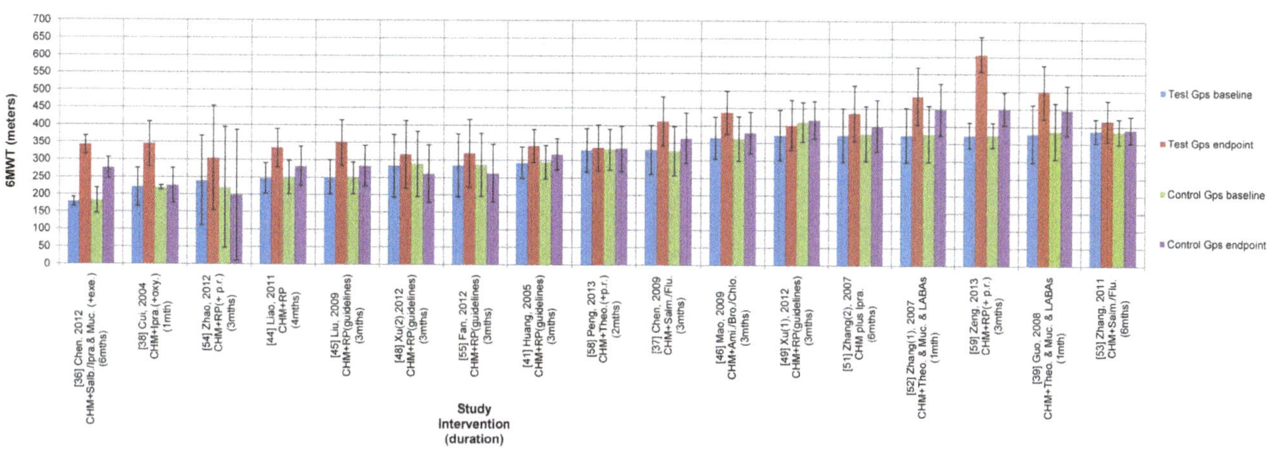

Figure 3. Mean 6MWT/D (meters) with SDs at baseline and end of treatment for 17 studies of CHM plus RP for stable COPD (showing type of intervention). Legend: SD: standard deviation, CHM: Chinese Herbal Medicine, RP: routine pharmacotherapy, mths: months, Gps: groups, Salb./Ipra.: salbutamol/ipratropium (inhaled), exe.: pulmonary exercise, Ipra.: ipratropium (inhaled), oxy.: oxygen therapy, RP(+p.r.): routine pharmacotherapy (pharmacotherapy plus pulmonary rehabilitation), RP (guidelines): routine pharmacotherapy (adjusted for severity according to guidelines), Theo.(+p.r.): oral theophylline (plus pulmonary rehabilitation), Salm./Flu.: salmeterol/fluticasone (inhaled), Ami./Bro./Chlo.: compound oral medication which contained aminophylline, bromhexine and chlorphenamine, Theo.: theophylline (oral), Muc.: Mucosolvan (oral), LABAs: long-acting β2 agonists (inhaled), Salb.: salbutamol (inhaled).

Study or Subgroup	Test Mean	Test SD	Test Total	Control Mean	Control SD	Control Total	Weight	Mean Difference IV, Fixed, 95% CI
13.1.1 CHM plus Ipra. vs Ipra.								
[42] Jian, 2012	4.14	0.97	33	4.82	0.76	34	31.2%	-0.68 [-1.10, -0.26]
Subtotal (95% CI)			33			34	31.2%	-0.68 [-1.10, -0.26]
Heterogeneity: Not applicable								
Test for overall effect: Z = 3.19 (P = 0.001)								
13.1.2 CHM plus Salb. vs Salb.								
[40] Hu, 2012	5.41	2.65	51	6.62	2.87	50	4.7%	-1.21 [-2.29, -0.13]
Subtotal (95% CI)			51			50	4.7%	-1.21 [-2.29, -0.13]
Heterogeneity: Not applicable								
Test for overall effect: Z = 2.20 (P = 0.03)								
13.1.3 CHM plus Theo. vs Theo.								
[47] Shan, 2011	2.03	1.27	29	3.11	1.34	28	11.9%	-1.08 [-1.76, -0.40]
Subtotal (95% CI)			29			28	11.9%	-1.08 [-1.76, -0.40]
Heterogeneity: Not applicable								
Test for overall effect: Z = 3.12 (P = 0.002)								
13.1.4 CHM plus Theo. (+p.r.) vs Theo.(+p.r.)								
[58] Peng, 2013	2.04	1.84	28	2.07	1.57	27	6.7%	-0.03 [-0.93, 0.87]
Subtotal (95% CI)			28			27	6.7%	-0.03 [-0.93, 0.87]
Heterogeneity: Not applicable								
Test for overall effect: Z = 0.07 (P = 0.95)								
13.1.5 CHM plus Salm./Flu. vs Salm./Flu.								
[37] Chen, 2009	3.66	2.21	30	4.87	2.26	30	4.3%	-1.21 [-2.34, -0.08]
[60] Yang, 2013	2.87	1.07	54	3.48	1.18	40	25.4%	-0.61 [-1.07, -0.15]
Subtotal (95% CI)			84			70	29.6%	-0.70 [-1.13, -0.27]
Heterogeneity: Chi² = 0.93, df = 1 (P = 0.34); I² = 0%								
Test for overall effect: Z = 3.18 (P = 0.001)								
13.1.6 CHM plus RP (guidelines) vs RP (guidelines)								
[49] Xu(1), 2012	2.12	2.03	17	1.47	1.55	15	3.5%	0.65 [-0.59, 1.89]
[50] Yu, 2011	2.13	1.57	44	2.91	1.83	43	10.6%	-0.78 [-1.50, -0.06]
Subtotal (95% CI)			61			58	14.1%	-0.42 [-1.04, 0.20]
Heterogeneity: Chi² = 3.81, df = 1 (P = 0.05); I² = 74%								
Test for overall effect: Z = 1.33 (P = 0.18)								
13.1.7 CHM plus RP (+ p.r.) vs RP (+ p.r.)								
[54] Zhao, 2012	4	2.7	26	6.4	3.5	23	1.7%	-2.40 [-4.17, -0.63]
Subtotal (95% CI)			26			23	1.7%	-2.40 [-4.17, -0.63]
Heterogeneity: Not applicable								
Test for overall effect: Z = 2.66 (P = 0.008)								
Total (95% CI)			312			290	100.0%	-0.71 [-0.94, -0.47]
Heterogeneity: Chi² = 13.24, df = 8 (P = 0.10); I² = 40%								
Test for overall effect: Z = 5.94 (P < 0.00001)								
Test for subgroup differences: Chi² = 8.50, df = 6 (P = 0.20), I² = 29.4%								

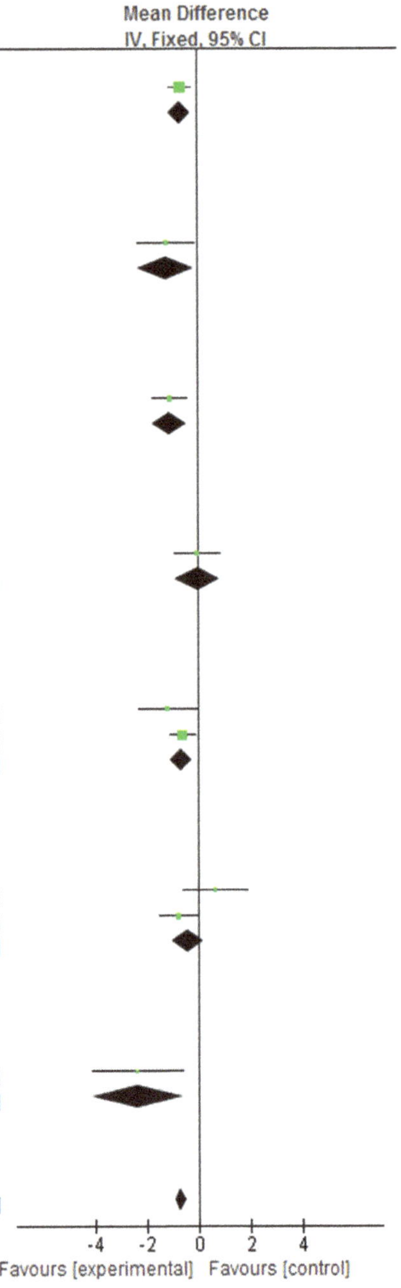

Figure 4. Forest plot comparing CHM plus RP group (Test) to RP group (Control) in terms of BODE Index scores in stable COPD at end of treatment. Legend: CHM: Chinese Herbal Medicine, RP: routine pharmacotherapy, SD: standard deviation, CI: confidence interval, Ipra.: ipratropium (inhaled), Salb.: salbutamol (inhaled), Theo.: theophylline (oral), Theo.(+p.r.): oral theophylline (plus pulmonary rehabilitation), Salm./Flu.: salmeterol/fluticasone (inhaled), RP (guidelines): routine pharmacotherapy (adjusted for severity according to guidelines), RP(+p.r.): routine pharmacotherapy (pharmacotherapy plus pulmonary rehabilitation).

One study used a placebo CHM combined with unspecified RP plus pulmonary rehabilitation (p.r.) in the control group. The baseline mean BODE Index was 6.1 in each group. After three months the RP group remained relatively stable (MD 0.30) but there was a significant improvement in the CHM plus RP group (MD −2.10). At EoT there was a clinically significant benefit in favour of the CHM plus RP group (MD −2.40) [54] (Figure 4, Table S4).

One study used oral theophylline combined with p.r. in patients with a mean BODE Index of 2.2. After two months, there were non-significant decreases in BODE Index in the control group (MD −0.15) and in the test group (MD −0.25). There was no difference between groups at EoT [58] (Figure 4, Table S4).

Based on study duration, the pooled data for the four studies that used CHM plus RP for 3 months showed a decrease in BODE Index from baseline of −1.59 (95%CI −2.06, −1.13, $I^2 = 43\%$, FEM) [37,49–51]. For the two studies that lasted 6 months, the change was −1.44 (95%CI −1.99, −0.90, $I^2 = 0\%$, FEM) [40,47]. The between-groups results were −0.83 for 3

Table 2. Meta-analysis of BODE Index at end of treatment and sensitivity analysis.

CHM plus RP groups versus the RP groups	BODE score (MD+95%CI) Model
Pooled data for two studies of CHM+Sal./Flu.[37,60]	−0.70 [−1.13, −0.27], I^2 = 0% FEM*
	−0.70 [−1.13, −0.27], I^2 = 0% REM*
Pooled data for four 3-mth studies[37,49–51]	−0.76 [−1.28, −0.24], I^2 = 66% FEM*
	−0.83 [−1.81, −0.16], I^2 = 66% REM
Pooled data for two 6-mth studies[40,47]	−1.12 [−1.69, −0.54], I^2 = 0%FEM*
	−1.12 [−1.69, −0.54], I^2 = 0%REM*
Pooled data for 5 studies of AM formulae[37,40,49,58,60]	−0.54 [−0.89, −0.19], I^2 = 55.5% FEM*
	−0.51 [−1.07, −0.05], I^2 = 55.5% REM
Pooled data for all 9 studies[37,40,42,47,49,50,54,58,60]	−0.71 [−0.94, −0.47], I^2 = 40% FEM*
	−0.72 [−1.06, −0.39], I^2 = 40% REM*
Pooled data for 8 studies[37,40,42,47,49,50,58,60] after excluding the English-language study[54]	−0.68 [−0.91, −0.44], I^2 = 27% FEM*
	−0.67 [−0.97, −0.38], I^2 = 27% REM*
Pooled data for 8 studies exclusively indexed in Chinese databases [37,40,42,47,49,50,58,60]	−0.68 [−0.91, −0.44], I^2 = 27% FEM*
	−0.67 [−0.97, −0.38], I^2 = 27% REM*
Pooled data for 7 studies[37,40,42,47,49,50,60] after excluding studies of pulmonary rehabilitation[54,58]	−0.72 [−0.97, −0.48], I^2 = 20% FEM*
	−0.73 [−1.02, −0.44], I^2 = 20% REM*
Pooled data for 6 studies[37,40,42,47,58,60] after excluding studies of undefined RP[49,50,54]	−0.72 [−0.97, −0.47], I^2 = 2% FEM*
	−0.72 [−0.98, −0.46], I^2 = 2% REM*
Pooled data for 3 studies in which mean BODE was greater than 4 at baseline[37,40,54]	−1.40 [−2.12, −0.69], I^2 = 0% FEM*
	−1.40 [−2.12, −0.69], I^2 = 0% REM*
Pooled data for 5 studies in which mean BODE was less than 4 at baseline[47,49,50,58,60]	−0.59 [−0.90, −0.29], I^2 = 47% FEM*
	−0.53 [−0.98, −0.07], I^2 = 47% REM*

*Significant difference, CHM: Chinese Herbal Medicine, RP: routine pharmacotherapy, MD: mean difference, CI: confidence interval, mth: month, REM: random effect model, FEM: fixed effect model, AM: Astragalus membranaceus, Salm./Flu.: salmeterol/fluticasone (inhaled).

months and −1.12 points for 6 months in favour of the CHM plus RP groups, both of which were significant (Table 2).

For all nine studies, the use of CHM plus RP was associated with a significant decrease in the BODE Index compared with RP alone (MD −0.71, 95%CI −0.94, −0.47, I^2 = 40%, FEM) [37,40,42,47,49,50,54,58,60] (Figure 4). Sensitivity analysis using REM yielded nearly identical results (Table 2). After excluding the single study that was indexed in PubMed a significant decline (MD −0.68) remained, with lower heterogeneity (I^2 = 27%) [54]. The two studies [54,58] that used p.r. in addition to RP were excluded from the meta-analysis, since p.r. has been reported to independently improve BODE Index in a controlled study [63] so it may have been a major contributor to the pooled result. The resultant MD was −0.72 (95%CI −0.97, −0.48) and I^2 was reduced to 20% (FEM). Analysis of data only from the six studies with clearly defined RP also found a similar result (MD −0.86) with low heterogeneity (Table 2) [37,40,42,47,58,60]. For the three studies of patients whose mean BODE Index was greater than 4 at baseline, there was a clinically significant benefit for CHM plus RP of −1.40 points (95%CI −2.12, −0.69, I^2 = 0%, FEM) [37,40,54]. For the five studies of less severe patients, whose mean scores were less than 4 at baseline, there was less benefit (MD −0.59) (Table 2) [47,49,50,58,60].

Regarding the CHMs used in the test groups, five contained *A. membranaceus* (AM) [37,40,49,58,60]. Compared to baseline, the BODE Index reduced by 1.18 points (95%CI −1.91, −0.44, I^2 = 68%, REM) in the AM plus RP groups and −0.43 points (95%CI −0.80, −0.05, I^2 = 0%, REM) in the RP groups. At EoT there was a relative benefit of −0.54 points (95%CI −0.89, 0.19, I^2 = 48% REM) in favour of the AM plus RP groups (Table 2).

6MWT/D. Twenty-two studies used the 6MWT/D [36–46,48,49,51–59] but the data in five studies were inadequate for meta-analysis [40,42,43,56,57]. The mean 6MWD and SDs are presented in Figure 3 and numerical results for the meta-analyses are in Figure 5, Table 3 and Table S5.

When studies were pooled according to duration, for the 3 studies of one month the relative benefit for the addition of the CHM was 68.49 meters (95%CI 22.91, 114.07, I^2 = 85%, REM) [38,39,52]. For the ten studies of 3 or 4 months, there was a relative benefit of 59.66 meters (95%CI 24.63, 94.69, I^2 = 93%, REM) [37,41,44–46,48,49,54,55,59]. When the three six-month studies were pooled, the benefit was 43.10 meters (95%CI 15.16, 71.04, I^2 = 83%, REM) at EoT [36,51,53] (Table 3). However, the heterogeneity was high in each of these pools. When the study that was the most notable outlier in the funnel plot was excluded [59], the heterogeneity was reduced to 51% for the 3–4 month studies and the benefit was reduced to 46.45 meters (95%CI, 31.19, 61.71) but this was still clinically significant.

When studies were pooled according to type of RP, ten groups of studies were identified.

1. Salmeterol/Fluticasone plus CHM

Two studies used salmeterol/fluticasone as RP, one for 6 months and one for 3 months [37,53]. After 6 months there was a small non-significant increase in walking distance in the RP group of 5.06 meters. In the CHM plus RP group the

Study or Subgroup	Test Mean	Test SD	Test Total	Control Mean	Control SD	Control Total	Weight	Mean Difference IV, Random, 95% CI
17.2.1 CHM plus Salm./Flu. vs Salm./Flu.								
[37] Chen, 2009	412.11	70.33	30	364.47	71.82	30	5.7%	47.64 [11.67, 83.61]
[53] Zhang, 2011	415.75	58.3	43	390.48	38.8	45	6.4%	25.27 [4.48, 46.06]
Subtotal (95% CI)			73			75	12.1%	31.44 [11.84, 51.04]
Heterogeneity: Tau² = 25.55; Chi² = 1.11, df = 1 (P = 0.29); I² = 10%								
Test for overall effect: Z = 3.14 (P = 0.002)								
17.2.2 CHM plus Theo. (+p.r.) vs Theo. (+p.r.)								
[58] Peng, 2013	335.73	65.81	28	333.4	64.01	27	5.8%	2.33 [-31.98, 36.64]
Subtotal (95% CI)			28			27	5.8%	2.33 [-31.98, 36.64]
Heterogeneity: Not applicable								
Test for overall effect: Z = 0.13 (P = 0.89)								
17.2.3 CHM plus Theo.& Muc.& LABAs vs Theo.& Muc.& LABAs								
[39] Guo, 2008	498	76	50	446	74	50	6.0%	52.00 [22.60, 81.40]
[52] Zhang(1), 2007	486	82	60	448	74	60	6.1%	38.00 [10.05, 65.95]
Subtotal (95% CI)			110			110	12.2%	44.65 [24.39, 64.90]
Heterogeneity: Tau² = 0.00; Chi² = 0.46, df = 1 (P = 0.50); I² = 0%								
Test for overall effect: Z = 4.32 (P < 0.0001)								
17.2.4 CHM plus Ami./Bro./Chlo. vs Ami./Bro./Chlo.								
[46] Mao, 2009	437.8	61.5	50	380.2	58.8	50	6.3%	57.60 [34.02, 81.18]
Subtotal (95% CI)			50			50	6.3%	57.60 [34.02, 81.18]
Heterogeneity: Not applicable								
Test for overall effect: Z = 4.79 (P < 0.00001)								
17.2.5 CHM plus Ipra.(+oxy.) vs Ipra.(+oxy.)								
[38] Cui, 2004	345	64	20	226	50	20	5.7%	119.00 [83.41, 154.59]
Subtotal (95% CI)			20			20	5.7%	119.00 [83.41, 154.59]
Heterogeneity: Not applicable								
Test for overall effect: Z = 6.55 (P < 0.00001)								
17.2.6 CHM plus Ipra. vs Ipra.								
[51] Zhang(2), 2007	436	80	60	401	74	60	6.1%	35.00 [7.43, 62.57]
Subtotal (95% CI)			60			60	6.1%	35.00 [7.43, 62.57]
Heterogeneity: Not applicable								
Test for overall effect: Z = 2.49 (P = 0.01)								
17.2.7 CHM plus Salb./Ipra.& Muc.(+exe.) vs Salb./Ipra.& Muc.(+exe.)								
[36] Chen, 2012	342	26.72	40	276.92	29.67	40	6.7%	65.08 [52.71, 77.45]
Subtotal (95% CI)			40			40	6.7%	65.08 [52.71, 77.45]
Heterogeneity: Not applicable								
Test for overall effect: Z = 10.31 (P < 0.00001)								
17.2.8 CHM plus RP (guidelines) vs RP (guidelines)								
[41] Huang, 2005	340.7	46.69	32	316.63	45.28	31	6.3%	24.07 [1.36, 46.78]
[45] Liu, 2009	349	65	30	283	58	30	6.0%	66.00 [34.83, 97.17]
[48] Xu(2), 2012	315.6	97.2	45	260.3	82.4	45	5.7%	55.30 [18.07, 92.53]
[49] Xu(1), 2012	401.94	71.58	17	416.87	52.78	15	5.3%	-14.93 [-58.19, 28.33]
[55] Fan, 2012	318.8	97.1	90	262.4	82.5	90	6.2%	56.40 [30.08, 82.72]
Subtotal (95% CI)			214			211	29.5%	39.27 [14.45, 64.09]
Heterogeneity: Tau² = 537.66; Chi² = 12.90, df = 4 (P = 0.01); I² = 69%								
Test for overall effect: Z = 3.10 (P = 0.002)								
17.2.9 CHM plus RP vs RP								
[44] Liao, 2011	334	55	30	282	56	33	6.1%	52.00 [24.57, 79.43]
Subtotal (95% CI)			30			33	6.1%	52.00 [24.57, 79.43]
Heterogeneity: Not applicable								
Test for overall effect: Z = 3.72 (P = 0.0002)								
17.2.10 CHM plus RP(+ p.r.) vs RP(+ p.r.)								
[54] Zhao, 2012	304.1	149.4	26	198.6	187.8	23	2.9%	105.50 [9.64, 201.36]
[59] Zeng, 2013	606.48	50.69	60	450.46	46.69	60	6.5%	156.02 [138.58, 173.46]
Subtotal (95% CI)			86			83	9.4%	153.65 [132.71, 174.59]
Heterogeneity: Tau² = 40.60; Chi² = 1.03, df = 1 (P = 0.31); I² = 3%								
Test for overall effect: Z = 14.38 (P < 0.00001)								
Total (95% CI)			711			709	100.0%	54.61 [33.30, 75.92]
Heterogeneity: Tau² = 1729.28; Chi² = 177.60, df = 16 (P < 0.00001); I² = 91%								
Test for overall effect: Z = 5.02 (P < 0.00001)								
Test for subgroup differences: Chi² = 115.00, df = 9 (P < 0.00001), I² = 92.2%								

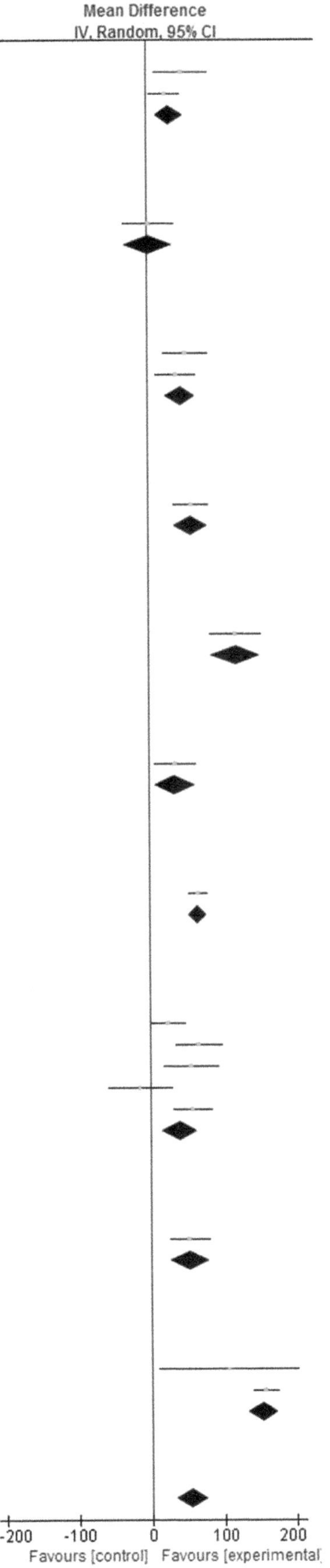

Figure 5. Forest plot comparing CHM plus RP group (Test) to RP group (Control) in terms of 6MWT/D (meters) in stable COPD at end of treatment. Legend: CHM: Chinese Herbal Medicine, RP: routine pharmacotherapy, SD: standard deviation, CI: confidence interval, Salm./Flu.: salmeterol/fluticasone (inhaled), Theo.(+p.r.): oral theophylline (plus pulmonary rehabilitation), Muc.: Mucosolvan (oral), LABAs: long-acting β2 agonists (inhaled), Ami./Bro./Chlo.: compound oral medication which contained aminophylline, bromhexine and chlorphenamine, Ipra.: ipratropium (inhaled), oxy.: oxygen therapy, Salb./Ipra.: salbutamol/ipratropium (inhaled), exe.: pulmonary exercise, RP (guidelines): routine pharmacotherapy (adjusted for severity according to guidelines), RP(+p.r.): routine pharmacotherapy (pharmacotherapy plus pulmonary rehabilitation).

increase of 28.27 meters was significant. At EoT there was a clinically significant difference between groups in favour of the test group (MD 25.27 m) [53]. In the three-month study, there was a significant improvement in both the RP and CHM plus RP groups. At EoT, the distance walked by those in the CHM plus RP group was significantly greater than in the group that only used salmeterol/fluticasone (MD 47.64 m) [37] (Table S5). The pooled data for this subgroup showed a clinically significant mean increase of 31.44 meters (95%CI 11.84, 51.04, $I^2 = 10\%$, REM) in the test groups compared to controls (Figure 5).

2. Theophylline (oral) plus pulmonary rehabilitation plus CHM

In the study that used this RP for two months, there was a small non-significant increase in 6MWT in both the CHM plus RP group (MD 6.47 m) and the RP group (MD 2.63 m). There was no significant difference between groups at EoT [58] (Table S5).

3. Theophylline (oral) plus Mucosolvan (oral) plus Long-acting beta2-agonist (LABA) (inhaled) plus CHM

Two studies used this RP for one month [39,52]. In one study, the test group achieved a significantly greater distance over baseline of 118.00 meters. The RP group achieved a lower but significant increase (MD 60.00 meters). At EoT, there was a clinically significant benefit in favour of the CHM plus RP group of 52.00 meters [39]. In the other study, there was a significant improvement in both the CHM plus RP group (MD 112.00 m) and the RP group (MD 70.00 m) compared to baseline. After one month, the CHM plus RP group achieved greater mean walking distance (MD 38.00 m) compared with the RP group [52]. There was a clinically significant benefit for adding CHM in this subgroup (44.65 m, $I^2 = 0\%$, FEM) [39,52] (Figure 5).

4. Aminophylline/Bromhexine/Chlorphenamine plus CHM

In the study that used this compound oral drug for three months, there was a non-significant increase in 6MWT in the control group of 17.50 meters. A significant increase was observed in the test group of 72.30 meters and there was a clinically significant difference between groups of 57.60 meters at EoT (Table S5) [46].

5. Inhaled Ipratropium plus oxygen therapy plus CHM

One study used inhaled ipratropium plus oxygen therapy as RP for one month. At EoT, the RP group remained relatively stable with a 6.00 meter increase but there was an improvement in the CHM plus RP group of 124.00 meters. At EoT, the addition of the CHM increased walking distance by 119 meters which was clinically significant (Table S5) [38].

6. Inhaled Ipratropium plus CHM

One study used this RP for 6 months. The baseline mean 6MWD was almost the same in each group (T: 374 m, C: 378 m). After treatment, there was non-significant increase in walking distance in the control group of 23.00 meters, while the CHM plus ipratropium group produced a significant improvement of 62.00 meters. The relative increase of 35 meters between groups at the end of the 6 months was clinically significant (Table S5) [51].

7. Inhaled Ipratropium/Salbutamol plus oral Mucosolvan plus exercise plus CHM

In one study, after six months treatment, walking distance significantly improved in both the control (MD 94.20 m) and CHM plus RP groups (MD 163.00 m). At EoT, the distance walked by those in the CHM plus RP group was greater by 65.08 meters than in the RP group which was clinically significant (Table S5) [36].

8. RP adjusted according to the guidelines plus CHM

Five studies used RP adjusted for the individual according to the guidelines for three months [41,45,48,49,55]. In one study, the mean walking distance declined in the control group (MD −28.40 m) while it increased in the test group (MD 32.10 m) but neither change was significant. However, a clinically significant improvement of 55.30 meters was observed between groups at three months [48]. In another study, there was a shorter mean walking distance in the test group compared to control group at the beginning of the study (MD −37.88 m) but the difference was not significant. After treatment, both groups achieved non-significant improvements (C: 5.90 m; T: 28.82 m), so there was no significant difference between groups at EoT [49]. In the third study, improvement was non-significant in the control group (MD 22.10 m) but significant in the test group (MD 47.56 m) after treatment. At EoT the test group showed a relative increase in walking distance of 24.07 meters compared to control [41]. In the fourth study, the mean walking distance declined in the control group (MD −24.10 m) while it increased significantly in the test group (MD 33.20 m). A clinically significant improvement of 56.40 meters was observed between groups at three months [55]. In the remaining study, there was a significant increase in walking distance in the control group over baseline of 35.00 meters. In the test group, the addition of the CHM produced an improvement of 98.00 meters over baseline. At EoT, there was a clinically significant difference between groups in favour of CHM plus RP (MD 66.00 m) [45] (Table S5). The pooled data of this subgroup demonstrated a clinically significant improvement in 6MWT of 39.27 meters (95%CI 14.45, 64.09, $I^2 = 69\%$, REM) in favour of the CHM plus RP groups (Figure 5, Table 3) [41,45,48,49,55]. When the single study of patients who could walk more than 300 meters at baseline was removed [49], the result remained clinically significant at 48.40 meters (95%CI 28.11, 68.69) with heterogeneity reduced to 50%.

9. Unspecified RP plus CHM

One study used CHM plus unspecified RP in the test group and showed clinically significant improvement within groups (C: 32.00 m; T: 87.00 m) as well as between groups (52.00 m, 95%CI 24.57, 79.43) after 4 months of treatment [44] (Table S5).

10. Unspecified RP with pulmonary rehabilitation plus CHM

Two studies used CHM combined with unspecified RP plus p.r. in the test group [54,59]. The greatest between-groups beneficial improvement was in the study that showed as an outlier in the funnel plot. The baseline mean walking

Table 3. Meta-analysis of 6MWT/D (meters) at end of treatment and sensitivity analysis.

CHM plus RP groups versus the RP groups	6MWT meters (MD+95%CI) Model
Pooled data for three 1-mth studies[38,39,52]	62.84 [45.23, 80.44], $I^2 = 85\%$ FEM*
	68.49 [22.91, 114.07], $I^2 = 85\%$ REM*
Pooled data for ten 3/4-mth studies[37,41,44–46,48,49,54,55,59]	74.20 [65.42, 82.98], $I^2 = 93\%$ FEM*
	59.66 [24.63, 94.69], $I^2 = 93\%$ REM*
Pooled data for three 6-mth studies[36,51,53]	52.12 [42.20, 62.04], $I^2 = 83\%$ FEM*
	43.10 [15.16, 71.04], $I^2 = 83\%$ REM*
Pooled data for 2 studies of CHM+Sal./Flu.[37,53]	30.87 [12.87, 48.87], $I^2 = 10\%$ FEM*
	31.44 [11.84, 51.04], $I^2 = 10\%$ REM*
Pooled data for 2 studies of CHM+Theo.& Muc.& LABA[39,52]	44.65 [24.39, 64.90], $I^2 = 0\%$ FEM*
	44.65 [24.39, 64.90], $I^2 = 0\%$ REM*
Pooled data for 5 studies of CHM+RP (guidelines)[41,45,48,49,55]	40.22 [26.93, 53.50], $I^2 = 69\%$ FEM*
	39.27 [14.45, 64.09], $I^2 = 69\%$ REM*
Pooled data for 2 studies of CHM+RP (+p.r.)[54,59]	154.40 [137.25, 171.56], $I^2 = 3\%$ FEM*
	153.65 [132.71, 174.59], $I^2 = 3\%$ REM*
Pooled data for 12 studies of AM formulae[36–38,41,44,45,48,49,53,55,58,59]	66.21 [59.40, 73.03], $I^2 = 93\%$ FEM*
	55.39 [27.29, 83.50], $I^2 = 93\%$ REM*
Pooled data for 2 studies of Ginseng formulae[39,52]	44.65 [24.39, 64.90], $I^2 = 0\%$ FEM*
	44.65 [24.39, 64.90], $I^2 = 0\%$ REM*
Pooled data for 5 studies of CS formulae[41,45,46,51,59]	82.96 [72.63, 93.29], $I^2 = 96\%$ FEM*
	68.11 [12.49, 123.72], $I^2 = 96\%$ REM*
Pooled data for 7 studies in which 6MWD was less than 300 meters at baseline [36,38,41,44,45,48,55]	37.69 [27.25, 48.14], $I^2 = 46\%$ FEM*
	37.05 [22.46, 51.64], $I^2 = 46\%$ REM*
Pooled data for 7 studies in which 6MWD was more than 300 meters at baseline [37,39,46,49,51–53]	59.79 [51.27, 68.30], $I^2 = 72\%$ FEM*
	60.73 [42.62, 78.84], $I^2 = 72\%$ REM*
Pooled data for All 17 studies[36–39,41,44–46,48,49,51–55,58,59]	62.36 [56.30, 68.42], $I^2 = 91\%$ FEM*
	54.61 [33.30, 75.92], $I^2 = 91\%$ REM*
Pooled data for 16 studies written in Chinese [36–39,41,44–46,48,49,51–53,55,58,59]	62.19 [56.11, 68.26], $I^2 = 92\%$ FEM*
	53.10 [31.42, 74.79], $I^2 = 92\%$ REM*
Pooled data for 15 studies exclusively indexed in Chinese databases[36,37,39,41,44–46,48,49,51–53,55,58,59]	60.48 [54.32, 66.65], $I^2 = 92\%$ FEM*
	48.99 [26.85, 71.12], $I^2 = 92\%$ REM*
Pooled data for 14 studies[36–39,41,44–46,48,49,51–53,55] after excluding studies of pulmonary rehabilitation[54,58,59]	50.96 [44.36, 57.56], $I^2 = 70\%$ FEM*
	48.86 [36.07, 61.64], $I^2 = 70\%$ REM*
Pooled data for 12 studies[37,39,41,44–46,48,49,51–53,55] after excluding studies of oxygen [38]& exercise [36] & pulmonary rehabilitation [54,58,59]	41.62 [33.63, 49.62], $I^2 = 41\%$ FEM*
	42.05 [31.46, 52.63], $I^2 = 41\%$ REM*
Pooled data for 6 studies[37,39,46,51–53] after excluding studies of oxygen [38]& exercise [36] & pulmonary rehabilitation [54,58,59] & undefined RP [41,44,45,48,49,55]	40.95 [30.19, 51.71], $I^2 = 0\%$ FEM*
	40.95 [30.19, 51.71], $I^2 = 0\%$ REM*

*Significant difference, CHM: Chinese Herbal Medicine, RP: routine pharmacotherapy, MD: mean difference, CI: confidence interval, mth: month, REM: random effect model, FEM: fixed effect model, Salm./Flu.: salmeterol/fluticasone (inhaled), Theo.: theophylline (oral), Muc.: Mucosolvan (oral), LABAs: long-acting β2 agonists (inhaled), RP(guidelines): routine pharmacotherapy (adjusted for severity according to guidelines), RP(+p.r.): routine pharmacotherapy (pharmacotherapy plus pulmonary rehabilitation), AM: *Astragalus membranaceus*, CS: *Cordyceps sinensis*.

distance was 375 meters in each group. After three months, a significant increase was observed in both the RP group (MD 75.34 m) and CHM plus RP group (MD 232.02 m). The test group showed a relative increase in walking distance of 156.02 meters compared to control at EoT [59]. In the other study, the baseline mean 6MWD was 20 meters further in the test group compared to control but this was not significant (Table S5). After three months the control showed a shorter mean walking distance of −21.40 meters whereas there was an improvement in the test group of 64.10 m but neither was significant. At EoT there was a significant benefit in favour of the CHM plus RP group of 105.50 meters [54]. The pooled effect at EoT was 153.65 meters in favour of the test groups which was significant with low heterogeneity (Figure 5, Table 3).

Overall, participants treated with CHM plus RP therapy achieved greater walking distances within 6 minutes compared to those treated with RP alone based on 17 studies (MD 54.61 m, 95%CI 33.30, 75.92, $I^2 = 91\%$, REM) but the heterogeneity was high [36–39,41,44–46,48,49,51–55,58,59] (Figure 5). Therefore, sensitivity analysis was undertaken (Table 3). Analysis of data from the sixteen studies written in Chinese and from the 15 studies exclusively indexed in Chinese databases found similar results (Table 3).

When the three studies that used p.r. were removed [54,58,59], the total benefit of adding CHM was 48.86 meters (95%CI 36.07, 61.64, $I^2 = 71\%$ REM). When the studies that used oxygen therapy [38], pulmonary exercise [36] and p.r. in addition to RP [54,58,59] were excluded from the meta-analysis, the mean difference decreased to 42.05 meters (95%CI 31.46, 52.63, REM) and I^2 was reduced to 41%. When the studies with undefined RP [41,44,45,48,49,55] were also excluded, the pooled benefit for the remaining six studies was 40.95 meters (95%CI 30.19, 52.89, $I^2 = 0\%$, FEM) which was clinically significant (Table 3).

When the seven studies of patients who could walk an average of 300 meters or more at baseline were considered separately [37,39,46,49,51–53], excluding two studies that used p.r. [58,59], the benefit was reduced to 37.05 meters (Table 3). Conversely, for the 7 studies of patients who could walk less than 300 meters at baseline [36,38,41,44,45,48,55], excluding the one that used p.r. [54], the pooled benefit was greater (MD 60.73, Table 3).

In terms of the CHMs, twelve studies used formulae that contained *A. membranaceus*. There was a non-significant increase in 6MWT/D in the control groups of 22.96 meters. A significant increase was observed in the test groups of 80.86 meters and there was a significant difference between groups of 55.39 meters at EoT but heterogeneity was high [36–38,41,44,45,48,49,53,55,58,59]. Removal of the outlier in the funnel plot reduced the benefit to 46.03 meters (95%CI 28.38, 63.67, $I^2 = 70\%$, REM) and removal of the four studies that used oxygen or p.r. as co-interventions [36,38,58,59] reduced the benefit to 39.89 meters (95%CI 24.45, 55.33, $I^2 = 55\%$ REM).

In the five studies that combined *A. membranaceus* with *A. macrocephala* the benefit for adding these CHMs was 49.56 meters (95%CI 32.08, 67.05, $I^2 = 60\%$, REM). When the study that also used p.r. [36] (Chen 12) was removed, the benefit remained clinically significant at 41.09 meters (95%CI 25.35, 56.84, $I^2 = 13\%$, REM).

For the five studies that contained cultured *C. sinensis* (CS) mycelia, the CHM plus RP groups achieved a significantly greater distance over baseline of 102.65 meters. The RP groups achieved a lower but significant increase of 35.56 meters. At EoT, there was a significant benefit in favour of the CS plus RP groups of 68.11 meters but heterogeneity was high [41,45,46,51,59]. When the outlier in the funnel plot [59] was removed the benefit was 44.56 meters (95%CI 25.37, 63.76, $I^2 = 54\%$, REM).

Two studies used the same formula with *Panax ginseng* as the main herb (Guo 2008 [39] and Zhang (1) 2007 [52]). The pooled effect for 6MWT was 44.65 meters in favour of the CHM plus RP groups after 1 month with no heterogeneity (Table 3).

Adverse events

Seventeen adverse events were reported in 3 studies [37,41,43], with 7 adverse events in the CHM plus RP groups. Among these 7 cases, one had abdominal distension [43], one had thirst [43], one had palpitations [43], one had constipation [43], one had insomnia [43], and two had thirst and abdominal distension [41]. There was no significant difference between CHM plus RP and RP groups in rate of AEs (RR 0.53, 95%CI 0.15, 1.93, $I^2 = 0\%$). There was no adverse event reported in 6 studies [44,50,54–56,58] and information on adverse events was not provided in 16 studies [36,38–40,42,45–49,51–53,57,59,60].

Discussion

This systematic review identified 25 randomized controlled trials of CHM plus RP versus RP for patients with stable COPD that included BODE Index and/or 6MWT/D as outcome measures. Meta-analysis found that compared with control groups that used RP, treatment that combined CHM plus the same RP produced a relative reduction in BODE Index in six out of seven studies. The pooled data showed a relative benefit of less than one point (−0.71) but four studies showed benefits of greater than one point [37,40,47,54]. Consistent with the correlations found for the baseline and EoT scores, the benefits were more pronounced when the COPD was worse at baseline. In the three studies of patients with mean BODE Indices greater than 4, the benefit for adding CHM to RP was a clinically significant reduction of 1.40 points.

A systematic review has reported that the combination of CHM plus RP could increase SGRQ scores compared with the RPs alone [18]. Since the BODE Index was found to correlate well with SGRQ scores in a large cohort study with 10 years follow-up [31], the results of this review are consistent with the previous review.

There was a relative increase in the 6MWT/D in favour of CHM plus RP in 15 out of 17 studies. In the pooled data, the mean increase was 54.61 meters but there was considerable heterogeneity in the analysis. When the pool was reduced to six studies, there remained a clinically significant increase of 40.95 meters with no heterogeneity. A greater benefit for the addition of the CHMs was found when the walking distances were shorter at baseline. Overall, 14 of the 17 studies showed relative increases of 25 meters or more and would appear to have produced clinically important gains in exercise tolerance [24].

The combination of the CHMs and RPs appeared to be well-tolerated by patients. The AE incidence was balanced between the CHM plus RP and the RP groups, and none of the reports were serious events. However, AEs were reported by only 9 out of 25 studies so the safety data is incomplete.

Limitations of the review

These promising observations should be interpreted with caution for several reasons. A range of methodological issues were identified. In particular, descriptions of the random sequence generation process and allocation concealment were lacking in the majority of studies. One study provided complete descriptions and used blind assessment but was not blind to patients and investigators [43]. It reported a significant benefit for 6MWT at EoT (6 months) and end of follow-up (18 months) but the data were presented as graphs and were not suitable for further analysis.

Overall, whether randomization and allocation concealment were effectively conducted in the majority of included studies remains unclear. Inadequate blinding may result in an overestimation of the effect in the test group. Only one study used an identical placebo to enable adequate blinding. This study found positive results for BODE Index and 6MWT in the combined CHM plus RP group, but the descriptions of randomisation and allocation concealment methods were not adequate and there was no assessment of the effectiveness of blinding, so the results may have been influenced by these methodological shortcomings [54].

The overemphasizing of positive effects arising from publication bias and language bias may be a limitation in this review. It includes only studies written in English or Chinese and all the included studies were conducted in China. Patients showed high compliance and may have expected a benefit from the addition of the CHM. This may have produced bias in patient performance or in measurement. Although the funnel plot for 6MWT/D showed a marked effect of the small studies, Egger's test was not suggestive of publication bias.

Interpretation of the results

Although these studies used the same overall study design and the same outcome measures, the meaningfulness of pooled data is limited by a number of factors including the RPs used, study duration, the CHMs used and the severity of the COPD.

A range of different RPs was used and a number of studies treated individual participants differently according to their COPD severity as per the guidelines [34,62]. Attempts were made to control for this source of variation by pooling studies that used the same specific RP.

For BODE Index, two studies used salmeterol/fluticasone (50 µg/500 µg) as RP [37,60]. Participants in Chen 2009 [37] had higher baseline scores (6.31) than those in Yang 2013 (3.75) [60]. A benefit of −1.44 was observed after 3 months in Chen 2009 but there was only a 0.27 decrease after 1 month in Yang 2013 in the RP groups. This may suggest an effect of baseline difference in the BODE Index. In addition, the CHMs used in Chen 2009 were quite different from those in Yang 2013. Therefore, even though the pooled data showed no heterogeneity, the meaningfulness of the relative benefit of 0.70 for the addition of the CHMs is limited by clinical differences including treatment duration, the CHMs used and baseline scores.

For 6MWT, in the two studies that used salmeterol/fluticasone (50 µg/500 µg) [37,53], Chen 2009 [37] found a benefit of 37.05 meters after 3 months but Zhang 2011 [53] found only a 5.06 meter increase after 6 months in the RP alone groups. These benefits were considerably lower than the 160 meter increase after 3 months using salmeterol/fluticasone (100 µg/250 µg) reported in a recent study from Iran [64]. However, the participants in each of these three studies had quite different exercise capacities at study commencement. In Mansori *et al* 2010 [64], the mean 6MWT at baseline was 300 meters, it was 327.42 meters in Chen 2009, and the patients in Zhang 2011 had the least impairment (385.42 m). These results suggest that greater benefits were evident in studies with lower exercise capacity at baseline. Consequently, even though the pooled benefit of 31.44 meters for this subgroup has low heterogeneity and the studies had the same duration, the patient groups were different.

For theophylline (oral) plus Mucosolvan (oral) plus LABA (inhaled), two studies were for one month [39,52]. The mean walking distances were similar at baseline (386 m vs 378 m respectively) and the majority of participants were at COPD stage II in both studies. So these studies were directly comparable in terms of RP, duration and participants. In Guo 2008 [39] the RPs produced a 60.0 meter increase while in Zhang (1) 2007 [52] the increase was similar at 70.0 meters. The pooled effect was 65.36 meters (95%CI: 45.17, 85.55, $I^2 = 0\%$). In this sub-group the relative benefit found in the pooled data of 44.65 meters ($I^2 = 0\%$) for the addition of the CHM is based on closely comparable studies.

In terms of the CHMs used in the above four studies, both Guo 2008 [39] and Zhang (1) 2007 [52] used the same CHM formula with the only difference being that Guo 2008 used a capsule while Zhang (1) 2007 used a decoction. Both studies produced clinically meaningful improvements in exercise tolerance. This strengthens the likelihood that the addition of this CHM to theophylline (oral) plus Mucosolvan (oral) plus LABA (inhaled) had real effects, over the short term at least. For the salmeterol/fluicasone group, Chen 2009 [37] and Zhang 2011 [53] used CHMs that showed distinct similarities in terms of their ingredients. Chen 2009 showed the greater benefit but due to the differences at baseline and the different study durations, it was not possible to determine whether the CHM used for 3 months in Chen 2009 was more effective than that used for 6 months in Zhang 2011.

Studies were also pooled when the RP was similar in that it was administered according to the COPD severity in accord with the GOLD or the CSRD guidelines. For BODE Index, there was no benefit for Xu (1) 2012 and a significant improvement in Yu 2011 but the pool produced a non-significant result with high heterogeneity ($I^2 = 74\%$). Both studies were for 3 months but RP was according to CSRD in Xu (1) 2012 and according to GOLD in Yu 2011. Xu (1) 2012 used two different CHMs according to syndrome differentiation and both these CHMs were quite different to the CHM used Yu 2011. This limits the meaningfulness of the pool.

For 6MWT, the pool included five studies each with durations of 3 months [41,45,48,49,55]. The pooled data showed a significant relative improvement of 39.27 meters but the heterogeneity was relatively high ($I^2 = 69\%$). Xu (1) 2012 [49] had a considerably longer mean walking distance at baseline (>411 m) than the other four studies (248 m–294 m) and this study was the major contributor to the heterogeneity. When removed, the pooled relative benefit was 48.0 meters ($I^2 = 50\%$). Within the remaining four studies, the greatest relative benefit was in Liu 2009 [45] (66.00 m). This study only included participants who conformed to the indications of the CHMs used, which may have produced a more targeted effect. However, it is difficult to compare the effects of this CHM with those used in the other three studies since Xu (2) 2012 [48] and Fan 2013 [55] included participants with different TCM syndromes while Huang 2005 [41] did not specify whether TCM syndrome differentiation was used in selection.

For the results of data pooling to be fully interpretable, studies of CHM plus RP need to be comparable in terms of not only the RP used and duration, but also the CHMs used and the appropriateness of the CHMs to the participant population. With regard to this aspect, thirteen of the 25 studies included TCM syndrome differentiation in participant selection. Of these, Li 2012 [43] and Xu (1) 2012 [49] allowed multiple syndromes and CHM selection according to syndrome. This more closely reflects actual practice but would appear to introduce additional sources of variation into a clinical trial. In the case of Xu (1) 2012, [49] large SDs were apparent for 6MWT and no significant differences were found over baseline for test or control groups at three months. Li 2012 [43] reported no significant benefit for the CHM at 3 months but found a benefit at 6 months of treatment which was still evident one year post-trial. However this study did not report data suitable for inclusion in the meta-analyses.

Effect of baseline values on outcomes

Significant negative correlations between baseline values and change at EoT were found for BODE Index and walking distance in both test and control groups. For 6MWT/D, the correlation found in the test groups was stronger than that in the control groups since there was decline in exercise tolerance in some studies and no change in others. Similarly, the correlation found in the test groups was twice that in the control groups for the BODE Index. In the case of the RP groups, in most studies it is not clear whether the participants had been using the same RP prior to the study or whether the RP was a new intervention. In the first case, it could be expected that most of the benefit for the RP would have been achieved prior to the trial and scores would not show much change during the trial, so this may account for some of the variability in the intervention effect found in the RP groups. Whether this effect holds for all types of interventions has not been further explored, but these correlations suggest that when BODE Index and 6MWT are used as outcome measures in clinical trials, the baseline values need to be considered when undertaking sample size calculations and when interpreting results.

Effects of the main herbs and main formulae

A previous review found that *Astragalus membranaceus* (AM) was the most frequently used herb in trials of CHM for COPD [18]. Similarly, it was frequently used in the studies that used BODE Index (n = 5) and 6MWT/D (n = 13) as outcomes. Significant benefits were found in the pooled data for studies of CHMs containing AM, with a decrease in the BODE Index of 0.62 points [37,40,49,58,60] and an increase in walking distance of 49.27 meters (Table 3) [36–38,41,44,48,49,53,55,58,59] for the test groups compared to the RP controls. This effect is supported by a recent review that found that oral Huangqi formulae had beneficial effects on lung function, quality of life, COPD symptoms, and incidence of exacerbations for patients with stable COPD [65].

The two studies that used *Panax ginseng* as the main herb showed a clinically significant 6MWD benefit of 44.65 meters in favour of the CHM plus RP groups [39,52]. This enhanced exercise tolerance is consistent with two recent reviews. One mentioned that *P. ginseng* may improve respiratory muscle strength and lung function [66]. Another review of ginseng-containing herbal formulae reported improvements in respiratory volume and quality of life [67].

The most commonly used formula (n = 5) contained cultured *Cordyceps sinensis* mycelia alone under the names 'Bailing Capsule' or 'Jinshuibao Capsule'. *C. sinensis* (CS) is a kind of fungus that is parasitic on the larvae of *Lepidoptera* species. It has been widely used as a time-honoured tonic food and herbal medicine in China [68]. Its production is so limited that it cannot be widely used and a cultured form is used instead. For the five studies that reported 6MWT, there was a relative benefit of 44.56 meters in the pooled data (Table 3) [41,45,46,51]. The one study in the BODE Index group reported a relative benefit of −1.21 points [40] in favour of the CS plus RP groups.

AM and CS are thought to strengthen the body's resistance to illness through effects on the immune system. Experimental studies have found that Astragalus polysaccharides (APS) extracted from AM had immunomodulatory activity by activating macrophages [14]. CS has been reported to have immunomodulatory [11–13] and anti-inflammatory activity [7–9]. In addition, effects on exercise have been investigated for these two herbs. Rats that received *A. membranaceus* flavonoids (AMF) showed higher endurance capacity in a swimming test when compared with those without AMF administration [69]. Also, CS supplementation, with or without exercise, was reported to improve exercise endurance capacity in rats by activating the skeletal muscle metabolic regulators [70].

The experimental studies suggest that each of the principal herbs, *A. membranaceus*, *P. ginseng* and *C. sinensis*, can benefit resistance to illness and improve exercise tolerance but it remains unclear whether these herbs are appropriate for all patients and whether particular combinations of herbs have additive effects in a clinical setting.

Conclusions

CHM appears to be a well-tolerated addition to routine pharmacotherapy for stable COPD. The meta-analysis results indicate that the addition of CHM to routine pharmacotherapies may produce additional benefits in terms of decreasing the BODE Index and increasing the 6MWD in stable COPD patients when used for up to six months. These potential benefits of CHM as a supportive intervention need to be further evaluated through trials that address the identified methodological deficiencies, have published protocols, provide quality-control data for both the CHM and control interventions and are of sufficient duration to assess any change. Trials should employ an identical placebo for the CHM in the control group to enable effective blinding. In order for outcomes to be fully interpretable, participants should have similar COPD severity at baseline, the PR should be standardised and the trial should investigate a single CHM intervention that is appropriate to the participant group.

Supporting Information

Figure S1 Funnel plot of 17 studies evaluating the effect of CHM plus RP for stable COPD on 6MWT/D. MD: mean difference, SE: standard error.
(TIF)

Table S1 Search terms used in PubMed. MeSH: MeSH terms, TW: text word.
(DOCX)

Table S2 Characteristics of the 25 studies of CHM plus RP for stable COPD. CHM: Chinese Herbal Medicine, RP: routine pharmacotherapy, mths: months, R/A: registration/analysis, M/F: male/female, yrs: years, CM: Chinese Medicine, NS: not stated, T: test group, C: control group, CVD: cerebrovascular disease. AE: acute exacerbation.
(DOCX)

Table S3 Interventions of the 25 studies of CHM plus RP for stable COPD. CHM: Chinese Herbal Medicine, RP: routine pharmacotherapy, Y: yes, N: no, CSRD: COPD Study Group of Chinese Society of Respiratory Disease: Treatment guidelines of COPD, GOLD: Global Initiative for Chronic Obstructive Lung Disease.
(DOCX)

Table S4 Results for individual studies: BODE Index (MD, 95%CI) for the CHM plus RP groups (T) and the RP groups (C) at baseline and end of treatment. *Significant difference, MD: mean difference, CI: confidence interval, CHM: Chinese Herbal Medicine, RP: routine pharmacotherapy, T: test group, C: control group, EoT: end of treatment, mths: months, Ipra.: ipratropium (inhaled), Salb.: salbutamol (inhaled), Theo.(+p.r.): oral theophylline (plus pulmonary rehabilitation), Theo.: theophylline (oral), Salm./Flu.: salmeterol/fluticasone (inhaled), RP (guidelines): routine pharmacotherapy (adjusted for severity according to guidelines), RP(+ p.r.): routine pharmacotherapy (pharmacotherapy plus pulmonary rehabilitation).
(DOCX)

Table S5 Results for individual studies: 6MWT/D (MD, 95%CI, meters) for the CHM plus RP groups (T) and the RP groups (C) at baseline and end of treatment. *Significant difference, CHM: Chinese Herbal Medicine, RP: routine pharmacotherapy, MD: mean difference, mths: months, CI: confidence interval, T: test group, C: control group, EoT: end of treatment, Salm./Flu.: salmeterol/fluticasone (inhaled), Theo.(+p.r.): oral theophylline (plus pulmonary rehabilitation),

Theo.: theophylline (oral), Muc.: Mucosolvan (oral), LABA: long-acting β2 agonist (inhaled), Ami./Bro./Chlo.: compound oral medication which contained aminophylline, bromhexine and chlorphenamine, Ipra.: ipratropium (inhaled), oxy.: oxygen therapy, Salb./Ipra.: salbutamol/ipratropium (inhaled), exe.: pulmonary exercise, RP(guidelines): routine pharmacotherapy (adjusted for severity according to guidelines), RP(+ p.r.): routine pharmacotherapy (pharmacotherapy plus pulmonary rehabilitation).
(DOCX)

Checklist S1 PRISMA checklist.
(DOC)

Author Contributions

Conceived and designed the experiments: XC. Performed the experiments: XC BM YD. Analyzed the data: XC BM YD. Wrote the paper: XC BM YD AZ CL CX LL. Reviewed the final manuscript: XC BM YD AZ CL CX LL. Approved the final manuscript: XC BM YD AZ CL CX LL.

References

1. Qaseem A, Wilt TJ, Weinberger SE, Hanania NA, Criner G, et al. (2011) Diagnosis and management of stable chronic obstructive pulmonary disease: a clinical practice guideline update from the American College of Physicians, American College of Chest Physicians, American Thoracic Society, and European Respiratory Society. Ann Intern Med 155: 179–191.
2. Murray CJ, Lopez AD (1997) Alternative projections of mortality and disability by cause 1990-2020: Global Burden of Disease Study. Lancet 349: 1498–1504.
3. George J, Ioannides-Demos LL, Santamaria NM, Kong DC, Stewart K (2004) Use of complementary and alternative medicines by patients with chronic obstructive pulmonary disease. Med J Aust 181: 248–251.
4. Hu J, Zhang J, Zhao W, Zhang Y, Zhang L, et al. (2011) Cochrane systematic reviews of Chinese herbal medicines: an overview. PLoS One 6: e28696.
5. Vickers A, Zollman C (1999) ABC of complementary medicine: herbal medicine. BMJ 319: 1050–1053.
6. Shin IS, Lee MY, Lim HS, Ha H, Seo CS, et al. (2012) An extract of Crataegus pinnatifida fruit attenuates airway inflammation by modulation of matrix metalloproteinase-9 in ovalbumin induced asthma. PLoS One 7: e45734.
7. Kim HG, Shrestha B, Lim SY, Yoon DH, Chang WC, et al. (2006) Cordycepin inhibits lipopolysaccharide-induced inflammation by the suppression of NF-kappaB through Akt and p38 inhibition in RAW 264.7 macrophage cells. Eur J Pharmacol 545: 192–199.
8. Rao YK, Fang SH, Tzeng YM (2007) Evaluation of the anti-inflammatory and anti-proliferation tumoral cells activities of Antrodia camphorata, Cordyceps sinensis, and Cinnamomum osmophloeum bark extracts. J Ethnopharmacol 114: 78–85.
9. Shahed AR, Kim SI, Shoskes DA (2001) Down-regulation of apoptotic and inflammatory genes by Cordyceps sinensis extract in rat kidney following ischemia/reperfusion. Transplant Proc 33: 2986–2987.
10. Denzler KL, Waters R, Jacobs BL, Rochon Y, Langland JO (2010) Regulation of inflammatory gene expression in PBMCs by immunostimulatory botanicals. PLoS One 5: e12561.
11. Koh JH, Yu KW, Suh HJ, Choi YM, Ahn TS (2002) Activation of macrophages and the intestinal immune system by an orally administered decoction from cultured mycelia of Cordyceps sinensis. Biosci Biotechnol Biochem 66: 407–411.
12. Kuo YC, Tsai WJ, Shiao MS, Chen CF, Lin CY (1996) Cordyceps sinensis as an immunomodulatory agent. Am J Chin Med 24: 111–125.
13. Kuo YC, Tsai WJ, Wang JY, Chang SC, Lin CY, et al. (2001) Regulation of bronchoalveolar lavage fluids cell function by the immunomodulatory agents from Cordyceps sinensis. Life Sci 68: 1067–1082.
14. Shao BM, Xu W, Dai H, Tu P, Li Z, et al. (2004) A study on the immune receptors for polysaccharides from the roots of Astragalus membranaceus, a Chinese medicinal herb. Biochem Biophys Res Commun 320: 1103–1111.
15. Chen N, Li H, Zhao LY, Liu JB, Huang Q, et al. (2009) [Therapy for clearing heat and resolving phlegm in treatment of systemic inflammatory response syndrome in acute deterioration stage of chronic obstructive pulmonary disease: a randomized controlled trial]. Zhong Xi Yi Jie He Xue Bao 7: 105–109.
16. Cui P, Wang YN, Gao TS, Qi TC, Mei L, et al. (2012) [Study on mechanism of traditional Chinese medicines reducing phlegm and resolving masses in treatment of goiter]. Zhongguo Zhong Yao Za Zhi 37: 3451–3456.
17. Chan E, Tan M, Xin J, Sudarsanam S, Johnson DE (2010) Interactions between traditional Chinese medicines and Western therapeutics. Curr Opin Drug Discov Devel 13: 50–65.
18. An X, Zhang AL, May BH, Lin L, Xu Y, et al. (2012) Oral Chinese herbal medicine for improvement of quality of life in patients with stable chronic obstructive pulmonary disease: a systematic review. J Altern Complement Med 18: 731–743.
19. Jones PW (2001) Health status measurement in chronic obstructive pulmonary disease. Thorax 56: 880–887.
20. Glaab T, Vogelmeier C, Buhl R (2010) Outcome measures in chronic obstructive pulmonary disease (COPD): strengths and limitations. Respir Res 11: 79.
21. Pinto-Plata VM, Cote C, Cabral H, Taylor J, Celli BR (2004) The 6-min walk distance: change over time and value as a predictor of survival in severe COPD. Eur Respir J 23: 28–33.
22. Brown CD, Wise RA (2007) Field tests of exercise in COPD: the six-minute walk test and the shuttle walk test. COPD 4: 217–223.
23. Wise RA, Brown CD (2005) Minimal clinically important differences in the six-minute walk test and the incremental shuttle walking test. COPD 2: 125–129.
24. Holland AE, Hill CJ, Rasekaba T, Lee A, Naughton MT, et al. (2010) Updating the minimal important difference for six-minute walk distance in patients with chronic obstructive pulmonary disease. Arch Phys Med Rehabil 91: 221–225.
25. Spruit MA, Polkey MI, Celli B, Edwards LD, Watkins ML, et al. (2012) Predicting outcomes from 6-minute walk distance in chronic obstructive pulmonary disease. Joural of the American Medical Directors Association 13: 291–297.
26. Cote CG, Casanova C, Marin JM, Lopez MV, Pinto-Plata V, et al. (2008) Validation and comparison of reference equations for the 6-min walk distance test. Eur Respir J 31: 571–578.
27. Celli BR, Cote CG, Marin JM, Casanova C, Montes de Oca M, et al. (2004) The body-mass index, airflow obstruction, dyspnea, and exercise capacity index in chronic obstructive pulmonary disease. N Engl J Med 350: 1005–1012.
28. Ong KC, Earnest A, Lu SJ (2005) A multidimensional grading system (BODE index) as predictor of hospitalization for COPD. Chest 128: 3810–3816.
29. Pinto-Plata V, Casanova C, Mullerova H, de Torres JP, Corado H, et al. (2012) Inflammatory and repair serum biomarker pattern. Association to clinical outcomes in COPD. Respir Res 13: 71.
30. Faganello MM, Tanni SE, Sanchez FF, Pelegrino NR, Lucheta PA, et al. (2010) BODE index and GOLD staging as predictors of 1-year exacerbation risk in chronic obstructive pulmonary disease. Am J Med Sci 339: 10–14.
31. Marin JM, Cote CG, Diaz O, Lisboa C, Casanova C, et al. (2011) Prognostic assessment in COPD: health related quality of life and the BODE index. Respir Med 105: 916–921.
32. Imfeld S, Bloch KE, Weder W, Russi EW (2006) The BODE index after lung volume reduction surgery correlates with survival. Chest 129: 873–878.
33. Shang Q, Xu H, Huang L (2012) Tanshinone IIA: A Promising Natural Cardioprotective Agent. Evid Based Complement Alternat Med 2012: 716459.
34. GOLD (2011) Global Strategy for Diagnosis, Management and Prevention of COPD The Global Initiative for Chronic Obstructive Lung Disease (GOLD).
35. Higgins JPT, Green S, eds (2011) Cochrane Handbook for Systematic Reviews of Interventions Version 5.1.0. The Cochrane Collaboration.
36. Chen GC, Li YX, Zhou ZY, Xue HR, Zhang YB (2012) Combination of Buzhong-Yiqi decoction and routine treatment for stable chronic obstructive pulmonary disease [in Chinese]. Shanghai Journal of Traditional Chinese Medicine 46: 42–44.
37. Chen Q, Hong XC, Cai Y, Ye L (2009) Clinical observation of integrated Chinese and western medicine treatment in patients with stable COPD [in Chinese]. Journal of Fujian University of Traditional Chinese Medicine 19: 12–14.
38. Cui CB, Yuan YD, Liu SH, Han DL, Gao XL, et al. (2004) Intervention effect of Tongfei mixture on nocturnal hypoxia in patients with chronic obstructive pulmonary disease [in Chinese]. Chinese Journal of Integrated Traditional and Western Medicine 24: 885–888.
39. Guo WX, Zhang FY, Yan GL (2008) Clinical observation of the therapeutic effect of Jianfei capsule on chronic obstructive pulmonary disease at stationary phase [in Chinese]. Hebei Journal of Traditional Chinese Medicine 30: 121–125.
40. Hu QG, Liu LL (2012) Clinical observation of Jinshuibao capsule combined with Bufeihuoxue capsule in treating patients with stable COPD [in Chinese]. Journal of Guiyang Collage of Traditional Chinese Medicine 34: 135–137.
41. Huang DH, Wu L, He DP, Lin L (2005) Clinical observation of tranquilization period of COPD treated by integration of traditional Chinese medicine and western medicine [in Chinese]. Journal of the Fourth Military Medical University 26: 1611–1613.
42. Jian XY, Huang SQ, Lai X, Chen WY, Jiang RB (2012) Influence of Pingchuan capsules on BODE indexes in patients with stable chronic obstructive pulmonary disease [in Chinese]. Journal of Beijing University of Traditional Chinese Medicine (TCM clinical edition) 19: 32–34.
43. Li SY, Li JS, Wang MH, Xie Y, Yu XQ, et al. (2012) Effects of comprehensive therapy based on traditional Chinese medicine patterns in stable chronic obstructive pulmonary disease: a four-center, open-label, randomized, controlled study. BMC Complement Altern Med 12: 197.

44. Liao YL, An W, Zhang W (2011) Stable COPD patients treated with Yupingfengsan in addition to routine therapy: 30 cases [in Chinese]. Guiding Journal of Traditional Chinese Medicine and Pharmacy 30: 63–66.
45. Liu CS (2009) Clinical observation on the treatment of 30 cases of chronic obstructive pulmonary disease at stable term by benefiting vital energy and promoting blood, resolving phlegm and dredging collaterals [in Chinese]. Guiding Journal of Traditional Chinese Medicine and Pharmacy 11: 10–12.
46. Mao R (2009) Clinical observation of Bailing capsules in treating stable COPD [in Chinese]. Chinese Journal of Integrated Traditional and Western Medicine 29: 362–367.
47. Shan LN, Liu XH, Zhong LH (2011) The effects of integrated Chinese and western medicine on prognostic indexes of patients with stable chronic obstructive pulmonary disease [in Chinese]. Journal of Guangzhou University of Traditional Chinese Medicine 28: 590–592.
48. Xu JZ, Fan DB, Qin XP, Yang L, Bai HH, et al. (2012) Clinical observation of Gujingao in the treatment of 45 participants with stable COPD [in Chinese]. Yunnan Journal of Traditional Chinese Medicine and Materia Medica 33: 31–32.
49. Xu TZ, Yao XL (2012) Effect observation on treating stable stage of COPD with therapy of Winter Disease In Summer [in Chinese]. Chinese archives of Traditional Chinese Medicine 30: 570–572.
50. Yu JY (2011) The effects of Gejiedingchuanjiaonang on BODE index in patients with stable chronic obstructive pulmonary disease [in Chinese]. Journal of Medical Information 4019.
51. Zhang FY, Liu YH, Li SF (2007) Effects of Bailing capsule combined with ipratropium bromide aerosol on the lung funtion and quality of life in patients with stable COPD [in Chinese]. Journal of Emergency in Traditional Chinese Medicine 19: 198–209.
52. Zhang FY, Wang YL, Li SF (2007) The effects of Basic Chinese Herbal Formula combined with conventional therapy for COPD patients and their exercise tolerence [in Chinese]. Shanxi Zhongyi Journal 28: 1594–1596.
53. Zhang RZ, Zheng SJ, Yan GZ (2011) Observation of the effects of Yupingfengsan combined with Jinshuiliujunjian treatment in patients with modrate COPD [in Chinese]. China Practical Medicine 6: 118–119.
54. Zhao YL, Song HR, Fei JX, Liang Y, Zhang BH, et al. (2012) The effects of Chinese Yam-Epimedium mixture on respiratory function and quality of life in patients with chronic obstructive pulmonary disease. Journal of Traditional Chinese Medicine 32: 203–207.
55. Fan BD, Qin XP, Xu JZ, Bai HH, Yu KS, et al. (2012) Clinical observation on the treatment of Bu-Fei-Jian-Pi-Yi-Shen decoction combined with western medicine for 90 patients with stable COPD [in Chinese]. Journal of Sichuan of Traditional Chinese Medicine: 83–85.
56. Liang AW, Tan YP, Liang W, Nong TQ, Su QJ, et al. (2013) The effect of Run-Fei-Jian-Pi-Bu-Shen decoction on improvement of symptoms and 6MWT of patients with stable COPD [in Chinese]. Journal of Emergency in Traditional Chinese Medicine: 1125–1127.
57. Lin YZ (2013) Clinical observation on integrated Chinese and western medicine treating stable COPD [in Chinese]. Chinese Manipulation and Rehabilitation Medicine: 103–105.
58. Peng ZQ (2013) The effect of No. 1-Bu-Fei decoction on patients with stable COPD of Lung Qi Deficiency syndrome and influence of MMP-9 [Master degree thesis in Chinese]: Fujian University of Traditional Chinese Medicine.
59. Zeng JQ, Liao ZC, Wang SM, Lin LS, Chen WY, et al. (2013) Clinical observation of modified Si-Jun-Zi granules in improving exercise tolerance of patients with COPD [in Chinese]. Journal of New Chinese Medicine: 32–34.
60. Yang CM, Lu YW, He YH (2013) Clinical observation of Tong-Qi-Pai-Yong decoction combined with Seretide for stable COPD [in Chinese]. Modern Journal of Integrated Traditional Chinese and Western Medicine: 729–730.
61. Society AT (1999) Pulmonary rehabilitation-1999. Am J Respir Crit Care Med 159: 1666–1682.
62. CSRD (2007) Chinese Society of Respiratory Disease (CSRD): guideline for diagnosis and management of chronic obstructive pulmonary disease (revision 2007). Chin J Inrern Med 46: 254–261.
63. Cote CG, Celli BR (2005) Pulmonary rehabilitation and the BODE index in COPD. Eur Respir J 26: 630–636.
64. Mansori F, Nemat Khorasani A, Boskabady MH, Boskabady M (2010) The effect of inhaled salmeterol, alone and in combination with fluticasone propionate, on management of COPD patients. Clin Respir J 4: 241–247.
65. Wu L, Chen YB, Xu YJ, Guo XF, Li XY, et al. (2013) Oral huangqi formulae for stable chronic obstructive pulmonary disease: a systematic review and meta-analysis. Evid Based Complement Alternat Med 2013: 705315.
66. Shergis JL, Zhang AL, Zhou W, Xue CC (2013) Panax ginseng in Randomised Controlled Trials: A Systematic Review. Phytother Res 27: 949–965.
67. An X, Zhang AL, Yang AW, Lin L, Wu D, et al. (2011) Oral ginseng formulae for stable chronic obstructive pulmonary disease: a systematic review. Respir Med 105: 165–176.
68. Li CY, Chiang CS, Cheng WC, Wang SC, Cheng HT, et al. (2012) Gene expression profiling of dendritic cells in different physiological stages under Cordyceps sinensis treatment. PLoS One 7: e40824.
69. Kuo YH, Tsai WJ, Loke SH, Wu TS, Chiou WF (2009) Astragalus membranaceus flavonoids (AMF) ameliorate chronic fatigue syndrome induced by food intake restriction plus forced swimming. J Ethnopharmacol 122: 28–34.
70. Kumar R, Negi PS, Singh B, Ilavazhagan G, Bhargava K, et al. (2011) Cordyceps sinensis promotes exercise endurance capacity of rats by activating skeletal muscle metabolic regulators. J Ethnopharmacol 136: 260–266.

18

Reporting Quality of Systematic Reviews/Meta-Analyses of Acupuncture

Yali Liu[1,2], Rui Zhang[1,3], Jiao Huang[1,3], Xu Zhao[1,4], Danlu Liu[1,2,3], Wanting Sun[1,4], Yuefen Mai[1,4], Peng Zhang[1,5], Yajun Wang[6], Hua Cao[7], Ke hu Yang[1,2,3]*

1 Evidence-Based Medicine Center, School of Basic Medical Sciences, Lanzhou University, Lanzhou, China, **2** Key Laboratory of Clinical Translational Research and Evidence-Based Medicine of Gansu Province, Lanzhou, China, **3** The First Clinical Medical College of Lanzhou University, Lanzhou, China, **4** The Second Clinical Medical College of Lanzhou University, Lanzhou, China, **5** Department of Cardiology, Qilu Hospital of Shandong University, Ji'nan, Shandong Province, China, **6** Acupuncture and Massage College, Gansu University of Traditional Chinese Medicine, Lanzhou, China, **7** Department of Neurology, Gansu Provincial Hospital of Traditional Chinese Medicine, Lanzhou, China

Abstract

Background: The QUOROM and PRISMA statements were published in 1999 and 2009, respectively, to improve the consistency of reporting systematic reviews (SRs)/meta-analyses (MAs) of clinical trials. However, not all SRs/MAs adhere completely to these important standards. In particular, it is not clear how well SRs/MAs of acupuncture studies adhere to reporting standards and which reporting criteria are generally ignored in these analyses.

Objectives: To evaluate reporting quality in SRs/MAs of acupuncture studies.

Methods: We performed a literature search for studies published prior to 2014 using the following public archives: PubMed, EMBASE, Web of Science, the Cochrane Database of Systematic Reviews (CDSR), the Chinese Biomedical Literature Database (CBM), the Traditional Chinese Medicine (TCM) database, the Chinese Journal Full-text Database (CJFD), the Chinese Scientific Journal Full-text Database (CSJD), and the Wanfang database. Data were extracted into pre-prepared Excel data-extraction forms. Reporting quality was assessed based on the PRISMA checklist (27 items).

Results: Of 476 appropriate SRs/MAs identified in our search, 203, 227, and 46 were published in Chinese journals, international journals, and the Cochrane Database, respectively. In 476 SRs/MAs, only 3 reported the information completely. By contrast, approximately 4.93% (1/203), 8.81% (2/227) and 0.00% (0/46) SRs/Mas reported less than 10 items in Chinese journals, international journals and CDSR, respectively. In general, the least frequently reported items (reported≤ 50%) in SRs/MAs were "protocol and registration", "risk of bias across studies", and "additional analyses" in both methods and results sections.

Conclusions: SRs/MAs of acupuncture studies have not comprehensively reported information recommended in the PRISMA statement. Our study underscores that, in addition to focusing on careful study design and performance, attention should be paid to comprehensive reporting standards in SRs/MAs on acupuncture studies.

Editor: Brett Thombs, McGill University, Canada

Funding: Project supported by the National Natural Science Foundation of China (Grant No. 81373882) http://www.nsfc.gov.cn/Portal0/default152.htm The funders had no role in study design, data collection and analysis, decision to publish, or preparation of the manuscript.

Competing Interests: The authors have declared that no competing interests exist.

* Email: kehuyangebm2006@126.com

Introduction

Systematic reviews (SRs) and meta-analyses (MAs) summarize large amounts of evidence and are a valuable tool for keeping clinicians up to date within their specialty [1,2]. As with all research, however, the value of SRs/MAs depends on how the analyses are performed, the actual findings, and the clarity of reporting [3]. If key information is reported poorly, the potential usefulness of the SRs/MAs is diminished.

Since 1987, numerous researchers have recognized the need to evaluate the quality of these types of reviews. For example, in 1987 Sacks and colleagues [4] evaluated reporting in SRs/MAs and found that it was inadequate. The Consolidated Standards of Reporting Trials (CONSORT) Group subsequently developed the Quality of Reporting of Meta-Analyses (QUOROM) statement to address suboptimal MA reporting. Ten years later, an updated QUOROM statement—entitled Preferred Reporting Items for Systematic Reviews and Meta-Analyses (PRISMA) statement—was developed and published [3]. The PRISMA statement consists of a checklist of 27 study reporting items such as title, abstract, methods, results, discussion, and funding sources. The checklist is intended to guide authors of SRs/MAs to improve the consistency and quality of reporting.

Acupuncture, a traditional medicine technique, has been widely used in clinical practice for thousands of years in China and many western countries. The number of published SRs/MAs of acupuncture studies has increased considerably in recent years. As the transparency and completeness of SRs/MAs in many fields is still not optimal [5–8], we examined how well SR/MA reporting standards have been followed in the field of acupuncture and compared adherence to these standards in acupuncture SRs/MAs published in three different types of journals/databases.

Methods

The protocol for this study was written in Chinese and has not been published. The study was not a classical systematic review, but we tried to report it according to PRISMA Checklist [3] (Text S1).

Inclusion/exclusion criteria

We included all SRs or MAs of acupuncture published in Chinese journals, international journals, and the Cochrane Database of Systematic Reviews (CDSR) prior to 2014. The experimental group of SRs/MAs of acupuncture studies was also compared with a control group of SRs/MAs of studies of other interventions, such as herbal medicine, massage and western medicine. Participants: human in any conditions, not animal; Intervention: acupuncture; Comparisons: sham acupuncture or other interventions, such as herbal medicine, massage, western medicine, etc; Outcomes: no limitations; Study design: SRs/MAs. We excluded SRs/MAs that focused primarily on traditional Chinese medicine (TCM) other than acupuncture (e.g., herbal medicine, massage).

Search strategy

We comprehensively and systematically searched the following literature archives for SRs/MAs published prior to 2014: CDSR, PubMed, EMBASE, Web of Science, Chinese Biomedical Literature Database (CBM), the TCM database, Chinese Journal Full-text Database (CJFD), Chinese Scientific Journal Full-text Database (CSJD), and the Wanfang database. Databases were searched three times: on March 24, 2011 for all entries submitted prior to March 2011, on June 12, 2012 for all entries submitted prior to January 2012 and on January 11, 2014 for all entries submitted prior to 2014. The search terms "acupuncture", "needling", "ear acupuncture", "electroacupuncture", "electro-acupuncture", "acupuncture points", "acupressure", "moxibustion", and "acupoint" were used with the terms "systematic review" or "meta-analysis". The search strategy is presented in Checklist S1.

Screening

The titles and abstracts of the studies were independently screened by at least two reviewers (Jiao Huang, Xu Zhao, or Rui Zhang) based on inclusion and exclusion criteria, and the full text of potentially suitable articles was retrieved for further assessment (Text S2).

Data extraction and analysis

Data were extracted independently by at least two reviewers (Rui Zhang, Jiao Huang, Xu Zhao, or Danlu Liu) in accordance with the PRISMA checklist and the assessment checklist for SRs/MAs of acupuncture studies developed for this study. Inconsistencies were subsequently resolved by discussion between the two reviewers or final decisions were made by the third principal investigator (Yali Liu). Data input utilized a standardized form and was done by trained data extractors (Wanting Sun, Pen Zhang, and Hua Cao). The form consisted of a general characteristics section (title, first author, funding source, study design, disease(s) examined, diagnostic criteria, intervention, and outcome) and a 27-item PRISMA information section (including title, abstract, introduction, method, results, discussion, and funding). Each item was assessed as "yes" if it was described in the paper or "no" if it was not (Text S3). Data were summarized with descriptive statistical analysis. For continuous data, the means ± SD was provided and one-way ANOVA was used. Data that followed a normal distribution were compared using the LSD- t test. Dichotomous data were summarized with descriptive statistical analysis (frequency, percentage). Pearson's χ^2 test and/or Fisher's exact test were used to assess differences in reporting among groups. P values less than 0.05 were considered significant. All statistical analyses were performed using Microsoft Excel (version 2007) and SPSS (version 13.0) software.

Results

Search

Our initial literature search identified 3993 potential SRs/MAs of acupuncture-related studies. After closer examination, 476 were chosen for inclusion in our analysis (Text S4). Of these, 203, 227, and 46 were published in Chinese journals, international journals, and CDSR, respectively. A flow chart of the literature search is shown in Figure 1.

General characteristics

General characteristics of the SRs/MAs analyzed are summarized in Table 1. The earliest acupuncture SRs/MAs in Chinese journals and international journals were published in 2002 and 1989, respectively. The number of acupuncture SRs/MAs in Chinese and international journals increased sharply after 2005, whereas the majority of acupuncture SRs/MAs in CDSR were published between 2008 and 2013 (Figure 2).

Acupuncture SRs/MAs in Chinese journals were conducted entirely by Chinese authors, whereas those published in international journals tended to be multinational collaborations, with Chinese first authors being most prevalent (27.31%, 62/227). Chinese authors were also most prevalent first authors in CDSR studies (34.78%, 16/46). The percentage of published acupuncture SRs/MAs in Chinese journals, international journals, and the CDSR that reported at least one funding source was 54.19% (110/203), 50.66% (115/227), and 89.13% (41/46), respectively, and the maximum number of funding sources reported was 5, 3, and 7, respectively.

The majority of SRs/MAs (95.37%, 454/476) included at least one randomized controlled trial (RCT). Nervous system diseases, musculoskeletal system diseases, and mental illness were most frequently examined (23.11, 18.91 and 13.44%, respectively). Approximately 38% (180/476) of the SRs/MAs reported western diseases or TCM syndromes in their diagnostic criteria. All acupuncture SRs/MAs examined described the interventions in detail. 39.92% (190/476) and 19.54% (93/476) SRs/MAs included adverse events and quality-of-life in the outcome which were reported as primary and/or secondary outcomes.

PRISMA information reporting

Comparison of PRISMA reporting among the three types of journals/databases (Table 2)

Among 476 SRs/MAs, only 3 reported the information completely. By contrast, approximately 4.93% (1/203), 8.81% (2/227) and 0.00% (0/46) SRs/MAs reported less than 10 items on the checklist in Chinese journals, international journals, and CDSR, respectively. In general, the least frequently reported items (reported≤50%) in SRs/MAs were item 5 ("protocol and

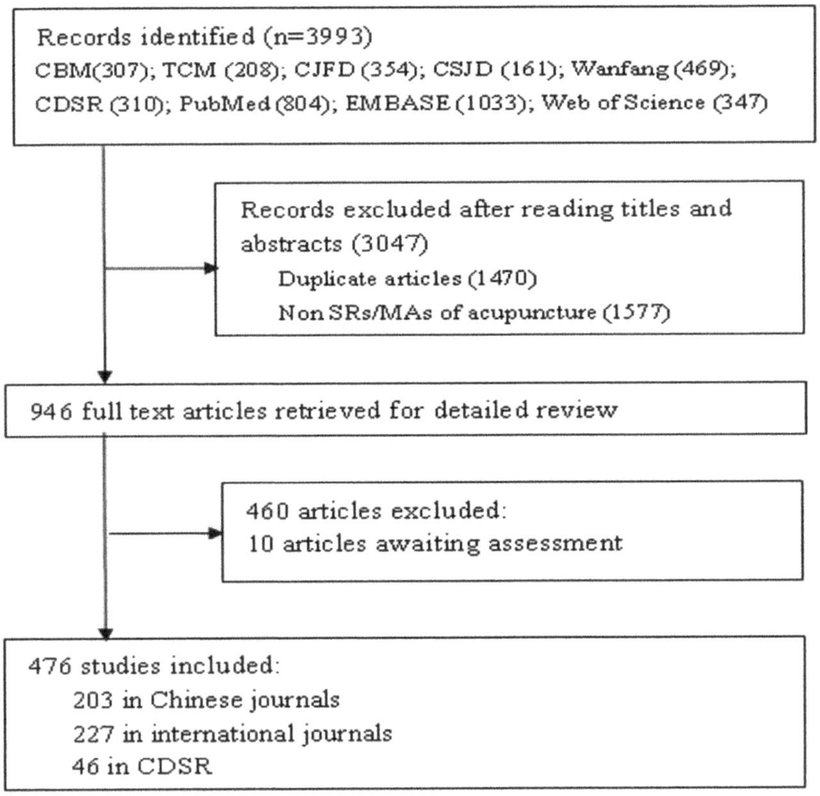

Figure 1. Flow chart of articles identified, included and excluded.

registration"), 15 and 22 ("risk of bias across studies"), and 16 and 23 ("additional analyses"). The remaining items on the checklist were adequately reported (i.e >90%), with the items listed in Table 2 being especially well reported.

Comparison of PRISMA reporting before and after release of the PRISMA statement (Table 3)

We found no statistical difference ($P>0.05$) for item 2 ("structured summary"), 5 ("protocol and registration"), 6 ("eligibility criteria"), 8 ("search"), 10 ("data collection process"), 11 ("data items"), 12 ("risk of bias in individual studies"), 16 ("additional analyses"), 17 ("study selection"), 18 ("study characteristics"), 23 ("additional analysis") and 27 ("funding") between SRs/MAs published prior to release of the PRISMA statement

Table 1. Characteristics of included studies.

Category	Characteristic	Chinese journals n = 203	International journals n = 227	CDSRs n = 46
Title	Systematic review	123 (122+1*)	167 (124+43*)	NA
	Meta analyses	66 (65+1*)	78 (35+43*)	NA
Author	The first author	203 (China)	62(China), 58(Korea), 39(England), 20(America)	16(China), 10(England), 9(Australia)
Funding source	Number of funded SRs/MAs	110 (54.19%)	110(48.46%)	40(86.96%)
Trial types	RCTs	193 (95.07%)	215(94.71%)	46 (100.0%)
Diseases	The first three	Nervous system 45 (22.17%), Musculoskeletal system 40 (19.70%), Mental illness 32 (15.76%)	Nervous system 57 (25.11%), Musculoskeletal system 42 (18.50%), Mental illness 27 (11.89%)	Musculoskeletal system 8 (17.39%), Nervous system 8 (17.39%), Mental illness 5 (10.87%)
Diagnostic criteria	Western medicine (diseases)	74(36.45%)	80(35.24%)	19(41.30%)
	Traditional medicine	44(21.67%)	6(2.64%)	0(0.00%)
Intervention		203(100.00%)	227 (100.00%)	46 (100%)
Outcome	Including adverse effect	54 (26.60%)	103 (45.37%)	33 (71.74%)
	Including quality of life	25 (12.31%)	45(19.82%)	23 (50.00%)

* Reported both "systematic review" and "meta-analysis".

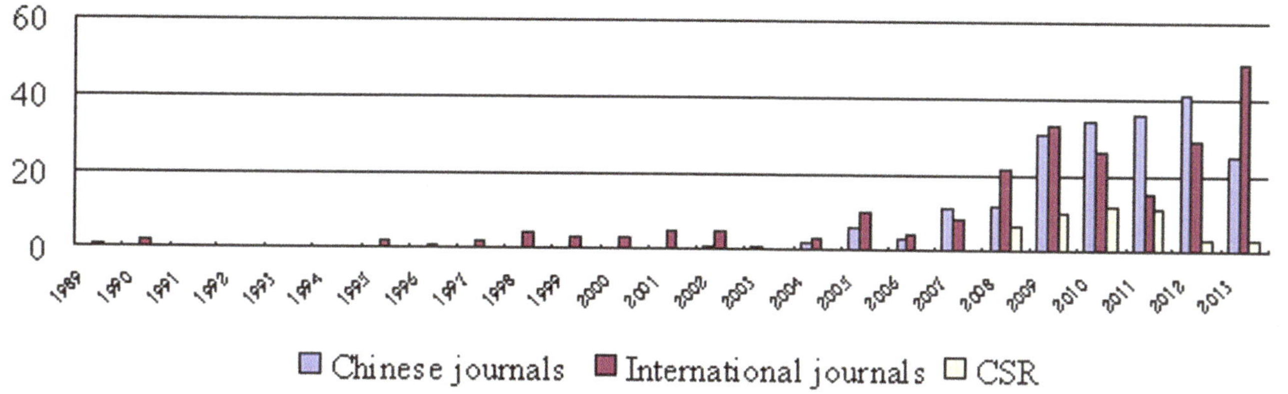

Figure 2. The number of included SRs MAs on acupuncture.

and those published after its release. Unfortunately, the rate of reporting of two items ("objective" and "information sources") had decreased in 2010–2013 compared with before 2010 ($P<0.001$).

Comparison of PRISMA reporting in Science Citation Index (SCI) and non-SCI journals (Table 3)

We found that PRISMA reporting in SRs/MAs in SCI journals was more complete overall than in non-SCI journals, especially for items 4 ("objective"), 5 ("protocol and registration"), 7 ("information sources"), 8 ("search"), 9 ("study selection"), 11 ("data items"), 23 ("additional analysis"), and 27 ("funding") ($P<0.001$).

Discussion

Over the last decade, numerous studies have assessed the quality of reporting in SRs/MAs by their compliance with assessment instruments such as the QUOROM and PRISMA statements [9–12]. These studies focused predominantly on SRs/MAs covering diagnostic research and critical care. Although some quality assessment studies have looked at acupuncture SRs/MAs [13–15], they have focused mainly on methodological diversity in database searching, risk of bias, and heterogeneity in search strategies among CDSR. Our study compared reporting quality and PRISMA compliance in acupuncture SRs/MAs between different journal types.

We found that the five PRISMA items, namely "Protocol and registration", "Risk of bias across studies" (both in the methods and results), and "Additional analyses" (both in the methods and results) in the methods and results, are not frequently reported, indicating that the overall quality of reporting in acupuncture SRs/MAs is far from adequate. Compared with SRs/MAs published in CDSR, those in Chinese and international journals were of inferior reporting quality. One possible explanation for the limited compliance may be that journals have failed to incorporate the PRISMA statement into their instructions to authors about submitting SRs/MAs [16]. We also found that SR/MA reporting was more complete in SCI journals than in non-SCI journals but that both require improvement in adherence to PRISMA standards.

Several studies have focused on the reporting quality of SRs/MAs covering the fields of TCM [17,18], physical therapy [19], orthopaedics [20], and oral implantology [21] field, which showed that the reporting quality was indeed poor. Although differences exist between these results and those we repot here, the reporting of major items in the PRISMA statement was similar to what we found in our present study. Additional, Fleming PS et al. [22] found that the quality of reporting was considerably better in reviews published in CDSR ($P<0.001$) than in non-CDSR.

Both the QUOROM and PRISMA statements encourage the use of specific terms in the titles of SRs/MAs, which help to identify these studies. Because of the special title format requirements of the CDSR, however, SRs/MAs published in this database cannot conform to the QUOROM/PRISMA recommendation.

Unequivocal descriptions of the scientific background and rationale for using acupuncture in the treatment of both western diseases and TCM syndromes provide the reader with a better understanding of the research context and rationale of SRs/MAs. In this respect, SRs/MAs in the CDSR were more explicit in their descriptions than those in international or Chinese journals.

The importance of protocol consistency and registration of SRs/MAs to the transparency of reporting is underscored by the fact that they are considered key aspects of the "reporting guidelines for systematic review protocols" in the international prospective register of systematic reviews (PROSPERO) [23,24]. We found that only SRs/MAs published in the CDSR provided protocol and registration details.

The PRISMA standards suggest that methodological details such as eligibility criteria, information sources, search strategies, study selection criteria, and data collection processes are necessary to judge the quality and accuracy of SRs/MAs. The majority of the SRs/MAs published in the CDSR adequately reported these items, whereas those published in Chinese and international journals did not. Eligibility criteria are an aspect of the PICOS criteria (participants, interventions, comparisons, outcomes, and study design) central to the PRISMA approach. We propose that it is equally important that search strategies be uniformly reported. Many international journals require information about search strategies in at least one database, and the flexibility of the CDSR layout allows reporting of search strategies for multiple databases. Chinese journals, however, rarely request search strategy information. There is also considerable need for more consistency in the databases obtain acupuncture studies. We propose that, AcuBriefs (www.acubriefs.com), AcuBase (www.acubase.fr), Acudoc2 RCT (www.acubriefs.com/), and the TCM database are the most systematic and comprehensive sources for acupuncture information. Chinese RCTs make up the highest proportion of primary studies included in acupuncture SRs/MAs. If methods for sequence generation, allocation concealment, and study blindness are not adequately described, low-quality studies [25] may mislead reviewers.

Table 2. Reporting of checklists for PRISMA statement.

Category		Item	Total n = 476	Chinese journals n = 203	International journals n = 227	CDSRs n = 46	*P* value
Title	1	Title	390(90.70%)[@]	188(92.61%)	202(88.99%)*	NA	NA
Abstract	2	Structured summary	446(93.70%)	199(98.03%)	201(88.55%)*	46(100.00%)[#]	0.000
Introduction	3	Rationale	380(79.83%)	152(74.88%)	182(80.18%)	46(100.00%)*[#]	0.001
	4	Objective	430(90.34%)	160(78.82%)	225(99.12%)*	45(97.83%)*	0.000
Methods	5	Protocol and registration	60(12.61%)	0(0.00%)	18(7.93%)	42(91.30%)*[#]	0.000
	6	Eligibility criteria	463(97.27%)	196(96.55%)	222(97.80%)	45(97.83%)	0.710
	7	Information sources	440(92.44%)	169(83.25%)	225(99.12%)*	46(100.00%)	0.000
	8	Search	282(59.24%)	87(42.86%)	156(68.72%)*	39(84.78%)	0.000
	9	Study selection	342(71.85%)	116(57.14%)	182(80.18%)*	44(95.65%)*	0.000
	10	Data collection process	411(86.34%)	159(78.33%)	207(91.19%)*	45(97.83%)	0.000
	11	Data items	270(56.72%)	59(29.06%)	170(74.89%)*	41(89.13%)*	0.000
	12	Risk of bias in individual studies	384(80.67%)	159(78.33%)	182(80.18%)	43(93.48%)	0.061
	13	Summary measures	387(81.30%)	182(89.66%)	164(72.25%)*	41(89.13%)	0.000
	14	Synthesis of results	402(84.45%)	191(94.09%)	167(73.57%)*	44(95.65%)[#]	0.000
	15	Risk of bias across studies	155(32.56%)	82(40.39%)	50(22.03%)*	23(50.00%)*[#]	0.000
	16	Additional analyses	191(40.13%)	77(37.93%)	76(33.48%)	38(82.61%)*[#]	0.000
Results	17	Study selection	430(90.34%)	188(92.61%)	197(86.78%)	45(97.83%)	0.024
	18	Study characteristics	431(90.55%)	176(86.70%)	209(92.07%)	46(100.00%)*[#]	0.012
	19	Risk of bias within studies	387(81.30%)	155(76.35%)	189(83.26%)	43(93.48%)*	0.016
	20	Results of individual studies	411(86.34%)	196(96.55%)	172(75.77%)*	43(93.48%)[#]	0.000
	21	Synthesis of results	389(81.72%)	192(94.58%)	156(68.72%)*	41(89.13%)[#]	0.000
	22	Risk of bias across studies	176(36.97%)	91(44.83%)	66(29.07%)*	19(41.30%)	0.003
	23	Additional analysis	165(34.66%)	49(24.14%)	75(33.04%)	41(89.13%)*[#]	0.000
Discussion	24	Summary of evidence	432(90.76%)	170(83.74%)	216(95.15%)*	46(100.00%)*	0.000
	25	Limitations	455(95.59%)	188(92.61%)	222(97.80%)	45(97.83%)	0.024
	26	Conclusions	464(97.48%)	193(95.07%)	226(99.56%)*	45(97.83%)	0.012
Funding	27	Funding	324(68.07%)	104(51.23%)	179(78.85%)*	41(89.13%)*	0.000

[@]n = 430;
* #: there were statistical differences compared with Chinese journals and international journals, respectively.

Table 3. The comparison for Reporting of checklists for SRs/MAs on PRISMA statement.

Category	Item		≦2009 year n = 186	>2009 year n = 290	*P* value	SCI n = 204	Non-SCI n = 272	*P* value
Title	1	Title	143(84.62%[$])	247(95.00%[#])*	0.022	145(92.36%[&])	245(90.07%)*	0.000
Abstract	2	Structured summary	171(91.94%)	275(94.83%)	0.205	188(92.16%)	258(94.85%)	0.231
Introduction	3	Rationale	113(60.75%)	268(92.41%)*	0.000	172(84.31%)	208(76.47%)*	0.035
	4	Objective	185(99.46%)	246(84.83%)*	0.000	201(98.53%)	229(84.19%)*	0.000
Methods	5	Protocol and registration	24(12.90%)	36(12.41%)	0.875	56(27.45%)	4(1.47%)*	0.000
	6	Eligibility criteria	184(98.92%)	279(96.54%)	0.076	199(97.55%)	265(97.43%)	0.933
	7	Information sources	179(96.24%)	261(90.00%)*	0.012	202(99.02%)	238(87.50%)*	0.000
	8	Search	110(59.14%)	172(59.31%)	0.971	160(78.43%)	122(44.85%)*	0.000
	9	Study selection	124(66.67%)	224(75.68%)*	0.011	173(84.80%)	169(62.13%)*	0.000
	10	Data collection process	165(88.71%)	245(84.48%)	0.193	187(91.67%)	224(82.35%)*	0.003
	11	Data items	98(52.69%)	171(58.97%)	0.178	153(75.00%)	117(43.01%)*	0.000
	12	Risk of bias in individual studies	143(76.88%)	240(82.76%)	0.115	172(84.31%)	212(77.94%)	0.081
	13	Summary measures	141(75.81%)	246(84.83%)*	0.014	160(78.43%)	227(83.46%)	0.164
	14	Synthesis of results	147(79.03%)	255(87.93%)*	0.009	162(79.41%)	240(88.24%)*	0.009
	15	Risk of bias across studies	39(20.97%)	118(40.69%)*	0.000	66(32.35%)	90(33.09%)	0.866
	16	Additional analyses	66(35.48%)	125(43.10%)	0.098	97(47.55%)	95(34.93%)*	0.005
Results	17	Study selection	162(87.10%)	268(92.41%)	0.055	183(89.71%)	247(90.81%)	0.687
	18	Study characteristics	165(88.71%)	266(91.72%)	0.273	193(94.61%)	238(87.50%)*	0.009
	19	Risk of bias within studies	140(75.27%)	247(85.17%)*	0.007	176(86.27%)	212(77.94%)*	0.020
	20	Results of individual studies	139(74.73%)	272(93.79%)*	0.000	169(82.84%)	242(88.97%)	0.054
	21	Synthesis of results	134(72.04%)	255(87.93%)*	0.000	154(75.49%)	235(86.40%)*	0.002
	22	Risk of bias across studies	49(26.34%)	129(44.48%)*	0.000	69(33.82%)	108(39.71%)	0.189
	23	Additional analysis	57(30.65%)	107(36.90%)	0.161	94(46.08%)	71(26.10%)*	0.000
Discussion	24	Summary of evidence	182(97.85%)	249(85.86%)*	0.000	193(94.61%)	239(87.87%)*	0.012
	25	Limitations	183(98.39%)	272(93.79%)*	0.017	198(97.06%)	257(94.49%)	0.176
	26	Conclusions	185(99.46%)	279(96.21%)*	0.033	202(99.02%)	262 (96.32%)	0.063
Funding	27	Funding	129(69.35%)	200(68.97%)	0.929	170(83.33%)	154(56.62%)*	0.000

[$]n = 169,
[#]n = 260,
[&]n = 157.
*: there were statistical differences compared with non-SCI journals/>2009 y and SCI journals/2009 y, respectively.

We found that there is also considerable inconsistency in reporting of study selection criteria. For example, many primary studies on acupuncture report a random allocation design but are not specific enough for the reader to determine if they are actual RCTs. We propose that these uncertainties should be clarified by contacting the primary authors to determine the appropriateness of including the studies in the SRs/MAs. Because it has been suggested that only 6.8% of acupuncture efficacy studies published in Chinese journals are based on actual RCTs [25], we strongly propose that authors of SRs/MAs verify this information prior to inclusion of studies.

Acupuncture is considered an alternative or complementary treatment to western medical interventions such as drugs and surgery, and it can be considered a separate specialty. Thus, SRs/MAs on acupuncture require not only compliance with general PRISMA reporting standards but also accurate reporting of acupuncture information. As a result, it is necessary to develop an extension of the PRISMA statement for acupuncture.

There are several limitations to our study. First, our analyses were limited to acupuncture-specific SRs/MAs and therefore may not be applicable to SRs/MAs in other fields. Second, our assessment process was not blinded, and therefore the outcomes may be influenced by publication date and other factors. Third, our assessment criteria (yes or no) did not allow partial information to be used. Fourth, our study focused primarily on acupuncture rather than other TCM. We failed to distinguish acupuncture from herbal medicine massage, or western medicine because individual SRs/MAs we included in our analysis often contained several control groups rather than one group.

In summary, SRs/MAs of acupuncture studies have not comprehensively reported the information recommended in the PRISMA statement. Our study underscores that, in addition to focusing on careful study design and performance, attention should be paid to comprehensive reporting standards when publishing SRs/MAs of acupuncture studies.

Supporting Information

Checklist S1 PRISMA Checklist.
(DOC)

Text S1 The English and Chinese databases search strategy.
(DOC)

Text S2 Inclusion Exclusion Section.
(DOC)

Text S3 Definitions of reporting items.
(DOC)

Text S4 476 SRs/MAs of acupuncture.
(DOC)

Acknowledgments

We thank Yongteng Xu, Xianxia Yan, Shengping Yang, Xin Tian, Yannan Zhou,Yiming Lu, Qingshan Guo (Lanzhou University) for previous work that contributed to the development in this study. We thank BiomEditor for providing assistance with final revision of the manuscript.

Author Contributions

Conceived and designed the experiments: YLL KHY. Performed the experiments: RZ JH XZ DLL WTS PZ HC. Analyzed the data: YFM JH. Contributed reagents/materials/analysis tools: YJW. Wrote the paper: YLL RZ.

References

1. Oxman AD, Cook DJ, Guyatt GH (1994) Users' guides to the medical literature. VI. How to use an overview. 238 Evidence-Based Medicine Working Group. JAMA 272:1367–1371.
2. Swingler GH, Volmink J, Ioannidis JP (2003) Number of published systematic 239 reviews and global burden of disease: database analysis. BMJ 327:1083–1084.
3. Moher D, Liberati A, Tetzlaff J, Altman DG, PRISMA Group (2009) Preferred reporting items for systematic reviews and meta-analyses: the PRISMA statement. BMJ 339: b2535.
4. Sacks HS, Berrier J, Reitman D, Ancona-Berk VA, Chalmers TC (1987) Meta-analysis of randomized controlled trials. New Engl J Med 316: 450–455.
5. Moher D, Tetzlaff J, Tricco AC, Sampson M, Altman DG (2007) Epidemiology and reporting characteristics of systematic reviews. PLoS Med 4:e78. [PMID: 17388659].
6. Kelly KD, Travers A, Dorgan M, Slater L, Rowe BH (2001) Evaluating the quality of systematic reviews in the emergency medicine literature. Ann Emerg Med 38:518–526.
7. Richards D (2004) The quality of systematic reviews in dentistry. Evid Based Dent 5:17.
8. Delaney A, Bagshaw SM, Ferland A, Manns B, Laupland KB, Doig CJ (2005) A systematic evaluation of the quality of meta-analyses in the critical care literature. Crit Care 9:R575–582.
9. Willis BH, Quigley M (2011) The assessment of the quality of reporting of meta-analyses in diagnostic research: a systematic review. BMC Med Res Methodol 11:163.
10. Delaney A, Bagshaw SM, Ferland A, Manns B, Laupland KB, Doig CJ (2005) A systematic evaluation of the quality of meta-analyses in the critical care literature. Crit Care 5:R575–82. [PMID: 16277721].
11. Moher D, Cook DJ, Eastwood S, Olkin I, Rennie D, et al (1999) Improving the quality of reports of meta-analyses of randomised controlled trials: the QUOROM statement. Quality of Reporting of Meta-analyses. Lancet 354: 1896–1900.
12. Delaney A, Bagshaw SM, Ferland A, Manns B, Laupland KB, et al (2005) A systematic evaluation of the quality of meta-analyses in the critical care literature. Crit Care 9: 575–582.
13. Sood A, Sood R, Bauer BA, Ebbert JO (2005) Cochrane systematic reviews in acupuncture: methodological diversity in database searching. J Altern Complement Med 11(4):719–722.
14. Liu Y, Yang S, Dai J, Xu Y, Zhang R, Jiang H, Yan X, Yang K (2011) Risk of Bias Tool in Systematic Reviews/Meta-Analyses of Acupuncture in Chinese Journals. PLoS One 6(12):e28130.
15. Lui S, Smith EJ, Terplan M (2010) Heterogeneity in search strategies among Cochrane acupuncture reviews: is there room for improvement? Acupunct Med 28(3):149–153.
16. Tao KM, Li XQ, Zhou QH, Moher D, Ling CQ, Yu WF (2011) From QUOROM to PRISMA: A Survey of High-Impact Medical Journals' Instructions to Authors and a Review of Systematic Reviews in Anesthesia. PLoS One 6(11):e27611.
17. Ma B, Guo JW, Qi GQ, , Li H, Peng J, Zhang Y, et al. (2011) Epidemiology, Quality and Reporting Characteristics of Systematic Reviews of Traditional Chinese Medicine Interventions Published in Chinese Journals. Plos One 6(5):e20185.
18. Ma B, Qi GQ, Lin XT, Wang T, Chen ZM, Yang KH (2012) Epidemiology, quality, and reporting characteristics of systematic reviews of acupuncture interventions published in Chinese journals[J]. J Altern Complement Med 18(9): 813–817.
19. Padula RS, Pires RS, Alouche SR, Chiavegato LD, Lopes AD, Costa LO (2012) Analysis of reporting of systematic reviews in physical therapy published in Portuguese. Rev Bras Fisioter 16(4):381–8.
20. Gagnier JJ, Kellam PJ (2013) Reporting and methodological quality of systematic reviews in the orthopaedic literature. J Bone Joint Surg Am 5, 95(11):e771–7.
21. Kiriakou J, Pandis N, Fleming PS, Madianos P, Polychronopoulou A (2013). Reporting quality of systematic review abstracts in leading oral implantology journals. J Dent 41(12):1181–7.
22. Fleming PS, Seehra J, Polychronopoulou A, Fedorowicz Z, Pandis N (2013) A PRISMA assessment of the reporting quality of systematic reviews in orthodontics. Angle Orthod 83(1): 158–163.
23. PROSPERO. international prospective register of systematic reviews. Available. http://www.crd.york.ac.uk/prospero/.
24. Moher D, Shamseer L, Clarke M, et al (2011) Reporting 270 Guidelines for Systematic Review Protocols. The19 Cochrane Colloquium.
25. Wu T, Li Y, Bian Z, et al (2009) Randomized trials published in some Chinese journals: how many are randomized?. Trials 10(1): 46.

19

Systems Pharmacology Dissection of Multi-Scale Mechanisms of Action for Herbal Medicines in Stroke Treatment and Prevention

Jingxiao Zhang[1], Yan Li[1]*, Xuetong Chen[2,3], Yanqiu Pan[1], Shuwei Zhang[1], Yonghua Wang[2,3]*

1 Key laboratory of Industrial Ecology and Environmental Engineering (MOE), Faculty of Chemical, Environmental and Biological Science and Technology, Dalian University of Technology, Dalian, Liaoning, China, **2** College of Life Sciences, Northwest A & F University, Yangling, Shaanxi, China, **3** Center of Bioinformatics, Northwest A & F University, Yangling, Shaanxi, China

Abstract

Annually, tens of millions of first-ever strokes occur in the world; however, currently there is lack of effective and widely applicable pharmacological treatments for stroke patients. Herbal medicines, characterized as multi-constituent, multi-target and multi-effect, have been acknowledged with conspicuous effects in treating stroke, and attract extensive interest of researchers although the mechanism of action is yet unclear. In this work, we introduce an innovative systems-pharmacology method that combines pharmacokinetic prescreening, target fishing and network analysis to decipher the mechanisms of action of 10 herbal medicines like *Salvia miltiorrhizae*, *Ginkgo biloba* and *Ephedrae herba* which are efficient in stroke treatment and prevention. Our systematic analysis results display that, in these anti-stroke herbal medicines, 168 out of 1285 constituents with the favorable pharmacokinetic profiles might be implicated in stroke therapy, and the systematic use of these compounds probably acts through multiple mechanisms to synergistically benefit patients with stroke, which can roughly be classified as preventing ischemic inflammatory response, scavenging free radicals and inhibiting neuronal apoptosis against ischemic cerebral damage, as well as exhibiting lipid-lowering, anti-diabetic, anti-thrombotic and antiplatelet effects to decrease recurrent strokes. Relying on systems biology-based analysis, we speculate that herbal medicines, being characterized as the classical combination therapies, might be not only engaged in multiple mechanisms of action to synergistically improve the stroke outcomes, but also might be participated in reducing the risk factors for recurrent strokes.

Editor: Robert Lafrenie, Sudbury Regional Hospital, Canada

Funding: The research is financially supported by the National Natural Science Foundation of China (Grant No. 11201049, 31170796 and 81373892). The funders had no role in study design, data collection and analysis, decision to publish, or preparation of the manuscript.

Competing Interests: The authors have declared that no competing interests exist.

* Email: yanli@dlut.edu.cn (YL); yh_wang@nwsuaf.edu.cn (YHW)

Introduction

Stroke is the second leading cause of death and the main cause of long-term disability in the world population. Annually, approximately 16 million first-ever strokes occur in the world, which results in nearly 6.2 million deaths [1]. And medication treatments both for acute stroke treatment and stroke prevention have changed over the years. Specifically, pharmacological treatments that are for the purposes of lysing clots and reestablishing blood flow, as well as those remedies that suppress apoptosis cascades after hypoxia-ischemia, inhibit ischemic inflammatory responses, prohibit excitatory neurotransmission or scavenge free radicals have all shown promising therapeutic potentials against stroke in animal models [2]. Meanwhile, preventive measures that aimed at controlling hypertension, atherosclerosis, hyperlipidemia, hyperglycemia, and other high risk factors can effectively reduce the incidence of stroke, as well as prevent recurrent stroke [3].

Researches show that cerebral ischemia can trigger an intricate series of biochemical and molecular mechanisms to impair the neurologic functions [4]; therefore, comparing with monotherapy, combination therapies have been identified as more promising strategies to improve stroke management [5]. Factually, more and more preclinical observations manifest that combining neuroprotective therapy with thrombolytic drugs is optimal, and this combination not only decreases reperfusion damage, but also inhibits downstream cascades of cell death [6]. And numerous combination therapies producing synergistic or additive effects have been reported when thrombolysis was used in conjunction with neuroprotective agents including anti-oxidants [7], MMP inhibitors [8], anti-thrombotic agents [9]. Additionally, considering the fact that various pathways implicated in cell death are triggered by cerebral ischemic, effective neuroprotective therapy might also require the combination of drugs in series which disturb distinct pathways during the evolution of ischemic damage [6]. Similarly, for stroke prevention, research shows that a combination strategy might reduce recurrent vascular events by 80% in patients with cerebrovascular disease [7]. Besides, the combinative therapy might reduce dosages for each agent, thereby decreasing the occurrence of adverse effects. However, in spite of these therapeutic benefits, effective and widely applicable medication treatments for stroke patients are still scarce.

Herbal medicines always contain combinations of bioactive ingredients which provide the synergistic effects, and thus have attracted more attentions in recent years. Fortunately, a large number of herbs have been widely used against cerebral stroke including *Salvia miltiorrhizae*, *Ginkgo biloba*, *Ephedrae herba*, *Erigeron breviscapus*, and so forth. Pharmacological studies have suggested that these herbal medicines or their corresponding products might dilate cardiocerebral vessels, suppress platelet aggregation, improve microcirculation in brain, protect against ischemic and reperfusion injury, possess neuroprotective properties or enhance the tolerance of ischemic tissue to hypoxia [10,11]. However, unlike conventional pharmacological drugs used in western medicine, bioactive ingredients of medicinal herbs often have not been specified and measured, although there have been some attempts to standardize these medicines by some governments. Meanwhile, the multiple components, targets and pathways involved in herbal medicines also complicate the pharmacological research.

Being an emerging area of pharmacology, systems pharmacology combines pharmacokinetic (the absorption, distribution, metabolism, excretion and toxicity properties of drugs) and pharmacodynamics models, as well as pathway and network analyses, to systematically analyze drugs, drug targets and effects [12], which provides a platform for identifying multi-scale mechanisms of action of herbal medicines. Among them, the study of pharmacokinetic characteristics of herbal medicines might help us to understand the molecular mechanisms of herbal active compounds. Considering the complexity of multiple constituents and targets involved in the therapeutic properties of herbal medicines, analyzing botanical herbs in the context of biological pathways and networks can facilitate a better understanding of multiple mechanisms of action of herbal medicines. In previous work, we have constructed a systems-pharmacology-based method which is specially designed for herbal medicines in drug discovery and in deciphering the therapeutic mechanisms. Combining with pharmacokinetics, pharmacology and network analyses, this method is devoted to evaluate the therapeutic effectiveness of herbs through identifying their active constituents and possible targets, and has been successfully used in dissecting the therapeutic mechanisms of herbal medicine in treatment of cardiovascular diseases [13] and influenza [14].

In this text, a modified systems-pharmacology method is employed to dissect the multiscale mechanisms of action of herbal medicine for improving stroke management, including providing pharmacological effects against cerebral stroke and offering preventive measures to reduce the primary and secondary stroke. Specifically, we firstly explored anti-stroke herbs and their corresponding constituents with a wide-scale text mining method. Then, based on the pharmacokinetic principles of drugs, we employed six ADME profiles (including aqueous solubility, lipophilicity, drug-likeness, oral bioavailability, Caco-2 permeability and blood-brain barrier (BBB)) to filter active ingredients with favorable pharmacokinetic properties from these anti-stroke herbs. Subsequently, target proteins of these active compounds were identified and validated through a systematic approach which effectively integrated abundant biological and pharmacological methods. Finally, based on pharmacology and network analyses, we interpreted the multi-scale mechanisms of action of herbs in stroke prevention and management.

Materials and Methods

Constructing herbs and ingredients database for stroke

We conducted a robust wide-scale text mining of PubMed and the clinical trial database (www.clinicaltrials.gov), and extracted the available anti-stroke herbs manually using the 'herbal medicine' and 'stroke' as search terms. Owning to diverse herbs with different research extents, P-value (as displayed in Eq.1) which had been described in our previous work [15] was employed to equilibrate this bias and further appraise the chance probability of co-occurrence of each herb and stroke [16].

$$P = 1 - \sum_{i=0}^{k-1} f(i) = 1 - \sum_{i=0}^{k-1} \frac{\binom{K}{i}\binom{N-K}{n-i}}{\binom{N}{n}} \quad (1)$$

where N represents the total number of papers in PubMed (22.8 million articles, until July 25th, 2013), K is the number of articles linked with stroke in PubMed (185,188 papers), n shows the number of articles of one herbal medicine, and k displays the number of articles about the effects of corresponding herb on stroke. Here, when P-value is less than 0.01, this herbal medicine is regarded as having significant correlation with stroke.

Subsequently, all constituents of these anti-stroke herbs were extracted from our own Traditional Chinese Medicine System Pharmacology Database and Analysis Platform (TCMSP, http://tcmspnw.com). Considering the fact that glycosides could be hydrolyzed to their aglycone forms before being absorbed, in this section, their corresponding aglycones were also added to the database for further research.

ADME screening

According to the pharmacokinetic models constructed in drug design, ADME properties can be roughly classified into two categories: "physicochemical" and "physiological" groups. The physicochemical ADME features like aqueous solubility (S) and lipophilicity are ruled by simple physical and chemical laws, while the physiological properties including *in vivo* pharmacokinetic properties (like Caco-2 permeability, et al) and *in vitro* ADME features (such as oral bioavailability (OB), etc.) are regulated by several physiological elements [17]. In this text, for filtering active compounds with favorable pharmacokinetic properties, six *in silico* physicochemical or physiological predictive profiles were considered, which consist of aqueous solubility (log$S$, the logarithm of aqueous solubility), lipophilicity (log$P$, logarithm of octanol-water partition coefficient), drug-likeness (DL), oral bioavailability, Caco-2 permeability and BBB penetration.

Aqueous solubility. Being one of the chief physicochemical properties to be optimized in drug discovery, aqueous solubility has been considered as an important factor in drug absorption and distribution. And one drug with adequate aqueous solubility is considered exempt from bioavailability problems [18]. Here, for filtering compounds with suitable aqueous solubilities from herbs, we calculated the log$S$ of each molecule using the ALOGPS 2.1 program [19]. This model was developed with 1291 molecules using ANN methodology and electrotopological state descriptors, resulting in an optimal predictive model with determination coefficient (R^2) = 0.91 and root mean squared error (RMS) = 0.62. Considering the fact that most drugs reveal a compromise between the polarities required for reasonable aqueous solubility and the hydrophobicities needed for satisfactory membrane passage [20], we set the threshold of log$S$ in the range of -5 to -1.

Lipophilicity. Molecular lipophilicity, another basic physicochemical property, plays an essential role in determining ADME properties and the overall suitability of drug candidates, hence controlling molecular lipophilic property within an optimal range can improve compound quality and the likelihood of therapeutic success [21]. In this text, molecular lipophilicity (expressed as a value of log*P*) was also predicted by ALOGPS 2.1 program, which developed the predictive model of lipophilicity on the basis of 64 neural networks, 12,908 compounds with experimental log*P* values from PHYSPROP database and 75 input parameters, providing an optimal model with $RMS = 0.49$ and standard mean error = 0.26 [22]. On the basis of Lipinski's rule of five, the compounds with log*P* less than 5 were selected for further analysis.

Drug-likeness. For the reason that medicinal properties of herbs depend on the presence of active constituents with drug-likeness features, in this study, we employed a robust self-constructed model preDruglike as described in our previous work [23] to calculate the drug-likeness index of each compound in herbs. This model is constructed based on the molecular descriptors and Tanimoto coefficient (as displayed in Eq.2).

$$T(A,B) = \frac{A \cdot B}{|A|^2 + |B|^2 - A \cdot B} \qquad (2)$$

where A shows the molecular properties of herbal ingredients, and B displays the average molecular properties of molecules in DrugBank database (http://www.drugbank.ca/) based on Dragon soft descriptors. Considering the fact that the average DL index for all 6511 molecules in DrugBank is 0.18, the molecule with suitable drug-likeness index (DL≥0.18) was chosen as candidate molecule for further research.

Oral bioavailability. Being an essential parameter in drug screening cascades, oral bioavailability was employed to determine the fraction of oral dose of compounds reaching systemic circulation in the TCM treatment. Here, a reliable *in silico* screening model OBioavail 1.1 constructed in our previous work [24] was engaged in OB value calculation of these herbal constituents. This model was constructed based on 805 structurally diverse drugs and drug-like molecules. Multiple linear regression, partial least square and support vector machine methods were employed during this model building, ending up with determination coefficient $(R^2) = 0.80$ and standard error of estimate $(SEE) = 0.31$ for test sets. Finally, the threshold of OB value is set to 30% by careful consideration of the following rules: 1) extracting information from the studied herbs should be as much as possible using the least number of molecules [13]; 2) the acquired model can be reasonably explicated by the existing pharmacological data [14].

Caco-2 permeability. For an orally administered drug, the majority of drug absorption occurs in the small intestine where the presence of villi and microvilli greatly increases the surface available for absorption [25]. A number of *in silico* drug absorption models using *in vitro* Caco-2 permeability have been widely established and used in drug discovery and development processes [26]. Here, we employed a robust *in silico* Caco-2 permeability prediction model preCaco2 [27] which was constructed by 100 drug molecules with satisfactory statistical results ($R^2 > 0.8$) to predict the drug absorption. Finally, we set the threshold of Caco-2 permeability to −0.4, for the reason that compound with Caco-2 value less than −0.4 is not permeable.

BBB penetration. Since blood-brain barrier is a protective fence between central nervous system (CNS) and systemic circulation to maintain the normal homeostasis of the CNS [28], predicting BBB permeability is regarded as an indispensible parameter in screening candidate compounds for stroke management. In this section, an updated and reliable BBB model preBBB which was constructed in our previous work [29] was employed to examine whether the constituents of herbal medicines pass through the BBB. The dataset of this model was composed of 190 related but chemically diverse compounds which are either penetrating or non-penetrating cross the BBB [23]. The statistical model was constructed by partial least squares discriminant analysis with two significant latent variables. In this model, compounds possessing BBB values greater than −0.3 were considered as penetrating, thus the threshold of BBB is set to −0.3.

Target fishing and validation

To identify molecular targets of these active ingredients, we proposed a systematic approach which effectively integrated data mining, chemogenomic, pharmacological and statistical methods. To be specific, first of all, information of target proteins for herbal ingredients was identified from Therapeutic Target Database (TTD, http://bidd.nus.edu.sg/group/ttd/) [30], DrugBank and HIT (Herbal Ingredients' Targets Database, http://lifecenter.sgst.cn/hit/) [31], and all compound-target interactions from these databases were known and supported by published literatures. Secondly, the efficient systemic analysis methods, including Similarity Ensemble Approach (SEA, http://sea.bkslab.org/) [32], information integration method (STITCH, http://stitch.embl.de/) [33] and omics-based Ligand-Target Chemogenomic model (LTC) [34], were implemented to predict the potential target proteins of herbal ingredients. Finally, for better defining the role of herbs in stroke prevention and treatment, TTD, PharmGKB (http://www.pharmgkb.org) [35] and Comparative Toxicogenomics Database (CTD, http://ctdbase.org/) were employed to eliminate the noise in the two previous steps, providing a more complete and greater accuracy view on compound-target associations.

For improving the reliability of predicted target results, molecular docking program was employed in this section using GOLD5.1 software, which utilizes an evolutionary genetic algorithm to optimize the docked pose of the ligand within the receptor [36]. 3D crystallographic structures of these targets were downloaded from the RCSB Protein Data Bank (http://www.pdb.org/) or constructed by the Swiss-Model Automated Mode Serve (http://swissmodel.expasy.org/) if the 3D structures were not obtainable. Prior to performing the docking process, crystallographic ligands were extracted and mixed into docking database for re-dock, and hydrogen atoms were added. The default genetic algorithm parameters were used and *GoldScore* scoring function was selected. Eventually, the predicted compound-target interactions with Gold dock scores greater than 40 were taken into account for further research.

Network construction

For further probing the multi-scale mechanisms of action of herbal medicines in stroke prevention and treatment, presently we constructed two kinds of networks: 1) Compound-Target network (C-T network). We used active compounds and their corresponding targets to generate a bipartite graph of compound-target interactions in which a compound and a target are linked with each other if the protein is a known or validated target of this compound, giving rise to the C-T network. 2) Target-Pathway network (T-P network). We firstly extracted the canonical pathways that were highly associated with stroke from KEGG database (http://www.genome.jp/kegg/), and then all target proteins attempted to be mapped onto these pathways, resulting in a target-pathway network. All these visualized networks were constructed by Cytoscape 2.8.1, an open source software project for biological network visualization and data integration [37].

Results and Discussion

Extensive experiences and abundant clinical data reveal that, comparing with conventional FDA-approved drugs, medicinal herbs, featured as multiple constituents, targets and actions, have been reported exhibiting notable benefits in preventing and treating stroke although the mechanism of action remains unclear, which makes the efforts for deciphering the pharmacological mechanism of herbal medicines even more imperative [10]. Meanwhile, it is worth noting that, during the decoding process, there are several valuable resources available for drug development, such as discovering bioactive molecules with therapeutic effects in stroke, designing multi-target drugs or combination drugs, as well as expanding the structural diversity of small molecules for stroke. In this study, based on the application of bioinformatics resources and methodologies, we present a systematic analysis framework which integrates active ingredients filtering, target identification and network construction to decode the mechanisms of action of herbal medicines in stroke management and prevention.

Anti-stroke herbs

Statistical results show that 10 herbs, as displayed in Table 1, are documented possessing significant correlations with stroke, like *S. miltiorrhiza*, *G. biloba*, *E. herba*, etc. Among them, *S. miltiorrhiza* obtains the optimal *P*-value (2.73E-16), indicating that anti-stroke may be one of the key therapeutic effects found so far for this herb. Factually, this herb has been documented exhibiting anti-atherosclerosis, anti-platelet aggregation, anti-oxidative and anti-inflammatory effects [38] which are all effective strategies in preventing and treating stroke. Analogously, *G. biloba* which possesses a favorable *P*-value (4.36E-15) has been widely used in treatment of acute ischemic stroke in China and occasionally in Europe [39].

Surprisingly, further research exhibits that these 10 herbal medicines or their corresponding herbal constituents are widely participated in Traditional Chinese Patent Medicine (TCPM) for treating stroke in China. For instance, Dan Shen agents [11] (consisted by the main components of *S. miltiorrhiza*) with eligible clinical trials are commonly used in treating ischemic stroke through dilating cerebral vessel, suppressing aggregation of platelets, refining blood circulation, removing blood stasis, as well as defending against ischemic reperfusion injury [40]. Notably, the same situation occurs in Deng Zhan Xi Xin infection (the extractive of *E. breviscapu*), *Ginkgo biloba* agents and Ligustrazine injection (the major constituent of *R. chuanxiong*). Additionally, herbs including *G. elata*, *R. chuanxiong*, *P. notoginseng* and et al. are frequently applied as the major ingredients of Chinese medicinal formulae, such as Xiaoshuan Tongluo and She Xiang Kang Shuang Tablets, to against ischemia stroke, as well as hemiplegia and aphasia after stroke.

After eliminating the overlapped compounds among herbs, a total of 1285 compounds (as displayed in Table S1 in Supporting Information S1) are finally extracted from these 10 medicinal herbs, including 1234 herbal constituents and 51 aglycones (the hydrolysis products of 97 glycosides). Among them, *G. biloba* is found having the largest numbers of chemical components (256 molecules), following by *E. herba* with 236 chemicals and *S. miltiorrhiza* having 206 compounds.

Screening active ingredients for anti-stroke

Before an orally administered drug exerting a pharmacological effect, this drug should hold satisfactory pharmacokinetic properties to overcome different barriers to reach its target. In this article, for screening the active pharmaceutical ingredients from these anti-stroke herbs, we introduced six ADME parameters: log*P*, log*S*, drug-likeness, Caco-2 cell permeability, oral bioavailability, blood-brain barrier permeability. As a result of these filters, 190 out of 1285 ingredients (as shown in Table S2 in Supporting Information S1) are demonstrated possessing satisfactory pharmacokinetic properties, among them, the representative compounds including their ADME parameters and structural information are displayed in Figures 1–4. Here, in order to illuminate clearly, three representative herbal medicines are specified in detail to interpret these filtering principles.

Uncaria rhynchophylla. In medicinal herb *U. rhynchophylla*, 41 out of 92 compounds are found meeting the screening criteria. Among them, plenty of indole alkaloids with satisfactory ADME properties have already been demonstrated exerting significant protective effects against several diseases. For example, the major constituents of this herb rhynchophylline ($\log P = 2.85$, $\log S = -3.66$, $DL = 0.57$, Caco-2 = 0.70, OB = 47.86% and BBB = 0.38) and isorhynchophylline ($\log P = 2.47$, $\log S = -3.36$, $DL = 0.52$, Caco-2 = 0.29, OB = 49.31% and BBB = −0.21) have been reported showing neuroprotective, vasodilatory and antiarrhythmia effects [41,42], thus becoming the candidate compounds for treating cardiovascular and central nervous system diseases.

Table 1. Statistics and association analysis between herbs and stroke.

Herb Name	*n*	*k*	*P*-value
Salvia miltiorrhizae (S. miltiorrhiza)	1716	55	2.73E-16
Ginkgo biloba (G. biloba)	2574	67	4.36E-15
Ephedrae herba (E. herba)	565	24	2.51E-10
Gastrodia elata (G. elata)	191	11	9.19E-07
Panax notoginseng (P. notoginseng)	581	19	9.45E-07
Erigeron breviscapus (E. breviscapu)	95	9	1.37E-07
Rhizoma chuanxiong (R. chuanxiong)	375	12	1.10E-04
Panax ginseng (P. ginseng)	3591	50	6.56E-04
Uncaria rhynchophylla (U. rhynchophylla)	102	6	2.48E-04
Scutellaria baicalensis (S. baicalensis)	848	15	6.89E-03

ID	Compound	Structure	OB (%)	Caco-2	DL	BBB	Log*P*	Log*S*	*Herb*
M_001	Vanillic acid	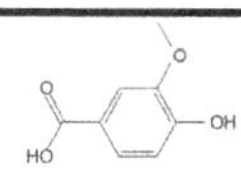	59.94	0.39	0.04	0.12	1.70	-1.47	*R. chuanxiong G. elata, G. biloba*
M_007	Ligustilide	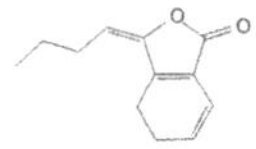	51.30	1.31	0.07	1.28	3.48	-2.58	*R. chuanxiong*
M_011	3 α - hydroxytanshinone IIa	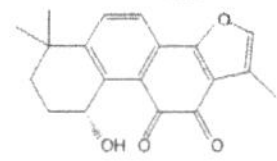	50.10	0.52	0.44	0.22	3.14	-3.97	*S. miltiorrhiza*
M_014	Salvianolic acid B	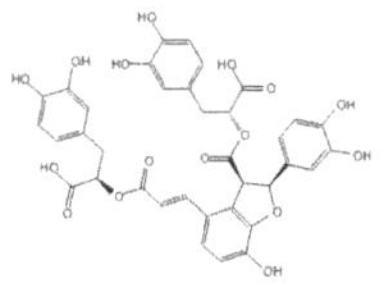	3.01	-1.68	0.41	-2.52	3.93	-4.51	*S. miltiorrhiza*
M_018	Cryptotanshinone	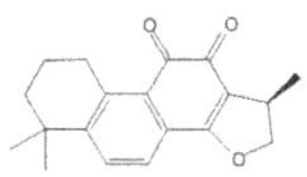	57.44	0.95	0.40	0.51	4.32	-4.48	*S. miltiorrhiza*
M_020	Isocryptotanshinone	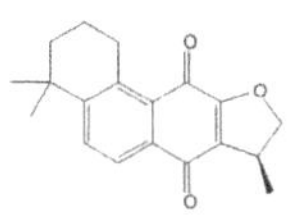	60.08	0.93	0.39	0.34	4.18	-4.42	*S. miltiorrhiza*
M_021	Isotanshinone IIb	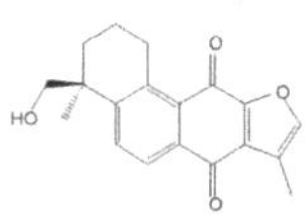	61.64	0.37	0.45	-0.33	3.10	-3.86	*S. miltiorrhiza*
M_022	Isotanshinone IIa	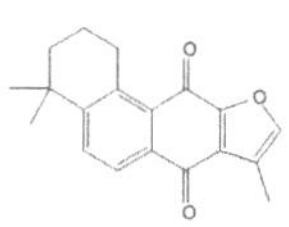	55.09	1.02	0.40	0.45	4.11	-4.34	*S. miltiorrhiza*
M_025	Salvianic acid A	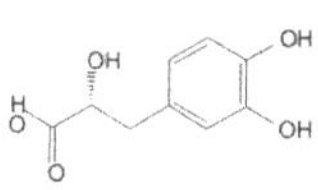	78.22	-0.27	0.06	-0.62	0.77	-1.47	*S. miltiorrhiza*
M_027	Tanshinone IIa	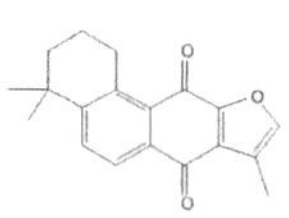	20.32	1.04	0.40	0.70	4.10	-4.45	*S. miltiorrhiza*
M_028	Tanshinone IIb	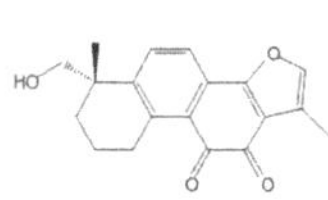	70.19	0.43	0.45	-0.30	3.31	-4.01	*S. miltiorrhiza*
M_029	Tanshinone I	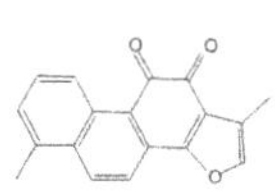	29.32	1.04	0.36	0.53	3.38	-4.38	*S. miltiorrhiza*
M_032	Caffeic acid	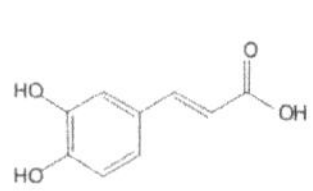	45.99	0.24	0.05	-0.13	1.67	-2.05	*S. miltiorrhiza, R. chuanxiong, G. biloba, E. breviscapu*
M_033	Ferulic acid	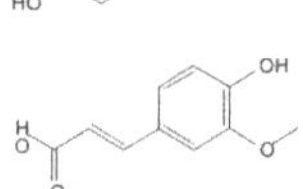	55.14	0.41	0.06	0.00	1.58	-2.33	*R. chuanxiong G. biloba, E. breviscapu*

Figure 1. Representative active constituents of anti-stroke herbs and their corresponding ADME parameters (Part 1).

Furthermore, isorhynchophylline also exhibits inhibitory effects on platelet aggregation and thrombosis, which mechanism may be at least partly due to the increase of intraplatelet cAMP generation [42,43]. It is noteworthy that two bioactive compounds kaempferol ($\log P = 1.23$, $\log S = -2.47$, DL = 0.24, Caco-2 = 0.28, OB = 42.30% and BBB = 0.02) and quercetin ($\log P = 1.07$, $\log S = -2.42$, DL = 0.28, Caco-2 = 0.03, OB = 42.24% and BBB = 0.00), being the common flavones existed in several herbs

ID	Compound	Structure	OB (%)	Caco-2	DL	BBB	Log*P*	Log*S*	*Herb*
M_034	Scutellarin*	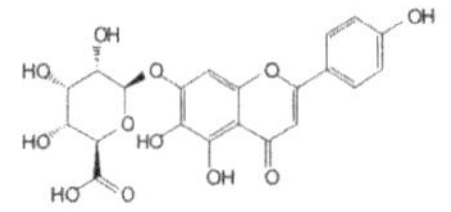	45.56	0.31	0.21	-0.36	2.22	-2.97	*E. breviscapu, S. baicalensis*
M_038	Naringenin	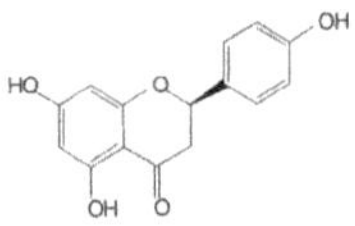	39.62	0.34	0.21	-0.21	2.47	-3.11	*E. breviscapu*
M_041	4'- hydroxybaicalein	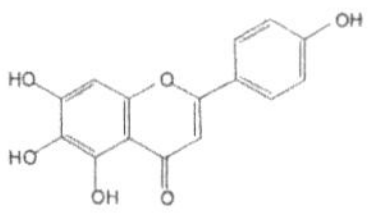	59.56	0.31	0.24	-0.43	2.22	-2.97	*E. breviscapu*
M_046	L-e picatechin	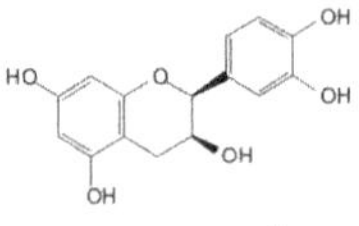	53.89	0.01	0.24	-0.65	1.02	-2.65	*U. rhynchophylla, G. biloba*
M_051	Rhynchophylline A	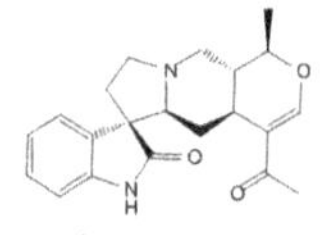	37.15	0.40	0.69	-0.15	2.29	-3.19	*U. rhynchophylla*
M_054	Rhynchophylline	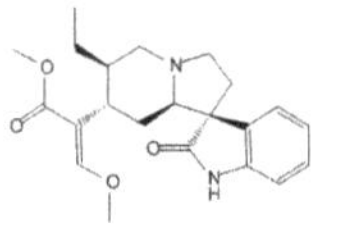	47.86	0.70	0.57	0.38	2.85	-3.66	*U. rhynchophylla*
M_059	Hirsuteine	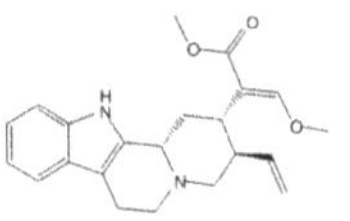	56.27	0.92	0.64	0.61	3.33	-4.04	*U. rhynchophylla*
M_060	Kaempferol	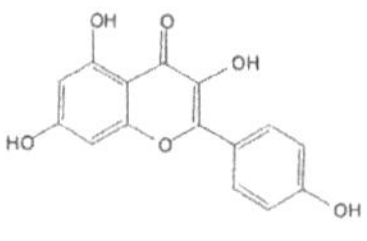	42.30	0.28	0.24	0.02	1.23	-2.47	*E. herba, E. breviscapu, U. rhynchophylla, G. biloba*
M_063	Isorhynchophylline	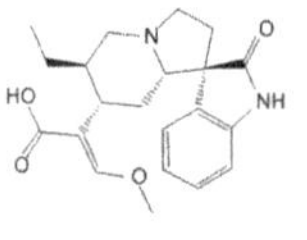	49.31	0.29	0.52	-0.21	2.47	-3.36	*U. rhynchophylla*
M_066	Quercetin	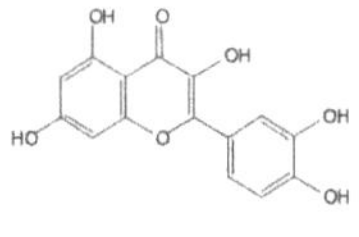	42.24	0.03	0.28	0.00	1.07	-2.42	*U. rhynchophylla, P. notoginseng, E. herba, E. breviscapu, G. biloba*
M_072	Ginsenoside CK	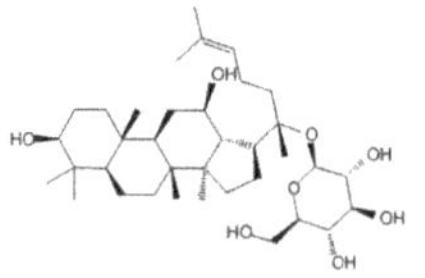	6.51	-3.39	0.04	-0.44	3.73	-4.62	*P. notoginseng*
M_076	Acacetin	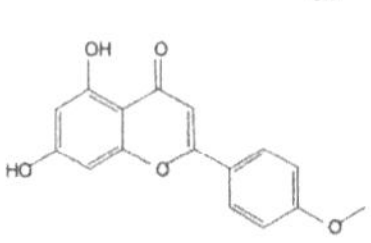	34.93	0.62	0.35	0.00	2.95	-3.51	*S. baicalensis*
M_078	Dihydrobaicalin*	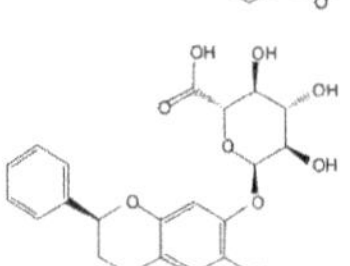	40.24	0.55	0.75	0.18	2.66	-2.98	*S. baicalensis*

Figure 2. Representative active constituents of anti-stroke herbs and their corresponding ADME parameters (Part 2). The sign * represents the molecule after deglycosylation.

ID	Compound	Structure	OB (%)	Caco-2	DL	BBB	Log*P*	Log*S*	*Herb*
M_089	Oroxylin A	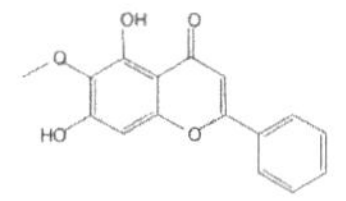	45.59	0.77	0.44	0.13	3.01	-3.34	*S. baicalensis*
M_091	Wogonin	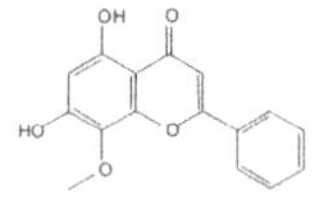	20.71	0.79	0.02	0.10	2.97	-3.36	*S. baicalensis*
M_092	Baicalein	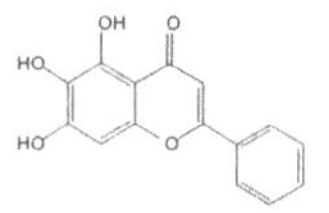	23.77	0.58	0.44	-0.05	2.66	-2.98	*S. baicalensis, E. breviscapu*
M_093	Baicalin	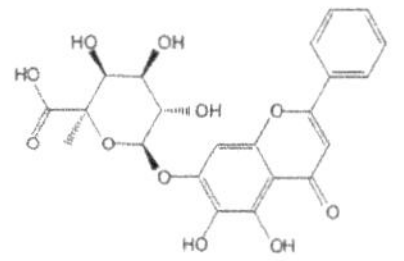	13.16	-1.05	0.23	-1.97	0.55	-2.23	*S. baicalensis, S. miltiorrhiza*
M_103	Ganhuangenin	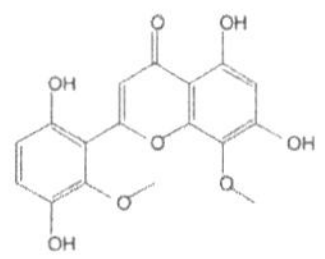	47.07	0.26	0.37	-0.39	2.19	-3.13	*S. baicalensis*
M_111	Skullcapflavone II	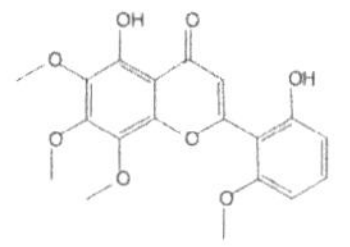	61.22	0.63	0.44	0.00	1.76	-3.45	*S. baicalensis*
M_119	Ephedrine	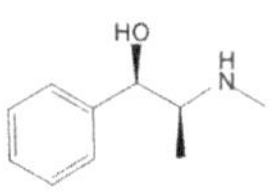	45.21	1.02	0.03	1.11	1.00	-1.30	*E. herba*
M_121	Ligustrazine	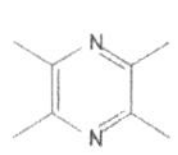	29.64	1.19	0.03	1.06	1.46	-0.96	*E. herba, R. chuanxiong*
M_124	Leucopelargonidin	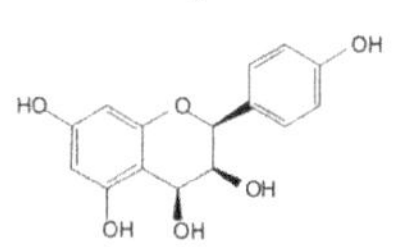	58.03	-0.14	0.24	-0.62	0.62	-2.20	*E. herba*
M_125	Herbacetin	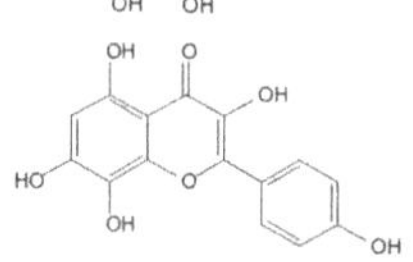	37.54	0.13	0.27	-0.74	1.08	-2.37	*E. herba*
M_133	Protopine	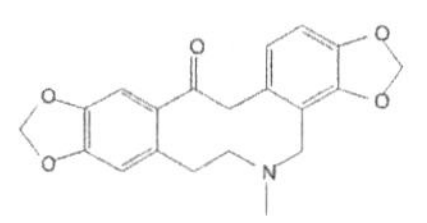	57.53	0.84	0.78	0.21	1.95	-3.24	*P. ginseng*
M_135	Beta-s antalol	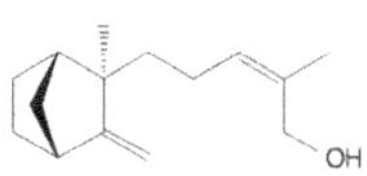	35.30	1.28	0.76	1.25	4.42	-3.91	*P. ginseng*
M_139	Ginsenoside Rd	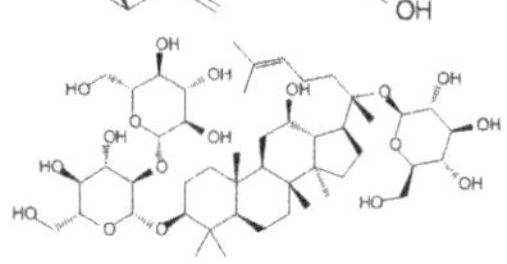	5.42	-2.88	0.09	-4.20	0.73	-3.39	*P. ginseng, P. notoginseng*
M_143	Glycyrrhizin	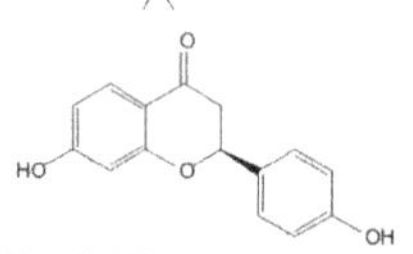	35.00	0.51	0.18	-0.22	2.79	-3.28	*P. notoginseng*

Figure 3. Representative active constituents of anti-stroke herbs and their corresponding ADME parameters (Part 3).

ID	Compound	Structure	OB (%)	Caco-2	DL	BBB	Log*P*	Log*S*	*Herb*
M_144	Protopanaxatriol	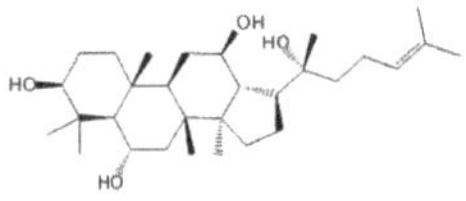	12.65	0.05	0.78	-0.65	4.21	-4.48	*P. notoginseng*
M_145	Protopanoxadiol	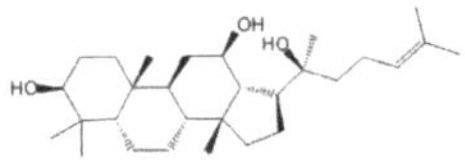	29.61	0.42	0.78	-0.29	4.74	-5.00	*P. notoginseng*
M_149	Cymbinodin A	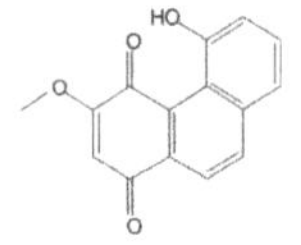	50.26	0.71	0.21	0.28	3.04	-3.70	*G. elata*
M_152	Diosmetin	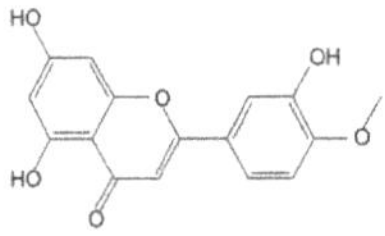	50.41	0.36	0.27	-0.50	2.52	-3.34	*G. biloba*
M_153	Epigallocatechin	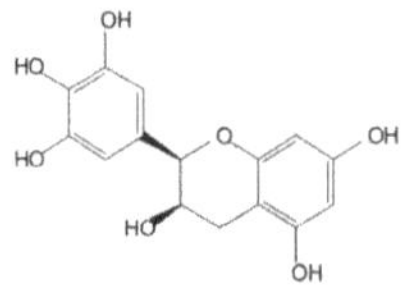	64.07	-0.22	0.27	-0.82	0.71	-2.55	*G. biloba*
M_155	Ginkgolide B	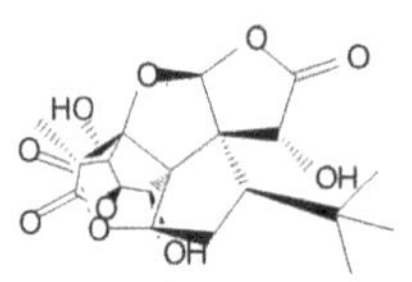	44.38	-1.22	0.73	-1.55	0.49	-1.91	*G. biloba*
M_157	Luteolin	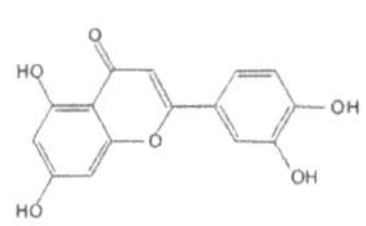	62.76	0.20	0.25	-0.75	2.15	-2.90	*G. biloba, S. miltiorrhiza, E. breviscapu*
M_160	Myricetin	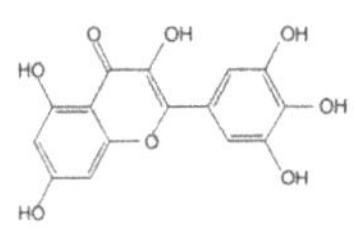	9.80	-0.25	0.31	-0.91	0.89	-2.43	*G. biloba*
M_161	Carthamidin	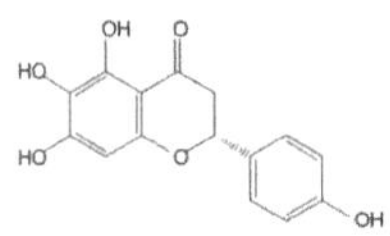	43.78	0.16	0.72	-0.42	2.22	-2.97	*S. baicalensis*
M_176	Rhynchophylline E	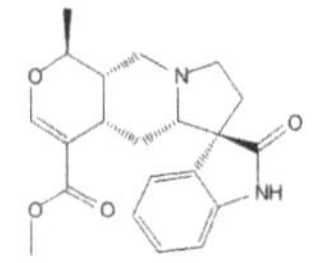	79.92	0.28	0.75	-0.24	2.31	-3.06	*U. rhynchophylla*
M_179	Angustoline	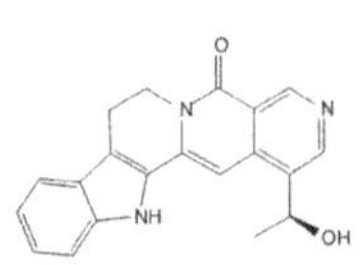	33.15	0.41	0.77	-0.31	1.84	-3.28	*U.rhynchophylla*
M_188	4- hydroxybenzyl alcohol	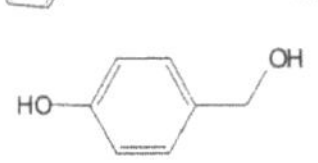	55.21	0.60	0.02	0.34	0.53	-0.32	*G. elata*
M_189	Isoferulic acid	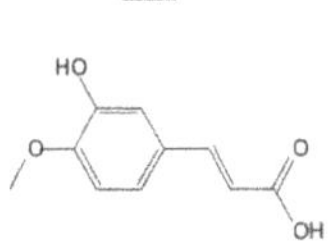	67.69	0.50	0.06	0.08	1.56	-2.35	*S. miltiorrhiza*

Figure 4. Representative active constituents of anti-stroke herbs and their corresponding ADME parameters (Part 4).

like *U. rhynchophylla* and *G. biloba*, also show satisfactory pharmacokinetic properties.

As we know, unlike allopathic western medicine, herbal medicine characterized as holistic treatment emphasizes on maintaining the integrity of human body. Factually, medicinal herb *U. rhynchophylla* not only acts on the central nervous system to produce anti-inflammation, anti-apoptosis and free radical scavenging activities [44], but also exhibits antiplatelet and anti-hypertensive effects on the cardiovascular system [45]. These phenomena prove that, as a typical holistic therapy, herb *U. rhynchophylla*, besides providing benefits in stroke treatment, shows preventive effects in primary and secondary stroke prevention. Therefore, compounds which have suitable pharmacokinetic properties but low BBB values are also considered as potential active compounds, such as L-epicatechin ($\log P = 1.02$, $\log S = -2.65$, DL = 0.24, Caco-2 = 0.01, OB = 53.89% and BBB = −0.65) and angustoline ($\log P = 1.84$, $\log S = -3.28$, DL = 0.77, Caco-2 = 0.41, OB = 33.15% and BBB = −0.31).

Scutellaria baicalensis. For herb *S. baicalensis*, 56 out of 111 constituents pass through the filtering criteria, and the majority of them (46 out of 56 active compounds) are flavonoids, such as oroxylin A ($\log P = 3.01$, $\log S = -3.34$, DL = 0.44, Caco-2 = 0.77, OB = 45.59% and BBB = 0.13) and acacetin ($\log P = 2.95$, $\log S = -3.51$, DL = 0.35, Caco-2 = 0.62, OB = 34.93% and BBB = 0.00). Surprisingly, most flavonoids in this herb have been proven to possess various biological activities. For instance, oroxylin A shows memory ameliorative activity in memory impaired mice [46], and also has neuroprotective effect against ischemic/reperfusion-induced brain damage [47]; acacetin exhibits anti-neuroinflammation effect through regulating the response to LPS stimuli *in vitro* and *in vivo*, and is also considered as a potential therapeutic agent for brain diseases [48].

Besides these, those constituents which have high contents in herb but low OB indexes such as baicalin (OB = 13.16%), baicalein (OB = 23.77%) and wogonin (OB = 20.71%) should attract our more attention. For example, baicalin obtains a poor OB index, however, the content of this flavone in *S. baicalensis* is extremely high (8.12% of dry root mass) [48], which significantly increase its absolute OB value. Actually, baicalin has been documented exhibiting powerful pharmacological activities, including protective effect against cerebrovascular dysfunction and inhibitory effect on brain inflammatory response [49]. Therefore, these bioactive ingredients with high contents in herb are also added into active ingredients database, although they have low OB values.

Salvia miltiorrhiza. After ADME prescreening, 35 constituents from *S. miltiorrhiza* have desirable physicochemical and physiological properties, including many documented bioactive compounds such as cryptotanshinone ($\log P = 4.32$, $\log S = -4.48$, DL = 0.40, Caco-2 = 0.95, OB = 57.44% and BBB = 0.51) and tanshinone IIb ($\log P = 3.31$, $\log S = -4.01$, DL = 0.45, Caco-2 = 0.43, OB = 70.19% and BBB = −0.30) which have been reported to show neuroprotective [50], antidiabete [51], anti-atherosclerosis [52] and anti-inflammatory [53] effects. Two bioactive compounds tanshinone IIa and tanshinone I as the major constituents of *S. miltiorrhiza* are also put into the active ingredient database due to their *in vitro* and *in vivo* biological activities [54]. One exception is salvianolic acid B which obtains the low OB (3.01%), caco-2 (−1.68) and BBB (−2.52), however, several *in vitro* studies indicate that salvianolic acid B displays significant pharmacological activities: protection of local cerebral ischemia-reperfusion injury [55], inhibition of platelet aggregation [56] and low density lipoprotein oxidation [57], as well as improving regional cerebral blood flow. In fact, several investigations have proposed that the bioactive effects of salvianolic acid B may not only be due to itself but also its metabolites, like isoferulic acid ($\log P = 1.56$, $\log S = -2.35$, DL = 0.06, Caco-2 = 0.50, OB = 67.69% and BBB = 0.08) and salvianic acid A ($\log P = 0.77$, $\log S = -1.47$, DL = 0.06, Caco-2 = −0.27, OB = 78.22%, BBB = −0.62) [58,13]. Therefore, these metabolites are also added into active ingredients database for further research.

Target proteins of anti-stroke herbal ingredients

In order to further decipher the underlying molecular mechanism of these herbal medicines, target proteins of those active ingredients were identified based on the comprehensive method. As a result, 196 candidate targets are identified for 185 compounds, while other 5 ingredients have no related targets. For increasing the reliability of target fishing, the predicted compound-target interactions are validated using docking program. As displayed in the Table S3 in Supporting Information S1, 183 targets linked with 168 molecules are reserved. The results also display that the majority of active herbal ingredients (129 out of 168 molecules) are linked with more than one target, exhibiting their promiscuous actions. For instance, compound luteolin which is shared by herbs *S. miltiorrhiza*, *G. biloba* and *E. breviscapu* not only serves as an inhibitors of xanthine dehydrogenase/oxidase (XDH) [59] and interleukin-4 (IL4) [60], but also acts as an antagonist of peroxisome proliferator-activated receptor gamma (PPARG) [61]; flavonoid compound kaempferol (shared by four herbs like *E. herba*) has interactions with tens of target proteins like arachidonate 5-lipoxygenase (ALOX5), and the same phenomenon also occur in quercetin, another common flavonoid compound shared by five herbal medicines.

As we know, during cerebral ischemic injury, several mechanisms can lead to neurons damage such as oxidative and nitrosative stress, inflammation and apoptotic-like cell death [6]. Hence, enzyme systems like pro-inflammatory cascades, caspases, nitric oxide synthases (NOSs), superoxide dismutases (SODs) and matrix metalloproteinases (MMPs) all have the prospect of becoming the therapeutic targets for stroke. Additionally, owing to the fact that diabetes, hypertension, dyslipidemia and atherosclerosis are all the main risk factors of stroke, a modest controlling of these factors can significantly reduce the frequency of primary and secondary stroke. Thus, appropriate antihypertensive, lipid-lowering, anti-diabetic and antiplatelet therapies have the promise of developing into remedies for preventing stroke. Based on the above strategies, 94 targets (as displayed in Table 2–4) that are implicated in stroke prevention and treatment are retrieved from 183 target validated proteins; meanwhile 168 compounds linked with these 94 targets are also extracted for further analysis.

For further elucidating the relationships between herbal ingredients and stroke, these 94 targets are sent to TTD and PharmGKB for discovering their corresponding diseases, which are then roughly classified into two categories: for stroke treatment (marked in bold in Tables 2–4) and for stroke prevention (others in the tables). As displayed in Tables 2–4, herbal medicines, featured as the typical multicomponent regimens, might simultaneously regulate multiple molecular components which are involved in the pathogenesis of stroke to exhibit the therapeutic or prophylactic effects. Factually, for stroke treatment and prevention, there exist many overlapping features in their pathologic and therapeutic processes. For example, inflammation involved in blood vessel wall and cerebral parenchyma contributes to tissue injury after ischemia and also to stroke risk [6]; recent observation confirms that a PPARG agonist pioglitazone being a prescription drug with hypoglycemic action to treat diabetes can decrease the incidence of stroke in patients with diabetes, and mediation of intracerebral

Table 2. The stroke-related targets of herbs and their corresponding diseases (Part 1).

ID	Protein Name	UniProt ID	Gene Name	Related Diseases
T_01	Tyrosine-protein phosphatase non-receptor type 1	P18031	PTPN1	Diabetes
T_02	**Prostaglandin G/H synthase 2**	**P35354**	**PTGS2**	**Stroke, Inflammation, Nervous system diseases, Myocardial infarction**
T_03	**Prostaglandin G/H synthase 1**	**P23219**	**PTGS1**	**Inflammation, Cardiovascular disease**
T_04	**Nitric-oxide synthase, endothelial**	**P29474**	**NOS3**	**Coronary artery disease, Heart diseases, Hypertension, Thromboembolism**
T_05	**Glycogen synthase kinase-3 beta**	**P49841**	**GSK3B**	**Diabetes, Ischemia, Brain injury, Nervous system diseases**
T_06	**Alpha-1D adrenergic receptor**	**P25100**	**ADRA1D**	**Hypertension**
T_07	**Nitric oxide synthase, inducible**	**P35228**	**NOS2**	**Ischemia reperfusion injury, Hypertension**
T_08	**Matrix metalloproteinase-9**	**P14780**	**MMP9**	**Atherosclerosis, Multiple sclerosis, Coronary artery disease, Heart failure**
T_09	Mitogen-activated protein kinase 1	P28482	MAPK1	Nervous system diseases
T_10	**Coagulation factor X**	**P00742**	**F10**	**Atrial fibrillation, Thromboembolism, Coronary artery disease**
T_11	Beta-1 adrenergic receptor	P08588	ADRB1	Hypertension
T_12	**Glycine receptor subunit alpha-1**	**P23415**	**GLRA1**	**Nervous system diseases**
T_13	**Superoxide dismutase [Cu-Zn]**	**P00441**	**SOD1**	**Ischemic injury**
T_14	**Tumor necrosis factor**	**P01375**	**TNF**	**Brain Diseases, Diabetes, Inflammation**
T_15	**Transcription factor p65**	**Q04206**	**RELA**	**Embolic focal cerebral ischemia, Ischemic renal injury, Thrombosis, Inflammation, Atherosclerosis**
T_16	Glycogen phosphorylase, muscle form	P11217	PYGM	Diabetes
T_17	**Coagulation factor VII**	**P08709**	**F7**	**Thromboembolism, Cardiovascular diseases**
T_18	**Caspase-3**	**P42574**	**CASP3**	**Venous thrombosis**
T_19	**Apoptosis regulator Bcl-2**	**P10415**	**BCL2**	**Nervous system diseases, Neoplasms**
T_20	**Apoptosis regulator BAX**	**Q07812**	**BAX**	**Neoplasms**
T_21	3-hydroxy-3-methylglutaryl-coenzyme A reductase	P04035	HMGCR	Myocardial infarction, Hyperlipidemias, Cardiovascular diseases, Arteriosclerosis, Hypertension
T_22	TGF-beta receptor type-1	P36897	TGFBR1	Cardiovascular diseases, Hypertension
T_23	Peroxisome proliferator-activated receptor gamma	P37231	PPARG	Hypertension, Cardiovascular diseases, Hyperlipidemias
T_24	Peroxisome proliferator-activated receptor delta	Q03181	PPARD	Venous thrombosis, Hyperlipidemias, Diabetes, Inflammation
T_25	Phospholipase A2, membrane associated	P14555	PLA2G2A	Myocardial infarction, Coronary artery disease, Atherosclerosis
T_26	Glucocorticoid receptor	P04150	NR3C1	Hypertension, Cardiovascular diseases, Diabetes

PPARG might also provide neuroprotective effect against brain ischemic injury [62].

Specifically, as displayed in Tables 2 and 3, proteins like PTGS2, AKT1, NOS2, MMP9, SOD1 and CASP3 can be regulated by herbal ingredients, and then may produce anti-inflammatory, anti-oxidant and anti-apoptosis effects against ischemic cerebral damage. For example, target PTGS2 is documented to be involved in pathogenic events that take place in both the early and late stages of cerebral ischemia, including attenuation of glutamate neurotoxicity [63], and abrogation of deleterious effects of postischemic inflammation [64]. Therefore, inhibition of PTGS2 has developed into an attractive therapeutic strategy of stroke due to the following advantages: 1) targeting both "early" and "later" components of ischemic injury; 2) relatively safe and well tolerated. For stroke prevention, herbal constituents that interact with series of targets like ACE, PPARG, ESR1, NR3C1, ADRA2A and PYGM, might exhibit lipid-lowering, anti-diabetic, anti-thrombotic and antiplatelet effects, subsequently lowering the risk of stroke. For instance, epidemiological evidence shows that blood pressure level is directly and continuously related with the ischemic stroke and intracerebral hemorrhage [65], and recently, an ACE inhibitor perindopril (a well-established antihypertensive agent)-based therapy is reported to reduce the risks of both ischemia and hemorrhagic stroke [66].

Network analysis of molecular mechanism for anti-stroke herbs

C-T network: elucidating the combining and additive strategies for herbal medications in stroke therapy and prophylaxis. As displayed in Figure 5, C-T network is generated based on 641 associations between 168 herbal ingredients (magenta circle nodes) and their corresponding 94 targets. As outlined above, we distinguish the potential targets into stroke therapy (limegreen circle nodes) and prophylaxis (limegreen diamond ones). Network analysis results show that the average number of targets per compound is 3.9. Nearly two thirds compounds (105 out of 168 compounds) are linked with more than one target, showing the multi-target properties of herbal ingredients. Among them, compound quercetin possesses the highest number of target interactions (degree = 42), following by apigenin with 26 targets and luteolin having 25 linked targets.

Table 3. The stroke-related targets of herbs and their corresponding diseases (Part 2).

ID	Protein Name	UniProt ID	Gene Name	Related Diseases
T_27	Mineralocorticoid receptor	P08235	NR3C2	Hypertension, Hyperlipidemias, Brain injury
T_28	**72 kDa type IV collagenase**	**P08253**	**MMP2**	**Nervous system diseases**
T_29	Thrombomodulin	P07204	THBD	Thrombosis
T_30	**E-selectin**	**P16581**	**SELE**	**Hypertension**
T_31	Protein kinase C, beta type	P05771	PRKCB	Diabetes
T_32	**Tissue-type plasminogen activator**	**P00750**	**PLAT**	**Nervous system diseases**
T_33	Vascular endothelial growth factor receptor 2	P35968	KDR	Hypertension
T_34	**Intercellular adhesion molecule 1**	**P05362**	**ICAM1**	**Multiple sclerosis, Inflammation**
T_35	**Prothrombin**	**P00734**	**F2**	**Myocardial infarction, Thromboembolism**
T_36	Cathepsin K	P43235	CTSK	Atherosclerosis
T_37	**BCL2-like 1**	**Q07817**	**BCL2L1**	**Neoplasms**
T_38	Oxysterols receptor LXR-alpha	Q13133	NR1H3	Cardiovascular diseases, Hypertension, Coronary artery disease, Atherosclerosis
T_39	Cell division protein kinase 4	P11802	CDK4	Diabetes
T_40	**Caspase-9**	**P55211**	**CASP9**	**Nervous system diseases**
T_41	Peroxisome proliferator activated receptor alpha	Q07869	PPARA	Hypertension, Coronary artery disease, Hyperlipidemias, Cardiovascular diseases
T_42	Thyroid hormone receptor beta-1	P10828	THRB	Hyperlipidemia
T_43	Transforming growth factor beta-1	P01137	TGFB1	Multiple sclerosis, Neoplasms
T_44	Integrin beta-3	P05106	ITGB3	Myocardial infarction, Cardiovascular disease
T_45	Endothelin-1 receptor	P25101	EDNRA	Hypertension, Cardiovascular disease
T_46	**Xanthine dehydrogenase**	**P47989**	**XDH**	**Hypertension**
T_47	**P-selectin**	**P16109**	**SELP**	**Stroke, Inflammation**
T_48	**Arachidonate 5-lipoxygenase**	**P09917**	**ALOX5**	**Cerebrovascular disorders, Inflammation**
T_49	Solute carrier family 2, facilitated glucose transporter member 4	P14672	SLC2A4	Diabetes
T_50	**Plasminogen activator inhibitor 1**	**P05121**	**SERPINE1**	**Thromboembolism, Inflammation**
T_51	Interstitial collagenase	P03956	MMP1	Myocardial infarction
T_52	Insulin receptor	P06213	INSR	Diabetes
T_53	**Interleukin-4**	**P05112**	**IL4**	**Inflammation**
T_54	**Interleukin-13**	**P35225**	**IL13**	**Inflammation**
T_55	Interferon gamma	P01579	IFNG	Multiple sclerosis
T_56	Heme oxygenase 1	P09601	HMOX1	Atherosclerosis, Cardiovascular diseases
T_57	**Hypoxia-inducible factor 1-alpha**	**Q16665**	**HIF1A**	**Stroke, Cardiovascular diseases**
T_58	Glucose-6-phosphatase	P35575	G6PC	Hyperglycemia
T_59	CD40 ligand	P29965	CD40LG	Atherosclerosis
T_60	**RAC-alpha serine/threonine-protein kinase**	**P31749**	**AKT1**	**Stroke, Brain ischemic insult, Diabetes**
T_61	**Monoamine oxidase A**	**P21397**	**MAOA**	**Nervous system diseases**
T_62	**Interleukin-6**	**P05231**	**IL6**	**Inflammation**
T_63	**C-C motif chemokine 2**	**P13500**	**CCL2**	**Atherosclerosis, Inflammation, Cardiovascular diseases**

As mentioned above, several pathways that lead to cell death are triggered by cerebral ischemia; therefore effective neuroprotective strategy might require a combination of drugs which act on distinct pathways during the progression of ischemic damage. Fortunately, by further analysis of the C-T net, we conclude that, in one herb, several compounds may bind to different points of same signaling pathway or different targets of different signaling cascades to exhibit the synergistic therapeutic actions. As an illustration, herb *Ginkgo biloba* (as displayed in Figure 6) was specified in detail to interpret the combination principle. During ischemia and reperfusion injury, overactivation of PPAR1 can induce translocation of AIF (apoptosis-inducing factor) from mitochondria to nucleus, which results in subsequent cell death [67]. Fortunately, compounds quercetin and myricetin of *G. biloba* which are identified as significant inhibitors of PPAR1 [68] collectively mediate the caspase-independent pathway, and have the potential to exhibit the additive anti-apoptosis effects. Moreover, compounds ginkgolide B and bilobalide of this herb

Table 4. The stroke-related targets of herbs and their corresponding diseases (Part 3).

ID	Protein Name	UniProt ID	Gene Name	Related Diseases
T_64	Angiotensin-converting enzyme	P12821	ACE	Arteriosclerosis, Hypertension, Heart failure, Hypokinesia, Stroke, Thromboembolism
T_65	Alpha-2A adrenergic receptor	P08913	ADRA2A	Hypertension, Heart failure, Cardiovascular diseases
T_66	Estrogen receptor	P03372	ESR1	Hyperlipidemia, Coronary artery diseases
T_67	**5-hydroxytryptamine receptor 1D**	**P28221**	**HTR1D**	**Nervous system diseases**
T_68	**5-hydroxytryptamine receptor 2A**	**P28223**	**HTR2A**	**Nervous system diseases, Diabetes**
T_69	Phosphatidylinositol-4,5-bisphosphate 3-kinase catalytic subunit, gamma isoform	P48736	PIK3CG	Myocardial infarction, Cardiovascular diseases
T_70	**Poly [ADP-ribose] polymerase 1**	**P09874**	**PARP1**	**Cardiovascular diseases**
T_71	**Myeloperoxidase**	**P05164**	**MPO**	**Nervous system diseases**
T_72	**Interleukin-1 beta**	**P01584**	**IL1B**	**Inflammation**
T_73	**Tissue factor**	**P13726**	**F3**	**Myocardial ischemia**
T_74	**C-X-C motif chemokine 10**	**P02778**	**CXCL10**	**Inflammation**
T_75	**Caspase-8**	**Q14790**	**CASP8**	**Nervous system diseases**
T_76	**Interleukin-1**	**P22301**	**IL10**	**Inflammation**
T_77	**Monoamine oxidase B**	**P27338**	**MAOB**	**Nervous system diseases**
T_78	**Ornithine decarboxylase**	**P11926**	**ODC1**	**Inflammation**
T_79	**Adenosine receptor A2a**	**P29274**	**ADORA2A**	**Ischemia reperfusion injuries, Inflammation, Nervous system diseases**
T_80	**Mitogen-activated protein kinase 14**	**Q16539**	**MAPK14**	**Inflammation, Nervous system diseases**
T_81	**Macrophage migration inhibitory factor**	**P14174**	**MIF**	**Arteriosclerosis, Inflammation**
T_82	Sodium-dependent serotonin transporter	P31645	SLC6A4	Dyslipidemias, Nervous system diseases
T_83	Stromelysin-1	P08254	MMP3	Myocardial infarction, Nervous system diseases
T_84	Alpha-1A adrenergic receptor	P35348	ADRA1A	Hypertension
T_85	**Acetylcholinesterase**	**P22303**	**ACHE**	**Brain ischemia, Nervous system diseases**
T_86	**Beta-2 adrenergic receptor**	**P07550**	**ADRB2**	**Multiple sclerosis, Hypertension, Inflammation**
T_87	**Histamine H1 receptor**	**P35367**	**HRH1**	**Cardiovascular diseases, Nervous system diseases, Ischemia**
T_88	**D(2) dopamine receptor**	**P14416**	**DRD2**	**Nervous system diseases**
T_89	**Arachidonate 12-lipoxygenase**	**P1854**	**ALOX12**	**Nervous system diseases**
T_90	**Integrin beta-2**	**P05107**	**ITGB2**	**Ischemic stroke**
T_91	**Interleukin-8**	**P10145**	**IL8**	**Nervous system diseases, Inflammation**
T_92	**Gamma-aminobutyric-acid receptor subunit alpha-5**	**P31644**	**GABRA5**	**Central Nervous system diseases**
T_93	Acyl coenzyme A:cholesterol acyltransferase	P23141	CES1	Atherosclerosis, Dyslipidemias, Cardiovascular disease, Nervous system diseases
T_94	Fatty acid binding protein adipocyte	P159	FABP4	Atherosclerosis

can block neuronal apoptosis by attenuating the activation of caspase-3 [69]; meanwhile myricetin can directly bind to the active site of caspase-3 to inhibit its activity [70]. All of these document that this herb is possible to regulate the caspase-independent pathway to display the synergistic inhibition of neuronal cell apoptosis. Therefore, we speculate that herb *G. biloba* might provide an effective therapeutic approach for the treatment of cerebral ischemia through synergistic inhibition of both the caspase-dependent and independent pathways.

Further analysis of the C-T net shows that, besides those combination therapies, several active ingredients in one herb can act on one common target, which might exhibit additive effects for improving the stroke outcome. For instance, after ischemia develops, NOS2 which produces NO contributes to the evolution of the cerebral injury [71], because of the fact that NOS2 is expressed in the setting of the inflammation response after cerebral ischemia. Then, inhibition of NOS2 expression or activity has potential to develop into an attractive therapeutic strategy for stroke. Fortunately, 39 herbal ingredients (as shown in Figure 5) like kaempferol, quercetin, ginkgolide B, ginsenoside C-K and oroxylin A all have interactions with NOS2, and might contribute to the anti-stroke effect of herbal medicines. Just for herb *S. baicalensis*, 12 constituents such as oroxylin A, acacetin and eugenol work together on protein NOS2, and might provide additive effects to reduce the infarct volume and ischemia brain damage.

Owing to the pathophysiology of stroke involved in multiple mechanisms, the use of combinations for improving the stroke outcome is especially rational. Facts have proven that therapies that eliminate the clot, restore blood flow, inhibit excitatory

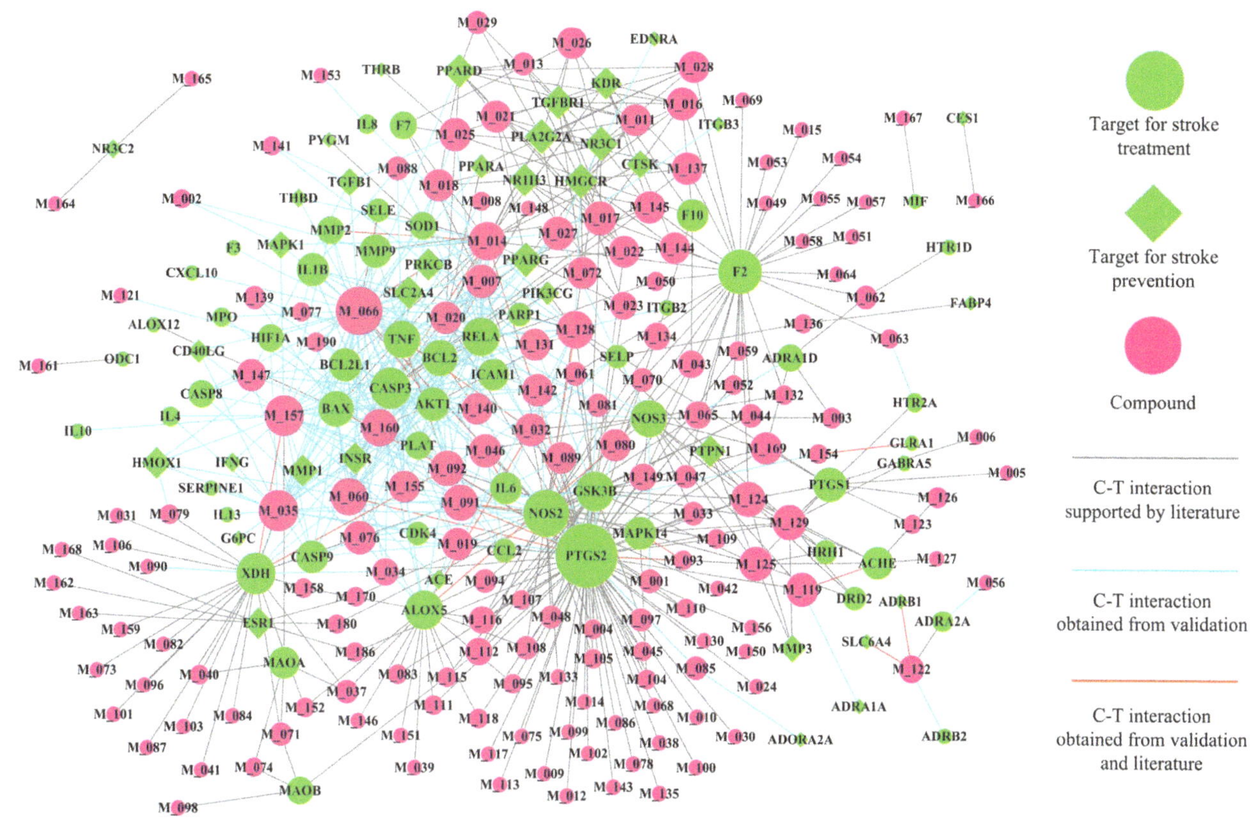

Figure 5. Compound-target network of anti-stroke herbs. Node size is proportional to its degree.

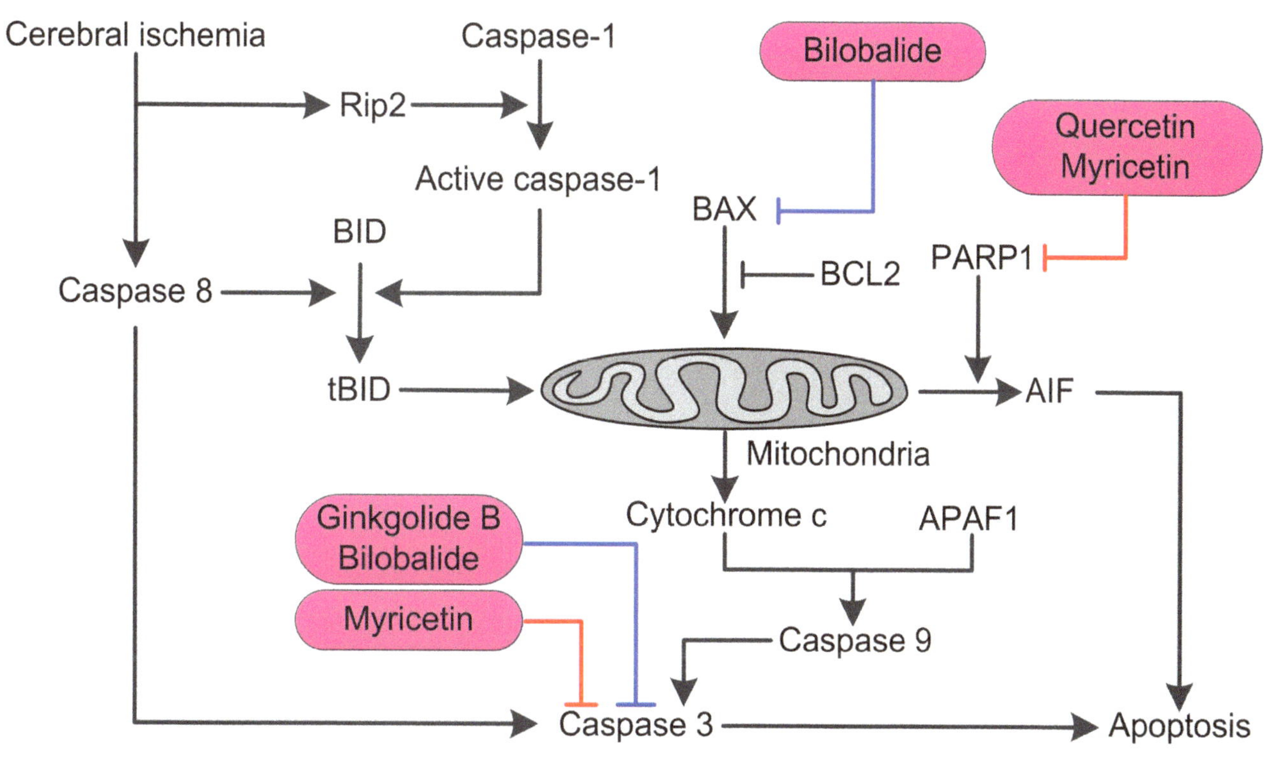

Figure 6. Illustrating the synergistic actions of anti-apoptosis of *Ginkgo biloba*.

neurotransmission, reduce inflammatory response following ischemia/reperfusion, or scavenge free radicals all have promising therapeutic potentials in animal models of stroke [72,73]. Luckily, in the C-T network of anti-stroke herbs (Figure 5), several high degrees of correlations of targets for anti-inflammation (like NOS2, ALOX5 and PPARG), anti-oxidant (including XDH and HMOX1) and anti-apoptosis (such as BAX, BCL2 and caspse-3), neuroprotection (for instance: AKT1, MMP9 and MMP2) are regulated by herbal ingredients, which might display a combination of multiple mechanisms for effective long-term treatment for stroke patients.

Furthermore, as we know, the incidence of stroke can be reduced with appropriate preventive measures like blood pressure lowering, as well as lipid-lowering, anti-diabetic, anti-thrombotic and antiplatelet therapies. In the C-T network of Figure 5, besides those potential therapies for stroke treatment, series of target proteins of herbal constituents are also engaged in diabetes mellitus (such as PPARG and NR3C1), atherosclerosis (for instance: PLA2G2A, NR1H3 and F10), hypertension (including ADRB1, NOS3 and ACE), dyslipidemia (like NR1H2, PPARD and HMGCR), which may be implicated in the primary and secondary stroke preventions.

In summary, as displayed in the C-T net, botanical medicines are engaged in multiple mechanisms of stroke to synergistically improve outcome, which are roughly classified into preventing inflammatory response, suppressing apoptosis, scavenging free radicals, inhibition of platelet aggregation, as well as modifying diabetes mellitus, hypertension, dyslipidemia and other stroke risk factors. And several ingredients in one herb might act on one the same target to display an additive effect, or bind at the different points of the same signaling pathway or at different targets of several pathways, and then have the potential to exhibit the synergistic therapeutic actions for stroke therapy and prophylaxis.

T-P network: holistic mechanisms of anti-stroke medicinal herbs. For better elaborating the major pathways involved in herbal medicines for stroke therapy, we extract the canonical pathways that are highly associated with stroke from KEGG database (http://www.genome.jp/kegg/), resulting in 30 canonical pathways including PI3K-Akt signaling pathway, TNF signaling pathway, neuroactive ligand-receptor interaction, calcium signaling pathway and metabolic pathways. For example, being a central mediator in signal transduction pathways modulating cell growth, metabolism and survival, the PI3K-Akt signaling pathway can mediate the neuroprotective activity of vascular endothelial growth factor and induce BBB permeability after focal cerebral ischemia [74]; MAPK signaling pathway transduces a large number of external signals, resulting in a large-scale cellular responses which contain cell proliferation, differentiation, inflammation and apoptosis, and now it is becoming obvious that this pathway plays a significant role in mediating cell survival following brain ischemia.

Subsequently, all target proteins from target fishing and validation attempt to be mapped onto these 30 pathways, generating a bipartite target-pathway network graph as displayed in Figure 7. Results show that after discarding 9 target proteins without participating in these pathways, this T-P network consists of 119 nodes (85 targets and 30 pathways) and 280 edges. And these pathways are linked with target proteins intensively, such as the TNF signaling pathway which exhibits the largest number of interactions with targets (degree = 17), neuroactive ligand-receptor interaction (degree = 16), PI3K-Akt signaling pathway (degree = 16) and HIF-1 signaling pathway (degree = 14). Actually, plenty of compounds in medicinal herbs are involved in these pathways, which maybe provide basis for stroke treatment and prevention strategies as well. For example, 62 herbal ingredients like ephedrine, corynantheine, ginkgolide A and pseudoephedrine are involved in mediating the major components of neuroactive ligand-receptor interaction pathway including ADRA2A, DRD2 and GABRA2, and might provide neuroprotective strategies to cerebral ischemia reperfusion injury. Analogously, the activation of PI3K-Akt signaling pathway has been proved essential for preventing the neuronal apoptosis and protecting the brain from cerebral ischemia/reperfusion injury [75]. And herbal ingredients like salvianolic acid B [76], cryptotanshinone [50] and ferulic acid [77] have been documented to regulate the PI3K-Akt signaling pathway in cerebral ischemia, thereby exhibiting protective effects against brain injury. Additionally, it is worth noting that several other pathways such as PPAR signaling pathway, arachidonic acid metabolism, insulin signaling pathway and TGF-beta signaling pathway can also be observed in this T-P network, and these pathways are closely related with glucose homeostasis, lipid profile, platelet coagulation and blood pressure. Therefore, we speculate that herbal medicines probably mediate these pathways to exhibit the anti-diabetes, antihypertensive, anti-platelet and anti-hyperlipidemia properties, and thereby might provide a combining system for stroke prevention.

Consequently, we deduce that herbal ingredients mainly target on proteins such as PTGS2, NOS, GSK3B, F2 and CASP3, and thereby have the potential to regulate the pathways like TNF signaling pathway, neuroactive ligand-receptor interaction, PI3K-Akt signaling pathway and HIF-1 signaling pathway to show the anti-apoptosis, anti-oxidant, anti-inflammatory, as well as other neuroprotective effects. Besides these, constituents of these ant-stroke herbs might also disturb PPAR signaling pathway, arachidonic acid metabolism, insulin signaling pathway and other pathways via regulating PPARG, MAPK1, PTGS1 and so forth, and then display anti-diabetes, antihypertensive, anti-platelet and anti-hyperlipidemia properties against recurrent stroke.

Conclusion

The lack of widely applicable and effective pharmacological therapies for stroke patients results in a growing interest in traditional herbal medications, for which extensive experience and plentiful clinical data on herbal medications in stroke have been accumulated over the past thousands of years. However, unlike conventional pharmacological medications used in western medicine, bioactive compounds and mechanisms of action of herbal medications have not been specified and measured precisely. Therefore, in this paper, we introduced systems pharmacology-based approach, which combines the use of computational modeling and wide-scale text-mining methods, to elucidate the mechanisms of action of the most widely studied medicinal herbs for the stroke treatment and prevention. The main findings are summarized as follows:

(1) Based on large-scale text mining method, 10 medicinal herbs such as *S. miltiorrhiza*, *G. biloba*, *E. herba*, etc. have been identified exhibiting significant correlations with stroke, and all these herbs or their corresponding herbal constituents are widely involved in TCPM for stroke treatment in China.

(2) After ADME prescreening, 168 compounds with satisfactory pharmacokinetic profiles have the potential to participate in stroke therapy, and the systematic use of these compounds might offer valuable clues on the combination therapies for stroke treatment and prevention.

(3) In target fishing, the results display that these 10 anti-stroke herbal medicines probably acts on 94 target proteins, and

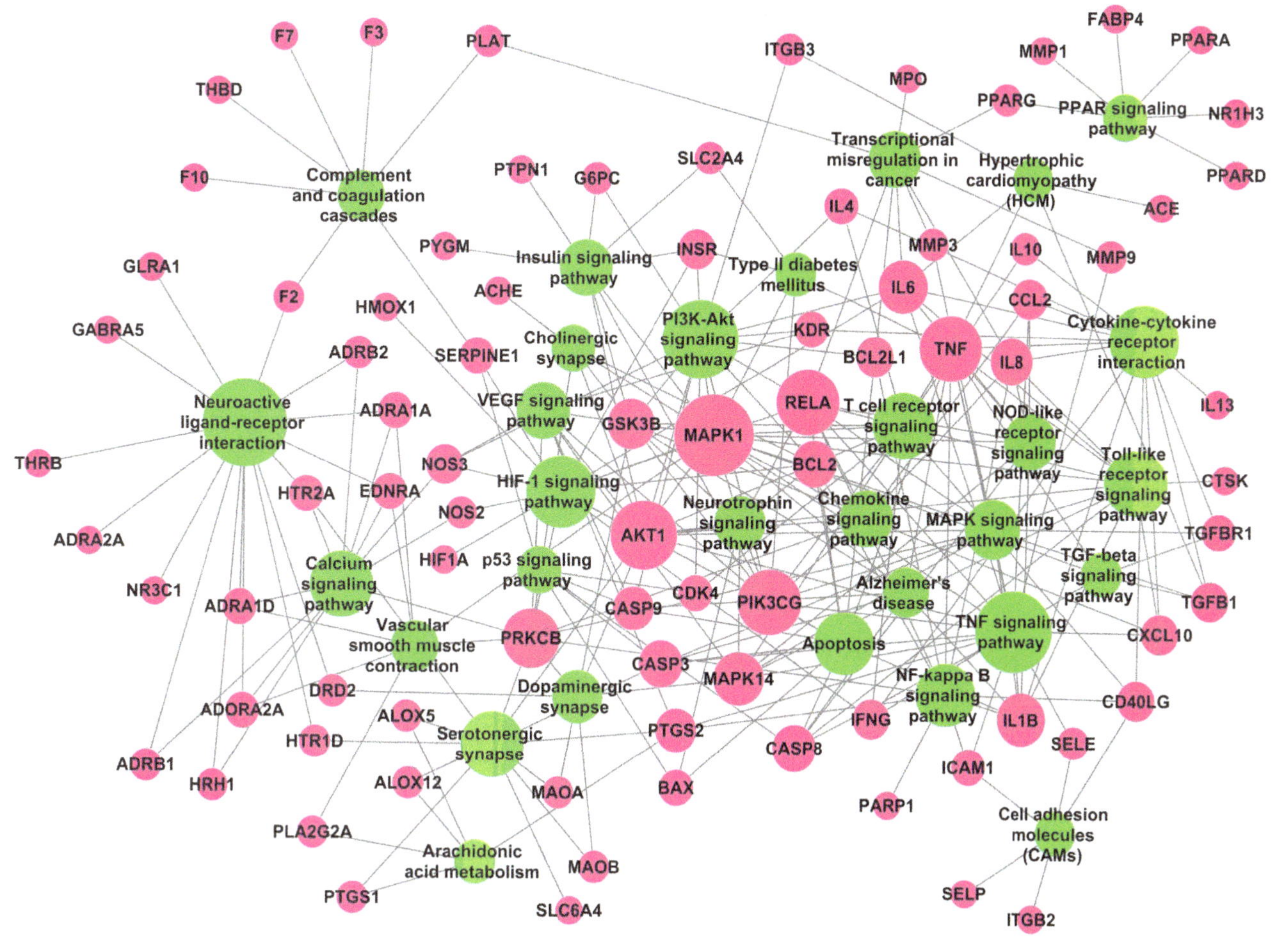

Figure 7. Target-pathway network of anti-stroke herbs where magenta nodes represent the targets and limegreen nodes signify pathways. Node size is proportional to its degree.

then exhibit the potential therapeutic benefits in stroke treatment and prevention through the following ways: producing anti-inflammation, anti-oxidant and anti-apoptosis effects against ischemic brain damage, and exhibiting lipid-lowering, anti-diabetic, anti-thrombotic and antiplatelet effects to reduce the risk factors of stroke.

(4) The results of C-T network indicate that medicinal herbs exhibit the therapeutic or prophylactic effects against stroke probably through synergistic and additive actions on multiple molecular components involved in the pathogenesis of stroke.

(5) The T-P network of anti-stroke herbs constructed in our work demonstrates that herbal medicines might simultaneously target several pathways like PI3K-Akt, TNF and calcium signaling pathways, and thereby exhibit synergistic benefits in stroke treatment and prevention.

Supporting Information

Supporting Information S1 Table S1, All compounds in ten anti-stroke herbs and the corresponding pharmacokinetics parameters. Table S2, Active constituents of anti-stroke herbs and their corresponding ADME parameters. Table S3, The detailed information of docking validation.
(DOCX)

Author Contributions

Conceived and designed the experiments: YL JXZ YHW XTC. Performed the experiments: JXZ YL XTC YHW. Analyzed the data: JXZ XTC SWZ YHW. Contributed reagents/materials/analysis tools: YL YHW YQP SWZ. Wrote the paper: JXZ YL YHW.

References

1. Mendis S, Puska P, Norrving B (2011) Global atlas on cardiovascular disease prevention and control: World Health Organization.
2. Gong X, Sucher NJ (1999) Stroke therapy in traditional Chinese medicine (TCM): prospects for drug discovery and development. Trends in Pharmacological Sciences 20: 191–196.
3. Broussalis E, Killer M, McCoy M, Harrer A, Trinka E, et al. (2012) Current therapies in ischemic stroke. Part A. Recent developments in acute stroke treatment and in stroke prevention. Drug Discovery Today 17: 296–309.
4. Mehta SL, Manhas N, Raghubir R (2007) Molecular targets in cerebral ischemia for developing novel therapeutics. Brain Research Reviews 54: 34–66.
5. O'Collins VE, Macleod MR, Donnan GA, Howells DW (2012) Evaluation of combination therapy in animal models of cerebral ischemia. Journal of Cerebral Blood Flow & Metabolism 32: 585–597.
6. Lo EH, Dalkara T, Moskowitz MA (2003) Mechanisms, challenges and opportunities in stroke. Nature Reviews Neuroscience 4: 399–415.
7. Asahi M, Asahi K, Wang X, Lo EH (2000) Reduction of tissue plasminogen activator-induced hemorrhage and brain injury by free radical spin trapping

after embolic focal cerebral ischemia in rats. Journal of Cerebral Blood Flow & Metabolism 20: 452–457.
8. Sumii T, Lo EH (2002) Involvement of matrix metalloproteinase in thrombolysis-associated hemorrhagic transformation after embolic focal ischemia in rats. Stroke 33: 831–836.
9. Shuaib A, Yang Y, Nakada MT, Li Q, Yang T (2002) Glycoprotein IIb/IIIa antagonist, murine 7E3 F(ab') 2, and tissue plasminogen activator in focal ischemia: evaluation of efficacy and risk of hemorrhage with combination therapy. Journal of Cerebral Blood Flow & Metabolism 22: 215–222.
10. Feigin VL (2007) Herbal medicine in stroke: does it have a future? Stroke 38: 1734–1736.
11. Wu B, Liu M, Liu H, Li W, Tan S, et al. (2007) Meta-analysis of traditional Chinese patent medicine for ischemic stroke. Stroke 38: 1973–1979.
12. Zhao S, Iyengar R (2012) Systems pharmacology: network analysis to identify multiscale mechanisms of drug action. Annual Review of Pharmacology and Toxicology 52: 505–521.
13. Li X, Xu X, Wang J, Yu H, Wang X, et al. (2012) A system-level investigation into the mechanisms of Chinese Traditional Medicine: Compound Danshen Formula for cardiovascular disease treatment. PLoS One 7: e43918.
14. Wang X, Xu X, Li Y, Li X, Tao W, et al. (2013) Systems pharmacology uncovers Janus functions of botanical drugs: activation of host defense system and inhibition of influenza virus replication. Integrative Biology 5: 351–371.
15. Huang C, Zheng C, Li Y, Wang Y, Lu A, et al. (2013) Systems pharmacology in drug discovery and therapeutic insight for herbal medicines. Brief Bioinform.
16. Tavazoie S, Hughes JD, Campbell MJ, Cho RJ, Church GM (1999) Systematic determination of genetic network architecture. Nature Genetics 22: 281–285.
17. Hou T, Xu X (2002) ADME evaluation in drug discovery. 1. Applications of genetic algorithms to the prediction of blood-brain partitioning of a large set of drugs. J Mol Model 8: 337–349.
18. Wang J, Krudy G, Hou T, Zhang W, Holland G, et al. (2007) Development of reliable aqueous solubility models and their application in druglike analysis. Journal of Chemical Information and Modeling 47: 1395–1404.
19. Tetko IV, Tanchuk VY, Kasheva TN, Villa AE (2001) Estimation of aqueous solubility of chemical compounds using E-state indices. J Chem Inf Comput Sci 41: 1488–1493.
20. Jorgensen WL, Duffy EM (2002) Prediction of drug solubility from structure. Adv Drug Deliv Rev 54: 355–366.
21. Arnott JA, Planey SL (2012) The influence of lipophilicity in drug discovery and design. Expert Opin Drug Discov 7: 863–875.
22. Tetko IV, Bruneau P (2004) Application of ALOGPS to predict 1-octanol/water distribution coefficients, logP, and logD, of AstraZeneca in-house database. J Pharm Sci 93: 3103–3110.
23. Liu H, Wang J, Zhou W, Wang Y, Yang L (2013) Systems approaches and polypharmacology for drug discovery from herbal medicines: an example using licorice. J Ethnopharmacol 146: 773–793.
24. Xu X, Zhang W, Huang C, Li Y, Yu H, et al. (2012) A novel chemometric method for the prediction of human oral bioavailability. International journal of molecular sciences 13: 6964–6982.
25. Pang KS (2003) Modeling of intestinal drug absorption: roles of transporters and metabolic enzymes (for the Gillette Review Series). Drug Metab Dispos 31: 1507–1519.
26. González-Álvarez I, Bermejo M, Mangas Sanjuan V, Centelles I, Garrigues TM, et al. (2011) In Silico Prediction of Caco-2 Cell Permeability by a Classification QSAR Approach. Molecular Informatics 30: 376–385.
27. Li L, Li Y, Wang Y, Zhang S, Yang L (2007) Prediction of human intestinal absorption based on molecular indices. Journal of molecular science 23: 286–291.
28. Kam A, Li KM, Razmovski-Naumovski V, Nammi S, Chan K, et al. (2012) The protective effects of natural products on blood-brain barrier breakdown. Curr Med Chem 19: 1830–1845.
29. Li L, Li Y, Wang Y, Zhang S (2007) Prediction of BBB permeation based on molecular indices. Chinese journal of medicinal chemistry 17: 221–228.
30. Zhu F, Shi Z, Qin C, Tao L, Liu X, et al. (2012) Therapeutic target database update 2012: a resource for facilitating target-oriented drug discovery. Nucleic Acids Res 40: D1128–1136.
31. Ye H, Ye L, Kang H, Zhang D, Tao L, et al. (2011) HIT: linking herbal active ingredients to targets. Nucleic Acids Res 39: D1055–1059.
32. Keiser MJ, Roth BL, Armbruster BN, Ernsberger P, Irwin JJ, et al. (2007) Relating protein pharmacology by ligand chemistry. Nat Biotechnol 25: 197–206.
33. Kuhn M, Szklarczyk D, Franceschini A, von Mering C, Jensen LJ, et al. (2012) STITCH 3: zooming in on protein-chemical interactions. Nucleic Acids Res 40: D876–880.
34. Yu H, Chen J, Xu X, Li Y, Zhao H, et al. (2012) A systematic prediction of multiple drug-target interactions from chemical, genomic, and pharmacological data. PLoS One 7: e37608.
35. Whirl-Carrillo M, McDonagh EM, Hebert JM, Gong L, Sangkuhl K, et al. (2012) Pharmacogenomics knowledge for personalized medicine. Clin Pharmacol Ther 92: 414–417.
36. Jones G, Willett P, Glen RC, Leach AR, Taylor R (1997) Development and validation of a genetic algorithm for flexible docking. Journal of Molecular Biology 267: 727–748.
37. Shannon P, Markiel A, Ozier O, Baliga NS, Wang JT, et al. (2003) Cytoscape: a software environment for integrated models of biomolecular interaction networks. Genome Res 13: 2498–2504.
38. Lin TH, Hsieh CL (2010) Pharmacological effects of Salvia miltiorrhiza (Danshen) on cerebral infarction. Chinese Medicine 5: 22.
39. Zeng X, Liu M, Yang Y, Li Y, Asplund K (2005) Ginkgo biloba for acute ischaemic stroke. Cochrane Database Syst Rev: CD003691.
40. Wu B, Liu M, Zhang S (2004) Dan Shen agents for acute ischaemic stroke. Cochrane Database Syst Rev: CD004295.
41. Zhou J, Zhou S (2010) Antihypertensive and neuroprotective activities of rhynchophylline: the role of rhynchophylline in neurotransmission and ion channel activity. J Ethnopharmacol 132: 15–27.
42. Zhou JY, Zhou SW (2012) Isorhynchophylline: A plant alkaloid with therapeutic potential for cardiovascular and central nervous system diseases. Fitoterapia 83: 617–626.
43. Chen CX, Jin RM, Li YK, Zhong J, Yue L, et al. (1992) Inhibitory effect of rhynchophylline on platelet aggregation and thrombosis. Zhongguo Yao Li Xue Bao 13: 126–130.
44. Suk K, Kim SY, Leem K, Kim YO, Park SY, et al. (2002) Neuroprotection by methanol extract of Uncaria rhynchophylla against global cerebral ischemia in rats. Life Sci 70: 2467–2480.
45. Shi JS, Yu JX, Chen XP, Xu RX (2003) Pharmacological actions of Uncaria alkaloids, rhynchophylline and isorhynchophylline. Acta Pharmacol Sin 24: 97–101.
46. Lee S, Kim DH, Lee DH, Jeon SJ, Lee CH, et al. (2010) Oroxylin A, a flavonoid, stimulates adult neurogenesis in the hippocampal dentate gyrus region of mice. Neurochem Res 35: 1725–1732.
47. Jeon SJ, Rhee SY, Seo JE, Bak HR, Lee SH, et al. (2011) Oroxylin A increases BDNF production by activation of MAPK-CREB pathway in rat primary cortical neuronal culture. Neuroscience Research 69: 214–222.
48. Ha SK, Moon E, Lee P, Ryu JH, Oh MS, et al. (2012) Acacetin attenuates neuroinflammation via regulation the response to LPS stimuli in vitro and in vivo. Neurochem Res 37: 1560–1567.
49. Chang CP, Huang WT, Cheng BC, Hsu CC, Lin MT (2007) The flavonoid baicalin protects against cerebrovascular dysfunction and brain inflammation in experimental heatstroke. Neuropharmacology 52: 1024–1033.
50. Zhang F, Zheng W, Pi R, Mei Z, Bao Y, et al. (2009) Cryptotanshinone protects primary rat cortical neurons from glutamate-induced neurotoxicity via the activation of the phosphatidylinositol 3-kinase/Akt signaling pathway. Experimental Brain Research 193: 109–118.
51. Kim EJ, Jung SN, Son KH, Kim SR, Ha TY, et al. (2007) Antidiabetes and antiobesity effect of cryptotanshinone via activation of AMP-activated protein kinase. Molecular Pharmacology 72: 62–72.
52. Suh SJ, Jin UH, Choi HJ, Chang HW, Son JK, et al. (2006) Cryptotanshinone from Salvia miltiorrhiza BUNGE has an inhibitory effect on TNF-alpha-induced matrix metalloproteinase-9 production and HASMC migration via down-regulated NF-kappaB and AP-1. Biochem Pharmacol 72: 1680–1689.
53. Jin DZ, Yin LL, Ji XQ, Zhu XZ (2006) Cryptotanshinone inhibits cyclooxygenase-2 enzyme activity but not its expression. Eur J Pharmacol 549: 166–172.
54. Wang X, Morris-Natschke SL, Lee KH (2007) New developments in the chemistry and biology of the bioactive constituents of Tanshen. Medicinal Research Reviews 27: 133–148.
55. Chen YH, Du GH, Zhang JT (2000) Salvianolic acid B protects brain against injuries caused by ischemia-reperfusion in rats. Acta Pharmacol Sin 21: 463–466.
56. Li M, Zhao C, Wong RN, Goto S, Wang Z, et al. (2004) Inhibition of shear-induced platelet aggregation in rat by tetramethylpyrazine and salvianolic acid B. Clinical Hemorheology and Microcirculation. 31: 97–103.
57. O K, Lynn EG, Vazhappilly R, Au-Yeung KK, Zhu DY, et al. (2001) Magnesium tanshinoate B (MTB) inhibits low density lipoprotein oxidation. Life Sci 68: 903–912.
58. Gao DY, Han LM, Zhang LH, Fang XL, Wang JX (2009) Bioavailability of salvianolic acid B and effect on blood viscosities after oral administration of salvianolic acids in beagle dogs. Arch Pharm Res 32: 773–779.
59. Choi MY, Song HS, Hur HS, Sim SS (2008) Whitening activity of luteolin related to the inhibition of cAMP pathway in alpha-MSH-stimulated B16 melanoma cells. Arch Pharm Res 31: 1166–1171.
60. Kawai M, Hirano T, Higa S, Arimitsu J, Maruta M, et al. (2007) Flavonoids and related compounds as anti-allergic substances. Allergology International 56: 113–123.
61. Mueller M, Lukas B, Novak J, Simoncini T, Genazzani AR, et al. (2008) Oregano: a source for peroxisome proliferator-activated receptor gamma antagonists. J Agric Food Chem 56: 11621–11630.
62. Culman J, Zhao Y, Gohlke P, Herdegen T (2007) PPAR-gamma: therapeutic target for ischemic stroke. Trends Pharmacol Sci 28: 244–249.
63. Seibert K, Masferrer J, Zhang Y, Gregory S, Olson G, et al. (1995) Mediation of inflammation by cyclooxygenase-2. Agents and Actions Supplements 46: 41–50.
64. Iadecola C, Niwa K, Nogawa S, Zhao X, Nagayama M, et al. (2001) Reduced susceptibility to ischemic brain injury and N-methyl-D-aspartate-mediated neurotoxicity in cyclooxygenase-2-deficient mice. Proceedings of the National Academy of Sciences of the United States of America 98: 1294–1299.

65. Di Napoli M, Papa F (2003) Angiotensin-converting enzyme inhibitor use is associated with reduced plasma concentration of C-reactive protein in patients with first-ever ischemic stroke. Stroke 34: 2922–2929.
66. Anderson C (2003) Blood pressure-lowering for secondary prevention of stroke: ACE inhibition is the key. Stroke 34: 1333–1334.
67. van Wijk SJ, Hageman GJ (2005) Poly(ADP-ribose) polymerase-1 mediated caspase-independent cell death after ischemia/reperfusion. Free Radic Biol Med 39: 81–90.
68. Geraets L, Moonen HJ, Brauers K, Wouters EF, Bast A, et al. (2007) Dietary flavones and flavonoles are inhibitors of poly(ADP-ribose)polymerase-1 in pulmonary epithelial cells. J Nutr 137: 2190–2195.
69. Shi C, Liu J, Wu F, Yew DT (2010) Ginkgo biloba extract in Alzheimer's disease: From action mechanisms to medical practice. Int J Mol Sci 11: 107–123.
70. Kuo PL (2005) Myricetin inhibits the induction of anti-Fas IgM-, tumor necrosis factor-alpha- and interleukin-1beta-mediated apoptosis by Fas pathway inhibition in human osteoblastic cell line MG-63. Life Sci 77: 2964–2976.
71. Iadecola C (1997) Bright and dark sides of nitric oxide in ischemic brain injury. Trends in Neurosciences 20: 132–139.
72. Meldrum BS (1995) Cytoprotective therapies in stroke. Current Opinion in Neurology 8: 15–23.
73. Gong X, Sucher NJ (1999) Stroke therapy in traditional Chinese medicine (TCM): prospects for drug discovery and development. Trends Pharmacol Sci 20: 191–196.
74. Kilic E, Kilic U, Wang Y, Bassetti CL, Marti HH, et al. (2006) The phosphatidylinositol-3 kinase/Akt pathway mediates VEGF's neuroprotective activity and induces blood brain barrier permeability after focal cerebral ischemia. FASEB J 20: 1185–1187.
75. Lu C, Liu L, Chen Y, Ha T, Kelley J, et al. (2011) TLR2 ligand induces protection against cerebral ischemia/reperfusion injury via activation of phosphoinositide 3-kinase/Akt signaling. Journal of Immunology 187: 1458–1466.
76. Liu CL, Xie LX, Li M, Durairajan SS, Goto S, et al. (2007) Salvianolic acid B inhibits hydrogen peroxide-induced endothelial cell apoptosis through regulating PI3K/Akt signaling. PLoS One 2: e1321.
77. Gim SA, Sung JH, Shah FA, Kim MO, Koh PO (2013) Ferulic acid regulates the AKT/GSK-3beta/CRMP-2 signaling pathway in a middle cerebral artery occlusion animal model. Lab Anim Res 29: 63–69.

Serum Metabonomic Analysis of Protective Effects of *Curcuma aromatica* Oil on Renal Fibrosis Rats

Liangcai Zhao[1], Haiyan Zhang[1], Yunjun Yang[3], Yongquan Zheng[1], Minjian Dong[1], Yaqiang Wang[1], Guanghui Bai[2], Xinjian Ye[2], Zhihan Yan[2*], Hongchang Gao[1,2*]

1 Institute of Metabonomics & Medical NMR, School of Pharmaceutical Sciences, Wenzhou Medical University, Wenzhou, China, **2** Radiology Department of the Second Affiliated Hospital, Wenzhou Medical University, Wenzhou, China, **3** Department of Radiology, the first Affiliated Hospital, Wenzhou Medical University, Wenzhou, China

Abstract

Background: *Curcuma aromatica* oil is a traditional herbal medicine demonstrating protective and anti-fibrosis activities in renal fibrosis patients. However, study of its mechanism of action is challenged by its multiple components and multiple targets that its active agent acts on.

Methodology/Principal Findings: Nuclear magnetic resonance (NMR)-based metabonomics combined with clinical chemistry and histopathology examination were performed to evaluate intervening effects of *Curcuma aromatica* oil on renal interstitial fibrosis rats induced by unilateral ureteral obstruction. The metabolite levels were compared based on integral values of serum ^{1}H NMR spectra from rats on 3, 7, 14, and 28 days after the medicine administration. Time trajectory analysis demonstrated that metabolic profiles of the agent-treated rats were restored to control levels after 7 days of dosage. The results confirmed that the agent would be an effective anti-fibrosis medicine in a time-dependent manner, especially in early renal fibrosis stage. Targeted metabolite analysis showed that the medicine could lower levels of lipid, acetoacetate, glucose, phosphorylcholine/choline, trimethylamine oxide and raise levels of pyruvate, glycine in the serum of the rats. Serum clinical chemistry and kidney histopathology examination dovetailed well with the metabonomics data.

Conclusions/Significances: The results substantiated that *Curcuma aromatica* oil administration can ameliorate renal fibrosis symptoms by inhibiting some metabolic pathways, including lipids metabolism, glycolysis and methylamine metabolism, which are dominating targets of the agent working *in vivo*. This study further strengthens the novel analytical approach for evaluating the effect of traditional herbal medicine and elucidating its molecular mechanism.

Editor: Rupesh Chaturvedi, Jawaharlal Nehru University, India

Funding: This work was supported by the National Natural Science Foundation of China (Nos. 21175099 and 81100598), the Zhejiang Provincial Project of Key Scientific Group (2010R50042), the Zhejiang Provincial Natural Science Foundation of China (No. Y13H070016), and the Scientific Research Foundation for the Talents, Wenzhou Medical University (QTJ13004 and QTJ08008). The funders had no role in study design, data collection and analysis, decision to publish, or preparation of the manuscript.

Competing Interests: The authors have declared that no competing interests exist.

* Email: zhihanyan@hotmail.com (ZY); gaohc27@gmail.com (HG)

These authors contributed equally to this work.

Introduction

Renal interstitial fibrosis (RIF) is the common end of progressive chronic renal disease. It is a complex pathologic process involving inflammation, lipid peroxidation, oxidative stress, hypoxia, also is characterized by cellular infiltration, fibroblast differentiation, increased extracellular matrix protein deposition, and tubule atrophy [1]. Once renal disease progresses to end-stage renal disease, patient survival will only depend on dialysis and kidney transplantation, which bring enormous physical and psychological pain, not to mention high economic burden. Thus, blocking or reversal of the progressive course of renal fibrosis is a key to the prevention of the disease advancing to end-stage. Although numerous efforts have been exerted to develop therapeutic strategies, such as angiotensin converting enzyme inhibitors and angiotensin II receptor blockers, fibrotic renal disease has remained a major unresolved problem in the clinical therapy of renal disease.

Traditional herbal medicines have been gaining more attention worldwide due to their intrinsic unique advantages, such as a holistic approach to examining the function and dysfunction of living organisms, different from the so-called "Western" medicine [2]. Our previous study proved that *Curcuma aromatica* oil (CAO), the volatile oil substances of the medicine, significantly attenuated total collagen of renal fibrosis rats after a 14-day treatment [3]. The agent was also found to ameliorate symptoms of diabetic nephropathy in rats [4]. Utilizing molecular biology technology, crystallization ingredients of *Curcuma aromatica* were certified to demonstrate protective activities against renal fibrosis through the up-regulation of heme oxygenase [5] and through the Nrf2-Keap1 signal transduction pathway [6]. As a traditional

Table 1. Serum clinical chemistry parameters.

	3 d			7 d			
	SO	UUO	CAO-UUO	SO	UUO	CAO-UUO	CAO-SO
LDL (mM/L)	1.68±0.58	2.38±0.87*	1.61±0.46#	1.25±0.26	2.62±0.46**	1.89±0.33#	1.27±0.62
HDL (mM/L)	0.40±0.17	0.93±0.56*	0.92±0.37	0.30±0.12	1.52±0.58**	1.12±0.48	0.27±0.08
TG (mM/L)	0.69±0.33	0.68±0.24	0.85±0.47	0.51±0.12	0.77±0.37	0.71±0.35	0.70±0.26
BUN (mM/L)	8.47±2.36	8.87±2.10	8.45±1.45	10.56±1.98	8.55±1.80	11.36±3.18#	9.85±3.45
SCr (umol/L)	79.23±9.37	102.90±27.67*	47.59±14.45*#	70.73±26.18	99.80±17.13**	30.78±7.35*##	28.10±6.15*
	14 d			**28 d**			
	SO	**UUO**	**CAO-UUO**	**SO**	**UUO**	**CAO-UUO**	
LDL (mM/L)	1.51±0.57	2.16±0.45*	1.54±0.28#	1.35±0.91	2.09±0.29*	1.93±0.25	
HDL (mM/L)	0.53±0.11	1.89±0.40**	1.05±0.67#	0.33±0.13	1.95±1.21*	1.39±0.47	
TG (mM/L)	0.69±0.42	0.91±0.36*	0.57±0.22##	0.61±0.31	0.61±0.37	0.56±0.23	
BUN (mM/L)	7.14±2.68	9.78±2.72*	7.11±2.75#	8.97±1.08	11.60±0.88**	6.13±2.28##	
SCr (umol/L)	73.47±24.34	79.93±21.67	46.40±10.07*#	96.15±9.39	104.23±25.44	42.22±7.38*##	

Data are expressed as mean ± SD (n = 6–8 for each group). LDL, low density lipoproteins; HDL, high density lipoproteins; TG, triglycerides; BUN, blood urea nitrogen; SCr, serum creatinine.
*P<0.05,
**p<0.01, compared with SO rats.
#P<0.05,
##p<0.01, compared with UUO rats.

herbal medicine, *Curcuma aromatica* is gaining more attention worldwide due to its long history of use in clinical practice. However, as *Curcuma aromatica* usually operates in the body through multiple components, multiple pathways, and multiple targets, not to mention the complex pathological process of renal fibrosis itself, the study of its anti-fibrosis mechanism is challenging.

Metabonomics technology, a non-targeted analysis of tissues or biofluids for organic low-molecular metabolite, provides entire metabolic profiles of organisms undergoing medical intervention and offers novel insight on the understanding of pharmacological mechanism [7]. Metabonomic analysis has been applied to evaluate therapeutic effects of many traditional herbal medicines, including *Rhizoma drynariae* extracts [8], berberine [9], *Shuang-long* formula [10], and *Liuwei Dihuang* pills [11]. Using NMR-based metabonomics, we previously evaluated the therapeutic effect of *Zhibai Dihuang* pill in the treatment of diabetic nephropathy rats [12]. These previous studies illustrated that metabonomics analysis is an effective approach for evaluating the effects of and for elucidating the mechanism behind traditional herbal medicine [13,14].

In this work, we used unilateral ureteral obstruction (UUO)-induced rats as a RIF model developing renal injury similar to clinical human renal fibrosis [15]. NMR-based metabonomics was applied to analyze the metabolic profile changes in the serum of the control, UUO, and CAO-treated RIF rats at different time points. We sought to determine (*i*) whether the metabolic profiles of RIF rats could be ameliorated by CAO treatment, (*ii*) which of the metabolic pathways disturbed in RIF rats could be intervened in by CAO treatment, and (*iii*) how the metabolic mechanism of CAO acts on holistically *in vivo*. The results of our study can facilitate the understanding of the regulation of traditional Chinese medicine, as well as its molecular mechanisms.

Materials and Methods

Subjects and materials

CAO was produced by the Tian Rui Medicine Co., Ltd. (Zhejiang, China). Adult male Sprague-Dawley rats (8 weeks age, 220±15 g), obtained from Shanghai SLAC Laboratory Animal Co. Ltd. (Shanghai, China), were kept in specific pathogen-free (SPF) colony of Laboratory Animal Center of Wenzhou Medical University, with regulated temperature and humidity and a 12/12 h light-dark cycle with lights on at 08:00 am. The animal production licenses are No. SCXK 2007-0005. During the whole experimental process, rats were fed with standard rat chow and tap water.

Ethics statement

The protocol for the animal experiment was approved by the Institutional Animal Committee of Wenzhou Medical University. All animals received care in accordance to the 'Guide for the Care and Use of Laboratory Animals'. Procedures using rats were approved by the Institutional Animal Care and Use Committee of Wenzhou Medical University (document number: wydw2012-0083).

Experimental design and sample collection

After acclimation of one week prior to conducting experiments, the rats were randomly divided into three groups: sham-operation control group (SO group), UUO model group (UUO or RIF group) and CAO-treated RIF group (CAO group), $n = 8$ for each group and 6–8 serum samples were obtained at each time point (3 d, 7 d, 14 d, and 28 d after UUO model was founded). In addition, to conclude that CAO treatment effect on serum profile is specific to renal fibrosis and to assist understanding the effect of CAO on the healthy rats, we also performed one sham-operated CAO-treated control group (CAO-SO group). The UUO and CAO rats were conducted to UUO model according to the operating procedure described previously [16]. Rats were anesthetized by i.p. injection of 10% chloral hydrate (3 mL/Kg), then, the left ureter was isolated and completely ligated with 4-0 silk sutures. The SO and CAO-SO rats underwent an identical surgical procedure without ureteral ligation. Rats were allowed to recover from anesthesia and were housed in standard rodent cages with ad libitum access to water and food until sacrificed. Solid food was withdrawn 12 h before and after surgery.

Three different doses of CAO treatment on RIF rats (100 mg/kg, 200 mg/kg, 300 mg/kg body weight, *i.p.*) were utilized in order to determine its optimal usage. The biochemical analysis and histopathology, as shown in Table S1 and Figure S1, suggest obvious amelioration of biochemical parameters and histopathology damages in RIF rats at the two high doses. Interestingly, negligible difference was found between higher doses, i.e. 200 mg/kg versus 300 mg/kg. And, refer to our previous study [3], we chose the dosage of 200 mg/kg in the subsequent studies, in which the drug-treated rats were administrated with CAO (200 mg/kg, *i.p.*) every 3 days for the following 28 days. The UUO and SO rats were administrated with the same volume of vehicle.

1.5 mL blood samples were drawn from the suborbital vein at days 3, 7, 14 and 28 post-operation under 10% chloral hydrate induced anesthesia. The sera were separated after centrifugation at 3 000 g for 10 min at 4°C and then stored at −80°C until NMR and clinical chemical analysis. Before sacrifice, the left kidneys were removed from the anesthetic rats and immersed in 10% (w/v) neutral buffered formalin solution for histological analysis.

Clinical chemistry and histopathology analysis

The clinical chemistry analysis of serum was carried out for the measurement of biochemical parameters including serum creatinine (SCr), blood urea nitrogen (BUN), triglycerides (TG), low density lipoproteins (LDL), and high density lipoproteins (HDL) by using Automatic Analyzer (BECKMAN-COULTER LX-20, USA). Histopathological changes in kidney tissues were assessed in at least 25 randomly selected tissue sections from each group under study. Sections were stained with Mayer's haematoxylin and eosin (HE) staining for light microscopic observation.

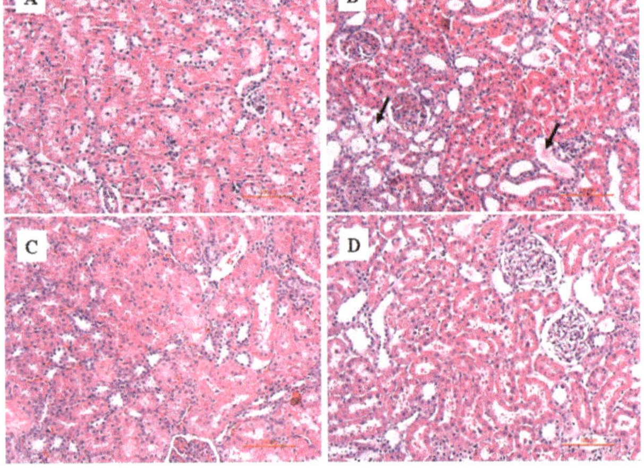

Figure 1. Representative HE-stained sections (200 fold) of kidneys from SO (A), UUO (B), CAO rats on 7 d (C) and 28 d (D), respectively. The SO rats exhibit no abnormal histopathological changes, whereas UUO rats display loss of brush border, tubular swelling atrophy and cystic dilation. Meanwhile, CAO rats display the different therapeutic effects of the agent.

Preparation of samples and acquisition of ^{1}H NMR spectra

Prior to NMR analysis, serum samples were thawed and 200 μL of each was diluted by 400 μL of phosphate buffer (0.2 mM Na_2HPO_4/NaH_2PO_4, pH 7.4) to minimize variations in pH and 60 μL D_2O for a field frequency lock. The mixed serum samples were centrifuged at 12 000 g for 10 min at 4°C to separate any precipitate. Aliquots of 500 μL of the supernatants were transferred to 5 mm NMR tubes. The detailed protocol refers to our previous work [17].

All NMR spectra were recorded at 298 K on a Bruker AVANCE III 600 NMR spectrometer operating at 600.13 MHz ^{1}H frequency and equipped with a triple resonance probe. The CPMG (Carr-Purcell-Meiboom-Gill) pulse sequence was used to attenuate the broad NMR signals from slowly tumbling molecules such as proteins and retain those from low-molecular weight compounds and some lipid components with a fixed relaxation delay $2n\tau$ of 120 ms. Typically, 128 scans were collected into 64 K data points over a spectral width of 12 000 Hz with a relaxation delay of 4 s and an acquisition time of 2.65 s. An exponential line-broadening of 0.3 Hz was applied to the FID prior to Fourier transformation. All spectra were carefully phased and baseline corrected and referenced to the methyl peak of lactate (CH_3, δ1.33) [18].

Multivariate pattern recognition

Following phase and baseline correction, each spectrum was segmented into chemical shift regions of equal width of 0.0015 ppm (buckets) corresponding to the region of δ 10.0 to 0.4 using the Bruker Topspin 2.1 software package. The region of δ 5.2 to 4.4 (containing the residual peak from the suppressed water resonance) was set to the zero integral in the analysis. The remaining spectral segments for each NMR spectrum were normalized to the total sum of the spectral intensity to partially compensate for differences in concentration of the many metabolites in the samples, and the normalized integral values were entered into SIMCA-P+12.0 software (Umetrics, Umeå, Sweden) for principal component analysis (PCA) and partial least squares-discriminant analysis (PLS-DA).

PCA is unsupervised multivariable statistical method, in which data are visualized by plotting the scores of the first two principal components (PC1 and PC2) to provide the most efficient 2D representation of the information, where the position of each point along a given axis in the scores plot is influenced by variables in the same axis in the loading plot. As a supervised multivariable statistics, PLS-DA revealed differences in the different groups, which is necessary to eliminate outliers and enhance the quality of the PCA model. Leave-one-out cross validation and permutation tests (200 cycles) were conducted to measure the robustness of the model obtained because of the small number of samples. The quality of the PCA and PLS-DA model is described by R^2 and Q^2 values. R^2 is defined as the proportion of variance in the data explained by the model, indicating goodness of fit. Q^2 is defined as the proportion of variance in the data predicted by the model, indicating predictability [19]. Loading plots were used to identify the metabolites responsible for the separation of groups. Significant differences among metabolites in PLS-DA were assessed by the absolute value of correlation coefficient, $|r|$, which was calculated in a Java environment.

Statistical analysis

To detect significant differences between metabolic changes, the normalized integral values of 0.0015 ppm were input into SPSS

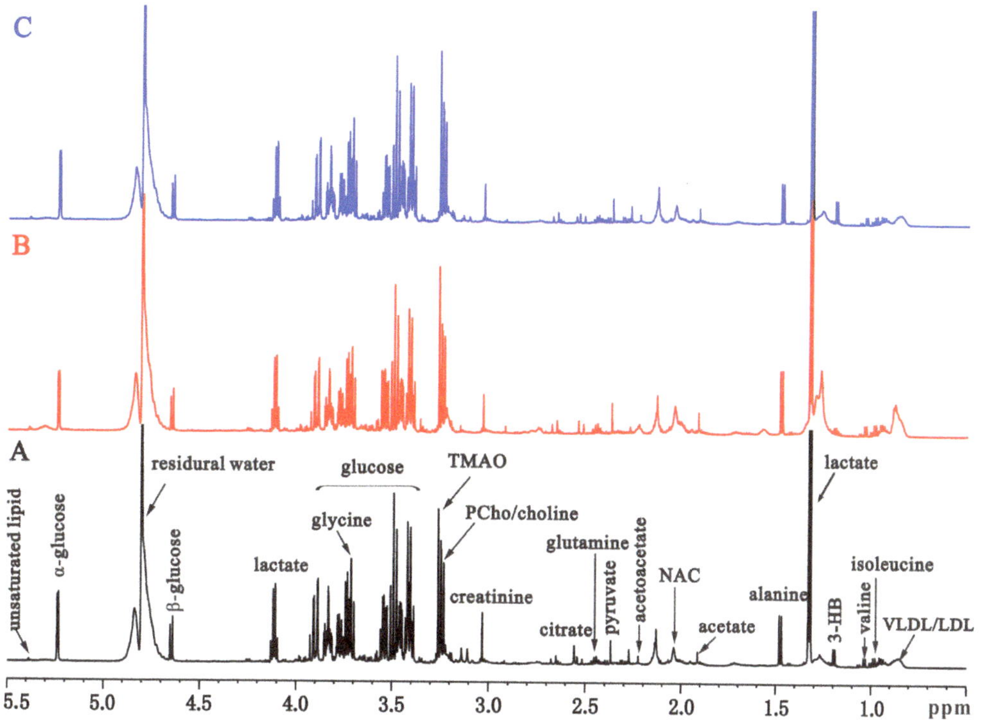

Figure 2. Representative ^{1}H CPMG spectra of serum obtained from the SO (A), UUO (B) and CAO (C) rats on day 7, respectively. NAC, N-acetylglycoproteins; TMAO, trimethylamine-N-oxide; 3-HB, 3-hydrobutyrate.

software (version 13.0, SPSS Inc, USA) for statistical analysis. Data were first analyzed using one-way analysis of ANOVA followed by the Dunnett's test (two-tailed). *P* value of less than 0.05 was considered statistically significant.

Results

Clinical chemical analysis and histopathology

Results of the biochemical analysis are depicted in **Table 1**. Compared with SO rats, distinct increase in serum LDL and HDL of UUO rats was observed at all investigated time points. For CAO rats, serum LDL concentration was significantly reduced by more than 50% of the level of UUO rats, whereas HDL concentration remained stable. Especially, after drug treatment for 7 days, almost all lipid indexes returned nearly to control levels, including TG. Indicators of renal (glomerular) function, SCr, and BUN levels were ameliorated markedly in CAO rats compared with UUO rats. While, these serum biochemical parameters were almost kept unchanged in CAO-SO rats. This suggested that renal function could be recovered by CAO agent dosage and the CAO treatment effect is specific to renal fibrosis. Interestingly, the SCr levels in CAO treated rats decreased significantly compared with the SO rats, which suggests that CAO modifying the creatinine metabolism might contribute a part of the mechanisms associated with CAO ameliorating renal fibrosis symptoms.

Figure 1 shows the representative images of the histological examination of HE-stained sections of kidneys from three groups of rats. SO rats does not exhibit abnormal histopathological changes (**Figure 1A**), whereas UUO rats display, to some extent, loss of brush border, interstitial inflammation, tubular swelling atrophy, and cystic dilation at both time points (**Figure 1B**). These findings suggested tubular injuries and fibrotic process in the kidney tissues from the rats during the whole experimental period. Meanwhile, CAO treatment significantly attenuated tubular damages in RIF rats on day 7, with the subjects showing no signs of tubular denaturation or necrosis, similar to the normal organizational structure of SO rats (**Figure 1C**). Interestingly, an apparent increase in tubular lesions and interstitial myofibroblasts were observed in CAO rats on day 28, similar to RIF rats (**Figure 1D**). Significant differences of the recovery trends among CAO-administrated rats illustrated the time-dependent therapeutic effects of CAO on RIF rats.

Time-dependent effects of CAO on the metabolic pattern of RIF rats

Representative ^{1}H NMR spectra of the serum samples obtained from SO, UUO, and CAO groups are shown in **Figure 2**. Resonance assignments were performed based on two-dimensional ^{1}H-^{1}H COSY and TOCSY spectra (data not shown) and our previous studies [20,21]. Firstly, to access changes of the metabolites concentration over time, the integral levels of serum samples from all the groups of the rats on days 3, 7, 14, and 28 were compared in **Table 2**. On both time points of day 7 and day 14, UUO rats showing increased levels of low-density lipoproteins/very low-density lipoproteins (LDL/VLDL), valine, leucine, isoleucine, alanine, acetate, trimethylamine-N-oxide (TMAO), creatine, and phosphatidylcholine/choline (PCho/choline), as well as decreased levels of 3-hydrobutyrate (3-HB), pyruvate, and glycine, comparing to the SO rats. Disturbances in endogenous metabolite levels were different between the earlier and later stages of RIF, and the trends were in good agreement with our previous results [22]. Interestingly, after CAO administration, disturbances in endogenous metabolite levels of UUO rats were almost recovered towards the control levels, especially on day 7 and day 14 timepoints. The results were supported by clinical

Table 2. Summary of change trends of metabolites significantly increased/decreased compared to SO or UUO groups in relative integral levels.

δ[1]H (ppm)	Metabolite	3 d		7 d		14 d		28 d	
		U vs. S	C vs. U	U vs. S	C vs. U	U vs. S	C vs. U	U vs. S	C vs. U
0.86,1.26	LDL/VLDL	↑*	—	↑*	↓*	↑*	↓*	↑*	↓*
0.94	Isoleucine	—	—	↑*	—	↑*	—	↑*	—
1.04	Valine	—	—	↑*	—	↑*	—	↑*	—
1.19	3-HB	↓*	—	↓*	↑*	↓*	↑*	↑*	↓*
1.32,4.10	Lacate	↓*	—	↓*	↑*	↑*	↓*	↑*	↓*
2.14	Acetoacetate	—	—	↑*	↓*	↑*	↓*	↑*	↓*
2.34	Pyruvate	—	↓*	↓*	↑*	↓*	↑*	↑*	↓*
2.52	Citrate	↓*	—	—	—	—	—	↑*	—
3.22	Pcho/choline	—	—	↑*	↓*	↑*	↓*	↓*	↓*
3.26	TMAO	↑*	↓*	↑*	↓*	↑*	↓*	↓*	—
3.54	Glycine	—	—	↓*	↑*	↓*	↑*	↓*	—
3.70–3.90	Glucose	—	↓*	↑*	↓*	↑*	↓*	↑*	↓*
5.30	Unsaturated lipid	↑*	—	↑*	↓*	↑*	↓*	↑*	↓*

S, sham-operation control group; U, unilateral ureteral obstruction group; C, Curcuma aromatica oil-treated group. 3-HB, 3-hydrobutyrate; TMAO, trimethylamine-N-oxide. Marks indicate the direction of the change, i.e. ↓ for decrease, ↑ for increase, – for no change.
*$P<0.05$ and
**$P<0.01$.

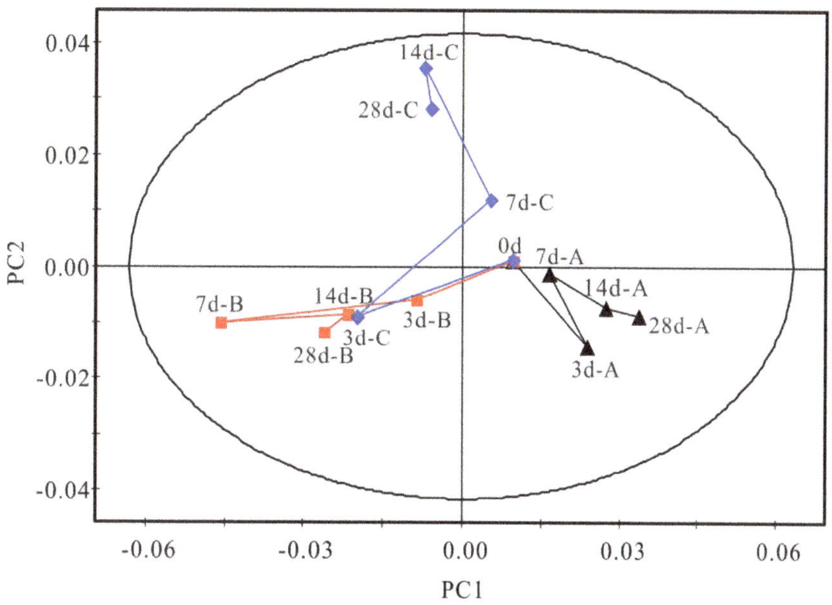

Figure 3. Time trajectory plot of mean data of serum ^{1}H CPMG spectra from SO (▲A), UUO (■B) and CAO (◆C) rats, respectively. The plot suggests time-dependent metabolic characteristics of different group rats.

chemistry and histopathology data, which substantiated that a time-dependent therapeutic effect of the agent in the body.

Then, to further evaluate the time-dependent interventional effect of CAO on renal fibrosis, average integral values of ^{1}H NMR spectra of all the serum samples were subjected to PLS-DA (**Figure 3**, $R^2X = 0.844$, $Q^2 = 0.738$), by which a pairwise day-to-day comparison can provide more details on the pathological process of the RIF. In the plot, a clear separation of trajectory diagrams of the UUO and SO groups was displayed, and the CAO group was almost located separated from UUO and SO groups. On day 7, the metabolic pattern of CAO rats ultimately approached to the region of SO rats, which suggested that the CAO treatment effect is significant to renal fibrosis on that timepoint. Interestingly, on days 14 and 28, while still located between the UUO and SO rats, the spot of CAO rats shifted farther from SO rats than that on day 7. All the data illustrated the renal fibrosis symptom of the RIF rats was prevented and alleviated by CAO treatment, and that maximum therapeutic efficacy of the agent was achieved after the drug administration for 7 days.

Metabonomic analysis of the CAO effect to RIF rats on day 7

To further explore the differences in the metabolic profiles of the treated groups, we subjected the samples of day 7 to PCA (**Figure 4**). We found that serum samples of CAO treated-SO rats were mixed in the cluster of SO rats, demonstrating that CAO treatment did not obviously alter the serum profile of SO rats. And CAO treated-UUO rats were clustered in the SO group, and separated with UUO group obviously (**Figure 4A**, $R^2X = 0.93$, $Q^2 = 0.835$), suggesting that dosage of the agent induced the metabolic profiles of the RIF rats to recover toward that of the control. This is in good agreement with the data of clinical biochemical analysis displayed above. **Figure 4B** shows the validation plot of permutation tests showed that the PCA model is robust and credible. **Figure 4C** illustrates the corresponding loading plot with color-coded correlation coefficients ($|r|$) of metabolites between different groups and shows the variables responsible for the separation of them. The weight of a variable in the discrimination is given by the square of its correlation coefficient, which is color-coded from zero in blue to high values in red. The negative regions in the loading plot corresponded to metabolites that increased in quantity in the serum of the rats, whereas positive regions corresponded to metabolites that decreased in quantity in the serum of rats.

To further verify the observed restoring effects of CAO treatment on RIF rats, box plots for typical metabolites concentration of serum samples on day 7 are displayed in **Figure 5**. Compared with that in UUO rats, most metabolites revealed manifest tendencies of recovery toward SO level in CAO rats, except for citrate, valine, leucine, and isoleucine (data not shown). Then the variations of metabolites allowed us to explore some important information about the mechanisms involved in molecular mechanism of the agent acting on renal fibrosis. **Figure 6** illustrates the altered metabolic pathways during the development of the disease, and drug-regulated targets based on the KEGG database (http://www.genome.jp/kegg/pathway.html).

Discussion

As a traditional herbal medicine, *Curcuma aromatica* has been widely used to treat arthritic pain, gastrointestinal, fibrosis, cancer in Asian countries such as India, Thailand, and China for a long time [23]. Modern medical research have demonstrated that *Curcuma aromatica* contains anti-inflammation, anti-oxidation, anti-viral, and anti-carcinogenic ingredients [23,24]. However, due to the multiple substances that comprise *Curcuma aromatica*, the detailed molecular mechanism of the active component in the body remains unclear. Metabonomics is an effective approach for evaluating the therapeutic effects of traditional herbal medicine. By identifying global metabolite levels and metabolic pathways after agent intervention, the approach opens up the possibility of studying the effect of multiple mixtures in complex biological systems, thereby bridging systems biology and traditional herbal

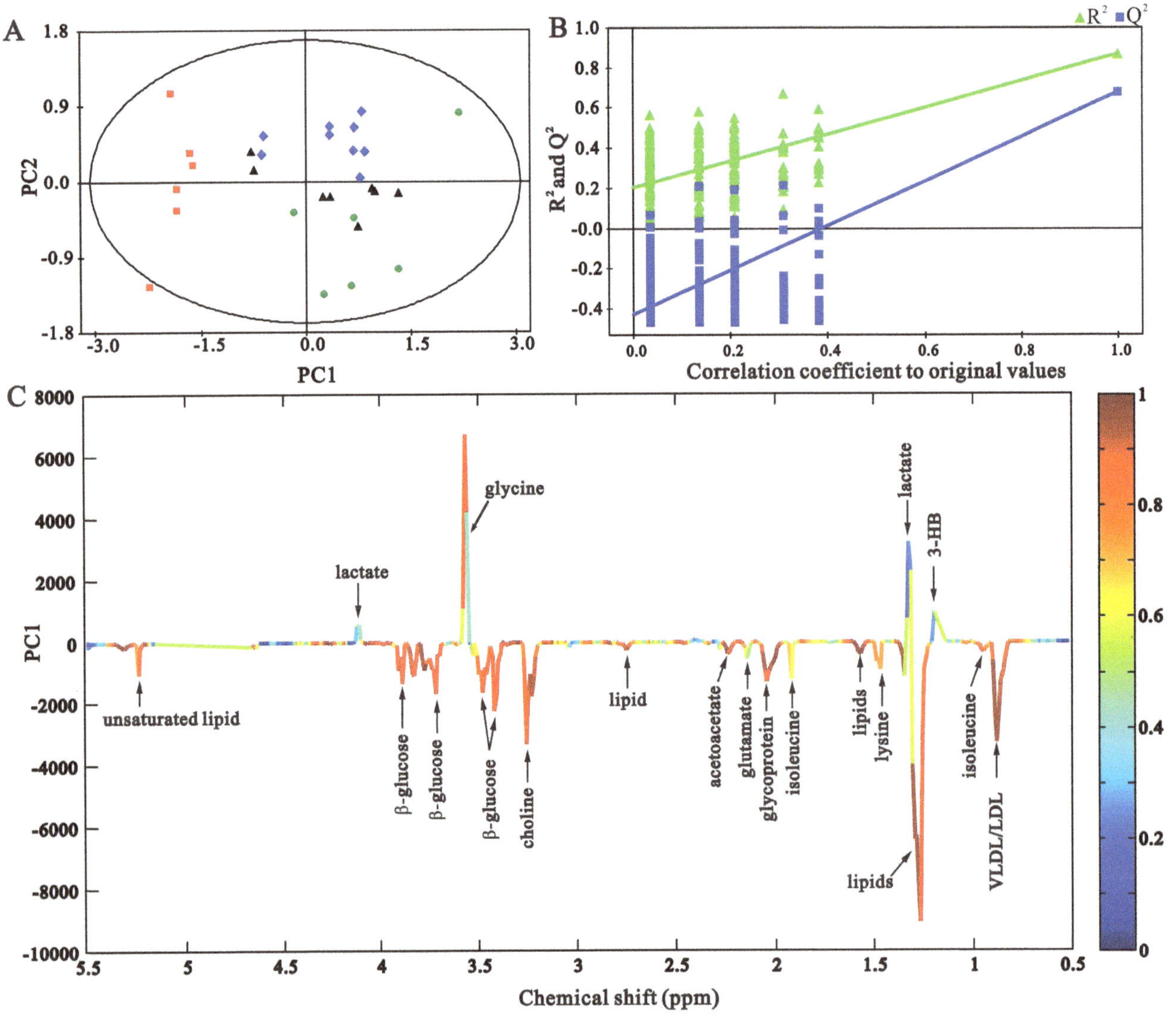

Figure 4. PCA scores plot (A), validation plot (B) and coefficient-coded loading plot (C) based on the ^{1}H CPMG spectra of control (▲), UUO (■), CAO-UUO (◆) and CAO-SO (●) rats on day 7. The coefficient-coded loading plot corresponding to PCA revealing the metabolites with large intensities responsible for the discrimination of the corresponding score plots.

medicine [2]. Thus, in this study, we applied quantitative metabonomics analysis to evaluate the therapeutic effect of CAO on RIF rats and to elucidate its underlying molecular mechanism.

In this study, the histopathological and metabolic analyses described above showed that treatment of CAO can prevent renal tissues from fibrosis injury in the early stage of RIF. Furhtermore, a pairwise day-to-day comparison by PLS-DA confirmed that CAO has the most manifest therapeutic effect on day 7 timepoint when the renal damage is mild. The metabolites altered and related pathways that appear to be regulated by CAO may represent potential metabolic biomarkers for disease diagnosis and provide clues to elucidate the molecular mechanism of the agent acting on renal fibrosis (**Figure 6**).

Lipids metabolism

Renal interstitial fibrosis is a multistep process involving inflammation, lipid nephrotoxicity, hypoxia, and oxidative stress. In this study, both biochemical and NMR analyses showed elevated concentration of VLDL/LDL, acetate, and triglycerides, as well as reduced level of 3-HB and acetoacetate (ketone body metabolism), in UUO rats. Excessive lipid accumulation in the blood of UUO rats stimulates the conversion of fatty acids into acetyl-CoA through the process of β-oxidation. As an important intermediate product of glucose and lipid metabolism, acetyl-CoA enters the TCA cycle or condenses into ketone bodies through which it is oxidized to supply the body with energy. Increased levels of VLDL/LDL and TG in the blood may be related to the reduction pathways of ketone bodies and TCA cycle metabolism in disease state. It was confirmed that hyperlipidemia had a profibrotic function in the pathogenesis of RIF [25]. In addition, as markers of medullar injury in the pathogenesis of kidney disease, increased PCho/choline and TMAO concentrations suggest enhanced N-oxidation of fatty acids in UUO rats [26]. The results of the study demonstrated that CAO dosage decreased the levels of TMAO, PCho/choline, and lipid metabolites in the

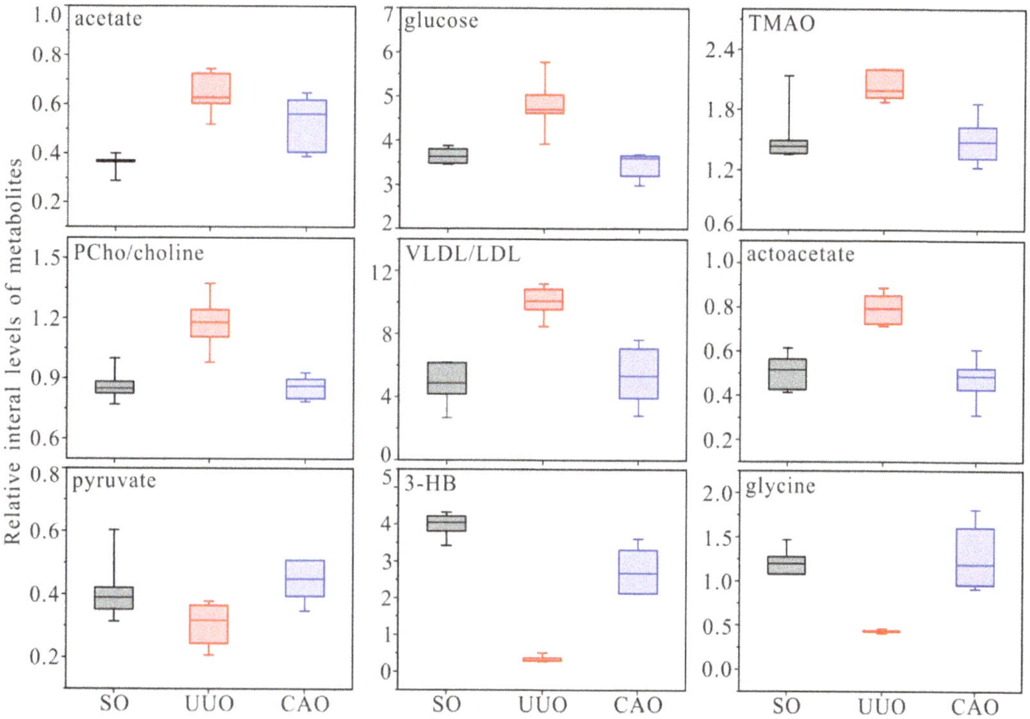

Figure 5. Box plots of relative integral levels of metabolites in serum samples of different groups of rats on day 7. The plots show that most of metabolic levels altered in UUO rats, are recovered to control level after CAO treatment.

serum, indicated that CAO may provide additional beneficial effects on renal injuries by lowering lipids levels in RIF rats.

Glucose metabolism

In earlier stages of RIF, the increased concentrations of glucose and lactate, as well as the decreased levels of pyruvate and citrate in the serum, are indicative of enhanced glycolysis and inhibited glucose oxidation process in model rats. Pyruvate, an important intermediate product of glycolysis and TCA cycle, is frequently associated with glycometabolism. It can be used to produce acetyl-CoA by the pyruvate dehydrogenase complex, after which it enters the TCA cycle, or it could be converted into alanine via alanine aminotransferase, into lactate via lactate dehydrogenase. It was reported that in the case of RIF, a large amount of acetyl-CoA was generated, which would exert a negative feedback on the activity of pyruvate dehydrogenase complex, thus inhibiting the pathway

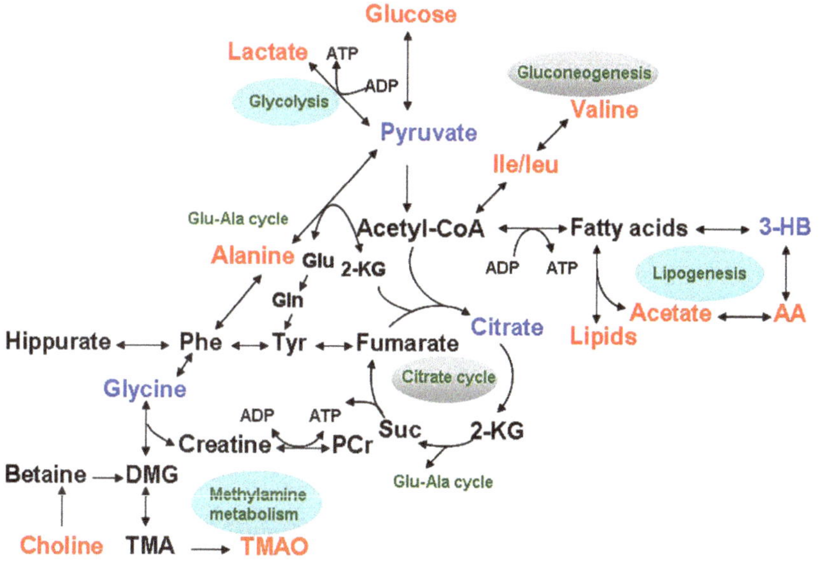

Figure 6. Disturbed metabolic pathways in serum of RIF rats treated with CAO. In UUO rats metabolites with increased and decreased levels compared to control rats are indicated in red and blue.

of TCA cycle and allowing the domination of two other outputs (lactate and glucogenic amino acids) [27]. Also the inhibited TCA cycle may be related to an impaired mitochondrial function in the proximal tubule of the RIF rats [28,29].

The enhanced pathway of the glycogenic amino acids (e.g., leucine, isoleucine and valine) metabolism possibly suggests tubular damage-induced protein degradation or disturbed protein synthesis [30]. In this study, decreased levels of pyruvate and citrate and elevated levels of lactate and certain glycogenic amino acids in earlier UUO stage indicate that glucose aerobic oxidation was inhibited and that the energy consumption pattern may have shifted to glycolysis and gluconeogenesis in response to RIF. Interestingly, after CAO treatment, the levels of glucose, lactate, and pyruvate recovered to control levels, whereas the concentration of citrate and glycogenic amino acids exhibited no change. These results suggest that CAO operates *in vivo*, probably by affecting the glycolysis pathway as opposed to the glucose oxidation and gluconeogenesis pathways.

Methylamine metabolism

Functioning as a conjugation acid of acetyl-CoA synthetase, glycine can protect renal cells from ATP depletion-induced injury [31,32] and keep proximal tubules from suffering from hypoxia, inflammation, and interstitial fibrosis [33]. The reduced level of glycine, and elevation of SCr and BUN in UUO rats as revealed by biochemical examination indicate the dysfunction of tubular reabsorption and perturbation in the methylamine metabolism pathway. Several other pivotal product concentrations, such as choline, creatine and TMAO discussed above, were enhanced in the serum of UUO rats. The increased levels of metabolites in the methylamine pathway in the disease state were restored toward control levels after CAO treatment, which supports the protective effects of the agent on renal tubular function by regulating the methylamine metabolism pathway.

Conclusions

In this work, NMR-based serum metabonomics analysis was applied to evaluate the effects of CAO dosage on RIF rats and to elucidate the underlying protective molecular mechanism. CAO treatment was found to significantly ameliorate renal fibrosis symptoms in time-dependent manner, especially in earlier RIF stage, by intervening in some dominating metabolic pathways, including glycolysis, lipid metabolism and methylamine metabolism. However, the other metabolic pathways altered in UUO rats, such as the gluconeogenesis and TCA cycle, were not ameliorated correspondingly in CAO-treated rats. Our results identified the main targets of the *Curcuma aromatica* agent that worked in the body, which need to be further studied with other complementary approaches including molecular biology and enzyme activity determination. This work also contributes to the evaluation of metabonomic technology on the efficacy of traditional herbal medicine and its underlying molecular mechanism.

Supporting Information

Figure S1 Representative HE-stained sections (200 fold) of kidneys from UUO (A), CAO doses of 100 mg/kg (B), 200 mg/kg (C) and 300 mg/kg (D) for 7 days, respectively. The UUO rats display clearly loss of brush border, tubular swelling atrophy and cystic dilation, while such histopathology damages were somewhat ameliorated in the CAO rats.
(EPS)

Table S1 Serum clinical chemistry parameters of different dosages of CAO on RIF rats for 7 days.
(DOCX)

Author Contributions

Conceived and designed the experiments: HG ZY YY. Performed the experiments: HZ YZ MD XY. Analyzed the data: HZ LZ GB. Contributed reagents/materials/analysis tools: YY ZY YW. Wrote the paper: HG LZ HZ.

References

1. Liu Y (2006) Renal fibrosis: new insights into the pathogenesis and therapeutics. Kidney Int 69: 213–217.
2. Wang M, Lamers RJ, Korthout HA, van Nesselrooij JH, Witkamp RF, et al. (2005) Metabolomics in the context of systems biology: bridging traditional Chinese medicine and molecular pharmacology. Phytother Res 19: 173–182.
3. Liao S, Gao HC, Li XK (2011) A preliminary study on the effect of curcuma aromatics on the renal fibrosis model rats. J Wenzhou Medical College 41: 3.
4. Hong JY, Sato EF, Kira Y, Nishikawa M, Shimada K, et al. (2006) Curcuma aromatica inhibits diabetic nephropathy in the rat. J Food Sci 71: S626–S632.
5. Gaedeke J, Noble NA, Border WA (2005) Curcumin blocks fibrosis in anti-Thy 1 glomerulonephritis through up-regulation of heme oxygenase 1. Kidney Int 68: 2042–2049.
6. Soetikno V, Sari FR, Lakshmanan AP, Arumugam S, Harima M, et al. (2012) Curcumin alleviates oxidative stress, inflammation, and renal fibrosis in remnant kidney through the Nrf2-keap1 pathway. Mol Nutr Food Res 57: 1649–1659.
7. Shyur LF, Yang NS (2008) Metabolomics for phytomedicine research and drug development. Curr Opin Chem Biol 12: 66–71.
8. Lu X, Xiong Z, Li J, Zheng S, Huo T, et al. (2010) Metabonomic study on 'Kidney-Yang Deficiency syndrome' and intervention effects of Rhizoma Drynariae extracts in rats using ultra performance liquid chromatography coupled with mass spectrometry. Talanta 83: 700–708.
9. Gu Y, Zhang Y, Shi X, Li X, Hong J, et al. (2010) Effect of traditional Chinese medicine berberine on type 2 diabetes based on comprehensive metabonomics. Talanta 81: 766–772.
10. Liang X, Chen X, Liang Q, Zhang H, Hu P, et al. (2011) Metabonomic study of Chinese medicine Shuanglong formula as an effective treatment for myocardial infarction in rats. J Proteome Res 10: 790–799.
11. Xie B, Gong T, Gao R, Liu J, Zuo J, et al. (2009) Development of rat urinary HPLC-UV profiling for metabonomic study on Liuwei Dihuang Pills. J Pharmaceut Biomed 49: 492–497.
12. Zhao L, Gao H, Zhao Y, Lin D (2012) Metabonomic analysis of the therapeutic effect of Zhibai Dihuang Pill in treatment of streptozotocin-induced diabetic nephropathy. J Ethnopharmacol 142: 647–656.
13. Wang M, Lamers RJAN, Korthout HAAJ, van Nesselrooij JHJ, Witkamp RF, et al. (2005) Metabolomics in the context of systems biology: bridging traditional Chinese medicine and molecular pharmacology. Phytother Res 19: 173–182.
14. Qiu J (2007) Traditional medicine: A culture in the balance. Nature 448: 126–128.
15. Chevalier RL, Forbes MS, Thornhill BA (2009) Ureteral obstruction as a model of renal interstitial fibrosis and obstructive nephropathy. Kidney Int 75: 1145–1152.
16. Grgic I, Kiss E, Kaistha BP, Busch C, Kloss M, et al. (2009) Renal fibrosis is attenuated by targeted disruption of KCa_3. 1 potassium channels. P Natl Acad Sci USA 106: 14518–14523.
17. Gao H, Dong B, Liu X, Xuan H, Huang Y, et al. (2008) Metabonomic profiling of renal cell carcinoma: high-resolution proton nuclear magnetic resonance spectroscopy of human serum with multivariate data analysis. Anal Chim Acta 624: 269–277.
18. Nicholson JK, Foxall PJD, Spraul M, Farrant RD, Lindon JC (1995) 750 MHz ^1H and ^1H-^{13}C NMR spectroscopy of human blood plasma. Anal Chem 67: 793–811.
19. Lindon JC, Nicholson JK (2008) Spectroscopic and statistical techniques for information recovery in metabonomics and metabolomics. Annu Rev Anal Chem 1: 45–69.
20. Gao H, Dong B, Liu X, Xuan H, Huang Y, et al. (2008) Metabonomic profiling of renal cell carcinoma: high-resolution proton nuclear magnetic resonance spectroscopy of human serum with multivariate data analysis. Anal Chim Acta 624: 269–277.
21. Garrod S, Humpfer E, Spraul M, Connor SC, Polley S, et al. (1999) High-resolution magic angle spinning ^1H NMR spectroscopic studies on intact rat renal cortex and medulla. Magn Reson Med 41: 1108–1118.

22. Zhang H, Jia J, Cheng J, Ye F, Li X, et al. (2012) ^{1}H NMR-based metabonomics study on serum of renal interstitial fibrosis rats induced by unilateral ureteral obstruction. Mol Biosyst 8: 595–601.
23. Jayaprakasha G, Jagan Mohan Rao L, Sakariah K (2005) Chemistry and biological activities of C. longa. Trends Food Sci Tech 16: 533–548.
24. Roth GN, Chandra A, Nair MG (1998) Novel bioactivities of Curcuma longa constituents. J Nat Prod 61: 542–545.
25. Khovidhunkit W, Kim MS, Memon RA, Shigenaga JK, Moser AH, et al. (2004) Effects of infection and inflammation on lipid and lipoprotein metabolism: mechanisms and consequences to the host. J Lipid Res 45: 1169–1196.
26. Bell JD, Lee JA, Lee HA, Sadler PJ, Wilkie DR, et al. (1991) Nuclear magnetic resonance studies of blood plasma and urine from subjects with chronic renal failure: identification of trimethylamine-N-oxide. Biochim Biophys Acta 1096: 101–107.
27. Song X, Wang J, Wang P, Tian N, Yang M, et al. (2013) ^{1}H NMR-based metabolomics approach to evaluate the effect of Xue-Fu-Zhu-Yu decoction on hyperlipidemia rats induced by high-fat diet. J Pharm Biomed Anal 78–79C: 202–210.
28. Wetmore DR, Joseloff E, Pilewski J, Lee DP, Lawton KA, et al. (2010) Metabolomic profiling reveals biochemical pathways and biomarkers associated with pathogenesis in cystic fibrosis cells. J Biol Chem 285: 30516.
29. Psihogios NG, Kalaitzidis RG, Dimou S, Seferiadis KI, Siamopoulos KC, et al. (2007) Evaluation of tubulointerstitial lesions' severity in patients with glomerulonephritides: An NMR-Based metabonomic study. J Proteome Res 6: 3760–3770.
30. Brosnan JT, Man KC, Hall DE, Colbourne SA, Brosnan ME (1983) Interorgan metabolism of amino acids in streptozotocin-diabetic ketoacidotic rat. Am J - Physiol 244: E151–158.
31. Kasuya F, Igarashi K, Fukui M (1999) Characterization of a renal medium chain acyl-CoA synthetase responsible for glycine conjugation in mouse kidney mitochondria. Chem-Biol Interact 118: 233–246.
32. Pan C, Bai X, Fan L, Ji Y, Li X, et al. (2005) Cytoprotection by glycine against ATP-depletion-induced injury is mediated by glycine receptor in renal cells. Biochem J 390: 447.
33. Yin M, Zhong Z, Connor HD, Bunzendahl H, Finn WF, et al. (2002) Protective effect of glycine on renal injury induced by ischemia-reperfusion in vivo. Am J Physiol-Renal 282: F417–423.

21

Chinese Proprietary Herbal Medicine Listed in 'China National Essential Drug List' for Common Cold

Wei Chen[1], George Lewith[2], Li-qiong Wang[1], Jun Ren[1], Wen-jing Xiong[1], Fang Lu[1], Jian-ping Liu[1]*

1 Centre for Evidence-Based Chinese Medicine, Beijing University of Chinese Medicine, Beijing, China, **2** Primary care and population Sciences, Medical School, University of Southampton, Southampton, United Kingdom

Abstract

Objective: Chinese proprietary herbal medicines (CPHMs) have long history in China for the treatment of common cold, and lots of them have been listed in the 'China national essential drug list' by the Chinese Ministry of Health. The aim of this review is to provide a well-round clinical evidence assessment on the potential benefits and harms of CPHMs for common cold based on a systematic literature search to justify their clinical use and recommendation.

Methods: We searched CENTRAL, MEDLINE, EMBASE, SinoMed, CNKI, VIP, China Important Conference Papers Database, China Dissertation Database, and online clinical trial registry websites from their inception to 31 March 2013 for clinical studies of CPHMs listed in the 'China national essential drug list' for common cold. There was no restriction on study design.

Results: A total of 33 CPHMs were listed in 'China national essential drug list 2012' for the treatment of common cold but only 7 had supportive clinical evidences. A total of 6 randomised controlled trials (RCTs) and 7 case series (CSs) were included; no other study design was identified. All studies were conducted in China and published in Chinese between 1995 and 2012. All included studies had poor study design and methodological quality, and were graded as very low quality.

Conclusions: The use of CPHMs for common cold is not supported by robust evidence. Further rigorous well designed placebo-controlled, randomized trials are needed to substantiate the clinical claims made for CPHMs.

Editor: Chang-Qing Gao, Central South University, China

Funding: This work is supported by a research capacity establishment grant from the State Administration of Chinese Medicine (201207007), the Program for Innovative Research Team of Beijing University of Chinese Medicine (2011-CXTD-09), and research fund for the outstanding young teachers of Beijing University of Chinese Medicine. The funders had no role in study design, data collection and analysis, decision to publish, or preparation of the manuscript.

Competing Interests: The authors have declared that no competing interests exist.

* Email: jianping_l@hotmail.com

Introduction

Common cold is often caused by rhinovirus [1]. Common symptoms include cough, sore throat, runny nose, fever, and etc. It is one of the most widespread illnesses in the world. On average, adults have two to three infections a year [2] and children have six to twelve a year [3]. The common cold is a mild and self-limiting illness that almost always resolves spontaneously. To date there is no effective treatment for common cold and the routine use of antibiotics for the common cold is not recommended [4]. Some alternative treatments are used for common cold; however, there is insufficient scientific evidence to support their use [3]. The recommended first line treatment for common cold is usually medication for symptom control to avoid the unnecessary prescription of antibiotics and the consequent risk of adverse drug reactions and antimicrobial resistance.

Chinese herbal medicines have long history in China for the treatment of common cold. It was recorded more than 2000 years ago in 'Inner Canon of Huangdi', the most acknowledged classics of TCM, that 'pathogenic wind can cause cold' [5]. Traditional Chinese medicine (TCM) practitioners and general public have deep belief that herbal medicines are effective in alleviating symptoms and shortening the duration of the common cold. Chinese proprietary herbal medicine (CPHMs) is an important component of Chinese herbs. It refers to Chinese herbs that mainly produced by modern manufacturing methods. CPHMs include different formulations such as powder, granule, pastille, tablet, and capsule, and are widely accepted by the Chinese population due to the convenience of application. Until now, More than two hundreds CPHMs have been authorized and listed in the 'China national essential drug list' (EDL), which is approved by the Chinese Ministry of Public Health and is regarded as the accepted reference point for the medicines used in medical institutions in China.

The World Health Organization (WHO) strategy calls for evidence-based TCM. In order to ensure evidence-based practice, we conducted systematic evaluation of all the CPHMs listed in the EDL 2012 for the treatment of common cold. Although RCT was acknowledged as the gold standard for therapeutic evaluation, we didn't want to neglect other designs because they might accounts for a large part of the clinical evidence. Our aim was to provide a well-round clinical evidence assessment of CPHMs for common cold based on a systematic literature search.

Methods

Inclusion criteria

Children and adults with the common cold were included. Typical symptoms include cough, sore throat, runny nose, sneezing, fever, and etc. Colds caused by influenza, acute bronchitis developing from a case of common cold, upper respiratory tract infection caused by bacteria, and patients concurrently suffering from other infectious or febrile diseases were excluded. There was no restriction on age and sex.

The interventions were confined to CPHMs listed in EDL 2012 for common cold. There was no restriction on study design. Systematic reviews (SR), randomized controlled trial (RCT), quasi-randomized controlled trial (Q-RCT), non-randomized controlled trial (NRCT), controlled before-and-after study (CBA), prospective cohort study (PCS), retrospective cohort study (RCS), historically controlled trial (HCT), nested case-control study (NCC), case-control study (CC), cross-sectional study (XS), before-and-after comparison (BA), case reports (CR), and case series (CS) were all identified. In order to reduce misclassification and inconsistencies, we used explicit study design features (as shown in Table S1) to facilitate our judgement on study design. Before assessment, two evaluators (WC, LQW) were trained to apply these standards consistently. Disagreement was resolved by discussion and consensus was reached through a third party (JPL).

For RCT, Q-RCT, NRCT, CBA, PCS, RCS, HCT, NCC, and CC studies, CPHMs compared with no treatment, placebo or conventional medication were included. Studies compared CPHM plus other interventions with other interventions alone were also included. CPHM combined with other TCM therapies (including acupuncture) compared with non-TCM therapies were excluded. Studies that compared different CPHMs were excluded. There was no restriction on language and publication type. Literatures that reported same data were be regarded as multiple publications and excluded.

Search strategy and study selection

The CENTRAL (2012, Issue 12) (http://www.cochrane.org/editorial-and-publishing-policy-resource/cochrane-central-register-controlled-trials-central), MEDLINE (http://www.ncbi.nlm.nih.gov/pubmed/), EMBASE (http://www.elsevier.com/online-tools/embase), SinoMed (Chinese Biomedical Literature Service System) (http://www.sinomed.ac.cn/), Chinese VIP information (VIP) (http://www.cqvip.com/), Chinese National Knowledge Infrastructure (CNKI) (http://www.cnki.net/),, China Important Conference Papers Database (http://www.cnki.net/), and China Dissertation Database (http://www.cnki.net/) were searched from their inception to 31 March 2013. The following search terms were used individually or combined: 'cold', 'nasopharyngitis', 'acute viral rhinopharyngitis', 'acute coryza', 'shang feng (cold in Chinese)', 'wai gan (cold in Chinese)', and 'feng han (cold in Chinese)'.

Website of the clinical trials registry including Chinese clinical trial registry (http://www.chictr.org/) and international clinical trial registry by U.S. national institutes of health (http://clinicaltrials.gov/) were also searched for ongoing registered clinical trials.

Two authors conducted the literature search (LQW, JR), study selection (WJX, FL) and data extraction (WC, LQW) independently. We extracted authors' name and title of study, year of publication, study design (detail of randomization if the study was RCT), sample size, demographic characteristics of the participants, name and component of CPHM, treatment process, detail of the control interventions, outcome and adverse effect for each study. Double check was conducted to reduce inconsistencies. Disagreement was resolved by discussion or through a third party (JPL).

Quality assessment

Two authors (WC, LQW) evaluated the quality of included studies independently. The quality of included RCTs were assessed by using the risk of bias tool according to the 'Cochrane Handbook of Systematic Reviews of Interventions' (Chapter 8) to address the following five criteria: random sequence generation, allocation concealment, blinding of participants and personnel, blinding of outcome assessment, incomplete outcome data, and selective reporting [6]. The quality of all the included trials was categorized to low/unclear/high risk of bias.

For the other study designs, different criteria were used. AMSTAR (A Measurement Tool to Access Reviews) [7] were used to assess the quality of SR, MINORS (Methodological Index for Non-Randomized Studies) [8] was used for NRCT, and NOS (Newcastle-Ottawa Scale) [9] was used for cohort and case-control studies. Due to the lack of acknowledged tool or scale for CR and CS, the quality assessment of these two studies was based on the explicit diagnostic criteria, detailed description of demographic characteristics, intervention, and acknowledged outcome measurements.

Data analysis

SPSS 19.0 statistics software (480c9826941a904069d8) was used for data analyses. Data were summarized using relative risk (RR) with 95% confidence intervals (CI) for binary outcomes or mean difference (MD) with 95% CI for continuous outcomes.

Results

Description of studies

Thirty-three CPHMs were listed in EDL 2012 for the treatment of common cold (the compositions, indications, and dosage of the 33 CPHMs were shown in Table S2). After primary searches, 83 citations were identified. The majority was excluded due to obvious ineligibility (for example, animal experiment, influenza, bacterial infection of the upper respiratory tract, and etc), 46 full text papers were retrieved and 13 studies [10–22] fulfilled the inclusion criteria (Figure 1). The excluded studies and reason for exclusion were listed in Table S3.

Search results showed that only 7 CPHMs had published supporting clinical evidence. These CPHMs were Chaihu injection (5 CSs, 1 RCT), Qingre Jiedu granules (1 CS, 1 RCT), Huoxiang Zhengqi liquid (1 CS), Ganmao Qingre granules (1 RCT), Shuanghuanglian oral liquid (1 RCT), Xiaoer Baotaikang granules 1 RCT), and Xiaoer Resuqing oral liquid (1 RCT). A total of 6 RCTs and 7 CSs were included. No other study design was identified. All the studies were conducted in China, and published in Chinese between 1995 and 2012. The first RCT was published in 1997 [21] and the rest were all published after 2007. No studies report on informed consent or on whether they were properly approved by an IRB. Only one trial [10] revealed funding sources (Taizhou Municipal Science and Technology Project).

The characteristics of included studies were listed in Table S4. A total of 2643 participants with common cold were involved, ranging from 20 to 1560 per study. Eight studies included children [10,11,13,16,19,20,22], 1 study included adults [17], and 4 studies

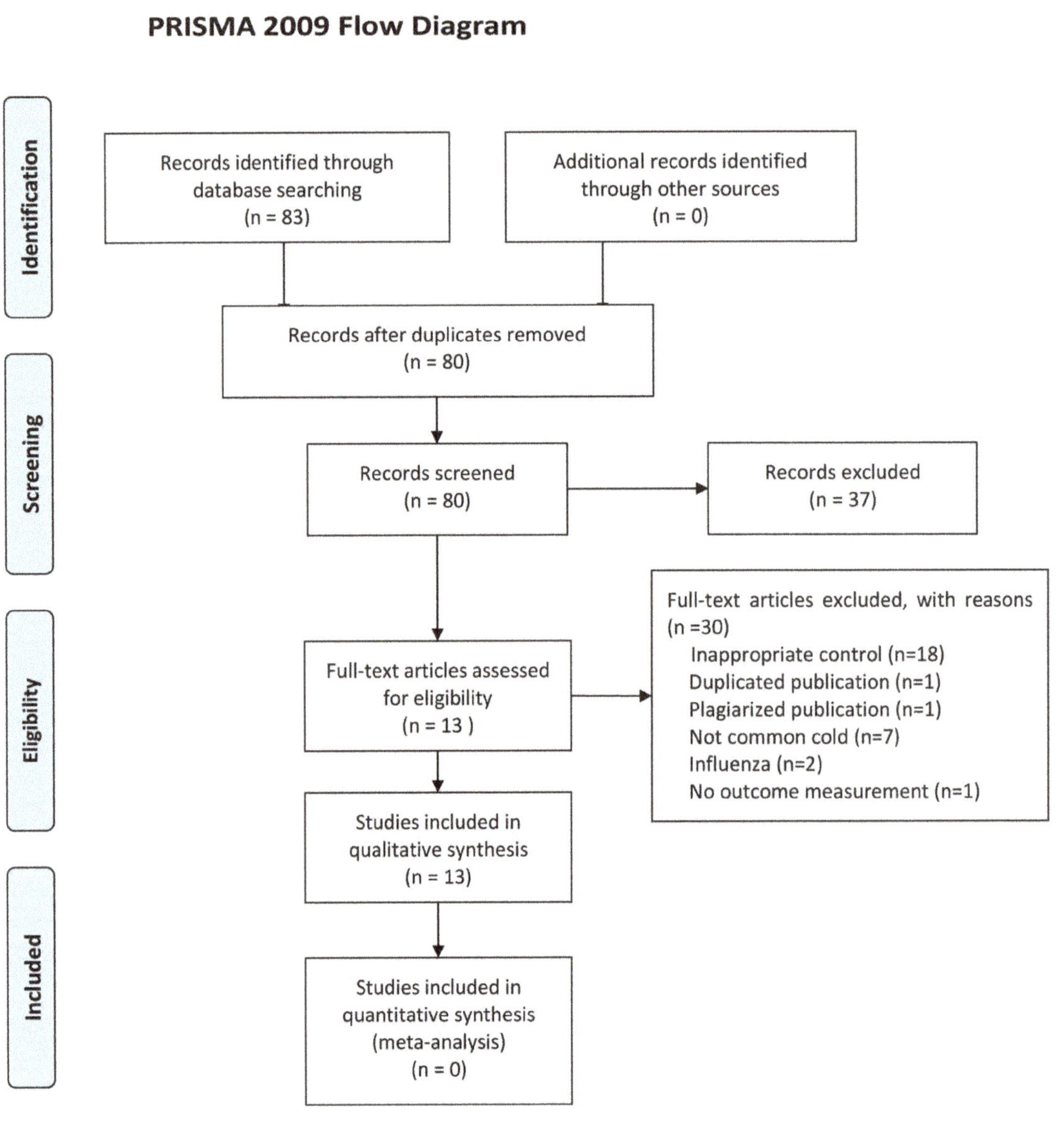

Figure 1. PRISMA 2009 Flow Diagram.

included both children and adults [12,14,15,18]. Five studies provided information on patients' syndrome differentiation (*Bianzheng*, TCM diagnosis) [16–19,21]. One trial used the diagnostic criterion for common cold of textbook 'practical paidonosology' [10], 1 trial used the diagnostic criterion of the China State Administration of Traditional Chinese Medicine, and the other 6 studies did not report their diagnostic criteria [11–15,20].

The routes of administration for CPHMs were quite diverse including oral intake, acupuncture point injection, intramuscular injection, retention enema, and nasal dripping. The treatment period was 3 to 5 days [11,14–17,19,21,22]. Four studies did not provide treatment period [12,13,18,20]. The reported outcomes were duration of fever, body temperature, or clinical symptoms improvement rate within a particular time. Clinical symptoms improvement rate was a composite measurement including a number of symptoms, of which body temperature was the vital one. Adverse events were reported in only 2 studies [12,18]. In Li 1997 [12], no allergic reaction was found. In Jiang 2012 [18], skin flushes, dizziness, and bitter taste in mouth were reported. While in the other 11 studies, the researchers did not reported whether or not they had monitored adverse events.

Therapeutic effects

Because common cold was a mild and self-limiting illness, we could not discriminate its spontaneous recovery with therapeutic effects by using the design of CSs. Therefore, we only calculated the therapeutic effects of CPHMs of RCTs (shown in Table S5). Results showed that Chaihu injection given at acupuncture point (LI 11) could shorten fever duration, Qingre Jiedu granules, Shuanghuanglian oral liquid, and Xiaoer Baotaikang granules had better clinical symptoms improvement rate within 3 days, and that Xiaoer Resuqing oral liquid had better clinical symptoms improvement rate within 5 days.

Methodological quality

Most of the included RCTs were of general poor methodological quality according to the predefined quality assessment criteria. Although 'random allocation' was mentioned in all RCTs, no trial described the methods for random sequence generation. We could not judge whether or not it was conducted properly due to the insufficient information. Allocation concealment and blinding were not reported in any RCT. No trial reported drop-outs or mentioned intention-to-treat analysis. Selective reporting was generally unclear in the RCTs due to the fact that all the RCT did not register before their start and we could not access to their trial protocol.

The included CSs were of very low quality. Most of the CSs did not reported diagnostic criterion, therefore it was possible that patients of influenza or upper respiratory tract infection caused by bacteria were included. Most of CSs did not provide a detailed description of baseline characteristics or treatment strategy. Moreover, most CSs used subjective outcome measurement such as cure rate, which was a self defined criteria and lacked unambiguous definition on outcome. Therefore made it difficult to interpret the effects even if the reported result was positive.

Discussion

In this review, only 7 CPHMs listed in EDL 2012 had clinical evidence to support their use for the common cold, and most of them only had one RCT or CS as supporting evidence. In addition, the evidence quality level of these 7 CPHMs were low due to the limitations in the design and implementation of studies. All studies had a very high likelihood of bias. Therefore the therapeutic effect of CPHM for the common cold should be taken in caution. More importantly, the fact that more than 80% of the CPHMs recommended in the EDL 2012 were not supported by clinical evidence revealed the enormous lack of evidence base that currently underpinned clinical use and policy making in China.

In August 2009, the 'Chinese national essential drug system' was officially launched and implemented. The 'Chinese national essential drug list' (2009 edition) has been issued in the same year [23]. The EDL was adjusted every 3 years and in the year 2012, the newest 2012 edition was published. The EDL 2012 contains 520 medicines, including 317 chemicals and biological products and 203 CPHMs. The CPHMs listed in EDL cover 137 kinds of internal medicine, 11 kinds of surgical medicine, 20 kinds of gynecological medicine, 7 kinds of ophthalmological medicine, 13 kinds of otorhinolaryngological medicine, and 15 kinds of orthopedics and traumatological medicine. The scope and number of CPHMs in the EDL 2012 was listed in Appendix S1. More than 3,100 medical and clinical experts had been assembled to evaluate the safety, effectiveness and economy of CPHMs. The selection process of medicine into EDL was strictly in accordance with the principle that they 'must be preventive and curative, safe and effective, affordable, easy to use, think highly of both Chinese and Western medicine' [24]. The detailed procedure for evaluation was not available because they were confidential files. However, our study demonstrated that they were less likely to be 'evidence-based' and revealed the sharp contrast between the policy and priority given to by the Chinese government to TCM.

In our review, the control interventions included antibiotics, antivirus drugs, and antipyretic and analgesic drugs. It was known that antibiotics had no effect against viral infections. Ribavirin and moroxydine were not recommended treatments for common cold. For mild and self-limiting illness which had no proved effective treatment, like common cold, randomized placebo controlled trial was the best study design to investigate the therapeutic effect. However, in this review, we did not find placebo controlled RCT. In addition, all the clinical studies were of poor methodology, which frequently happened for Chinese clinical studies. For RCTs, methodology such as randomisation, blinding and placebo controls were not used. No trial reported drop-out or withdrawal, or mentioned intention-to-treat analysis. Poor methodology suggested the positive interpretation of the therapeutic effect of CPHMs could be biased, so claims about their effectiveness should be interpreted with caution. For CSs, we could not discriminate spontaneous recovery with therapeutic effects using the design of CSs due to the lack of comparison. The positive result itself drawn from a CS was not reliable. In addition, all the included CSs had poor methodology quality which was embodied in lack of diagnostic criterion, inadequate description of baseline characteristics or treatment strategy, and inappropriate outcome measurement, and therefore downgraded the reliability of the positive results. We thought part of the reason for the poor quality of TCM studies was that the research training in evidence-based medicine and critical appraisal had only just begun in China. There remains urgent need to train Chinese researchers in conducting unbiased trials in the future. Recently the government had increased the investment in TCM research, and many research activities were on-going in academic institutions and universities. With increasing awareness of the international guidelines for reporting of clinical trials, we hope the picture may change in future.

In the era of EBM, we need better evidence for CPHMs, and to achieve this we need to do thoughtful, placebo-controlled trials with proper randomization and blinding and, above all else, we need to think carefully about inappropriate control and outcome assessment. In the literature searching, a total of 18 trials were excluded due to inappropriate control. As a control, the drug should be definite effective or definite ineffective, or was widely used in clinical practice. During the literature searching, we found lots of trials which compared CPHM with another Chinese herb. We could not prove that the Chinese herb used as control was effective for common cold because we could not find any previous placebo-controlled trials on the treatment of this Chinese herb. Therefore, we have to exclude them. Using two different Chinese herbs as mutual comparison was a common mistake in TCM clinical trials in China and future researchers should be aware of this and make the correction. In our review, all the Chinese studies were so dependent on the presence or absence of fever as opposed to other symptoms, and this was at odds with the way Western medicine tends to design its evaluation of upper and lower respiratory tract infections. Most of the studies used body temperature or duration of fever as the main or exclusive outcome. For the studies that used composite criteria such as 'clinical symptoms improvement rate', body temperature was also a vital component. However, fever is just one of the symptoms and by no means the primary outcome because simple respiratory infections caused a range of symptoms (sore throat, muscle aches, sometimes gastrointestinal upset, runny nose, etc). Our suggestion to the future researchers was to use well validated outcome measurements and to consider all the related symptoms. A patient-reported daily symptom diary including symptom variables giving each symptom a score would be a valuable approach. Patients could also completed Likert scales of how satisfied or concerned they were with different aspects of treatment. These Likert scales have previously been shown to be reliable, have good construct validity, and predict illness duration [25–27].

In our review, we searched all studies assessing the CPHMs for treatment of common cold regardless of study design. However, only CSs and RCTs were identified. The possible reasons might be that in China few TCM practitioners, researchers, and journal editors have received scientific research methodology training [28–30]. Articles based on case series were more acceptable during the 1990s and early 2000's as they were closer to clinical practice. Since the year of 2000, with the spread of evidence-based medicine, more and more TCM practitioners began to use RCTs because it was regarded as the gold standard for evaluating therapeutic effects. That was why we did not find other study designs.

In our review, all the included 13 studies were published in 12 different journals. The 12 journals were all legitimate Chinese medical journals. However, only 5 journals were rated as the core journals in China. The grade of journal was thought related to the quality of the trials it published. We suggest the editors of all TCM journals to be trained on clinical research methodology to ensure the scientific scrutiny for published researches.

The report of adverse events of CPHMs was not adequate. One study [12] reported that no allergic reaction was found; one study [18] reported skin flushes, dizzy and bitter taste. However, their reports were too brief to providing useful information. Turner observed that adverse events were often not well-reported in CAM RCTs [31]. In China, it was commonly believed that CPHMs was safer than western medicine. However, the increasing reports of adverse events associated with Chinese herbal medicines have excited attentions [32–34]. More and more TCM researchers began to investigate the specific mechanism of ingredient of Chinese herbs and its safety. TCM investigators for future study should be encouraged to monitor and report adverse events in clinical trials to GCP standards in order to evaluate the potential harms of CPHMs.

We have found that a systematic review titled 'Chinese medicinal herbs for the common cold' has been published in the Cochrane library in 2007 [35]. In this review, the author assessed the effect of Chinese medicinal herbs for the common cold. They only included RCT and included both CPHMs and individually prescribed herbal formulae. Our review is different from Zhang 2007 [35] not only in aim, but also in inclusion criteria, search strategy, analysis, and problem revealed. Our aim was to provide a well-round clinical evidence assessment of state authorized recommended CPHMs for common cold. Therefore we included all study designs and restricted CPHMs as those in the EDL.

The limitation of our review was that there were 6 studies that did not provided their diagnostic criteria, just mentioned that 'common cold patients were included'. We did not exclude them with the intent to providing more information in our review. Thereafter, possibility existed that participants with other acute respiratory infections such as influenza were recruited.

In summary, a confirmative conclusion on the beneficial effect of CPHMs for common cold still cannot be drawn. To ensure evidence-based clinical practice, further rigorous placebo-controlled, randomized trials are warranted. Further TCM researchers should pay more attention to reducing risks of bias and other limitations of trials, and improving the reporting quality by complying with international reporting standards such as the CONSORT [36], in addition, more emphasis should be paid on the selection of control intervention and outcome measurement. Too much dependent on the presence of absence of fever is not recommended.

The rough results of this review have been published in abstract form in the Journal of Alternative and Complementary Medicine as a conference paper for the 2014 International Research Congress on Integrative Medicine and Health [37].

Supporting Information

Table S1 List of study design features.
(DOCX)

Table S2 Compositions and indications of 33 CPHMs listed in 'China national essential drug list 2012' for common cold.
(DOCX)

Table S3 List of the excluded studies with reasons.
(DOCX)

Table S4 The characteristics of included studies.
(DOC)

Table S5 Effect estimations of CPHMs for treatment of common cold in included trials.
(DOCX)

Checklist S1 PRISMA 2009 checklist.
(DOC)

Appendix S1 The scope and number of CPHMs in the 'Chinese national essential drug list 2012'.
(DOCX)

Author Contributions

Conceived and designed the experiments: WC JPL. Performed the experiments: WC LQW JR WJX FL. Analyzed the data: WC LQW. Wrote the paper: WC. Revised the manuscript: GL.

References

1. Turner RB. (2001) The treatment of rhinovirus infections: progress and potential. Antiviral Research 49: 1–4.
2. Eccles R. (2005) Understanding the symptoms of the common cold and influenza. Lancet Infect Dis 5: 718–725.
3. Simasek M, Blandino DA. (2007) Treatment of the common cold. American Family Physician 75: 515–520.
4. Kenealy T, Arroll B. (2013) Antibiotics for the common cold and acute purulent rhinitis. Cochrane Database Syst Rev 6: CD000247.
5. Yang SS. (1965) Inner Canon of Huangdi·Taisu. Beijing: People's Medical Publishing House.
6. Higgins JPT, Altman DG, Sterne JAC. (editors) (2011) Chapter 8: Assessing risk of bias in included studies. In: Higgins JPT, Green S (editors). Cochrane Handbook for Systematic Reviews of Interventions Version 5.1.0 (updated March 2011). The Cochrane Collaboration, 2011. Available from www.cochrane-handbook.org.
7. Shea BJ, Grimshaw JM, Wells GA, Boers M, Andersson N, et al. (2007) Development of AMSTAR: a measurement tool to assess the methodological quality of systematic reviews. BMC Med Res Methodol 15: 10.
8. Slim K, Nini E, Forestier D, Kwiatkowski F, Panis Y, et al. (2003) Methodological index for non-randomized studies (minors): development and validation of a new instrument. ANZ J Surg 73: 712–716.
9. GA Wells, B Shea, D O'Connell, J Peterson, V Welch, et al. The Newcastle-Ottawa Scale (NOS) for assessing the quality of nonrandomised studies in meta-analyses. Available: http://www.ohri.ca/programs/clinical_epidemiology/oxford.asp. Accessed 24 October 2013.
10. Lv GQ. (2010) Chaihu injection acupoint block in treating pediatric cold and fever. Inner Mongol Journal of Traditional Chinese Medicine 29: 151–152.
11. Dai LH. (1995) Chaihu auricular point injection in treating pediatric cold and fever in 84 cases. Journal of Henan College of Traditional Chinese Medicine 10: 45.
12. Li ZX, Liu XP. (1997) Chaihu injection enema retention in treating cold and fever in 30 cases. Shanxi J of Traditional Chinese Medicine 13: 16.
13. Wang ZY. (2003) Chaihu injection enema retention in treating pediatric cold and fever in 26 cases. Journal of Emergency in Traditional Chinese Medicine 12: 503.
14. Zhang HY, Wang YF. (2009) Chaihu injection nasal dripping in treating cold and fever. Qingdao Medical Journal 36: 431–432.

15. Wang LZ. (1999) Chaihu injection in treating cold and fever. Shandong Journal of Traditional Chinese Medicine 18: 282.
16. Zhao MD. (2012) Clinical research on Qingre Jiedu granules in treating children with viral upper respiratory tract infection in 106 cases. Chinese Community Doctors 14: 223–224.
17. Xu HQ, Zhao JC. (2010) Clinical report of Qingre Jiedu granules in treating wind-heat type of common cold in 90 cases. Medical Journal of Chinese People's Health 22: 132.
18. Jiang XQ, Chen SQ, Yuan JX. (2012) Analysis of 1560 patients taking Huoxiang Zhengqi liquid in our hospital department of traditional Chinese medicine. Guangming Journal of Chinese Medicine 27: 386–387.
19. Di JH. (2012) Clinical observation of Ganmao Qingre granules in treating pediatric wind-cold type of common cold in 30 cases. Chinese Pediatrics of Integrated Traditional and Western Medicine 4: 277–278.
20. Wang HR, Wang YF. (1997) Clinical observation of Shuanghuanglian oral liquid in treating children with upper respiratory tract infection. Qingdao Medical Journal 29: 40.
21. Wu CF, Guan MC, Chi XW. (2012) Clinial observation of Xiaoer Baotaikang granules in treating children with upper respiratory tract infection. Strait Pharmaceutical Journal 24: 239–240.
22. Li QF, Song M. (2007) Clinical observation of Xiaoer Resuqing oral liquid in treating pediatric cold and fever. Shandong Medical Journal 47: 24.
23. The Central People's Government of the People's Republic of China (2009) Healthy ministry: Chinese project of establishing national essential drug system was officially launched. Available: http://www.gov.cn/gzdt/2009-08/18/content_1395565.htm. Accessed 12 May 2014.
24. National Health and Family Planning Commission of the People's Republic of China (2013) The 'Chinese national essential drug list' (2012 edition) has been published. Available: http://www.moh.gov.cn/mohywzc/s3582/201303/b058a4edf14e4dc9a1f6f0f0c71a2ccc.shtml. Accessed 12 May 2014.
25. Little P, Rumsby K, Kelly J, Watson L, Moore M, et al. (2005) Information leaflet and antibiotic prescribing strategies for acute lower respiratory tract infection: a randomized controlled trial. JAMA 293: 3029–3035.
26. Little P, Gould C, Williamson I, Moore M, Warner G, et al. (2001) Pragmatic randomised controlled trial of two prescribing strategies for childhood acute otitis media. BMJ 322: 336–342.
27. Williamson IG, Rumsby K, Benge S, Moore M, Smith PW, et al. (2007) Antibiotics and topical nasal steroid for treatment of acute maxillary sinusitis: a randomized controlled trial. JAMA 298: 2487–2496.
28. Zhang Y, An R, He LY, Chen LN, Liu SY, et al. (2010) Investigation and analysis on actuality and demands of scientific researchers in state clinical research facility of TCM. International Journal of Traditional Chinese Medicine 32: 523–524.
29. Han M, Tian N, Yang GY, Liu GH, Chen J, et al. (2013) Survey and Analysis on Basic Status of Clinical Scientific Researchers of the National Chinese Medicine Clinical Research Base. Modernization of Traditional Chinese Medicine-World Science and Technology 15: 1771–1775.
30. An R. (2011) Investigations and analysis of professional work building of the National Chinese Medicine Clinical Research Base. [Dissertation of Master's Degree]: Beijing university of Chinese Medicine.
31. Turner LA, Singh K, Garritty C, Tsertsvadze A, Manheimer E, et al. (2011) An evaluation of the completeness of safety reporting in reports of complementary and alternative medicine trials. BMC Complement Altern Med 11: 67.
32. Gottieb S. (2000) Chinese herb may cause cancer. BMJ 320: 1623.
33. Ishizaki T, Sasaki F, Ameshima S, Shiozaki K, Takahashi H, et al. (1996) Pneumonitis during interferon and/or herbal drug therapy in patients with chronic active hepatitis. European Respiratory Journal 9: 2691–2696.
34. Melchart D, Linde K, Weidenhammer W, Hager S, Shaw D, et al. (1999) Liver enzyme elevations in patients treated with traditional Chinese medicine. JAMA 282: 28–29.
35. Zhang X, Wu T, Zhang J, Yan Q, Xie L, et al. (2007) Chinese medicinal herbs for the common cold. Cochrane Database of Systematic Reviews Issue 1. Art. No.: CD004782. DOI: 10.1002/14651858.CD004782.pub2.
36. Moher D, Hopewell S, Schulz KF, Montori V, Gøtzsche PC, et al, for the CONSORT Group. (2010) CONSORT 2010 Explanation and Elaboration: updated guidelines for reporting parallel group randomised trial. BMJ 340: c869.
37. Chen W, Wang LQ, Liu JP. (2014) Chinese Patent Medicines Listed in China National Essential Drug List for Common Cold: An Evidence Synthesis. The Journal of Alternative and Complementary Medicine. 5: A128–A128.

Chinese Herbal Medicine Suppresses Invasion-Promoting Capacity of Cancer-Associated Fibroblasts in Pancreatic Cancer

Lianyu Chen[1,2], Chao Qu[1,2], Hao Chen[1,2], Litao Xu[1,2], Qi Qi[1,2], Jianmin Luo[2], Kun Wang[1,2], Zhiqiang Meng[1,2], Zhen Chen[1,2]*, Peng Wang[1,2]*, Luming Liu[1,2]*

1 Department of Integrative Oncology, Fudan University Shanghai Cancer Center, Shanghai, China, 2 Department of Oncology, Shanghai medical college, Fudan University, Shanghai, China

Abstract

Pancreatic cancer remains one of the leading causes of cancer-related deaths, due to aggressive growth, high metastatic rates during the early stage and the lack of an effective therapeutic approach. We previously showed that Qingyihuaji (QYHJ), a seven-herb Chinese medicine formula, exhibited significant anti-cancer effects in pancreatic cancer, associated with modifications in the tumor microenvironment, particularly the inhibition of cancer-associated fibroblast (CAF) activation. In the present study, we generated CAF and paired normal fibroblast (NF) cultures from resected human pancreatic cancer tissues. We observed that CAFs exhibited an enhanced capacity for inducing pancreatic cancer cell migration and invasion compared with NFs, while QYHJ-treated CAFs exhibited decreased migration and invasion-promoting capacities in vitro. The results of further analyses indicated that compared with NFs, CAFs exhibit increased CXCL1, 2 and 8 expression, contributing to the enhanced invasion-promoting capacities of these cells, while QYHJ treatment significantly suppressed CAF proliferation activities and the production of CAF-derived CXCL1, 2 and 8. These in vitro observations were confirmed in mice models of human pancreatic cancer. Taken together, these results suggested that suppressing the tumor-promoting capacity of CAFs through Chinese herbal medicine attenuates pancreatic cancer cell invasion.

Editor: Donald Gullberg, University of Bergen, Norway

Funding: This study was supported by National Science Fundation of China (81001061, 81370068, 81273953, 81173461); Shanghai Nature Science Fund, Shanghai, China (09ZR1406800); Doctoral Programs Foundation of Ministry of Education of China (20090071120076); Shanghai Science and Technology Committee Rising-Star Program (11QA1401300); Medical Talents Training Program of Health Bureau of Shanghai (XYQ2011008); and Fudan University Zhuo-Xue program. The funders had no role in study design, data collection and analysis, decision to publish, or preparation of the manuscript.

Competing Interests: The authors have declared that no competing interests exist.

* E-mail: llm1010@yahoo.com.cn (LL); wangp413@163.com (PW); cz.chenzhen@gmail.com (ZC)

These authors contributed equally to this work.

Introduction

Due to aggressive growth and a high metastatic rate during the early stage, pancreatic cancer remains a highly lethal malignant disease [1], and only approximately 10–20% of pancreatic cancer is resectable at the time of diagnosis [2]. Gemcitabine has been the standard treatment for advanced pancreatic cancer; however, the median survival is 5–6 months, with the frequent development of chemo-resistance during the treatment [3]. Thus, pancreatic cancer remains a dreadful disease, and there is an urgent need of further studies to reveal the molecular mechanisms of tumor invasion and metastasis to develop an effective therapeutic approach to prevent and/or treat of pancreatic cancer.

Cancer associated fibroblasts (CAFs), predominant components of the tumor stroma, have been extracted from several invasive human carcinomas, including pancreatic cancer [4,5,6]. Pancreatic ductal adenocarcinoma is characterized by an extensive stromal response called desmoplasia [7]. Within the tumor stroma, CAFs are the primary cell type, which play an important role in tumor progression [5]. CAFs secrete multiple factors, including CXC, CC chemokines, and other inflammatory mediators, that promote the proliferation, invasion, and metastasis of cancer cells. Moreover, accumulating evidence has demonstrated that CAFs play a key role in the acquisition of drug resistance in tumor therapy [8], which negatively impacts clinical outcomes [9,10]. Therefore, inhibiting the activation of CAFs might represent a potential therapeutic approach for pancreatic cancer treatment.

QYHJ, a seven-herb Chinese medicinal formula used for treating pancreatic cancer in China, inhibits both tumor growth and metastasis in nude mice models of pancreatic cancer [11,12,13]. In addition, the combined use of QYHJ with conventional Western medicine prolongs survival time in patients with liver metastases from pancreatic cancer [14]. However, the underlying molecular mechanism remains unclear.

Here, we demonstrated that CAFs exhibited an enhanced capacity for inducing pancreatic cancer cell migration and invasion compared with NFs, while QYHJ-treated CAFs exhibited decreased migration- and invasion-promoting capacities in vitro. In addition, we showed that compared with NFs, CAFs express high levels of CXCL1, 2 and 8, contributing to the enhanced invasion-promoting capacity of these cells. Thus, QYHJ treatment could suppress the proliferation activities and CXCL1, 2 and 8 expression levels in CAFs. Taken together, these results suggest that suppressing the tumor-promoting capacity of CAFs with Chinese herbal medicine attenuates pancreatic cancer cell invasion.

Materials and Methods

Ethics Statement

All animal experiments were conducted in accordance with the guidelines of the National Institutes of Health for the Care and Use of Laboratory Animals. The study protocol was also approved through the Committee on the Use of Live Animals in Teaching and Research, Fudan University, Shanghai. At the end of the study, all animals were decapitated through spinal cord separation at the nuchae to minimize suffering. The fibroblasts were isolated from resected tissues of two patients with pancreatic ductal adenocarcinomas (PDAC). Before sample collection, written informed consent was obtained from each patient in accordance with institutional guidelines, and the study was approved through the committees for the ethical review of research at the Fudan University Shanghai Cancer Center.

Cell Lines and Mice

The human pancreatic cancer cell line Capan1 and BxPC3 were obtained from the American Type Culture Collection, and cultured in Dulbecco's modified Eagle medium (DMEM; Gibco, Carlsbad, CA) supplemented with 10% fetal bovine serum (FBS; Gibco, Carlsbad, CA) at 37 °C with 5% CO_2. The morphology of the Capan1 cell line was regularly assessed, and the cells were tested for the absence of mycoplasma contamination (MycoAlert, Lonza, Rockland, ME, USA). The Capan1 and BxPC3 cell lines at the 30~40 passages were used in our study.

Female BALB/c-nu/nu nude mice aged 4–6 weeks were obtained from the Shanghai Institute of Materia Medica, Chinese Academy of Sciences (Shanghai, China), housed in laminar flow cabinets under specific pathogen-free conditions and provided food and water *ad libitum*.

Isolation of CAFs and paired NFs

Stromal fibrolasts were isolated as previously described [15]. Briefly, surgically resected pancreatic cancer tissues were obtained from two patients with pancreatic ductal adenocarcinoma. Written informed consent was obtained before tissue collection. The fresh pancreas tumor tissue and adjacent normal tissue (at least 2 cm from the outer tumor margin) were minced into 1–3 mm^3 fragments and digested with 0.25% trypsin at 37°C for 30 min. The resulting fragments were centrifuged at 600 xg for 5 min and washed once with DMEM containing 10% fetal bovine serum. The tissue fragments were subsequently plated and incubated at 37°C. The culture medium was changed twice a week for 3–4 weeks. Under these conditions, fibroblasts were explanted from tissue fragments while other cells were mostly retained in the tissue. Fibroblasts formed multi-layer colonies spreading on the culture dish. After 3–4 weeks cultured cells were roughly trypsinized and re-plated into T25 culture flasks (passage one). The fibroblasts were then sub-cultured for another 2–3 passages until the cultures were free of contamination of epithelial cells and subsequently maintained in DMEM supplemented with 10% fetal bovine serum, 2% penicillin and streptomycin (Invitrogen, Carlsbad, CA, USA). The cells were grown at 37°C in a humidified atmosphere containing 5% CO_2.NF and CAF strains were used at the 4–5 passages.

Immunohistochemistry and immunofluorescence

Immunohistochemistry (IHC) was performed as previously described [16]. Briefly, the tumor tissue samples were fixed in 10% formalin and embedded in paraffin wax. Unstained 3-μm sections were subsequently cut from the paraffin blocks for IHC analysis. The sections were stained with the following antibodies: rabbit anti-vimentin (1:200), rabbit anti-α-SMA (1:100), rabbit anti-CXCL1 (1:100), rabbit anti-CXCL2 (1:200), and rabbit anti-CXCL8 (1:25) at 4°C overnight. The sections were incubated with secondary antibodies, and the avidin-biotin peroxidase complex was used according to the manufacturer's instructions (Vector Laboratories, CA, USA). An immunoglobulin-negative control was used to rule out non-specific binding. Two independent investigators and one pathologist, all of whom were blinded to the model/treatment type for the series of specimens, performed all procedures. To quantitatively evaluate the CAF-induced proliferative activity in each group, we calculated the ratio of the area positive for vimentin and α-SMA staining to the total area in histological sections from ten fields under light microscopy (200×) [11].

For immunofluorescence staining, the cells were fixed with 4% paraformaldehyde and incubated with anti-Pan-CK (1:100), anti-α-SMA (1:100), anti-vimentin (1:100), anti-E-cadherin (1:100), anti-CD31(1:200) and anti-D2-40 (1:100) at 4°C overnight. The cells were subsequently incubated with fluorescence-conjugated secondary antibody for 1 h. After washing, the cells were mounted with mounting medium containing DAPI (Vector Laboratories). A negative control, in which the primary antibody was omitted, was used to test for antibody specificity. The images were captured using a confocal Leica fluorescence microscope.

Drugs and Reagents

QYHJ, a seven-herb Chinese medicinal formula, comprised *Scutellria barbata* (Ban zhi lian), *Heydyotis diffusa* (Bai hua she she cao), *Amorphophallus kiusianus* (She liu gu), *Coix lacryma-jobi* (Yi ren), *Gynostemma pentaphyllum* (Jiao gu lan), *Ganoderma luncidum* (Ling zhi) and *Amomum cardamomum* (Bai dou kou), was prepared as previously decribed [11,12,13]. Briefly, QYHJ powder was obtained from Jiang-yin Tianjiang Pharmaceutical Co, Ltd. To ensure standardization and maintain the interbatch reliability of QYHJ, a high performance liquid chromatography (HPLC) chromatographic fingerprint was developed for quality control. The fingerprint chromatograms of QYHJ formula are shown in our previous report [17]. The final decoction of QYHJ was prepared after dissolving the herbal powder in distilled water to the required concentration. The daily dosage for rabbit and nude mice was 15 g/kg and 18 g/kg, respectively, calculated according to the following human-rabbit or human-mouse transfer formula: Db = Da × (Rb/Ra) × (Wb/Wa)2/3, where D, R, and W represent dosage, shape coefficient, and body weight, respectively, and a and b represent human and mouse or rabbit, respectively. Human recombinant CXCL1, 2, and 8 were obtained from PeproTech (Rocky Hill, NJ, USA). The anti-CXCR1 blocking antibody was obtained from R&D Systems (Minneapolis, MN, USA). The CXCR2 inhibitor SB 225002 was obtained from Enzo Life Sciences, Inc. (Farmingdale, NY, USA). The following antibodies were used: anti-E-cadherin, anti-Vimentin, anti-α-SMA, anti-CXCL8, anti-CXCL1 (all from Epitomics, Burlingame, CA, USA), anti-Pan Cytokeratin (AE1/AE3) (Pan-CK; Ascend Biotechnology, Guangzhou, China), and anti-CXCL2 (Bioss, Beijing, China).

Preparation of QYHJ-Containing Serum

The QYHJ-Containing Serum was prepared as previously described [18]. Briefly, 20 female rabbits, weighing 1800±2200 g, were randomly divided into two groups: the QYHJ-Containing Serum group and the vehicle control group. The QYHJ-Containing Serum group was gavaged with intragastric QYHJ once a day for 7 consecutive days (12.5 g/kg body weight/time), and the vehicle control group was gavaged with intragastric deionized water. Blood was collected from the carotid artery within 2 h after the last administration and incubated at room temperature for 2 h. The serum from the whole blood was centrifuged (4,000 r/min for 10 min) and inactivated in a 56°C water bath for 30 min. The serum was stored at −80°C, and repeated freezing and thawing were avoided.

Migration and invasion assay

Cell migration and invasion were determined using transwell cell migration plates (Corning, NY, USA) and Matrigel invasion chambers (Matrigel-coated membrane, BD Biosciences, San Jose, CA, USA) as previously described [19]. Briefly, the cells (1.0×10^4) were seeded in serum-free medium into the upper chamber and allowed to invade toward 10% FCS in the lower chamber as a chemoattractant. After 12 h (for migration assays without matrigel coating) or 48 h (for invasion assays with matrigel coating), the cells that had invaded through the membrane and adhered to the underside of the membrane were counted as previously described [16].

Western Blot Analysis

Total protein was extracted from the cultured cells, and quantitated using the bicinchoninic acid assay kit (Pierce, Rockford, IL, USA). Western blotting was performed according to our previous report [16]. Equal amounts of protein from different samples were separated through 10% SDS-polyacrylate gel electrophoresis and transferred to a polyvinylidene fluoride membrane. Blocking buffer, containing 5% non-fat milk, was used to block and incubate the membranes with primary antibodies. The expression of the target proteins was examined using an enhance chemiluminescence (ECL) kit (Amersham Pharmacia Biotech, Uppsala, Sweden), and the quantitative analysis was performed using ImageJ software.

RNA isolation and real-time PCR

Total RNA was isolated from the cells using TRIzol Reagent (Invitrogen, San Diego, CA, USA), and reverse transcription PCR (RT-PCR) was performed according to the manufacturer's instructions (TakaRa). Quantitative real-time PCR measurements were performed using SYBR green I (Roche Diagnostics, Branchburg, NJ, USA). The primer sequences for CXCL1, 2, and 8 are listed in Table 1. GAPDH was used as an internal control. All experiments were performed in triplicate and repeated twice.

Conditioned medium (CM) preparation

CM from CAFs and NFs was obtained as previously described, with slight modifications [20]. Briefly, the cells were maintained in DMEM at 37°C for 48 h. The conditioned medium from CAFs or NFs was harvested. The conditioned medium was cleared through centrifugation, followed by 1:1 dilution with defined medium prior to treating the Capan 1 cells; the conditioned medium was freshly transferred without storage.

To obtain CM from QYHJ-treated CAFs, isolated CAFs were plated onto T25 flasks (1×10^6 cells) and cultured in DMEM containing 10% QYHJ-Containing Serum or Control-Containing Serum. Twenty-four hours later, the medium was removed and the cells were washed twice with PBS. Cells were subsequently incubated with 5 ml fresh DMEM medium for an additional 48 hours. The CM was subsequently harvested as described above.

Enzyme-Linked Immunosorbent (ELISA) assay

The serum CXCL1, 2, and 8 concentrations were measured using an ELISA as previously described [17]. The blood sample was stored at room temperature for 30 min, centrifuged (12000×g) for 15 min, and cryopreserved at -80°C. The concentrations were measured using a sandwich ELISA kit (DuoSet; R&D Systems, Minneapolis, MN, USA). To detect cytokine secretion in the culture medium, the cells were plated onto 6-well plates and treated as described above. After 48 h, the media were collected and stored at −80°C until further use.

Cell proliferation assay

The cell proliferation assay was performed as previously described [16]. Approximately 5×10^3 cells in 0.1 ml were plated in duplicate wells of 96-well plates. After overnight incubation, the suspension was removed and changed into different condition media. Subsequently, the indices of cell proliferation were assessed daily using the Cell Counting Kit-8 (CCK-8, Dojindo, Molecular Technologies, Inc, Gaithersburg, MD), and the growth curve was drawn according to the OD values obtain from CCK-8 assay.

Establishment of xenograft tumor models

Xenograft tumor models were established as previously described [16]. Briefly, Capan1 cells (2×10^6 in 0.2 ml) in logarithmic phase were injected subcutaneously into the right axilla of nude mice. The length and width of the tumors (in mm) were measured weekly using calipers. The tumor volume was calculated using the formula $(a\times b^2)\times0.5$, where a and b are the long and short dimensions, respectively. The mice were sacrificed when the tumors reached 1.5 cm in diameter. The tumors were removed and weighed. Each group consisted of at least six mice.

Statistical analysis

The data are expressed as the means ± standard deviation (SD). Statistical analyses were performed using analysis of variance (ANOVA) and Student's t-test. A P-value of <0.05 was considered statistically significant. All statistical analyses were performed using the SPSS 15.0 software package.

Results

Generation of cancer-associated fibroblast (CAF) cultures

We extracted fibroblasts from the resected specimens of two pancreatic ductal adenocarcinomas. The tumor masses were dissociated, and various cell types were separated to obtain populations of CAFs. We also isolated a second population of fibroblasts from a noncancerous region of the pancreas at least 2 cm from the outer tumor margin in each of the same two patients. We termed these cells "normal fibroblasts (NFs)." All experiments were performed through comparisons between CAFs and the corresponding NFs, thereby avoiding bias due to interindividual differences. The purity of the cultured fibroblast cells was verified through immunostaining using vimentin and PDGFR-β (mesenchymal cell marker) and E-cadherin and cytokeratin (CK) (epithelial cell marker). In addition, D31 and D2-40 were used to exclude the endothelial origin (Figure 1A and Figure S1). All cell cultures were vimentin and PDGFR-β positive

Table 1. Primers and annealing temperatures used for RT-PCR.

Gene		Primer sequence	Product size (bp)	Annealing (°C)
CXCL1	F	5′-TGAAGGCAGGGGAATGTATGTG-3′	226	60
	R	5′-AGCCCCTTTGTTCTAAGCCAGA -3′		
CXCL2	F	5′-AGATCAATGTGACGGCAGGGA-3′	235	60
	R	5′-CTCTCTGCTCTAACACAGAGGGAA-3′		
CXCL8	F	5′-AAGCCACCGGAGCACTCCATA-3′	170	60
	R	5′-CGGCCAGCTTGGAAGTCATGT-3′		
GAPDH	F	5′-GGGAGCCAAAAGGGTCATCATCTC -3′	353	60
	R	5′-CCATGCCAGTGAGCTTCCCGTTC -3′		

and 91% to 100% E-cadherin, cytokeratin, CD31 and D2-40 negative. Compared with NFs, the established CAFs expressed high levels of alpha smooth muscle actin (α-SMA), a marker of activated fibroblasts, typically expressed in CAF but not normal quiescent fibroblasts. These observations were further confirmed through Western blot analysis (Figure 1B). Taken together, our results indicated that we successfully established paired CAF and NF cultures from human PDAC.

Pancreatic cancer cells treated with conditioned media from QYHJ-treated CAFs showed reduced invasion

CAFs contribute to the invasive and metastatic process in human pancreatic cancer [5]. In this study, we examined the migration and invasion-inducing effects of CAF on human pancreatic cancer cells using transwell chambers with or without Matrigel coating. The transwell assays demonstrated that the conditioned medium (CM) from control-treated CAFs exhibited an enhanced capacity for inducing pancreatic cancer cell migration and invasion (Figure 2 and Figure S2). Next, we evaluated the effects of QYHJ on CAF-induced cell migration and invasion, the CM from QYHJ or control-treated CAFs were harvested and the effects of this medium on pancreatic cancer cell migration and invasion were also evaluated. We observed that CM from QYHJ-treated CAFs exhibited decreased migration and invasion-promoting capacities compared with that of control-treated CAFs (Figure 2 and Figure S2), these results suggested that

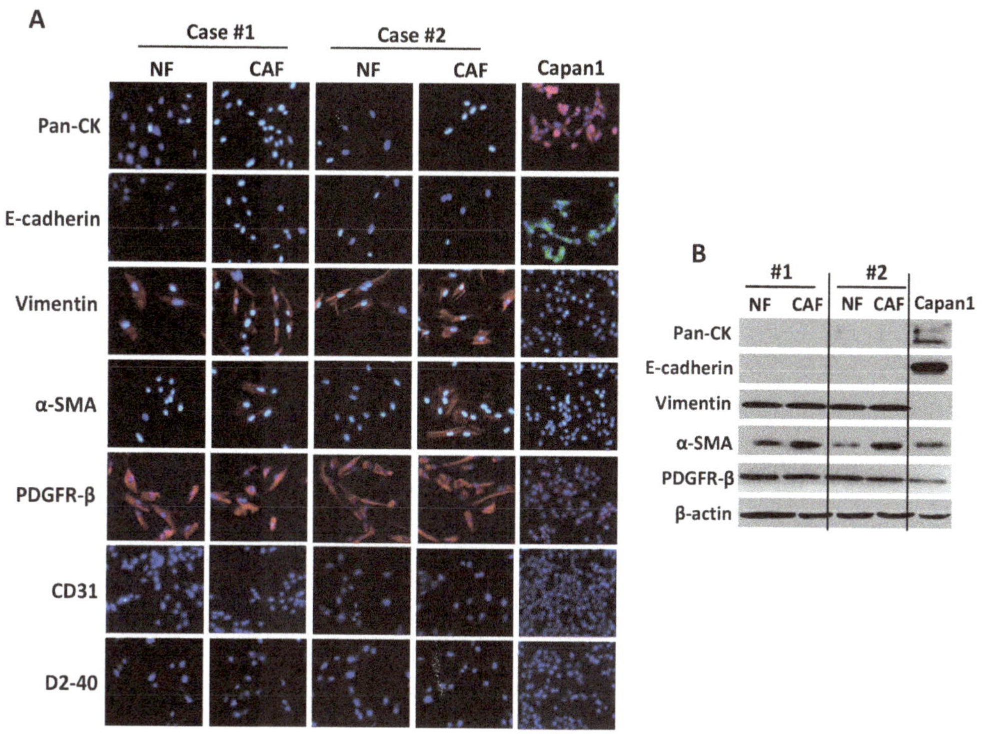

Figure 1. Generation and characterization of cancer-associated fibroblast cultures. A. Fibroblasts were extracted from the resected tissues of two pancreatic ductal adenocarcinomas. The purity of the cultured fibroblast cells was verified through immunofluorescence to detect Pan-CK (red), E-cadherin (green), vimentin (red), α-SMA (red), PDGFR-β (red), CD31 (red) and D2-40 (red). The cell nuclei were counterstained with DAPI (blue). Positive control tissues for CD31 and D2-40 immunostaining have been used (Figure S1). B. Western blot analysis confirmed the expression pattern of the markers used in A.

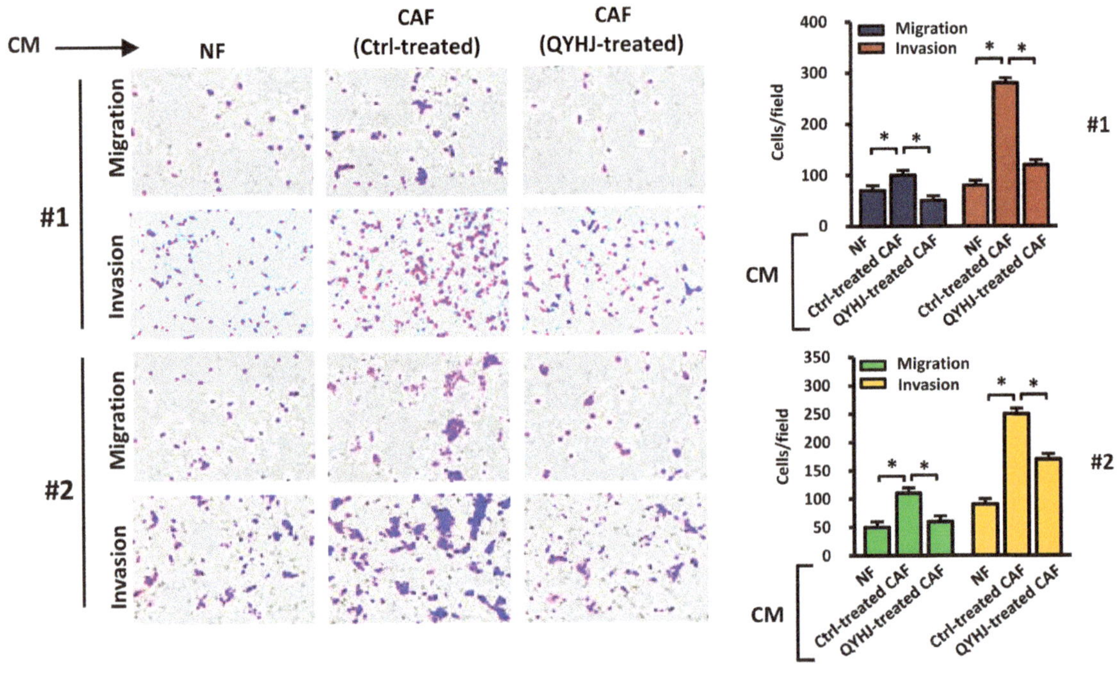

Figure 2. Pancreatic cancer cells treated using conditioned media from QYHJ-treated CAFs showed reduced invasion. The cell migration and invasion capacity of pancreatic cancer cells treated with conditioned media (CM) from NFs, Ctrl-treated CAFs and QYHJ-treated CAFs was compared using transwell chambers with or without Matrigel coating. The numbers of cells that traveled through the membrane were counted in 10 fields under a ×20 objective lens. Original magnification, ×200. The results represent the means ± SD of the values obtained in three independent experiments. Statistical significance was calculated using ANOVA. * $P<0.05$.

QYHJ treatment might suppress pancreatic cancer cell migration and invasion through targeting CAFs.

QYHJ inhibits the secretion of CXCL1, 2 and 8 form CAFs

CAFs directly stimulate tumor cell proliferation through various growth factors, hormones and cytokines in a context-dependent manner [5]. We previously showed that CAFs promote the migration and invasion of Capan1 cells in vitro, and this property was inhibited after treated with QYHJ. We next attempted to identify the potential molecules that mediate the correlation between fibroblasts and cancer cells. Previous studies have shown that the members of the CXC chemokine subfamilies, including GRO1 (CXCL1), GRO2 (CXCL2) and IL-8 (CXCL8), are among one of the most highly up-regulated genes identified in CAFs compared with NFs in pancreatic cancer [21]. Therefore, we examined the expression of these factors in CAFs and paired NFs. We observed that CAFs exhibit increased CXCL1, 2 and 8 mRNA and protein expression compared with NFs. In addition, we observed that QYHJ treatment significantly suppressed the expression of CXCL1, 2 and 8 in both CAF cell lines (Figure 3A-B). ELISA assay also confirmed that CAFs treated with QYHJ secreted lower levels of CXCL1, 2 and 8 into the medium (Figure 3C). Thus, these results suggested that QYHJ inhibits the expression of CXCL1, 2 and 8 in CAFs.

QYHJ inhibited CAF proliferation in vitro

Previous studies have indicated that the number of CAFs in the stroma is significantly associated with the poor differentiation and prognosis of cancers [22,23,24], and reduced CAF numbers were also observed when the tumor was treated[11]. We therefore hypothesized that QYHJ affects CAF proliferation. The in vitro proliferation assay indicated that QYHJ treatment inhibited the proliferation of CAFs in both cell lines (Figure 4), thereby contributing to the suppressed CXC chemokine secretion from CAFs.

CXCLs increased the migration and invasion of human pancreatic cancer cells

CXC chemokines have been associated with cancer cell invasion in many types of human cancers[25]. As we have observed that CAF exhibited increased CXC chemokines expression and secretion, we confirmed whether the upregulated secretion of CXC chemokines contributes to the enhanced capacity for inducing pancreatic cancer cell migration and invasion. We tested the effects of CXC chemokines on cell migration and invasion using transwell chambers with or without Matrigel coating. The addition of recombinant human CXCL1, 2 and 8 increased both the migration and invasion of Capan 1 cells in the transwell assays. Furthermore, the inhibition of CXC chemokine signaling using receptor antagonists significantly blocked CXC chemokine-induced cell migration and invasion (Figure 5 and Figure S3).

QHYJ treatment inhibit tumorigenesis and expression of CXCL1, 2, 8 in vivo.

To further confirm the effects of QYHJ on CAF proliferation activity and CXCLs production in vivo, we established mice xenograft models using Canpan1 cells. The mice were randomly divided into QYHJ and control groups, treated with QYHJ (0.2 ml, gavage, daily) or normal saline as a control, respectively. We observed that QYHJ treatment resulted in reduced tumor growth (Figure 6A). Consistent with the results of the in vitro analyses, QYHJ reduced CAF proliferation in tumors (Figure 6B). Moreover, IHC confirmed that tumors treated with QYHJ

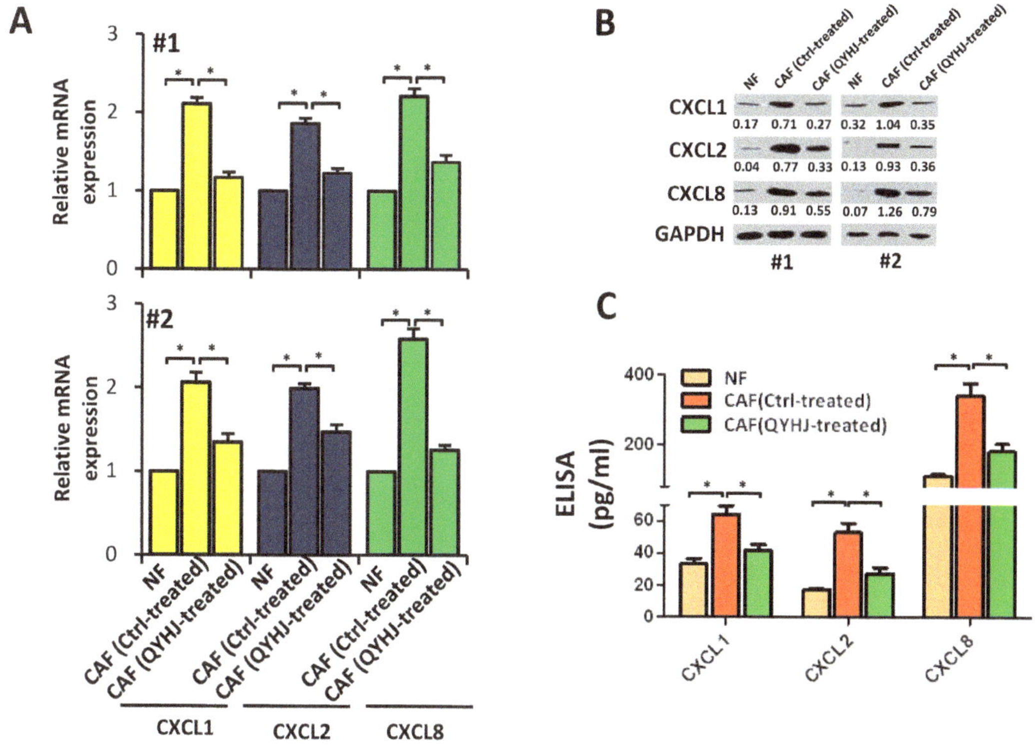

Figure 3. QYHJ suppressed CXCL production in CAFs. A–B. CAFs were treated with QYHJ-Containing Serum or Control-Containing Serum for 48 h. The cells were then harvested, and the expression of CXCL1, 2 and 8 was evaluated using real-time PCR (A) and western blotting (B). C. The isolated CAFs were plated in T25 flasks (1×10^6 cells) and cultured in DMEM containing 10% QYHJ-Containing Serum or Control-Containing Serum. Twenty-four hours later, the media were removed, and the cells were washed twice with PBS. The cells were subsequently incubated with 5 ml of fresh DMEM medium for an additional 48 hours. The medium was subsequently harvested, and the CXCL1, 2 and 8 concentrations were detected through ELISA. ANOVA was used to determine the statistical significance. * $P<0.05$.

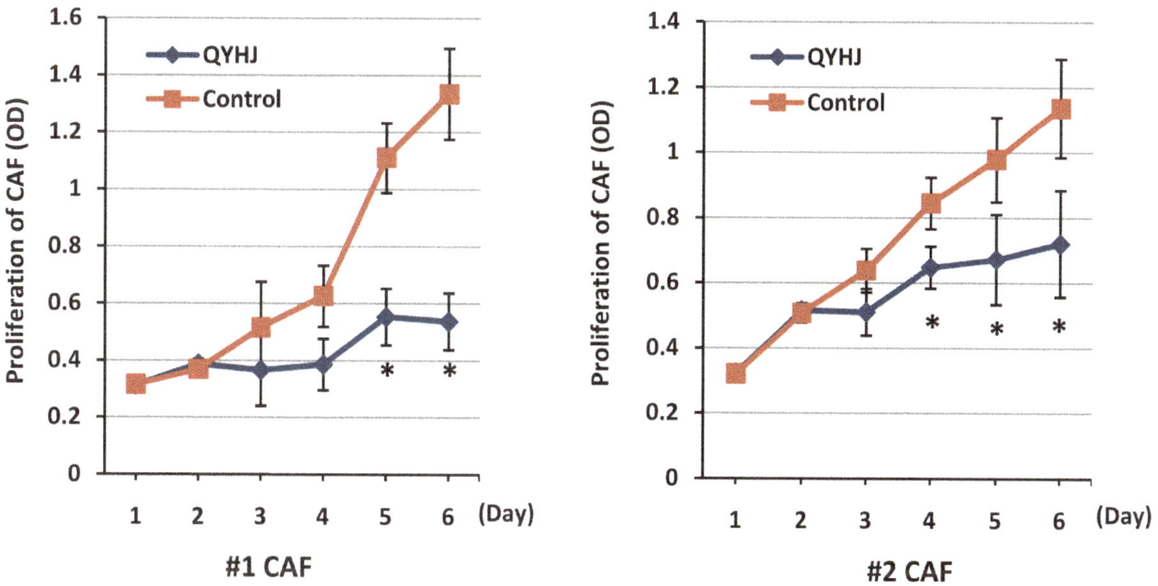

Figure 4. QYHJ inhibited CAF proliferation in vitro. Approximately 5×10^3 CAFs in 0.1 ml were plated in duplicate wells of 96-well plates. After overnight incubation, the suspension was removed and transferred to DMEM containing 10% QYHJ-Containing Serum or Control-Containing Serum. The cell proliferation indices were assessed daily using the Cell Counting Kit-8. The results are presented as the means ± SD of values obtained in three independent experiments. *$P < 0.05$.

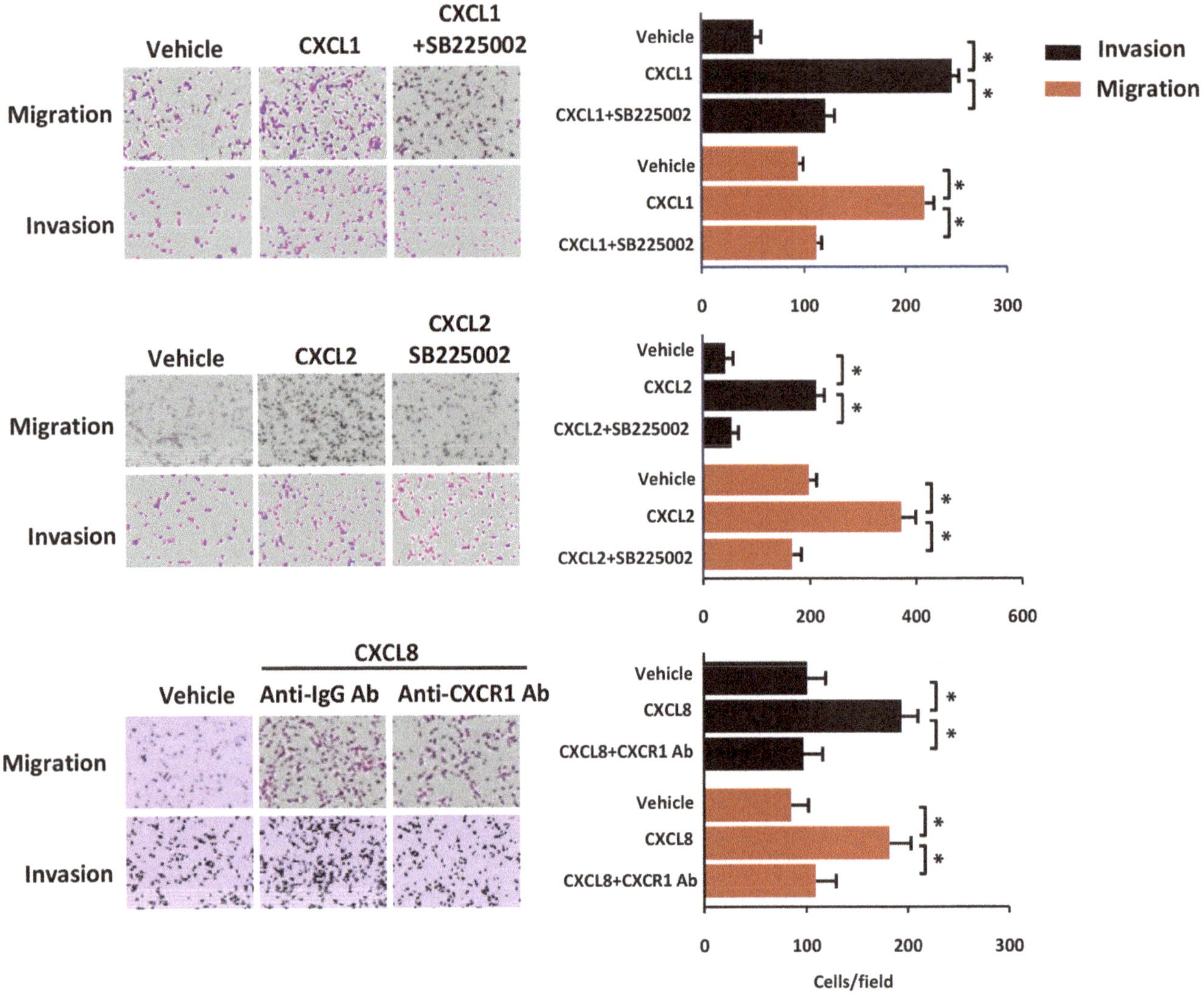

Figure 5. CXCLs increased the migration and invasion of human pancreatic cancer cells. Migration and invasion assays were performed on Capan1 cells treated with vehicle, 100 ng/ml CXCL1, 2, and 8, or their antognists 20 μg/ml anti-CXCR1 antibody and 400 nM SB 225002 as indicated, using transwell cell chambers. The number of cells that invaded the membrane was counted in 10 fields under the ×20 objective lens. Original magnification, ×200. The results are presented as the means±SD of values obtained in three independent experiments. The statistical significance was calculated using ANOVA. $^{*}P < 0.05$.

exhibited the reduced expression of CXCL1, 2, and 8 (Figure 6D). Therefore, our results suggested that QHYJ treatment inhibited CAF proliferation and the expression of CXCL1, 2, and 8, potentially reflecting the anti-cancer effects of QHYJ in pancreatic cancer.

Discussion

In this study we showed that the QYHJ inhibits pancreatic cancer cell invasion and metastasis by targeting CAFs, particularly the production of CXCL1, 2, and 8. These findings further confirmed our previous speculation that cells in the tumor microenvironment might serve as pivotal targets for Chinese herbal medicine[11].

Traditional Chinese medicine (TCM) is based on a unique theory formed in lone-term practical experience. For the last thousand years, TCM has been widely practiced in China, and more than 90% of modern Chinese cancer patients have received TCM therapy during treatment [26]. Recently, TCM has been used abroad and is well accepted in many countries, particularly for the treatment of oncology [27]. TCM is based on the concept of holism, considering the interrelationship of the human body and the surrounding environment on the macro level. At the microscopic scale, we consider the holistic relationship between cancer cells and the microenvironment. Indeed, recent studies have confirmed that tumor cells do not act in isolation, but rather subsist in a rich microenvironment provided by resident fibroblasts, inflammatory cells, endothelial cells, pericytes, leukocytes, and the extracellular matrix [28]. As the cancer progresses, the surrounding microenvironment is activated, coevolving through continuous paracrine communication, to support carcinogenesis [29]. Pancreatic cancer is characterized by an extensive stromal response called desmoplasia [7]. CAFs are the primary cell type in the tumor stroma, and the importance of a role for CAFs in tumor progression is well accepted [5]. Therefore, as cancer is no longer considered a discrete entity defined only through the traits of cancer cells within the tumor, eventually affecting the entire

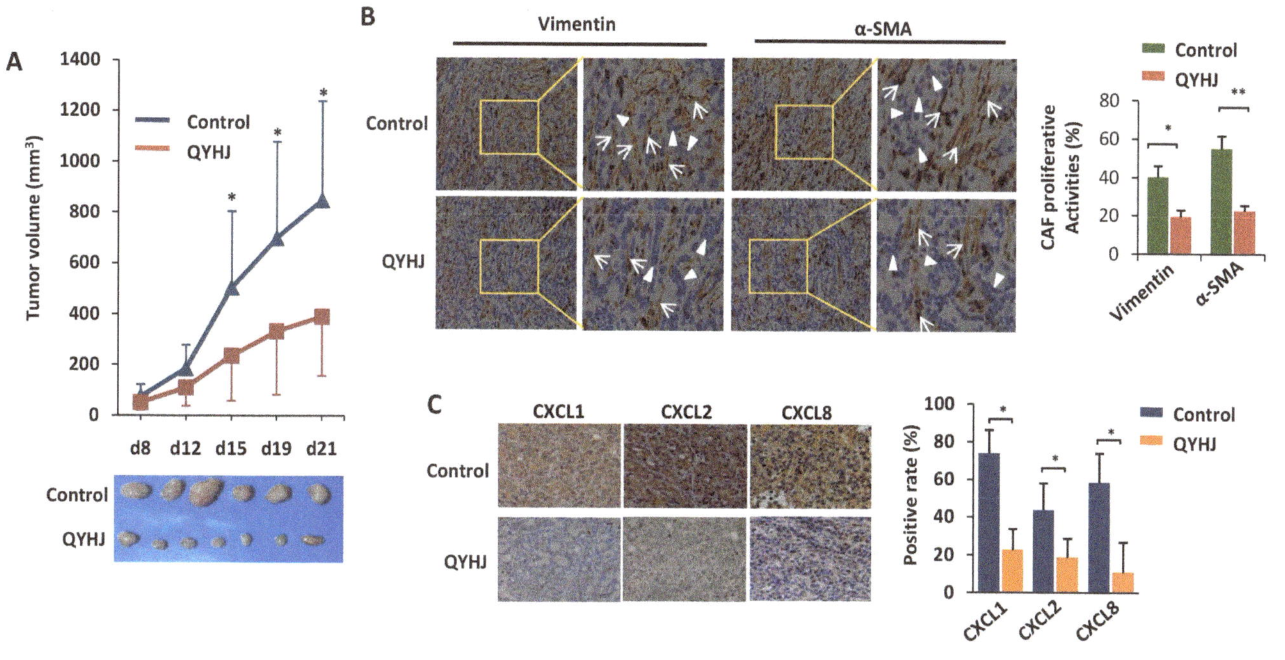

Figure 6. QHYJ treatment inhibited tumor growth and the expression of CXCL1, 2, and 8 in vivo. A. Effect of QYHJ on tumor growth in a subcutaneously transplanted tumor model. Capan1 cells (2×10^6cells in 200 ml) were injected subcutaneously into the right axilla of each BALB/c-nu/nu nude mouse. The next day, the mice were orally treated with or without QYHJ. The mean tumor volumes of vehicle-treated (saline water) and QYHJ-treated tumors were measured. The mean ±standard deviation was determined in each treatment group. The tumor growth curves are shown in the upper panel, and photographs of subcutaneously transplanted tumors from both groups are shown in the lower panel. Student's t-test was used to determine the statistical significance. *$P < .05$ compared with the QYHJ-treated group. B. IHC staining for vimentin and α-SMA on sections of tumors to evaluate CAF proliferative activities. A arrow indicates fibroblast and arrowhead indicates pancreatic cancer cell. Original magnification, 200×. CAF proliferative activities (right) were quantitatively evaluated after calculating the ratio of the vimentin or α-SMA antibody-positive staining area to the total area in each field, and the mean value from ten fields under 200× microscopy are indicated. *$P < 0.05$. C. IHC staining using anti-CXCL1, 2, and 8 antibodies was performed using sections of transplanted tumors. Original magnification, ×200. The positive rates of CXCL1, 2, and 8 in tumors are shown on the right. Student's t-test was used to determine the statistical significance. *$P < 0.05$.

organism, TCM offers a holistic approach to regulate the integrity of all body functions and the interaction between the humans and the surrounding environment. Targeting the tumor microenvironment might represent a potential therapeutic approach for pancreatic cancer treatment.

QYHJ is a seven-herb Chinese formula used in the treatment of pancreatic cancer in China. We previously showed that QYHJ inhibits both tumor growth and metastasis in nude mice with pancreatic cancer models [12,13]. The combination of QYHJ treatment with conventional Western medicine prolongs survival in patients with pancreatic cancer liver metastases [14].The exact mechanism underlying the effects of QYHJ in pancreatic cancer treatment remains unclear. Recent studies have indicated that QYHJ treatments dramatically alter the tumor microenvironment, observed through decreased CAF proliferation [11]. Therefore, in this study, we further evaluated the effects of QYHJ on CAF proliferation and the production of CAF-derived chemokines. We observed that QYHJ inhibited CAF proliferation both in vitro and in vivo. In addition, the inhibition of CXCL production through QYHJ treatment resulted in the reduced invasion of pancreatic cancer cells. Thus, this study was the first to identify a new target of pancreatic cancer cells using Chinese herbal medicine.

CXCL1, 2, and 8, produced primarily by mononuclear cells, macrophages and a smaller percentage of fibroblasts, endothelial cells, T and B lymphocytes, chondrocytes and amnion cells, are pleiotropic cytokines that induce tumor formation, promote tumor proliferation and facilitate tumor metastasis [30,31]. Increasing evidence has shown that CXCL1, 2, and 8 are frequently elevated in many types of human cancers [30,32,33,34], including pancreatic cancer [31]. In addition, therapies targeting CXCL1, 2, and 8 in the treatment of cancers have been reported [30,35,36], and the down-regulation of CXCL1, 2, and 8 inhibited the invasion of tumor cells [32] [35]. Using in vitro function assays, we demonstrated that CAFs exhibit increased CXCL1, 2 and 8 expression in pancreatic cancer, contributing to the enhanced invasion-promoting capacity of these cells. Therefore, targeting CXC chemokine signaling between CAF and cancer cells through pharmacological inhibition might provide a promising therapy for pancreatic cancer. The results obtained in the present study showed that Chinese herbal medicine QYHJ could significant suppress the production of CAF-derived CXCL1, 2 and 8, thereby preventing pancreatic cancer cell invasion.

Thus, in this study, we have demonstrated that CAFs exhibited an enhanced capacity for inducing pancreatic cancer cell migration and invasion compared with NFs, while QYHJ-treated CAFs exhibited decreased migration and invasion-promoting capacities in vitro. In addition, we showed that QYHJ significantly suppressed CAF proliferation activities and the production of CAF-derived CXCL1, 2 and 8. Taken together, these results suggested that suppressing the tumor-promoting capacity of CAFs through Chinese herbal medicine attenuates pancreatic cancer cell invasion.

Supporting Information

Figure S1 Positive control for CD31 and D2-40 immunostaining. (A) The positive control for CD31 is vascular

endothelium in pancreas. (B) The positive control for D2-40 is lymphatic endothelium in lymph node.
(TIF)

Figure S2 Pancreatic cancer cells BxPC3 treated using conditioned media from QYHJ-treated CAFs showed reduced invasion. The cell migration and invasion capacity of pancreatic cancer cells BxPC3 treated with conditioned media (CM) from NFs, Ctrl-treated CAFs and QYHJ-treated CAFs was compared using transwell chambers with or without Matrigel coating. The numbers of cells that traveled through the membrane were counted in 10 fields under a ×20 objective lens. Original magnification, ×200. The results represent the means ± SD of the values obtained in three independent experiments. Statistical significance was calculated using ANOVA. * $P<0.05$.
(TIF)

Figure S3 CXCLs increased the migration and invasion of human pancreatic cancer cells BxPC3. Migration and invasion assays were performed on BxPC3 cells treated with vehicle, 100 ng/ml CXCL1, 2, and 8, or their antognists 20 µg/ml anti-CXCR1 antibody and 400 nM SB 225002 as indicated, using transwell cell chambers. The number of cells that invaded the membrane was counted in 10 fields under the ×20 objective lens. Original magnification, ×200. The results are presented as the means±SD of values obtained in three independent experiments. The statistical significance was calculated using ANOVA. *$P < 0.05$.
(TIF)

Acknowledgments

We thank Dr Yi Qin (Fudan University Shanghai Cancer Center, Shanghai) for experimental technical help.

Author Contributions

Conceived and designed the experiments: PW. Performed the experiments: LC PW CQ HC LX KW QQ JL ZM ZC LL. Analyzed the data: LC CQ PW ZC LL. Contributed reagents/materials/analysis tools: ZC LL. Wrote the paper: LC CQ PW.

References

1. Hezel AF, Kimmelman AC, Stanger BZ, Bardeesy N, Depinho RA (2006) Genetics and biology of pancreatic ductal adenocarcinoma. Genes Dev 20: 1218–1249.
2. Li D, Xie K, Wolff R, Abbruzzese JL (2004) Pancreatic cancer. Lancet 363: 1049–1057.
3. Jemal A, Tiwari RC, Murray T, Ghafoor A, Samuels A, et al. (2004) Cancer statistics, 2004. CA Cancer J Clin 54: 8–29.
4. Tchou J, Kossenkov AV, Chang L, Satija C, Herlyn M, et al. (2012) Human breast cancer associated fibroblasts exhibit subtype specific gene expression profiles. BMC Med Genomics 5: 39.
5. Hwang RF, Moore T, Arumugam T, Ramachandran V, Amos KD, et al. (2008) Cancer-associated stromal fibroblasts promote pancreatic tumor progression. Cancer Res 68: 918–926.
6. Quiros RM, Valianou M, Kwon Y, Brown KM, Godwin AK, et al. (2008) Ovarian normal and tumor-associated fibroblasts retain in vivo stromal characteristics in a 3-D matrix-dependent manner. Gynecol Oncol 110: 99–109.
7. Merika EE, Syrigos KN, Saif MW (2012) Desmoplasia in pancreatic cancer. Can we fight it? Gastroenterol Res Pract 2012: 781765.
8. Martinez-Outschoorn UE, Lin Z, Ko YH, Goldberg AF, Flomenberg N, et al. (2011) Understanding the metabolic basis of drug resistance: therapeutic induction of the Warburg effect kills cancer cells. Cell Cycle 10: 2521–2528.
9. Tlsty TD, Coussens LM (2006) Tumor stroma and regulation of cancer development. Annu Rev Pathol 1: 119–150.
10. Kalluri R, Zeisberg M (2006) Fibroblasts in cancer. Nat Rev Cancer 6: 392–401.
11. Chen Z, Chen LY, Wang P, Dai HY, Gao S, et al. (2012) Tumor Microenvironment Varies under Different TCM ZHENG Models and Correlates with Treatment Response to Herbal Medicine. Evid Based Complement Alternat Med 2012: 635702.
12. Yin JH, Shi WD, Zhu XY, Chen Z, Liu LM (2012) Qingyihuaji formula inhibits progress of liver metastases from advanced pancreatic cancer xenograft by targeting to decrease expression of Cyr61 and VEGF. Integr Cancer Ther 11: 37–47.
13. Wang P, Chen Z, Meng ZQ, Luo JM, Lin JH, et al. (2010) Ski acts as therapeutic target of qingyihuaji formula in the treatment of SW1990 pancreatic cancer. Integr Cancer Ther 9: 50–58.
14. Ouyang H, Wang P, Meng Z, Chen Z, Yu E, et al. (2011) Multimodality treatment of pancreatic cancer with liver metastases using chemotherapy, radiation therapy, and/or Chinese herbal medicine. Pancreas 40: 120–125.
15. Walter K, Omura N, Hong SM, Griffith M, Goggins M (2008) Pancreatic cancer associated fibroblasts display normal allelotypes. Cancer Biol Ther 7: 882–888.
16. Wang P, Chen Z, Meng ZQ, Fan J, Luo JM, et al. (2009) Dual role of Ski in pancreatic cancer cells: tumor-promoting versus metastasis-suppressive function. Carcinogenesis 30: 1497–1506.
17. Zhang J, Wang P, Ouyang H, Yin J, Liu A, et al. (2013) Targeting Cancer-Related Inflammation: Chinese Herbal Medicine Inhibits Epithelial-to-Mesenchymal Transition in Pancreatic Cancer. PLoS One 8: e70334.
18. Feng Q, Gou XJ, Meng SX, Huang C, Zhang YQ, et al. (2013) Qushi Huayu Decoction Inhibits Hepatic Lipid Accumulation by Activating AMP-Activated Protein Kinase In Vivo and In Vitro. Evid Based Complement Alternat Med 2013: 184358.
19. Wang P, Chen L, Zhang J, Chen H, Fan J, et al. (2013) Methylation-mediated silencing of the miR-124 genes facilitates pancreatic cancer progression and metastasis by targeting Rac1. Oncogene.
20. Muerkoster S, Wegehenkel K, Arlt A, Witt M, Sipos B, et al. (2004) Tumor stroma interactions induce chemoresistance in pancreatic ductal carcinoma cells involving increased secretion and paracrine effects of nitric oxide and interleukin-1beta. Cancer Res 64: 1331–1337.
21. Sato N, Maehara N, Goggins M (2004) Gene expression profiling of tumor-stromal interactions between pancreatic cancer cells and stromal fibroblasts. Cancer Res 64: 6950–6956.
22. Ino Y, Yamazaki-Itoh R, Oguro S, Shimada K, Kosuge T, et al. (2013) Arginase II expressed in cancer-associated fibroblasts indicates tissue hypoxia and predicts poor outcome in patients with pancreatic cancer. PLoS One 8: e55146.
23. Kinoshita T, Ishii G, Hiraoka N, Hirayama S, Yamauchi C, et al. (2013) Forkhead box P3 regulatory T cells coexisting with cancer associated fibroblasts are correlated with a poor outcome in lung adenocarcinoma. Cancer Sci 104: 409–415.
24. Schoppmann SF, Jesch B, Riegler MF, Maroske F, Schwameis K, et al. (2013) Podoplanin expressing cancer associated fibroblasts are associated with unfavourable prognosis in adenocarcinoma of the esophagus. Clin Exp Metastasis 30: 441–446.
25. Zhu Q, Han X, Peng J, Qin H, Wang Y (2012) The role of CXC chemokines and their receptors in the progression and treatment of tumors. J Mol Histol 43: 699–713.
26. Chen Z, Gu K, Zheng Y, Zheng W, Lu W, et al. (2008) The use of complementary and alternative medicine among Chinese women with breast cancer. J Altern Complement Med 14: 1049–1055.
27. Chang KH, Brodie R, Choong MA, Sweeney KJ, Kerin MJ (2011) Complementary and alternative medicine use in oncology: a questionnaire survey of patients and health care professionals. BMC Cancer 11: 196.
28. Langley RR, Fidler IJ (2011) The seed and soil hypothesis revisited—the role of tumor-stroma interactions in metastasis to different organs. Int J Cancer 128: 2527–2535.
29. Pietras K, Ostman A (2010) Hallmarks of cancer: interactions with the tumor stroma. Exp Cell Res 316: 1324–1331.
30. Benelli R, Stigliani S, Minghelli S, Carlone S, Ferrari N (2013) Impact of CXCL1 overexpression on growth and invasion of prostate cancer cell. Prostate 73: 941–951.
31. Frick VO, Rubie C, Wagner M, Graeber S, Grimm H, et al. (2008) Enhanced ENA-78 and IL-8 expression in patients with malignant pancreatic diseases. Pancreatology 8: 488–497.
32. Bandapalli OR, Ehrmann F, Ehemann V, Gaida M, Macher-Goeppinger S, et al. (2012) Down-regulation of CXCL1 inhibits tumor growth in colorectal liver metastasis. Cytokine 57: 46–53.
33. Nishikawa R, Suzumori N, Nishiyama T, Nishikawa H, Arakawa A, et al. (2012) Clinical significance of serum growth-regulated oncogene alpha (GROalpha) in patients with gynecological cancer. Eur J Gynaecol Oncol 33: 138–141.
34. Dong QM, Zhang JQ, Li Q, Bracher JC, Hendricks DT, et al. (2011) Clinical significance of serum expression of GRObeta in esophageal squamous cell carcinoma. World J Gastroenterol 17: 2658–2662.
35. Killian PH, Kronski E, Michalik KM, Barbieri O, Astigiano S, et al. (2012) Curcumin inhibits prostate cancer metastasis in vivo by targeting the inflammatory cytokines CXCL1 and −2. Carcinogenesis 33: 2507–2519.
36. Kavandi L, Collier MA, Nguyen H, Syed V (2012) Progesterone and calcitriol attenuate inflammatory cytokines CXCL1 and CXCL2 in ovarian and endometrial cancer cells. J Cell Biochem 113: 3143–3152.

Permissions

All chapters in this book were first published in PLOS ONE, by The Public Library of Science; hereby published with permission under the Creative Commons Attribution License or equivalent. Every chapter published in this book has been scrutinized by our experts. Their significance has been extensively debated. The topics covered herein carry significant findings which will fuel the growth of the discipline. They may even be implemented as practical applications or may be referred to as a beginning point for another development.

The contributors of this book come from diverse backgrounds, making this book a truly international effort. This book will bring forth new frontiers with its revolutionizing research information and detailed analysis of the nascent developments around the world.

We would like to thank all the contributing authors for lending their expertise to make the book truly unique. They have played a crucial role in the development of this book. Without their invaluable contributions this book wouldn't have been possible. They have made vital efforts to compile up to date information on the varied aspects of this subject to make this book a valuable addition to the collection of many professionals and students.

This book was conceptualized with the vision of imparting up-to-date information and advanced data in this field. To ensure the same, a matchless editorial board was set up. Every individual on the board went through rigorous rounds of assessment to prove their worth. After which they invested a large part of their time researching and compiling the most relevant data for our readers.

The editorial board has been involved in producing this book since its inception. They have spent rigorous hours researching and exploring the diverse topics which have resulted in the successful publishing of this book. They have passed on their knowledge of decades through this book. To expedite this challenging task, the publisher supported the team at every step. A small team of assistant editors was also appointed to further simplify the editing procedure and attain best results for the readers.

Apart from the editorial board, the designing team has also invested a significant amount of their time in understanding the subject and creating the most relevant covers. They scrutinized every image to scout for the most suitable representation of the subject and create an appropriate cover for the book.

The publishing team has been an ardent support to the editorial, designing and production team. Their endless efforts to recruit the best for this project, has resulted in the accomplishment of this book. They are a veteran in the field of academics and their pool of knowledge is as vast as their experience in printing. Their expertise and guidance has proved useful at every step. Their uncompromising quality standards have made this book an exceptional effort. Their encouragement from time to time has been an inspiration for everyone.

The publisher and the editorial board hope that this book will prove to be a valuable piece of knowledge for researchers, students, practitioners and scholars across the globe.

List of Contributors

Takahiro Fujimaki, Etsu Tashiro, Mitsuhiro Kitagawa and Masaya Imoto
Department of Biosciences and Informatics, Faculty of Science and Technology, Keio University, Yokohama, Japan

Shinji Saiki, Daisuke Yamada and Nobutaka Hattori
Department of Neurology, Juntendo University School of Medicine, Bunkyo, Tokyo

Shiou-Huei Chao, Ying-Chieh Tsai and Ya-Huei Kang
Institute of Biochemistry and Molecular Biology, National Yang-Ming University, Taipei, Taiwan

Hui-Yu Huang
Department of Food Science, Nutrition and Nutraceutical Biotechnology, Shih Chien University, Taipei, Taiwan

Chuan-Hsiung Chang and Chih-Hsien Yan
Center for Systems and Synthetic Biology, National Yang-Ming University, Taipei, Taiwan
Institute of Biomedical Informatics, National Yang-Ming University, Taipei, Taiwan

Wei-Shen Cheng
Institute of Biomedical Informatics, National Yang-Ming University, Taipei, Taiwan

Koichi Watanabe
Yakult Central Institute for Microbiological Research, Tokyo, Japan

Ki-Ho Cho and Woo-Sang Jung
Department of Cardiovascular & Neurologic Diseases, College of Oriental Medicine, Kyung Hee University, Seoul, South Korea

Tae-Hun Kim
Department of Cardiovascular & Neurologic Diseases, College of Oriental Medicine, Kyung Hee University, Seoul, South Korea
Korea Institute of Oriental Medicine, Daejeon, South Korea

Myeong Soo Lee
Korea Institute of Oriental Medicine, Daejeon, South Korea

Jia-bo Wang, Xue-ru Zhang, Xiaohui Chu, Ping Zhang and Yan-ling Zhao
China Military Institute of Chinese Medicine, 302 Military Hospital, Beijing, China

Ling-na Zeng
China Military Institute of Chinese Medicine, 302 Military Hospital, Beijing, China,
Faculty of Life Science and Technology, Kunming University of Science and Technology, Kunming, China

Bao-cai Li
Faculty of Life Science and Technology, Kunming University of Science and Technology, Kunming, China

Qing-ce Zang
China Military Institute of Chinese Medicine, 302 Military Hospital, Beijing, China,
Pharmacy College, Jiangxi University of Traditional Chinese Medicine, Nanchang, China

Qian-feng Gong
Pharmacy College, Jiangxi University of Traditional Chinese Medicine, Nanchang, China

Xiao-he Xiao
Integrative Medicine Center, 302 Military Hospital, Beijing, China

Ping He and Yong Shen
Center for Advanced Therapeutic Strategies of Brain Disorders, Roskamp Institute, Sarasota, Florida, United States of America

Pengtao Li, Qian Hua and Yuan Liu
Department of Pathology, School of Preclinical Medicine, Beijing University of Chinese Medicine, Beijing, China

Matthias Staufenbiel
Novartis Pharm Ltd., Nervous System Research, Basel, Switzerland

Rena Li
Center for Hormone Advanced Science and Education, Roskamp Institute, Sarasota, Florida, United States of America

Jia-bo Wang, Yan-ling Zhao, Cheng Jin, Dao-jian Liu, Hong-juan Wang and Xiao-he Xiao
Integrative Medicine Center, 302 Military Hospital, Beijing, People's Republic of China

Hai-ping Zhao
Integrative Medicine Center, 302 Military Hospital, Beijing, People's Republic of China
Key Laboratory of Modern Preparation of Traditional Chinese Medicine, Ministry of Education, Jiangxi University of Traditional Chinese Medicine, Nanchang, People's Republic of China

Wei-jun Kong, Fang Fang and Lin Zhang
Integrative Medicine Center, 302 Military Hospital, Beijing, People's Republic of China
Chengdu University of Traditional Chinese Medicine, Chengdu, People's Republic of China

Ying-Hung Lu and Yi-Ling Chen
School of Pharmacy and Graduate Institute, College of Pharmacy, China Medical University, Taichung, Taiwan

Hsin-Hui Tsai
School of Pharmacy and Graduate Institute, College of Pharmacy, China Medical University, Taichung, Taiwan
Department of Pharmacy, China Medical University Hospital, Taichung, Taiwan

Hsiang-Wen Lin
School of Pharmacy and Graduate Institute, College of Pharmacy, China Medical University, Taichung, Taiwan
Department of Pharmacy, China Medical University Hospital, Taichung, Taiwan
Department of Pharmacy Administration, College of Pharmacy, University of Illinois at Chicago, Chicago, Illinois, United States of America

Gail B. Mahady
Department of Pharmacy Practice, College of Pharmacy, PAHO/WHO Collaborating Centre for Traditional Medicine, University of Illinois at Chicago, Chicago, Illinois,
United States of America

Shi Guang Li, Chen Sheng Ou-Yang and Zhen-Jiang Yang
Graduate School, Guangzhou University of Chinese Medicine, Guangzhou, China
Department of Oncology and Hematology, Shenzhen Hospital of Traditional Chinese Medicine, Shenzhen, Guangdong Province, China

Hai Yong Chen and Yao Tong
School of Chinese Medicine, Li Ka Shing Faculty of Medicine, The University of Hong Kong, Hong Kong SAR, China

Xi-Xin Wang
Shanxi Province Hospital of Traditional Chinese Medicine, Taiyuan, Shanxi Province, China

William C.S. Cho
Department of Clinical Oncology, Queen Elizabeth Hospital, Hong Kong SAR, China

Markus Helfer, Herwig Koppensteiner, Martha Schneider, Stephanie Rebensburg, Michael Schindler and Ruth Brack-Werner
Institute of Virology, Helmholtz Zentrum München - German Research Center for Environmental Health, Neuherberg, Germany

Sara Forcisi, Constanze Müller and Philippe Schmitt-Kopplin
Research Unit Analytical BioGeoChemistry, Helmholtz Zentrum Muünchen - German Research Center for Environmental Health, Neuherberg, Germany

Brandon J. Auerbach
Infectious Diseases Institute, College of Health Sciences, Makerere University, Kampala, Uganda
Harvard Medical School, Boston, Massachusetts, United States of America

David L. Thomas
Division of Infectious Diseases, Department of Medicine, School of Medicine, Johns Hopkins University, Baltimore, Maryland, United States of America

Thomas C. Quinn
Division of Intramural Research, National Institute of Allergy and Infectious Diseases, National Institutes of Health, Bethesda, Maryland, United States of America

Steven J. Reynolds
Division of Intramural Research, National Institute of Allergy and Infectious Diseases, National Institutes of Health, Bethesda, Maryland, United States of America

Division of Infectious Diseases, Department of Medicine, School of Medicine, Johns Hopkins University, Baltimore, Maryland, United States of America

Mohammed Lamorde
Infectious Diseases Institute, College of Health Sciences, Makerere University, Kampala, Uganda
Department of Pharmacology and Therapeutics, School of Medicine, University of Dublin, Trinity College, Dublin, Ireland

Concepta Merry
Infectious Diseases Institute, College of Health Sciences, Makerere University, Kampala, Uganda
Department of Pharmacology and Therapeutics, School of Medicine, University of Dublin, Trinity College, Dublin, Ireland
St James's Hospital, Dublin, Ireland

Collins Kukunda-Byobona
Department of Botany, Makerere University, Kampala, Uganda

Ponsiano Ocama
Harvard Medical School, Boston, Massachusetts, United States of America
Department of Medicine, College of Health Sciences, Makerere University, Kampala, Uganda

Aggrey S. Semeere
Infectious Diseases Institute, College of Health Sciences, Makerere University, Kampala, Uganda
Department of Medicine, College of Health Sciences, Makerere University, Kampala, Uganda

Anthony Ndyanabo, Iga Boaz, Valerian Kiggundu and Fred Nalugoda
Rakai Health Sciences Program, Entebbe, Uganda

Ron H. Gray and Maria J. Wawer
Rakai Health Sciences Program, Entebbe, Uganda
Department of Population, Family, and Reproductive Health, Bloomberg School of Public Health, Johns Hopkins University, Baltimore, Maryland, United States of America

Gregory D. Kirk
Department of Epidemiology, Bloomberg School of Public Health, Johns Hopkins University, Baltimore, Maryland, United States of America

Lara Stabinski
Division of Intramural Research, National Institute of Allergy and Infectious Diseases, National Institutes of Health, Bethesda, Maryland, United States of America
Department of Epidemiology, Bloomberg School of Public Health, Johns Hopkins University, Baltimore, Maryland, United States of America

Yao Tong, Hei Kiu Wong, Yi-Bin Feng and Di Wang
School of Chinese Medicine, Faculty of Medicine, the University of Hong Kong, Hong Kong, China

Zhang-Jin Zhang
School of Chinese Medicine, Faculty of Medicine, the University of Hong Kong, Hong Kong, China
Department of Psychiatry, Fourth Military Medical University, Xijing Hospital, Xi'an, Shaanxi, China

Qing-Rong Tan and Huai-Hai Wang
Department of Psychiatry, Fourth Military Medical University, Xijing Hospital, Xi'an, Shaanxi, China

Xue-Yi Wang
Mental Health Center, Hebei Medical University, Shijiazhuang, Hebei, China

Lai-Ming Ho
School of Public Health, the University of Hong Kong, Hong Kong, China

Roger Ng
Department of Psychiatry, Kowloon Hospital, Hong Kong, China

Grainne M. McAlonan
Department of Psychiatry, the University of Hong Kong, Hong Kong, China

Chuan-Yue Wang
Capital Medical University, Beijing Anding Hospital, Beijing, China

Vivian Taam Wong
Chinese Medicine Section, Hospital Authority, Hong Kong, China

Hyun-Woo Cho and Kwang-Ho Heo
Department of Rehabilitation Medicine of Korean Medicine, Spine and Joint Center, Pusan National University Korean Medicine Hospital, Yangsan, Republic of Korea

Eui-Hyoung Hwang and Byung-Cheul Shin
Department of Rehabilitation Medicine of Korean Medicine, Spine and Joint Center, Pusan National University Korean Medicine Hospital, Yangsan, Republic of Korea,
Division of Clinical Medicine, School of Korean Medicine, Pusan National University, Yangsan, Republic of Korea

Byungmook Lim
Division of Humanities and Social Medicine, School of Korean Medicine, Pusan National University, Yangsan, Republic of Korea

Jian-Ping Liu
Center for Evidence-Based Chinese Medicine, Beijing University of Chinese Medicine, Beijing, China

Kiichiro Tsutani
Department of Drug Policy and Management, Graduate School of Pharmaceutical Sciences, The University of Tokyo, Tokyo, Japan

Myeong Soo Lee
Brain Disease Research Center, Korea Institute of Oriental Medicine, Daejeon, Republic of Korea

Hitomi Hino, Yuka Suzuki and Eiichi Ishii
Department of Pediatrics, Ehime University Graduate School of Medicine, Shitsukawa, Toon, Ehime, Japan

Hisaaki Takahashi and Junya Tanaka
Department of Molecular and Cellular Physiology, Ehime University Graduate School of Medicine, Shitsukawa, Toon, Ehime, Japan
Ehime Proteo-Medicine Research Center, Department of Basic and Clinical Neuroscience, Ehime University, Toon, Ehime, Japan

Mitsumasa Fukuda
Department of Pediatrics, Ehime University Graduate School of Medicine, Shitsukawa, Toon, Ehime, Japan
Ehime Proteo-Medicine Research Center, Department of Basic and Clinical Neuroscience, Ehime University, Toon, Ehime, Japan

Wei Chen
Centre For Evidence-Based Chinese Medicine, Beijing University of Chinese Medicine, Beijing, China

Chi Eung Danforn Lim
Faculty of Medicine, South Western Sydney Clinical School, University of New South Wales, Sydney, Australia

Hong-Jun Kang
Intensive Care Unit, Chinese PLA General Hospital, Beijing, China

Jianping Liu
Centre For Evidence-Based Chinese Medicine, Beijing University of Chinese Medicine, Beijing, China
NAFKAM, University of Tromso, Tromso, Norway

Xun Li
Centre for Evidence-based Chinese Medicine, Beijing University of Chinese Medicine, Beijing, China
Centre for Complementary Medicine Research (CompleMED), University of Western Sydney, Sydney, New South Wales, Australia

Guoyan Yang, Xinxue Li and Jianping Liu
Centre for Evidence-based Chinese Medicine, Beijing University of Chinese Medicine, Beijing, China

Alan Bensoussan
Centre for Complementary Medicine Research (CompleMED), University of Western Sydney, Sydney, New South Wales, Australia

Yan Zhang, Jiu Chang and Xiaoxuan Sun
School of Preclinical Medicine, Beijing University of Chinese Medicine, Beijing, China

Jingli Yang
School of Management, Beijing University of Chinese Medicine, Beijing, China

Xiaoyun Zhou and Yu Guo
School of Acupuncture and Moxibustion, Beijing University of Chinese Medicine, Beijing, China

Yue Xu
School of Humanities, Beijing University of Chinese Medicine, Beijing, China

Junhua Zhang, Wei Zhao, Yongling Zhang, Li Zhang and Hongcai Shang
Research Institute of Traditional Chinese Medicine, Tianjin University of Traditional Chinese Medicine, Tianjin, China

Jing Hu
Research Institute of Traditional Chinese Medicine, Tianjin University of Traditional Chinese Medicine, Tianjin, China
Department of Epidemiology and Biostatistics, School of Public Health, Peking University, Beijing, China

Xiankun Chen
Evidence-Based Medicine & Clinical Research Service Group, Guangdong Provincial Academy of Chinese Medical Sciences, Guangzhou, China
Guangdong Provincial Hospital of Chinese Medicine, Guangzhou, China

Brian May, Yuan Ming Di and Anthony Lin Zhang
Traditional & Complementary Medicine Research Program, Health Innovations Research Institute, School of Health Sciences, RMIT University, Melbourne,Australia

Chuanjian Lu
Guangdong Provincial Hospital of Chinese Medicine, Guangzhou, China
Guangdong Provincial Academy of Chinese Medical Sciences, Guangzhou, China

Charlie Changli Xue
Guangdong Provincial Hospital of Chinese Medicine, Guangzhou, China
Traditional & Complementary Medicine Research Program, Health Innovations Research Institute, School of Health Sciences, RMIT University, Melbourne, Australia,
Guangdong Provincial Academy of Chinese Medical Sciences, Guangzhou, China

Lin Lin
Department of Respiratory Medicine, Guangdong Provincial Hospital of Chinese Medicine, Guangzhou, Guangdong Province, China

Yali Liu
Evidence-Based Medicine Center, School of Basic Medical Sciences, Lanzhou University, Lanzhou, China
Key Laboratory of Clinical Translational Research and Evidence-Based Medicine of Gansu Province, Lanzhou, China

Rui Zhang and Jiao Huang
Evidence-Based Medicine Center, School of Basic Medical Sciences, Lanzhou University, Lanzhou, China
The First Clinical Medical College of Lanzhou University, Lanzhou, China

Xu Zhao, Wanting Sun and Yuefen Mai
Evidence-Based Medicine Center, School of Basic Medical Sciences, Lanzhou University, Lanzhou, China
The Second Clinical Medical College of Lanzhou University, Lanzhou, China

Peng Zhang
Evidence-Based Medicine Center, School of Basic Medical Sciences, Lanzhou University, Lanzhou, China
Department of Cardiology, Qilu Hospital of Shandong University, Ji'nan, Shandong Province, China

Danlu Liu and Ke hu Yang
Evidence-Based Medicine Center, School of Basic Medical Sciences, Lanzhou University, Lanzhou, China,
Key Laboratory of Clinical Translational Research and Evidence-Based Medicine of Gansu Province, Lanzhou, China,
The First Clinical Medical College of Lanzhou University, Lanzhou, China

Yajun Wang
Acupuncture and Massage College, Gansu University of Traditional Chinese Medicine, Lanzhou, China

Hua Cao
Department of Neurology, Gansu Provincial Hospital of Traditional Chinese Medicine, Lanzhou, China

Jingxiao Zhang, Yan Li, Yanqiu Pan and Shuwei Zhang
Key laboratory of Industrial Ecology and Environmental Engineering (MOE), Faculty of Chemical, Environmental and Biological Science and Technology, Dalian University of Technology, Dalian, Liaoning, China

Xuetong Chen and Yonghua Wang
College of Life Sciences, Northwest A & F University, Yangling, Shaanxi, China
Center of Bioinformatics, Northwest A & F University, Yangling, Shaanxi, China

Liangcai Zhao, Haiyan Zhang, Yongquan Zheng, Minjian Dong and Yaqiang Wang
Institute of Metabonomics & Medical NMR, School of Pharmaceutical Sciences, Wenzhou Medical University, Wenzhou, China

Guanghui Bai, Xinjian Ye and Zhihan Yan
Radiology Department of the Second Affiliated Hospital, Wenzhou Medical University, Wenzhou, China

Hongchang Gao
Institute of Metabonomics & Medical NMR, School of Pharmaceutical Sciences, Wenzhou Medical University, Wenzhou, China
Radiology Department of the Second Affiliated Hospital, Wenzhou Medical University, Wenzhou, China

Yunjun Yang
Department of Radiology, the first Affiliated Hospital, Wenzhou Medical University, Wenzhou, China

Wei Chen, Li-qiong Wang, Jun Ren, Wen-jing Xiong, Fang Lu and Jian-ping Liu
Centre for Evidence-Based Chinese Medicine, Beijing University of Chinese Medicine, Beijing, China

George Lewith
Primary care and population Sciences, Medical School, University of Southampton, Southampton, United Kingdom

Lianyu Chen, Chao Qu, Hao Chen, Litao Xu, Qi Qi, Kun Wang, Zhiqiang Meng, Zhen Chen, Peng Wang and Luming Liu
Department of Integrative Oncology, Fudan University Shanghai Cancer Center, Shanghai, China
Department of Oncology, Shanghai medical college, Fudan University, Shanghai, China

Jianmin Luo
Department of Oncology, Shanghai medical college, Fudan University, Shanghai, China

Index